The Neurobiological Basis of Violence

The Neurobiological Basis of Violence:

Science and Rehabilitation

Edited by

Professor Sheilagh Hodgins
Department of Forensic Mental Health Science
Institute of Psychiatry at King's College London
London
UK

Doctor Essi Viding
Developmental Risk and Resilience Unit
Research Department of Clinical Educational and Health Psychology
Division of Psychology and Language Sciences
University College London
London
UK

Doctor Anna Plodowski
Department of Forensic Mental Health Science
Institute of Psychiatry at King's College London
London
UK

PHILOSOPHICAL
TRANSACTIONS
— OF —
THE ROYAL
SOCIETY

Originating from a Theme Issue first published in Philosophical
Transactions of the Royal Society B: Biological Sciences

http://publishing.royalsociety.org/philtransb

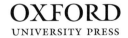

OXFORD
UNIVERSITY PRESS

OXFORD

UNIVERSITY PRESS

Great Clarendon Street, Oxford OX2 6DP

Oxford University Press is a department of the University of Oxford.
It furthers the University's objective of excellence in research, scholarship,
and education by publishing worldwide in

Oxford New York

Auckland Cape Town Dar es Salaam Hong Kong Karachi
Kuala Lumpur Madrid Melbourne Mexico City Nairobi
New Delhi Shanghai Taipei Toronto

With offices in

Argentina Austria Brazil Chile Czech Republic France Greece
Guatemala Hungary Italy Japan Poland Portugal Singapore
South Korea Switzerland Thailand Turkey Ukraine Vietnam

Oxford is a registered trade mark of Oxford University Press
in the UK and in certain other countries

Published in the United States
by Oxford University Press Inc., New York

A catalogue record for this title is available from the British Library
Data available

Library of Congress Cataloging in Publication Data
Data available

Typeset in Minion by Cepha Imaging Private Ltd., Bangalore, India
Printed on acid-free paper
by the MPG Books Group in the UK.

ISBN 978-0-19-954-3533

10 9 8 7 6 5 4 3 2 1

Acknowledgements

The editors would like to thank the authors for their important contributions to this volume. Their hard work, dedication to furthering understanding of persistent violence, and expertise is well reflected in their chapters. We would also like to thank Professor Sir Michael Rutter for his insightful comments on the volume. We are grateful to The Royal Society who hosted a two-day meeting on the topic of this book in October 2007. We would also like to thank Miss Gerry Costello for preparing the manuscript.

S. Hodgins holds a Royal Society Wolfson Merit Award and funding from the NIHR Biomedical Research Centre South London and Maudsley NHS Foundation Trust / Institute of Psychiatry at King's College London.

Contents

List of Contributors

Doctor Edward M Bernat Department of Psychology, University of Minnesota, Minneapolis, USA

Doctor Nigel J Blackwood Department of Forensic Mental Health Science, Institute of Psychiatry at King's College London, London,UK

Doctor R James R Blair Mood & Anxiety Program, National Institute of Mental Health, National Institutes of Health, Bethesda, Maryland, USA

Mr Joshua W Buckholtz Neuroscience Graduate Program and Department of Psychology, Vanderbilt University, Nashville, Tennessee, USA

Professor Mark R Dadds The University of New South Wales, Sydney, New South Wales, Australia; Child and & Adolescent Psychiatry, Institute of Psychiatry at King's College London, London, UK

Mr Stéphane A De Brito Department of Forensic Mental Health Science. Institute of Psychiatry at King's College London, London, UK

Professor Conor Duggan Professor of Forensic Mental Health, Division of Psychiatry, University of Nottingham, Nottingham, UK; Nottinghamshire Healthcare NHS Trust, Nottingham, UK

Doctor Graeme Fairchild Developmental Psychiatry Section, University of Cambridge, Cambridge, UK

Doctor Elly Farmer National Clinical Assessment and Treatment Service (NCATS), Fresh Start NSPCC, London, UK

Professor Paul J Frick Department of Psychology, University of New Orleans, New Orleans, USA

Miss Sarah L Gregory Department of Forensic Mental Health Science, Institute of Psychiatry at King's College London, London, UK

Professor Jonathan Hill Child Psychiatry Research Group, The University of Manchester, Manchester, UK

Professor Sheilagh Hodgins Department of Forensic Mental Health Science, Institute of Psychiatry at King's College London, London, UK

Doctor Alice P Jones Developmental Risk and Resilience Unit, Research Department of Clinical, Educational and Health Psychology, Division of Psychology and Language Sciences, University College London, London, UK

Doctor Henrik Larsson Department of Medical Epidemiology and Biostatistics, Karolinska Institutet, Stockholm, Sweden

Doctor Vicki Leidecker Division of Clinical Psychology, The University of Liverpool, Liverpool, UK

Professor Rolf Loeber Western Psychiatric Hospital and Clinic, University of Pittsburgh, Pittsburgh, USA

Doctor Eamon McCrory Developmental Risk and Resilience Unit, Research Department of Clinical, Educational and Health Psychology, Division of Psychology and Language Sciences, University College London, London, UK; and Fresh Start, NSPCC, London, UK

Professor James McGuire University of Liverpool, School of Population, Community and Behavioural Sciences, Division of Clinical Psychology, Liverpool, UK

Professor Andreas Meyer-Lindenberg Director, Central Institute of Mental Health, Department of Psychiatry and Psychotherapy, University of Heidelberg, Mannheim, Germany

Professor Lynne Murray Winnicott Research Unit, Department of Psychology, The Unversity of Reading, Reading, UK

Professor Candice L Odgers Department of Psychology and Social Behavior, University of California-Irvine, Irvine, USA

Professor Dustin Pardini Western Psychiatric Hospital and Clinic, University of Pittsburgh, Pittsburgh, USA

Professor Christopher J Patrick Director Clinical Science and Psychopathology Research Training Program, Department of Psychology, University of Minnesota, Minneapolis, USA

Ms Amelie Petitclerc School of Psychology, Université Laval, Québec, Canada

Doctor Anna Plodowski Department of Forensic Mental Health Science, Institute of Psychiatry at King's College London, London, UK

Ms Tracy Rhodes School of Psychology, The University of New South Wales, Sydney, New South Wales, Australia

Professor Michael Rutter Social, Genetic and Developmental Psychiatry Centre, Institute of Psychiatry at King's College London, London, UK

Doctor Helen Sharp Division of Clinical Psychology, The University of Liverpool, Liverpool, UK

Doctor Christina Stadler Department of Child and Adolescent Psychiatry, Johann Wolfgang Goethe University, Frankfurt Am Main, Germany

Doctor Phillipp Sterzer Department of Psychiatry, Charité Campus Mitte, Berlin, Germany

Professor Richard E Tremblay International Laboratory for Child and Adolescent Mental Health Development, Paris, France; University College, Dublin, Ireland; University of Montreal, Montreal, Canada

Professor Stephanie H M van Goozen School of Psychology, Cardiff University, Cardiff, UK

Doctor Essi Viding Developmental Risk and Resilience Unit, Research Department of Clinical, Educational and Health Psychology, Division of Psychology and Lanugage Sciences, University College London, London, UK

Introduction: The two-way interplay between neuroscience and clinical practice in the understanding of violence and of its remediation

Michael Rutter

The field of violence has rather suffered from a divide between basic laboratory neuroscience and clinical science using non-experimental research strategies. This volume seeks to bridge this divide and, in so doing, to highlight some of the key scientific challenges, as well as the dilemmas and difficulties in the translation of scientific findings (whether basic or clinical) into policy and practice applications.

The time is ripe for such a bridging endeavour because of the leverage provided by the new technologies of molecular genetics and both structural and functional brain imaging. But, also, there is the availability of multiple high quality long-term prospective longitudinal studies (which emphasize the developmental trends and the individual differences that require explanation). Equally, there has been the major expansion of systematic quantitative studies of intervention efficacy. The challenge is provided by the recognition that, up to now, there has been remarkably little cross-talk among these different research approaches. Thus, for example, most of the neuroscience has concerned adults and has mainly involved samples showing extreme behaviors. By contrast, the longitudinal evidence indicates the major age trends that have been found and the importance of dimensions of both risk and psychopathology. Equally, the efficacy studies have been very informative on what does, and does not, "work" with respect in the broad field of antisocial behavior, but has largely ignored the role of individual differences that result in different forms of intervention being needed for offenders with different characteristics. The chapters indicate what can be achieved in integrating neuroscience with clinical practice and policy. In the years ahead, it may be expected that there will be a new generation of research that brings biological measures into the mainstream of longitudinal research, that tackles the biological meaning of age trends, and that uses both of these to examine the mediating mechanisms underlying individual differences in responses to interventions.

The first chapter by Loeber and Pardini very usefully summarizes the range of causal questions that need to be addressed. For the most part, neurobiological research has tended to focus on individual differences in the liability to engage in violent behavior – the first causal question. The implication is that these individual differences are stable over the course of development, but longitudinal studies have been clear-cut in showing that substantial changes take place over time (see e.g. Sampson & Laub, 1993; Laub & Sampson, 2003). The second type of causal question, therefore, concerns the origins of general developmental trends – the rise in physical aggression in the early preschool years (Côté *et al.*, 2006), followed by the fall during middle and later childhood (Nagin & Tremblay, 1999), but then a peak in offending that includes serious violence in late adolescence (Rutter, Giller, & Hagell, 1998). As Loeber and Pardini note, on the whole, there is a tendency for a progression from minor aggression, through physical fighting, to very serious violence.

The third type of causal question also focuses on developmental trends but differs in focusing on individual differences in course as they relate to variations in life circumstances – as reflected, for example, in marriage (Sampson *et al.*, 2006), or being a member of a delinquent gang (Thornberry *et al.*, 1993). The findings (not considered in this volume) clearly point to the environmental influence of psychosocial features (Rutter, 2005; 2007). What they do not do, however, is determine whether neurobiological features affect individual susceptibility to such environmental forces.

A fourth, yet again different, causal question concerns group differences – such as the major sex difference in antisocial behavior (see Moffitt *et al.*, 2001) or the ethnic variations (see Rutter & Tienda, 2005). Do their origins reflect the same neurobiological or psychosocial influences that operate within these broad groups? Up to now there has been very little serious attempt to tackle that question. Somewhat comparable issues arise with respect to the very major secular changes in the overall rate of crime in the last half century or so (Rutter & Smith, 1995).

Finally, there are the situational influences on whether any particular individual engages in violence on this occasion (and not some other) or in that social circumstance (see Rutter, Giller, & Hagell, 1998). There has been a tendency to focus on psychosocial situational factors but the parallel neurobiological question concerns the possible role of alcohol or other drugs in predisposing to violence through the removal of inhibitions (see e.g. Ito *et al.*, 1996; Tonry & Wilson, 1990; White *et al.*, 2002). It is important to appreciate that mediation may lie either in the chemical effect of the substance or from the impulsive, reckless lifestyle of substance users.

It is often assumed that violent crime differs in its origins and meaning from non-violent acquisitive crime, such as theft (see Rutter, Giller, & Hagell, 1998 for a succinct discussion of the evidence). A key methodological problem is that most offenders commit a wide range of offences; specialization is the exception rather than the rule. It has been found that the greater the number of offences, the greater the likelihood that at least one will involve violence. Because of the substantial overlap between recidivist crime and violence, any study of violence needs to take that into account, and few have done so. As discussed in this volume, it is also crucial to appreciate that violent crime itself is heterogeneous – with the distinctions among instrumental aggression (i.e. to further some purpose such as theft), angry aggression (i.e. a response to a provoking situation), and "sadistic" aggression (i.e. violence that seems to be intrinsically rewarding) possibly particularly important.

Odgers, in the second chapter, mainly focuses on the long-term risks for violence and poor physical health associated with life-course-persistent (LCP) antisocial behavior as identified by Moffitt (1993). Numerous studies have shown that LCP begins in childhood and there has been the general assumption that the key driving force lies in an unusually early age of onset. However, Odgers' trajectory analyses were critically important in showing that childhood-limited (CL) antisocial behavior was very common – with only a third going on to follow a LCP path (Odgers, Caspi *et al.*, 2007). The key question is what drives the persistence into adult life. The findings showed that a range of childhood variables (including ADHD) were associated with LCP and was much less frequent in CL, but a family history of antisocial behavior or alcohol problems was also an important differentiator (Odgers,

Milne *et al.*, 2007). Accordingly, it may well be that the early onset is more likely to be a proxy indicator of some important liability, rather than a cause in its own right. At the very least, research needs to be undertaken to test that possibility.

There has sometimes been an assumption that one trajectory is sufficient to encompass the age trends evident in early life and those apparent in adolescent/adult life, but the evidence suggests that a dual trajectory may be more accurate (Nagin, Barker, Lacourse, & Tremblay, 2008). That is, the early trajectory does not adequately account for the later trajectory. Trajectory analyses need to be used both to examine the moderating turning point effects of later life experiences (such as from drug use or being part of a delinquent peer group) and whether later turning point effects apply to everyone or only to particularly vulnerable sub-groups.

Odgers usefully summarizes the evidence showing an association between antisocial behavior when young and poor physical health in early adult life. The association is strongest with LCP, but it also applies to adolescence-onset antisocial behavior. As Odger emphasizes, there are several rather different mechanisms by which this association could arise and the evidence to date does not yet provide an answer on mediation of risks.

Hodgins raises the important question of possible heterogeneity in antisocial behavior generally and in violence in particular. The issue derives from the well documented associations between schizophrenia and aggressive behavior. Most individuals with schizophrenia do not engage in serious violence but the proportion that do is greatly raised over the general population base rate. She discusses the possibility that part of the association derives from drug misuse, but mainly puts forward a tripartite typology. The first group consists of individuals with early onset antisocial behavior that precedes the onset of psychosis but yet persists. In this group, the antisocial behavior is part of the pattern of precursors for schizophrenia and the causal influences probably do not differ greatly from those for antisocial behavior in the absence of psychosis. The second group is different in that they did *not* show antisocial behavior in childhood and the third group was similar in that respect but differed in their callousness and lack of remorse. She queries whether the deficits associated with schizophrenia make it more difficult for the individuals to learn *not* to be aggressive.

Frick and Petitclerc, in the fourth chapter, summarize the evidence that within a childhood-onset group with antisocial behavior, those with a callous and unemotional affective style constitute a meaningfully distinctive sub-group equivalent to psychopathy as seen in adult life. They point to the, as yet still limited, body of evidence that this is not synonymous with the broader construct of antisocial behavior. The callous/unemotional (CU) style is particularly associated with violent offending. It may also be accompanied by poor effortful inhibitory control, although this is also found in young people with antisocial behavior but without CU traits. It is argued, however, that the combination of fearlessness and poor effortful inhibitory control may be particularly likely to foster the occurrence of CU traits. Frick and Petitclerc point to the twin study evidence that genetic influences are particularly important in the population variance in CU features, as well as the clinical evidence that children with CU traits may be particularly difficult to treat through interventions focussed on parenting.

Dadds and Rhodes (in the next chapter) directly take up the challenge of seeking a synergy between specific biological processes and psychological experiences as they unfold developmentally. They start by noting the extensive evidence that behavioral interventions focusing on parenting have a substantial effect in reducing violence and antisocial behavior, but go on to focus on the neglected question of heterogeneity in response associated with child characteristics. Their own work found that young boys with callous-emotional traits were less responsive to these parenting interventions. They argued that the reduced recognition of, and response to, fearful expression might be a function (at least in part) of failing to look at the eyes of stimulus faces. Strikingly, their findings supported this hypothesis. They went on to note the emerging data showing that manipulations of the serotonin system may directly influence facial emotion processing. Both human and animal studies seem to suggest that serotonergic dysfunction (which is associated with adverse experiences) is particularly related to thresholds for explosive violence, whereas low cortisol is associated with "cold", more predatory, violence.

Dadds and Rhodes conclude by seeking to bring these findings together in order to raise possibilities for innovative interventions. They argue that what is needed now is the use of neuroscience findings to consider both how specific parenting strategies might be adapted to deal with individual differences in emotional sensitivity, and how drugs might be employed to enhance psychological effectiveness. With respect to the latter, they instance the neuropeptide oxytocin (which enhances social recognition and approach behavior) and D-cycloserene (DCS) which strengthens extinction of learned fear memorics, thereby possibly enhancing their later retrieval. With respect to the former, they point to the possible value of helping emotionally callous children to focus on the salient aspects of emotional situations. The authors are explicit that these are futuristic approaches that have yet to be tried and tested but what they propose would serve to capitalize on the possibilities of integrating neuroscience and clinical science as applied to the remediation of violence.

Hill, Murray, Leidecker, and Sharp (in the following chapter) deal with emotional responses in a very different way in their longitudinal study, from 18 months to age 5 years, of the children of mothers with postnatal depression, together with a control group. Security of attachment was used at 5 years to assess intentionality (meaning an interpretation in terms of emotions); and conduct disorder symptoms were assessed by teachers' questionnaire at the same age. The findings showed that responding in the intentional stance in the high threat scenario had a significant effect in the postnatal depression group but not in the controls. Similarly, insecure attachment had effects only in the high threat condition. A mediation analysis showed that the lack of use of intentionality provided the route to conduct problems. The attempt to assess mediation was informative and the findings are compatible with a rather different emotional response to that associated with psychopathy. Caution is required because of the small sample size, the cross-sectional nature of the findings at 5 years, and the lack of any demonstrated connection with violence.

Blair, in chapter 7, examines the possible neurobiological basis of psychopathy. He argues that any neurobiological model would have to account for both the emotional dysfunction and the increased risk for reactive and instrumental aggression associated with psychopathy. He reports that the amygdala is crucial for responding to fearful emotional expressions that serve to reinforce stimulus-reinforcement learning, which is crucial for socialization. The ventromedial prefrontal cortex (VmPFC) is also critical for the representation of reinforcement information because impairment is likely to lead to impaired decision-making. There is substantial research (mainly with adults) that has given rise to findings that are compatible with this model and, without doubt, it constitutes a most valuable way of approaching the challenges. For the reasons already noted, however, key questions remain to be investigated.

In the following chapter, Plodowski, Gregory, and Blackwood provide a thoughtful discussion of the contribution of structural and functional imaging findings in adult men exhibiting violent antisocial behavior. Clearly, brain imaging carries the potential for testing the detailed neurobiological models of both reactive and instrumental violence, but they point out that the neural underpinning of the key processes has still to be accomplished. A major limitation in the published findings so far had been the lack of adequate consideration of comorbidity (especially substance use) and a failure to examine satisfactorily the key diagnostic differentiation (such as between those with and without psychopathy) and the possible moderating role of anxiety levels. The chapter concludes with a very helpful discussion of future research directions – not only with respect to imaging, but also in terms of the needed integration with other research approaches.

The next chapter by Sterzer and Stadler examines the more limited brain imaging findings in childhood and adolescence. They note the important heterogeneity of antisocial behavior and the importance of considering the particular role of deviant emotional processing in individuals with CU traits. The evidence from functional imaging studies suggests that the impaired processing of social distress cues is associated with reduced amygdala response to fearful facial expressions and reduced connectivity with frontal brain regions. The chapter ends with an important caveat on the need to differentiate between "state" and "trait" markers, to examine the degree to which such markers change as a consequence of therapeutic interventions, and to determine whether the brain features represent a cause or consequence of antisocial behavior.

The caveats are reinforced by de Brito and Hodgins in chapter 10, which considers executive functions shown by persistently violent offenders. They highlight the regrettable failure of most neuropsychological research to differentiate antisocial individuals with, and those without, CU traits. Nevertheless, such evidence as is available suggests that offenders with psychopathy do not show impairments in "cool" executive functioning (EF) (meaning the cognitive aspects of EF), whereas they might show deficits in "hot" (i.e. motivational aspects) EF. Because antisocial behavior is much commoner in males than females, and because there is a peak of crime in adolescence, commentators have often assumed that the pubertal surge of testosterone in males must play a role – especially in relation to violent aggression. The careful review by van Goozen and Fairchild (chapter 11) casts doubt on this seemingly plausible assumption. Insofar as there is an association, it is more likely to be due to prenatal organizational influences, rather than direct effects of male hormones in adolescence. It might be added that the finding that antisocial behavior shows more of a rise in adolescence in females than in males (Moffitt, Caspi, Rutter, & Silva, 2001) also raises doubts on the direct hormonal effect hypothesis. In addition, it is important to note the effects of experiences on testosterone levels. Thus, the victors in a competitive tennis match show a rise, and losers a fall, in testosterone levels (Booth, Shelley, Mazur, Tharp, & Kittok, 1989). This is not just a function of exercise because much the same was found with respect to winning and losing in chess competitions (Mazur, Booth, & Dabbs jr., 1992). Hormones influence behavior but so, also, behavior influences hormones.

Van Goozen and Fairchild go on to consider the evidence on cortisol and antisocial behavior. As with all research considered in this volume, there is the problem that so few studies differentiate between antisocial behavior that is, and that which is not, associated with CU traits. In addition, however, there are the considerations of the need to differentiate between the basal levels of cortisol and the response to stressors, between the causes of antisocial behavior, and between the HPA axis (hypothalamic-pituitary-adrenal axis) effects of the abuse/adversity that predisposes to antisocial behavior and the correlates of antisocial behavior as such. There is no doubt that stress, HPA axis, and aggression are inter-related, but the mediating mechanisms remain frustratingly obscure.

Patrick and Bernat, in the final chapter 12 on neurobiological models, provide an important additional perspective through their integrative review of psychophysiological studies.

They differentiate between *causal* studies (such as those by Caspi *et al.*, 2002), *biomarker* studies focusing on biological differences that distinguish between aggressive and non-aggressive individuals, and *process* studies that seek to identify how aggressive individuals may be distinctive in their biological (including psychological) processes of stimuli and events. Both functional magnetic resonance imaging (fMRI) and electrocortical response measures (such as provided by EEG and ERP – event-related potential responses) constitute important research strategies. They note the substantial evidence that aggressive individuals tend to show a lower than usual level of autonomic arousal combined with higher auto-nomic reactivity, but also the substantial evidence that markedly different results are found with individuals showing psychopathy. Up to now, process studies have tended to study psychopathy as a syndrome and, hence, have not examined separately the two components of emotional callousness and antisocial deviance (including aggression). Similarly, most research into aggression in individuals without aggression has not adequately differentiated between a vulnerability to a broad range of antisocial behavior, drug/alcohol problems and disinhibiting behavior and aggression per se. They argue that individuals who are impul-sively aggressive show lower levels of autonomic arousal at rest, but enhanced autonomic reactivity to immediate stressors. They suggest that these findings show the potential of pharmacologic agents to provide an adjunct to psychological treatments. Patrick and Bernat consider two alternative integrative conceptual models – one focusing on the variety of impulse control problems, and one based on a neurobiological model reflecting dysfunction in a set of interconnected brain systems. Clearly, the challenge is to bring these two approaches together.

Viding, Larsson and Jones (in chapter 13) use twin study findings to ask the question whether antisocial behavior needs to be subdivided into whether or not it is associated with psychopathy, as manifest in the form of callous-unemotional traits. Their findings show a higher heritability for antisocial behavior associated with psychopathy than for antisocial behavior that is not accompanied by these traits. They argue that because psychopathy involves a lack of response to others' distress, it may require different forms of intervention. Their paper is also important in noting that genetic influences may operate through either gene-environment correlations (rGE) or interactions (G x E), as well as through main effects.

The following chapter (14) by Buckholtz and Meyer-Lindenberg returns to this theme. Buckholtz and Meyer-Lindenberg refer to Caspi and colleague's (2002) finding that the "L" variant of the monoamine oxidase A (MAOA) gene, although not directly associated with antisocial behavior as such, did show a significant moderation of the impact of early life maltreatment on the development of antisocial behavior later in life (G x E). This effect held for four distinct measures of impulsively violent antisocial behavior. Subsequent studies, including a meta-analysis (Taylor & Kim-Cohen, 2007) have independently replicated and extended this finding in new cohorts and with additional measures of impulsive violence, although the predictive effect did not reach statistical significance in two studies.

Buckholtz and Meyer-Lindenberg note the human and animal studies that highlighted the likely importance of the MAOA gene and point to the confirmatory study in primates (Bennett, Lesch, Heils, Long, Lorenz *et al.*, 2002; Champoux, Bennett, Shannon, Higley, Lesch *et al.*, 2002). There are important methodological hazards to be overcome in studying G x E (see Rutter, 2008) but the findings are potentially very important in pointing to possible biological pathways that bring together the effects of G and of E (see Caspi & Moffitt, 2006; Rutter, 2007; 2008). Uncertainties remain on whether the G x E concerns responsivity to the environment or susceptibility to adverse environments (from an evolutionary perspective, the former seems more probable). Similarly it has yet to be established whether the G x E particularly concerns violence as such, rather than recidivist crime that just includes violence as one of many forms of antisocial behavior.

A further challenge is presented by the need for more direct studies of the neural effects. Meyer-Lindenberg and colleagues (2006) have shown how this can be achieved through structural and functional brain imaging. As Buckholtz and Meyer-Lindenberg explain, their own research was crucial in showing that these G x E effects applied in individuals *without* psychopathology. Interestingly, however, the G x E effect on neural structures and functions applied in men but not women. A path analysis showed that functional connectivity between the ventromedial prefrontal cortex and the amygdala (indicating the value of an intermediate phenotype approach) was greater in men with the MAOA-L genotype than in those with the H allele. Taken as a whole, the findings suggest that the MAOA-L allele specifically contributes to an impulsive/reactive dimension of aggression not linked with psychopathy. They conclude with the reminder that the MAOA-L is not a violence gene per se; on its own it is compatible with mental health; and the interest lies in the light thrown on the role of neural systems in aggression rather than in its predictive value as such (which is small).

McGuire (in chapter 15) echoes Loeber and Pardini's emphasis on both the range of causal questions that need addressing and the heterogeneity of aggressive behavior (including the massive number of killings associated with war and with genocide). In the biological investigation of individual differences, it is crucial not to lose sight of the fact that many people will resort to violence when there is intergroup conflict. Moreover, the deaths associated with war and genocide far outweighs the deaths due to personal violence. The risk factor for individual differences in propensity to engage in violence may, or may not, be the same in the two cases, but we must not neglect the powerful social forces predisposing to (and often used to justify) group violence. He argues that in order to understand violent offending, it is essential to construct a model that incorporates evolutionary predisposition to aggression in some interpersonal circumstances, individual differences in temperament, socialization influences, the level of economic adversity and stress, and the development of attitudes, expectations and coping styles.

Against that background, McGuire presents an authoritative overview of the evidence on the efficacy of interventions designed to reduce aggression and violence. He concludes that there is reasonably good evidence that emotional self-management, interpersonal skills training, problem-solving strategies and allied training approaches show mainly positive effects of a worthwhile kind. On the other hand, attention is drawn to the lack of attention to subgroup differences in responsiveness, such as those claimed to be associated with psychopathy. At least as seriously, relatively little is known on the factors mediating beneficial effects (or those mediating treatment resistance). By the same token, despite the general acceptance of multiple pathways to the same endpoint, very little research has investigated the different types of interplay among causal factors – including moderator and mediation effects (see Baron & Kenny, 1986; Kraemer *et al.*, 2001). The chapter concludes with an important reminder of the multiple elements involved in causality (see Academy of Medical Sciences, 2007).

McCrory and Farmer (chapter 16) provide a more detailed examination of different intervention approaches. Like others, they emphasize the heterogeneity in antisocial behavior and the need to consider both mediation mechanisms and moderator effects. They argue for the value of a multi-levels approach that recognizes the importance of the dynamic interplay between genes and environment across the course of development and the need for a focus on the specific active ingredients of each effective intervention, as well as the variations among individuals in their response.

   Duggan (in chapter 17) provides a dose of reality-testing by insisting that a considerable gap remains between scientific evidence and clinical practice – at least as viewed in relation to the pattern of antisocial personality disorder (ASPD). He argues that one of the problems lies in the breadth of the impairments associated with ASPD and the lack of consensus on how it should be conceptualized. Another problem concerns the leap required in moving from neuroscience to clinical need. Duggan suggests that a unifying theory is needed to bring together the clinical findings in order to identify mechanisms that address treatment-responsiveness variations. It is suggested that that should now be possible. Whether or not the clinical concept of personality disorder constitutes the best way forward in understanding violence is uncertain. Maybe the future should lie in examining the connections between brain functioning and individual differences in violent behavior. The final chapter by Tremblay focuses on prevention of the onset of physical aggression rather than its remediation once it has become established. Very reasonably, he argues that we need to differentiate between actual physical aggression and general disruptiveness, misbehavior and antisocial behavior. With respect to that distinction, the empirical evidence points to an onset of physical aggression within the preschool years. Tremblay suggests that the greatest interest, therefore, should be in the trajectories over time and the differences between those who learn *not* to aggress and those who continue to do so. Although that is indeed a pertinent issue, we should note that relatively stable differences remain over time among individuals. The largest difference lies between those who never exhibit aggression to any significant degree and those who persist in doing so throughout the whole of the developmental period. Tremblay argues that more attention needs to be paid to G x E and to the possibility of epigenetic effects by which experiences alter gene expression. Some researchers may query the assumption that most experiential effects operate through epigenetic mechanisms (clearly alternative possibilities need to be examined and tested), and other researchers will point to the limitation that gene expression tends to be tissue-specific. Lymphocyte studies may provide clues on methylation patterns, but extrapolation to the brain is tricky. That is, of course, where animal models could be informative. To what extent do methylation patterns in lymphocytes reflect patterns in the brain? More particularly, what would be lost by the inability to link methylation patterns to particular genes operating in particular parts of the brain? Nevertheless, there should be a general welcoming of Tremblay's plea for more use of experimental designs that can utilize intervention findings to test causal hypotheses.
   This volume provides much fruitful discussion on the challenges and solutions involved in integrating basic and applied neuroscience. The focus throughout is on violence and the problems associated with it. However, the background is provided by the general awareness of the need to consider what is meant by a "cause" when dealing with multifactorial traits or disorders, and of the ever present need to combine research strategies when seeking to identify component causes (Academy of Medical Sciences, 2007). There is important neuroscience that is potentially relevant to clinical practice and there are good clinical studies that highlight the heterogeneities that must be considered. It is not just a question of going from the bench to the bedside. Rather, what is required is a creative two-way iterative interplay among basic neurosciences, clinical science, and applications in the field (see Rutter & Plomin, 2008). This book provides a host of useful leads as to how this might proceed.

References

Academy of Medical Sciences (2007). *Identifying the Environmental Causes of Disease: How Should We Decide What to Believe and When to Take Action?* London: Academy of Medical Sciences.

Baron, R. M., & Kenny, D. A. (1986). The moderator-mediator variable distinction in social psycho-logical research: conceptual, strategic, and statistical considerations. *Journal of Personality and Social Psychology*, *51*, 1173–1182.

Bennett, A. J., Lesch, K. P., Heils, A., Long, J. C., Lorenz, J. G., Shoaf, S. E., *et al.* (2002). Early experience and serotonin transporter gene variation interact to influence primate CNS function. *Molecular Psychiatry*, *7*, 118–122.

Booth, A., Shelley, G., Mazur, A., Tharp, G., & Kittok, R. (1989). Testosterone, and winning and los-ing in human competition. *Hormones and Behaviour*, *23*, 556–571.

Caspi, A., McClay, J., Moffitt, T. E., Mill, J., Marin, J., Craig, I. W., *et al.* (2002). Role of genotype in the cycle of violence in maltreated children. *Science*, *297*, 851–854.

Caspi, A., & Moffitt, T. E. (2006). Gene-environment interaction research and neuroscience: a new partnership? *Nature Reviews Neuroscience*, *7*, 583–590.

Champoux, M., Bennett, A. J., Shannon, C., Higley, J. D., Lesch, K. P., & Suomi, S. J. (2002). Serotonin transporter gene polymorphism, differential early rearing, and behavior in rhesus monkey neo-nates, *Molecular Psychiatry*, *7*, 1058–1063.

Côté, S., Vaillancourt, T., LeBlanc, J. C., Nagin, D., & Tremblay, R. E. (2006). The development of physical aggression during childhood: a Nation Wide Longitudinal Study of Canadian Children. *The Journal of Abnormal Child Psychology*, *34*, 71–85.

Ito, T., Miller, N., & Pollock, V. E. (1996) Alcohol and aggression: a meta-analysis on the moderating effects of inhibitory cues, triggering events, and self-focused attention. *Psychological Bulletin*, *120*, 60–82.

Kraemer, H. C., Stice, E., Kazdin, A., Offord, D., & Kupfer, D. (2001). How do risk factors work together? mediators, moderators, and independent, overlapping, and proxy risk factors. *American Journal of Psychiatry*, *158*, 848–856.

Laub, J. H., & Sampson, R. J. (2003). *Shared Beginnings, Divergent Lives: Delinquent Boys to Age 70.* Cambridge, MA: Harvard University Press.

Mazur, A., Booth, A., & Dabbs jr., J. M. (1992). Testosterone and chess competition. *Social Psychology Quarterly*, *55*, 70–77.

Meyer-Lindenberg, A., Buckholtz, J. W., Kolachana, B., Hariri, A. R., Pezawas, L., Blasi, G., *et al.* (2006). Neural mechanisms of genetic risk for impulsivity and violence in humans. *Proceedings of the National Academy of Sciences of the USA*, *103*, 6269–6274.

Moffitt, T. E. (1993). Adolescence-limited and life-course-persistent antisocial behavior: a develop-mental taxonomy. *Psychological Review*, *100*, 674–701.

Moffitt, T. E., Caspi, A., Rutter, M., & Silva, P. A. (2001). *Sex Differences in Antisocial Behavior: Conduct Disorder, Delinquency, and Violence in the Dunedin Longitudinal Study.* Cambridge: Cambridge University Press.

Nagin, D., & Tremblay, R. E. (1999). Trajectories of boys' physical aggression, opposition, and hyper-activity on the path to physically violent and nonviolent juvenile delinquency. *Child Development*, *70*, 1181–1196.

Nagin, D. S., Barker, T., Lacourse, E., & Tremblay, R. E. (2008). The interrelationship of temporally distinct risk markers and the transition from childhood physical aggression to adolescent violent delinquency. In P. Cohen (ed), *Applied Data Analytic Techniques for Turning Points Research* (pp. 18–36). New York: Routledge.

Odgers, C. L., Caspi, A., Broadbent, J. M., Dickson, N., Hancox, R. J., Harrington, H., *et al.* (2007). Prediction of differential adult health burden by conduct problem subtypes in males. *Archives of General Psychiatry*, *64*, 476–484.

Odgers, C. L., Milne, B. J., Caspi, A., Crump, R., Poulton, R., & Moffitt, T. E. (2007). Predicting prognosis for the conduct-problem boy: can family history help? *Journal of the American Academy of Child and Adolescent Psychiatry*, *46*, 1240–1249.

Rutter, M. (2005). Environmentally mediated risks for psychopathology: research strategies and find-ings. *Journal of the American Academy of Child and Adolescent Psychiatry*, *44*, 3–18.

Rutter, M. (2007). Gene-environment interdependence. *Developmental Science*, *10*, 12–18.

Rutter, M. (ed) (2008). *Genetic Effects on Environmental Vulnerability to Disease.* London: Wiley.

Rutter, M., Giller, H., & Hagell, A. (1998). *Antisocial Behavior by Young People.* New York: Cambridge University Press.

Rutter, M., & Plomin, R., (2008). Pathways from science findings to health benefits. *Psychological Medicine*, *14*, 1–14.

Rutter, M., & Smith, D. (eds) (1995). *Psychosocial Disorders in Young People: Time Trends and Their Causes*. Chichester: Wiley.

Rutter, M., & Tienda, M. (eds) (2005). *Ethnicity and Causal Mechanisms*. New York: Cambridge University Press.

Sampson, R. J., & Laub, J. H. (1993). *Crime in the Making: Pathways and Turning Points Through Life*. Cambridge, MA: Harvard University Press.

Sampson, R. J., Laub, J. H., & Wimer, C. (2006). Does marriage reduce crime? a counterfactual approach to within-individual causal effects. *Criminology*, *44*, 465–508.

Taylor, A., & Kim-Cohen, J. (2007). Meta-analysis of gene-environment interactions in developmental psychopathology. *Development and Psychopathology*, *19*, 1029–1037.

Thornberry, T. P., Krohn, M. D., Lizotte, A. J., & Chard-Wiershem, D. (1993). The role of juvenile gangs in facilitating delinquent behavior. *Journal of Research in Crime and Delinquency*, *30*, 55–87.

Tonry, M., & Wilson, J. Q. (1990). Drugs and crime. In, *Crime and Justice: A Review of Research, Vol. 13*. Chicago: University of Chicago Press.

White, H. R., Tice, P. C., Loeber, R., & Sthouthamer-Loeber, M. (2002). Illegal acts committed by adolescents under the influence of alcohol and drugs. *Journal of Research in Crime and Delinquency*, *39*, 131–152.

1

Neurobiology and the development of violence: Common assumptions and controversies

Rolf Loeber and Dustin Pardini

Introduction

Violence and serious property crime continue to lead to high levels of personal injury and financial damage for victims (Welsh & Loeber, in press), and stimulate concerns about safety and increased costs for security, police, and preventive efforts. For example, in the year 2000 alone, the total costs resulting from non-fatal injuries and death attributable to violence were more than $70 billion in the United States (Corso *et al.*, 2007). Research on the victim costs of crime shows that the victim costs of an average chronic juvenile offender committing crime between ages 7 and 17 amounts to about $1.25 million (based on self-reported delinquency; Welsh *et al.*, in press).

Despite a substantial decrease in violence perpetration and victimization since about 1991–3 in the United States (e.g., Blumstein & Wallman, 2000; Baum, 2005), the American prison population quadrupled between 1980 and 2000 (Rosenfeld, 2004). Similarly, the British Crime Survey shows that in England and Wales violence has decreased since 1995 (Newburn, 2007), but the prison population has increased by two thirds between 1993 and 2005. Thus, in both countries, legislation and the courts have increased their emphasis on implementing punitive sanctions for crime rather than addressing the multiple causes—neurobiological, individual, social, economic, environmental processes—of criminal behaviour. Despite this practice, it is clear that furthering our understanding of the mechanisms through which neurobiological and other factors influence violence is the only way in which societies can develop and enact policies that will serve to maintain sustainable reductions in violent crime over time.

In the following text, in which we explore these issues in greater detail, *violence* refers to forcible robbery, attacking with intent to injure, sexual coercion, or rape; *aggression*, on the other hand, refers to lesser injurious acts, whereas *antisocial behaviour* is a general term encompassing aggression, violence, and non-violent forms of delinquency.

Modelling the neurobiological and social, individual, economic, and environmental influences on violence

To aid in the exploration of how neurobiological as well as social, individual, economic, and environmental factors influence the developmental progression of violence, Fig. 1.1 shows a basic heuristic model based on existing theoretical and empirical research in the area. This model represents the interrelationship between several broad-based factors believed to be important in the development of violence, including genetic, social, economic, and environmental influences, and the neurobiological factors of brain structure and function. In the model, social influences are posited to encompass interactions of the

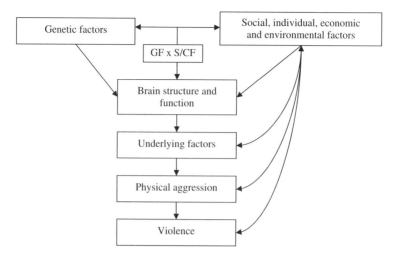

Fig. 1.1 Relationships between elements of neurobiological factors (GF) and social and contextual factors (S/CF) that influence the development of violence.

individual with parents, siblings, peers, and eventually, partners and co-workers. Individual factors are factors such as academic achievement and school motivation. Economic factors comprise factors such as family socio-economic status and welfare. Examples of environmental factors are neighbourhood disadvantage and school climate.

It is hypothesized that genetic and social as well as other factors and their interactions contribute to changes in neurobiological structure and function, which in turn influence a developmental cascade of behaviours that can eventually lead to violence. Specifically, brain structure and function are believed to influence early emerging underlying factors that increase one's propensity for violence (such as temperament), which in turn affect minor forms of aggression that then influence the probability of more serious violence. This cascade is also recursive, given that underlying factors, minor forms of aggression, and violence can serve to influence social and environmental factors over time, as well as being influenced by them. Although this heuristic model is thought to apply to both males and females, the nature of the factors contained within each broad-based category (i.e., genetic, social, individual, economic, and environmental factors) that are important for understanding the development of violence may differ by gender. Many neurobiological studies of violence often share a number of implicit or explicit assumptions about violence. These assumptions include the following:

- Individuals differ in their propensity to commit violence, and these differences are already present early in life.
- Aggression and violence have elements in common with personality traits that are presumed to be stable in individuals (e.g., Olweus, 1979).
- The underlying causes of aggression and violence are attributed to factors present early in life, especially neurobiological factors.

Although these assumptions are reasonable, the vast majority of the neurobiological studies of violence have been cross-sectional (or retrospective) rather than longitudinal and have concentrated on comparisons between offenders and non-offenders or between aggressive and non-aggressive youth (see Raine, 1993; Fishbein, 2000; Rowe, 2002). Even when studies are based on longitudinal data, the analyses are often focused on comparisons between deviant and non-deviant groups rather than comparisons between developmental types of offenders (e.g., early versus late onset offenders) or developmental change in offending (e.g., persistence in versus desistance from offending). Thus, neurobiological studies that treat the dependent variable of violence as a dynamic phenomenon are relatively rare.

Over the years, the number of longitudinal studies has increased and findings on the stability and change in offending have clarified individual differences in developmental growth of violence and the factors influencing such growth. Thus, we know much more about individual differences pertaining to the age–crime curve, developmental pathways to violence, desistance, and the types of individuals following different trajectories of violence. Also, we know more about underlying factors that are postulated to cause individual differences in the propensity for violent behaviour within populations. Some of these underlying factors—such as fearlessness and behavioural dysregulation—are thought to change with development. We pose that it is time to re-examine aggression and violence and underlying factors as dependent variables in neurobiological studies and ask ourselves which aspects of aggression, violence, and underlying factors are best explained by neurobiological factors.

Yet another aspect of neurobiological factors requires attention. Researchers agree that the impact of genetics, brain structure, and brain functioning on behaviour is not immutable but can be changed through human interactions (e.g., Taylor & Kim-Cohen, 2007). To what extent do social and other factors predict violence, and do they predict homicide as the most extreme expression of violence as well? How much is known about the degree to which neurobiological factors add to these predictors of violence, either as main effects or through interactions with social and environmental factors?

It is also important to recognize that the prevalence and incidence of violence in societies is rarely constant over decades. Instead, studies show large secular changes in violence in a matter of years. The causes of such secular changes have given rise to much speculation (e.g., Blumstein & Waldman, 2000), and have included population structural factors (such as the size of crime-prone cohorts, immigration), poverty, family disruption, violence in the media, gang membership, teenage childbearing, and many other factors. The question again is, to what extent do neurobiological factors explain secular changes in violence for populations of individuals as either main effects or in interaction with different population structural factors?

In this chapter, we address four controversies regarding neurobiological factors that explain violence:

1. Scholars often assume stability of individual differences in neurobiological factors pertaining to violence—yet much change occurs in aggression and violence during the life course.
2. Individual differences in aggression and violence reflect one or more of the underlying mechanisms that are believed to have neurobiological origins—yet there is little agreement about which underlying mechanisms apply best.
3. The development of aggression and violence can be explained to some degree by social and other factors—yet it is unclear to what extent neurobiological factors explain violence over and above the explanatory power of social and other factors. Also, the role of neurobiological factors in the escalation to, and desistence from, violence is poorly understood.
4. Violence waxes and wanes in society over time—yet the explanation of secular differences in violence by means of neurobiological and other factors is not clear.

These four topics are interrelated: knowledge of stability and change in violence is the dependent variable that neurobiological factors attempt to explain. Underlying mechanisms, neurobiological, social, and other factors constitute elements of models to explain violence. Lastly, these explanations when applied to successive age cohorts are relevant for the explanation of secular changes in violence. Part of this chapter is based on longitudinal analyses from the Pittsburgh Youth Study[1] and serves to illustrate the key points of these issues.

Developmental change in violence

Neurobiological, social, and other explanations of violence should take into account that there are at least four key sets of differences among individuals: the age–crime curve, desistance, developmental pathways, and developmental trajectories.

Age–aggression and age–violence curves

There are at least two age-related, normative curves relevant to the study of neurobiology of aggression and violence. The first curve is the *age–aggression curve* and indicates that aggression is high in childhood and decreases afterwards. For example, Nagin and Tremblay (2005) have provided evidence that physical aggression in childhood peaks around age 2 and then decreases (see also Kingston and Prior, 1995; NICHD Early Child Care Research Network, 2004). There are individual differences, however, in terms of the timing and rate of outgrowing aggression during the preschool years. We are not aware of neurobiological studies that explain why this is earlier for some children than for others.

The second normative curve is usually called the *age–crime curve* (Farrington, 1986). The age–crime curve for property crime and violence is a universally observed curve showing that the prevalence of offenders is low in late childhood and early adolescence, peaks in middle to late adolescence, and decreases subsequently (Farrington, 1986; Laub & Sampson, 2003; Tremblay & Nagin, 2005). The curve for violence is similar but tends to peak somewhat later (Loeber *et al.*, 2008). The curve is slightly earlier for girls than boys (Farrington, 1986; Elliott *et al.*, 2005), which is indicative of a higher proportion of late-onset cases during adolescence among boys than among girls.

The two age–antisocial behaviour curves pose a major challenge for the explanation of violence on the basis of neurobiological factors. Studies on neurobiological factors to date

---

[1] The Pittsburgh Youth Study (PYS) began in 1986 and comprised boys who were enrolled in the public schools in Pittsburgh. The sample is about evenly distributed between African-American and Caucasian boys. The young males have been regularly followed up over a period of thirteen years. The study consists of three age cohorts of boys, who were in 1st, 4th, or 7th grades of public schools at the time of the first assessment in 1987–88 (called the youngest, middle, and oldest cohorts). The participation rate of boys and their parents was about 85% of the eligible boys. On the basis of screening at the first assessment, antisocial boys were oversampled, but the final sample consisted of an additional sample of randomly selected non-deviant boys. The youngest cohort has been assessed 18 times between ages 7 and 19, and the oldest cohort has been assessed 16 times between ages 13 and 25. In contrast, the middle cohort was discontinued after 7 assessments and had a single follow-up assessment at about age 24. One of the strengths of the PYS is the availability of multiple informants (including parents and teachers) to enhance the validity of measurements; in addition, official records of delinquency were collected. Further details about the study are available elsewhere (Loeber *et al.*, 1998, 2008).

have not addressed why there is an increase, peaking, and a decrease in offending in the same individuals over many years and why there are individual differences in the upslope, peaking, and downslope of that curve. An exception is a study by Loeber *et al.* (2007) using data from the PYS, which in addition to social and other factors examined heart rate and galvanic skin response. Predictive analyses discriminating between desisters and persisters in delinquency between ages 17 and 20 showed that all of the significant predictors were either child or peer risk factors. None of the cognitive, physiological, parenting, or community factors significantly predicted desistance from delinquency. The results leave open the possibilities that other neurobiological factors can explain desistance in the downslope of the age–crime curve, a point we will return to when discussing underlying factors.

Desistance

Desistance refers to individuals' cessation of delinquent acts. The notion that desistance primarily takes place in the downslope of the age–crime curve (e.g., Moffitt, 1993) is a mistaken one because this is a prevalence curve and not a curve on the relative persistence of offending. Instead, desistance from antisocial behaviour and delinquency, including violence, takes place throughout childhood and adolescence (Tremblay *et al.*, 2004; Prinzie *et al.*, 2005; Loeber *et al.*, 2008). Longitudinal research also shows that there is discontinuity in violence for a proportion of violent offenders. For example, in the PYS, desistance processes relating to violence operated from at least late childhood onwards and were documented throughout adolescence and early adulthood (Loeber *et al.*, 2008). The probability of desistance from serious offending (which includes violence) is inversely related to age of onset (particularly, onset in late childhood is negatively associated with later desistance). Only one quarter of the early onset offenders desisted from serious offending later.

Developmental pathways

Scientists are interested in very-high-risk individuals who are likely to express violent behaviour years later. However, because violence as a rule emerges in mid-to-late adolescence, it is also necessary to focus on less serious forms of aggression that are developmental precursors to violence. Individuals differ in their development of different severity levels of aggression, with some developing minor aggression only while others progress to serious, repeated violence. Conceptually, this is often referred to as a *developmental pathway* to violence, with most individuals progressing very little on that pathway and a minority progressing to the most extreme forms of violence. Loeber and colleagues (1993, 1997, 2005) empirically charted pathways in the PYS that youngsters typically follow in a remarkably orderly progression from less to more serious problem behaviours and delinquency from childhood to adolescence. The development from minor antisocial behaviours to serious delinquency best fits a model of three incremental pathways (Fig. 1.2): (1) *overt pathway* starts with minor aggression, has physical fighting as a second stage, and severe violence as a third stage; (2) *covert pathway*, prior to age 15, starts with minor covert acts, has property damage as a second stage, and moderate to serious delinquency as a third stage; and (3) *authority conflict pathway*, prior to age 12, starts with stubborn behaviour, has defiance as a second stage, and authority avoidance (e.g., truancy) as a third stage. The pathways model has been documented in four longitudinal data sets (Tolan & Gorman-Smith, 1998; Loeber *et al.*, 1999; Tolan *et al.*, 2000) and largely applies to girls as well (Gorman-Smith & Loeber, 2005).

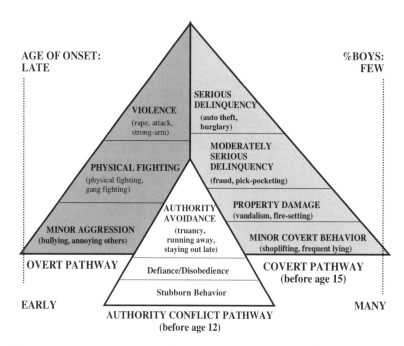

Fig. 1.2 Developmental pathways to violence, property crime, and authority conflict problems.

Some individuals are on a single pathway (e.g., some are only on the authority conflict pathway). The most affected individuals escalate on all three pathways. Escalation in either the overt or covert pathway is often preceded by an escalation by boys in the authority conflict pathway (Loeber *et al.*, 1993); in other words, conflict with authority figures is either a precursor or a concomitant of the escalation by boys in overt or covert acts. Also, an early age of onset of problem behaviour or delinquency, compared to a later onset, is more closely associated with the escalation by boys to more serious behaviours in the overt and covert pathways (Tolan *et al.*, 2000). The pathways model accounts for the majority of the most seriously affected boys—the self-reported high-rate offenders and court-reported delinquents (Loeber *et al.*, 1993, 1997). In summary, developmental pathways in antisocial behaviour and delinquency and developmental transitions between different disruptive diagnoses share a conceptualization of escalation in the severity of antisocial behaviours with development in certain individuals but not in others. The pathways model also represents selection processes, in that increasingly smaller groups of youth are at risk for more serious behaviours, comparable to a successive sieving process.

Developmental trajectories

The specification of developmental pathways can be contrasted with the identification of *developmental trajectories* (sometimes called *developmental types*), which are defined as the classification of individuals according to their pattern of deviant behaviour over time. The assumption is that a population of individuals 'is composed of a mixture of groups with distinct developmental trajectories' (Nagin & Tremblay, 2001, p. 21). Typically, trajectory analyses have been based on repeated measurements of a *single* indicator of problem behaviour. Usually, the results of trajectory analyses identify young males whose problem behaviour remains high over time, those whose problem behaviour remains low, those whose problem behaviour increases, and those whose problem behaviour decreases between childhood and early adulthood (e.g., Broidy *et al.*, 2003; Bushway *et al.*, 2003; Lacourse *et al.*, 2003; Piquero, in press). For example, Fig. 1.3 shows the developmental trajectories for violence in the oldest sample of the PYS (Loeber *et al.*, 2008). The results show four violence trajectories: no or low (51.76%), moderate declining (28.4%), high declining (5.6%), and late onset (5.6%). Thus, not all trajectories of violence started at the earliest measurement for this cohort (age 13): some emerged during adolescence. This late-onset trajectory also has been documented in other studies (e.g., Brame *et al.*, 2001) and presents a new view on the development of violence. We have not found studies in which neurobiological factors predicted late-onset violence.

Controversies about developmental change

We have briefly reviewed developmental change relevant to violence from four angles: the age–crime curve, desistance, developmental pathways, and categories of individuals with different developmental trajectories. Each of the four approaches indicates that stability in aggression and violence does occur. However, each of these approaches also elucidates the fact that there are major individual differences in aggression and violence that emerge over time, with some never escalating from minor forms of aggression to violence, some starting violence rather late, and others desisting from aggression and violence. These findings pose a considerable challenge for neurobiological studies based on the assumption that stable individual differences are trait-like for all aggressive or violent individuals and are already present early in life for *all* of those who eventually become violent. This is an oversimplification that runs counter to developmental data. The next generation of neurobiological studies can benefit from addressing stability and developmental change in all its different expressions, and by doing so, become more representative of the variety of developmental expressions of aggression and violence that actually occur in the early life course of males and females.

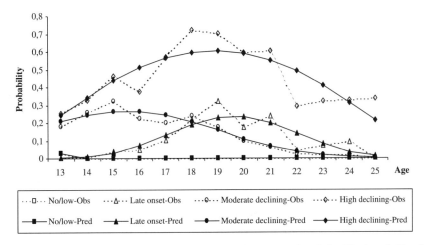

Fig. 1.3 Developmental trajectories of violence in the oldest sample of the Pittsburgh Youth Study. (From Loeber, R., Farrington, D. P., Stouthamer-Loeber, M., & White, H. R. (2008). *Violence and Serious Theft: Development and Prediction from Childhood to Adulthood.* New York: Routledge).

Identifying underlying factors

Research on the neurobiology of violence is based on the longstanding belief that certain individual difference characteristics play an important role in the development of violence. We refer to these characteristics as *underlying factors* because they are postulated to underlie individual differences in the propensity for violent behaviour within a population. Several of the assumptions made about underlying factors, either implicitly or explicitly in the research literature, make them relevant to the study of neurobiological factors. These assumptions are similar to those articulated in the introduction to this chapter and mainly pertain to the developmental origins and course of underlying factors. Perhaps the most common assumption is that underlying factors represent the behavioural manifestations of genetically driven differences in neurobiological functioning that subsequently lead to a predisposition for violent behaviour. Along these lines, underlying factors are often presumed to be stable and observable in early development (often referred to as *temperament*) well before the onset of violent behaviours. Additionally, these factors are frequently described as being useful for identifying a homogenous subgroup of individuals who have a common neurobiological risk factor for violence. Despite their inferred genetic and neurobiological underpinnings, a vast majority of the studies continue to assess underlying factors using indirect methods such as rating scales, behavioural observations, or performance-based tasks. As a result, there is often a fundamental disconnect between the theoretical conceptualization of underlying factors and the operationalization of these constructs.

Although it is commonly accepted that no single underlying factor accounts for individual differences in the propensity towards violence, there is considerable disagreement among scholars on which underlying factors are the most important for understanding the development of violence. Most contemporary models posit that there are two or more causal pathways to violence that are at least partially driven by underlying factors (Frick & Morris, 1994; Raine, 2002; Lahey & Waldman, 2003; Blair *et al.*, 2006). However, the relative importance placed on specific underlying factors varies greatly across developmental models, and there is continued debate about the relative utility of specific underlying factors for understanding the development of violence. Despite these complexities, three broad categories of underlying factors have received considerable attention in the theoretical and empirical literature: emotional and behavioural dysregulation, cognitive impairments, and deficient processing of aversive stimuli. The empirical evidence linking these broad-based categories to early conduct problems and violence are briefly reviewed here to provide a foundation from which to discuss the ongoing controversies and implications for neurobiological research. Readers interested in more extensive discussions of the putative neurobiological mechanisms associated with these underlying factors are referred to subsequent chapters, as well as previously published reviews (Frick & Morris, 1994; Raine, 2002; Lahey & Waldman, 2003; Blair *et al.*, 2006).

Emotional and behavioural dysregulation

General problems related to emotional and behavioural dysregulation have long been implicated as underlying factors in the development of violence. Many studies characterize problems with emotional dysregulation as frequent experiences of negative affect (particularly irritability and anger), sudden mood swings, and intense negative emotional reactivity with very little provocation (Lahey & Waldman, 2003). On the other hand, behavioural dysregulation has been characterized by overactivity, poor inhibitory control, impulsivity, restlessness, and inattention (Lynam, 1996; Waschbusch, 2002). Although developmental studies on antisocial behaviour have clustered aspects of both emotional and behavioural dysregulation into a single construct referred to as a *difficult* (Giancola *et al.*, 2006) or *undercontrolled* temperament (Henry *et al.*, 1996), this practice has largely been abandoned as evidence suggests that these features are distinct constructs that may uniquely contribute to the development of psychopathology (for discussion, see Rothbart, 2004).

Studies have consistently linked emotional dysregulation (particularly irritability and anger) to conduct problems and violence in children and adolescents. Features of emotional dysregulation have been associated with childhood aggressive behaviour across several cultures (Rothbart *et al.*, 1994; Chang *et al.*, 2003; Oldehinkel *et al.*, 2004). Moreover, this association has been found using several different assessment methods, including measuring emotional dysregulation using parent-report scales (Olson *et al.*, 2000), behavioural observations (Owens & Shaw, 2003), social cognitive measures (Orobio de Castro *et al.*, 2002; Vitale *et al.*, 2005), physiological measures of vagal reactivity (Beauchaine *et al.*, 2007), and functional magnetic resonance imaging (fMRI) measures of neural reactivity to provocation (Coccaro *et al.*, 2007; Eisenberger *et al.*, 2007). In addition, there is evidence that the covariation between emotional dysregulation and aggression is influenced by shared genetic factors (Gjone & Stevenson, 1997) and that emotional dysregulation predicts the development of aggression in children even after controlling for features of behavioural dysregulation (Rothbart *et al.*, 1994).

Several studies have also found a consistent association between early behavioural dysregulation and childhood conduct problems (Rothbarth *et al.*, 1994; Gjone & Stevenson, 1997; Lemery *et al.*, 2002). It is well documented that conduct problems co-occur with difficulties related to behavioural dysregulation (Angold *et al.*, 1999; Waschbusch, 2002), with changes in attention deficit/hyperactivity disorder (ADHD) symptoms paralleling fluctuations in conduct disorder symptoms over time (Lahey *et al.*, 2002). However, studies exploring the prospective relationship between problems with behavioural dysregulation and later antisocial and violent behaviour have provided somewhat mixed results (Lahey *et al.*, 1995, 2002; Lynam, 1996; Waschbusch, 2002; Broidy *et al.*, 2003). Specifically, after appropriately controlling for initial levels of antisocial behaviour, the majority of the recent longitudinal investigations have found non-significant associations between features of childhood behavioural dysregulation and later antisocial behaviour (Lahey *et al.*, 1995, 2002; Broidy *et al.*, 2003). As a result, the ability of measures of behavioural dysregulation to provide unique information about the developmental course of antisocial and violent behaviour is questionable.

Cognitive impairments

Another broad set of underlying factors implicated in the development of violence includes performance-based measures of cognitive abilities, particularly those related to intelligence and executive functioning (Lahey & Waldman, 2003). In terms of the former, studies have consistently found that children and adolescents who exhibit antisocial and violent behaviour exhibit lower intellectual abilities than healthy controls (for reviews, see Henry & Moffitt, 1997; Lahey & Waldman, 2002; Nigg & Huang-Pollock, 2003). Longitudinal evidence suggests that lower intellectual abilities are associated with antisocial and aggressive behaviour even after controlling for co-occurring problems with behavioural dysregulation (Séguin *et al.*, 2004; Raine *et al.*, 2005). However, recent studies have found that deficits in intellectual abilities may not distinguish between children who exhibit chronic delinquent behaviour and those who desist from delinquent behaviour in late adolescence and early adulthood (Raine *et al.*, 2005; Loeber *et al.*, 2007).

Cognitive impairments related to the executive functions of working memory and response modulation have also been implicated in the development and maintenance of violence (for review, see Morgan & Lilienfeld, 2000). Longitudinal evidence suggests that difficulties with working memory may be particularly pronounced in childhood-onset physical aggression, and that this association may not be accounted for by low intellectual abilities or problems with behavioural dysregulation (Séguin *et al.*, 1999, 2004). Moreover, fMRI evidence suggests that antisocial men with a history of violent behaviour exhibit functional neurobiological differences in the prefrontal regions subserving working memory, in comparison to healthy controls of normal intelligence (Kumari *et al.*, 2006). In terms of response modulation, several studies have found that children and adults exhibiting antisocial behaviour tend to perseverate in responding to previously rewarded cues, even after the contingencies change and the response results in a punishment (for review, see Wallace *et al.*, 2000). However, recent longitudinal evidence suggests that problems with response modulation may be characteristic of children who exhibit transient aggression, not those who exhibit persistent aggression across time (Séguin *et al.*, 2001).

Deficient processing of aversive stimuli

Deficits in affectively responding to aversive stimuli have also been implicated as an underlying factor in the development of violence. One influential model in this area suggests that low levels of fearfulness to threatening stimuli may underlie serious and chronic forms of violent behaviour. Along these lines, low levels of fearfulness have been related to chronic childhood behaviour problems (Shaw *et al.*, 2003), childhood aggression (Rothbart *et al.*, 1994), the onset of delinquent behaviour (Tremblay *et al.*, 1994), and the commission of serious violence (Pardini, 2006). In addition, physiological (Levenston *et al.*, 2000; Raine, 2002) and neurological (Birbaumer *et al.*, 2005) markers of fearlessness have been associated with severe and persistent forms of antisocial and violent behaviour.

There is some evidence suggesting that fearlessness leads to the development of serious violence by inhibiting the development of guilt and empathy (Pardini, 2006). Along these lines, Blair and colleagues (2001, 2006) have found evidence indicating that persistent forms of psychopathic violence are associated with an inability to effectively identify social distress cues in others, particularly fearful and sad faces. However, it is important to note that neuroimaging studies have found that severe antisocial behaviour in children and adults is associated with an abnormal neural responsiveness to a wide variety of negatively valenced stimuli (Kiehl *et al.*, 2001; Flor *et al.*, 2002; Sterzer *et al.*, 2005), not just features of distress in others. As a result, the nature of the association between low affective arousal to aversive stimuli and violence is still unclear.

Controversies regarding underlying factors

Although a rapidly growing body of research has implicated several underlying factors in the development of violent behaviour, several controversies regarding the nature of these associations and the potential implications for understanding the neurobiological underpinnings of violence remain. Some of the key issues that need further study are as follows:

- The specificity of the proposed underlying factors for understanding the development of violent behaviour is unclear. Although theoretical models often propose an underlying factor as a driver of violent behaviour, rather than a driver of antisocial behaviour in general, this hypothesis is rarely empirically tested. More importantly, several of the underlying factors described in the preceding text have been empirically linked to psychopathology other than antisocial behaviour, such as internalizing problems (Geurin *et al.*, 1997), substance use disorders (Cloninger *et al.*, 1996), and schizophrenia (Morgan & Lillienfeld, 2000). However, it is not clear why individuals with the same underlying factor would develop divergent forms of psychopathology.

- Underlying factors are often assumed to index specific aspects of neurobiological functioning, but they are frequently measured using behavioural rating scales. This practice is problematic given that the correlations between behavioural rating scales of underlying factors and aspects of neurobiological functioning are often counter-intuitive and differ depending on the rating scale used (e.g., Horn *et al.*, 2003).

- Underlying factors are often conceptualized as relatively immutable characteristics, even though emerging evidence suggests that aspects of temperament can be influenced by social factors such as parenting (Rapee, 2002). Moreover, it is now apparent that the brain structures believed to subserve several underlying factors continue to mature into early adulthood (Gogtay *et al.*, 2004). As a result, greater attention needs to be paid to the dynamic nature of underlying factors as well as the neurobiological factors believed to subserve them.

- Studies need to examine more critically the ability of underlying factors to predict the developmental course of violent and antisocial behaviour, including escalation and desistence. Longitudinal studies frequently do not control for prior levels of antisocial behaviour or environmental factors when looking at the predictive utility of underlying factors. In addition, many studies have not examined which underlying factors are the most important for predicting violence after controlling for their co-occurrence.

- Measures of underlying factors sometimes include behaviours consistent with early forms of aggression and conduct problems, especially measures of emotional and behavioural dysregulation. Future studies should make clear empirical and theoretical distinctions between early forms of violent behaviour (e.g., hitting, threatening) and the underlying factors placing youth at risk for developing these behaviours (e.g., irritable mood).

- Researchers should begin breaking complex underlying factors into component pieces in order to better understand their relationship with violence (for discussion, see Rothbart, 2004). For example, as researchers have dismantled the construct of emotional dysregulation, it has become clear that anger is associated with increased levels of aggression (Rothbart *et al.*, 1994), whereas increased fear seems to be negatively related to violence (Pardini, 2006).

- The seemingly contradictory finding that violent behaviour is associated with both emotional dysregulation and low arousal to aversive stimuli needs to be more thoroughly examined. Although models have suggested that this apparent paradox indicates the presence of different subgroups of violent individuals (e.g., Frick & Morris, 2004; Blair *et al.*, 2006; Pardini, 2006), developmental research in this area is still limited.

- The possibility that different underlying factors may interact to produce an increased risk for violent behaviour needs to be more thoroughly examined. In support of this practice, Colder *et al.*, (2002) found that lower levels of infant fearfulness were associated with increases in externalizing problems across early childhood only for those children with high levels of behavioural dysregulation. Similarly, more studies are needed to examine which environmental factors may protect children who exhibit underlying factors from developing violent behaviour over time.

Causes of violence and homicide

As shown in Fig. 1.1, we conceptualize that underlying factors and behavioural manifestations of violence are the result of neurobiological, social, individual, economic, and environmental causes. There is a voluminous literature on the neurobiological, social, and other causes of violence (e.g., Hawkins *et al.*, 1998; Lipsey & Derzon, 1998). For the following text, we draw from several major reviews on predictors of violence, delinquency, and Conduct Disorder (Lipsey & Derzon, 1998; Loeber & Farrington, 1998, 2001; Burke *et al.*, 2002) as well as from the PYS. In the PYS, we found that 51 factors significantly predicted violence in young men (Loeber *et al.*, 2005). Fig. 1.4 shows a prediction index for violence constructed on the basis of the eleven strongest predictors (Loeber *et al.*, 2005): truancy, low school motivation, onset of delinquency before age 10, cruelty to people, depressed mood, physical aggression, callous or unemotional behaviour, low family socio-economic status, family on welfare, high parental stress, and bad (i.e., disadvantaged) neighbourhood (parent-reported). The higher the individuals score on the index the more likely it is that they will commit violence later (odds ratio [OR] = 6.0 for four or more risk factors). Remarkably, the range of probabilities for future violence in the Pittsburgh data is from 3% at zero risk factors to 100% at nine or more risk factors.

Another important issue to be determined is whether homicide, as the most extreme form of violence, can be predicted among violent offenders, and whether there is a dose–response association between the number of risk factors and later homicide. Loeber *et al.* (2005) found the following predictors of homicide among the violent offenders: high risk score (of disruptive behaviour) at screening, positive attitude to substance use, Conduct Disorder by age 13, carrying a weapon, gang fighting, selling hard drugs, peer delinquency, repeating grade(s), and family on welfare. The results showed that the higher the number of risk factors, the higher the probability of homicide. The probability of homicide is low for zero to three risk factors, but after that it almost linearly increases to about 15% at six or more risk factors. The OR, based on four or more risk factors, amounted to 14.5. Because genetic factors (and other neurobiological factors measured at a young age) were not available in

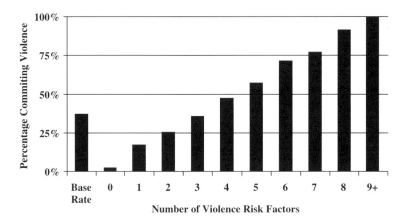

Fig. 1.4 Proportion of boys committing violent offences for different levels of risk in the Pittsburgh Youth Study. (From Loeber, R., Pardini, D. A., Homish, D. L., Wei, E. H., Crawford, A. M., Farrington, D. P., *et al.* (2005). The prediction of violence and homicide in young men. *Journal of Consulting and Clinical Psychology*, 73, 1074-1088.) .

this study, it remains to be seen to what extent neurobiological factors can contribute to the prediction of violence and homicide (genetic information is likely to be collected for these cohorts in the near future.)

Controversies regarding causation

The prediction results, and those of several other studies (e.g., Farrington, 1997; Hawkins *et al.*, 1998; Lipsey & Derzon, 1998), indicate a robust association between the number of social and other risk factors and the probability of later violence. However, we want to emphasize the following controversies:

- There is only a single study of the prediction of homicide in a population sample (i.e., Loeber *et al.*, 2005). Studies still have to demonstrate that neurobiological factors uniquely predict violence if a large range of known social and other factors are taken into account.
- The effect of neurobiological factors could be mediated through various individual difference characteristics represented by one or more underlying factors. For example, neurobiological problems associated with the processing of fear stimuli could lead to callous-unemotional behaviour, which in turn is related to violence (Pardini, 2006). Thus, future studies need to explain both underlying factors and different manifestations of aggression and violence as these phenomena develop over the life course.
- Further, although there is increasing evidence that gene–environment interactions are important (Taylor & Kim-Cohen, 2007), the range of social and other factors that are documented in these interactions is large. Therefore, there is a need to better understand the mechanism(s) by which gene–environment interactions operate.

Causes of secular changes in violence and causes of cohort differences in violence

Over the past century, the United States has seen a much higher rate of violence than most European countries, but it is far less known that this does not apply to all forms of violence, and that Europe at one time had a higher homicide rate than the United States. Data from the United States and a few European countries for the years 1980–99 (Farrington & Jolliffe, 2005) clearly show that the rate of homicide and rape is substantially higher in the United States compared to England and Wales, Switzerland, and the Netherlands. However, the rate of robbery and burglary in the United States, based on victim surveys, are similar compared to several European countries, especially since the 1990s.

The crime rates between 1981 and 1999 have varied a great deal. Major increases and decreases in crime have taken place, such as decreases in homicide, rape, robbery, and burglary in the United States, increases in burglary and rape in England and Wales, and increase in robbery in the Netherlands. Over a longer period of observation, the rate of homicide in Europe after the year 1200 was much higher than the rate of homicide in the United States in the last century, but the European rate has decreased dramatically since the early middle ages. The current rate of homicide in the United States is similar to the rate that was common in Europe around the year 1700 (Eisner, 2004). The bottom line is that there are secular changes in violence rates of countries and cities, and that some of these secular changes have been large over time. The fact, however, is that secular changes are not necessarily taking place across countries at the same time. For these and other reasons, it is important to address the causes of secular changes in violence.

There is a voluminous literature with numerous hypotheses about the causes of secular changes in crime and violence (e.g., Blumstein & Wallman, 2000). We propose that secular changes in violence pose a unique challenge to studies on the neurobiology of violence. Are there neurobiological factors that either solely or in conjunction with social, individual, economic, and environmental factors influence secular changes in violence, and if so, by what mechanism(s)? As far as we know, there are no studies that have proved that one or more neurobiological factors can sufficiently explain secular changes in violence. Part of the problem in identifying any cause, neurobiological or otherwise, of secular changes in violence is the ecological fallacy (the assumption that all members of a group exhibit character-istics seen in aggregate statistics collected on the group at large). Another problem is that the causes of changes in the prevalence of violence in populations are not necessarily directly linked to changes in individuals' propensity to violence. We argue that the latter is an essen-tial step, especially because neurobiological factors are thought to reside in individuals rather than in populations.

The annual community rate of violence in a population over time is actually the sum of the violent offending rates of individuals of different ages, represented by an aggregation of successive age–crime curves of different age cohorts. Thus, over a period of, say, 1990–2000, the violence of some individuals may be represented in 1995 and 1996, whereas a younger generation's violence is represented in 1997 and 1998. The years in which their violence is most represented in the graphs are their peak years of violence (in the age–crime curve, about ages 15 to 22), which then show up markedly in population graphs of violence. Our approach to better address the origins of secular changes is to decompose these changes in the violence rate of populations into a series of age–crime curves for successive age cohorts of individuals whose violence contributes to secular levels of crime in the whole population.

Opening this avenue of inquiry has the advantage of making use of longitudinal studies with multiple cohorts. We argue that such studies allow us to identify the causes of violence for one cohort and compare these with the causes of violence for another cohort. This approach is particularly valuable when there are large cohort differences in violence. Fig. 1.5 illustrates this point with the youngest and oldest cohorts in the PYS (who were on average six years apart). The oldest compared to the youngest cohort had a substantially different age–crime curve: the curve was higher and appeared to have a larger base for the oldest cohort, suggesting that desistance processes in the downslope of the age–crime curve in the oldest cohort took place about five years later than in the youngest cohort. Even during the period in which the two cohorts overlapped (ages 13 to 19), there were major differences in violence-related outcomes, including gang membership and gun carrying. For example, gang membership decreased from a peak of 6% at age 15 to less than 2% at age 19 in the youngest cohort, but increased from 6% at age 13 to 9% at age 19 in the oldest cohort. In addition, gun carrying decreased from a peak of 8% at age 16 to 5% at age 19 in the youngest cohort, whereas gun carrying increased in the oldest cohort from 2% at age 13 to 17% at age 19. Two lessons can be learned from these results: (1) even with age cohorts just six years apart, there can be major changes in the age–crime curve; and (2) differences between cohorts in violence were accompanied by activities—gang membership and gun carrying—that directly fuel violence. Thus, if successive age cohorts display unusually high levels of violence, this will create a sequence of age–crime curves that are higher and broader than the typical curves. In aggregate these successive, high age–crime curves will translate into higher

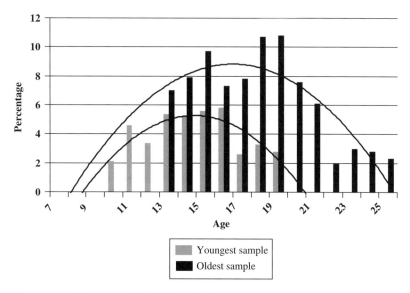

Fig. 1.5 Different age-crime curves for violence in the youngest and oldest sample of the Pittsburgh Youth Study.

rates of violence in communities where the cohorts reside and/or are active, thus contributing to secular changes in violence over time.

We translate this line of thinking in a shift from the question 'what are the causes of secular changes in violence?' to the question 'what are the causes of cohort differences in violence?' (see also Jacobson *et al.*, 2000) The advantage of this approach is that it brings us closer to the investigation of causes for individuals that in aggregate can represent the causes of violence in populations. For example, Fabio *et al.* (2006) examined predictors of the differences between the two cohorts in the PYS for self-reported violence and found that cohort differences did not contribute to the regression equation once individual factors (gun carrying, gang membership, drug dealing, hard drug use), race, family socio-economic status, and period effects (factors manifest during a specific period that affect all cohorts) had been taken into account.

Controversies regarding secular changes in violence

• It remains to be seen which, if any, of the individual factors that predict secular differences in violence are related to one or more neurobiological factors.
• It is also unclear to what extent mixtures of neurobiological and non-biological factors differ for boys and girls in the explanation of cohort differences and, down the line, secular differences in violence.

Conclusions

We began by specifying several common assumptions in neurobiological studies and pointed to four controversial areas relevant in the investigation of neurobiological factors and the development of violence. The majority of the investigations of neurobiological factors have been cross-sectional (or retrospective). As a consequence, conceptualizations about the dependent variable of aggression and violence in neurobiological studies have been mostly static rather than dynamic and have not reflected individuals' developmental changes in aggression and violence during the life course as evident from longitudinal studies. Although we agree that it is useful to search for neurobiological, social, and other factors to explain stable individual differences in aggression and violence, longitudinal investigations on the neurobiology of violence need to address key questions about change as well. Examples of such questions are: Why do most children outgrow aggression in the first years of life? Why do some violent youth desist in violence? Why do some youth but not others progress along a pathway from minor forms of aggression to serious violence and homicide? Why do some individuals have a late onset of violence? Why are there categories of individuals with different trajectories of violence during childhood and adolescence? Answers to all of these questions can enrich the search for neurobiological underpinnings of violence, deepen theoretical explanations, and eventually improve prevention and intervention problems targeting violence.

We also made a case that most of the conceptualizations of neurobiological, social, and other causes interpose underlying factors as necessary links between neurobiological factors and aggression and violence. We illustrated the large variety of underlying factors that have been proposed, and the comparative lack of information about which of the underlying factors is most valid and can be measured most reliably. Although many scholars agree about the need to link neurobiological factors to underlying factors, they tend to disagree about which underlying factors are the most valid and reliable and do not pay sufficient attention to the possible relationships between underlying factors. Neurobiological studies often do not recognize that underlying factors may change and are possibly key elements of the explanation of the age–aggression and age–crime curves. Finding out which neurobiological factors (in conjunction with social and other factors) influence changes in underlying factors appears to be of the highest priority.

We illustrated that although the predictive power of social, individual, economic, and environmental factors in the prediction of violence and homicide is considerable, we do not sufficiently know what the additional explanatory power is of neurobiological factors. Even though progress has been made in the study of gene–environment interactions (Moffitt, 2005; Taylor & Kim-Cohen, 2007), these findings should be interpreted with caution. Environmental risk variables tend to occur in concert rather than singly. For instance, Koot *et al.* (in press) stressed that most findings on gene–environment interactions for a wide range of antisocial outcomes have been based on childhood maltreatment as an environmental risk factor. However, maltreatment may serve as an index of adverse familial conditions. Taylor and Kim-Cohen's (2007) meta-analysis showed that the interaction between genetic and environmental factors results in a risk that is far higher than the sum of the individual risk factors. However, a close examination of the results shows little agreement among the studies about the observed interaction mechanisms.

Finally, we showed that the explanation of secular changes in violence poses yet another series of challenges to neurobiological studies. If secular changes occur within years, it will be difficult to test which neurobiological factors are elements in the explanation of secular change. We argue that longitudinal studies with multiple cohorts are essential in this quest, because cohort differences in violence are a building block for secular changes in population violence.

Our experience lies in the developmental aspects of aggression and violence and to some extent in the study of neurobiological causes (e.g., see the work of our collaborators such as Eaves *et al.*, 1997; McBurnett *et al.*, 1997; Raine *et al.*, 2005). We hope, however, that researchers of the neurobiology of violence can see the merits of the avenues for investigation that we have proposed and that this will eventually lead to improved knowledge about the causes of violence.

Acknowledgments

The research on this chapter was supported by grant 2005-JK-FX-0001 from the Office of Juvenile Justice and Delinquency Prevention, grants numbers 50778 and 51091 from the National Institute of Mental Health, and grant number 411018 from the National Institute on Drug Abuse. The work of D. Pardini was supported by grant K01 MH078039 from the National Institutes of Mental Health. Points of view or opinions are those of the authors and do not necessarily represent the official position or policies of the US Department of Justice, the National Institute of Mental Health, and the National Institute of Drug Abuse.

References

Angold, A., Costello, E. J., & Erkanli, A. (1999). Comorbidity. *Journal of Child Psychology and Psychiatry*, *40*, 57–87.

Baum, K. (2005). Juvenile victimization and offending, 1993–2003, Bulletin NCJ 209468. Washington, DC: US Department of Justice, Office of Juvenile Justice Programs, Bureau of Justice Statistics. Available at: http://www.ojp.usdoj.gov/bjs/abstract/jvo03.htm.

Beauchaine, T. P., Gatzke-Kopp, L., & Mead, H. K. (2007). Polyvagal theory and developmental psychopathology: emotion dysregulation and conduct problems from preschool to adolescence. *Biological Psychology*, *74*, 174–184.

Birbaumer, N., Veit, R., Lotze, M., Erb, M., Hermann, C., Grodd, W., & Flor, H. (2005). Deficient fear conditioning in psychopathy: a functional magnetic resonance imaging study. *Archives of General Psychiatry*, *62*, 799–805.

Blair, R. J. (2001). Neurocognitive models of aggression, the antisocial personality disorders, and psychopathy. *Journal of Neurology, Neurosurgery, and Psychiatry*, *71*, 727–731.

Blair, R. J., Peschardt, K. S., Budhani, S., Mitchell, D. G., & Pine, D. S. (2006). The development of psychopathy. *Journal of Child Psychology and Psychiatry*, *47*, 262–276.

Blumstein, A., & Wallman, J. (2000). *The Crime Drop in America*. New York: Cambridge University Press.

Brame, B., Nagin, D. S., & Tremblay, R. E. (2001). Developmental trajectories of physical aggression from school entry to late adolescence. *Journal of Child Psychology and Psychiatry*, *42*, 503–512.

Broidy, L. M., Nagin, D. S., Tremblay, R. E., Bates, J. E., Brame, B., Dodge, K. A., *et al.* (2003). Developmental trajectories of childhood disruptive behavior and adolescent delinquency: a six-site, cross-national study. *Developmental Psychology*, *39*, 222–245.

Burke, J. D., Loeber, R., & Birmaher, B. (2002). Oppositional defiant disorder and conduct disorder: a review of the past 10 years, Part II. *Journal of the American Academy of Child & Adolescent Psychiatry*, *41*, 1275–1293.

Bushway, S. D., Thornberry, T. P., & Krohn, M. S. (2003). Desistance as a developmental process: a comparison of static and dynamic approaches. *Journal of Quantitative Criminology*, *19*, 129–153.

Chang, L., Schwartz, D., Dodge, K. A., & McBride-Chang, C. (2003). Harsh parenting in relation to child emotion regulation and aggression. *Journal of Family Psychology*, *17*, 598–606.

Cloninger, C. R., Sigvardsson, S., & Bohman, M. (1996). Type I and type II alcoholism: an update. *Alcohol Health and Research World*, *20*, 18–23.

Coccaro, E. F., McCloskey, M. S., Fitzgerald, D. A., & Phan, K. L. (2007). Amygdala and orbitofrontal reactivity to social threat in individuals with impulsive aggression. *Biological Psychiatry*, *62*, 168–178.

Colder, C. R., Mott, J. A., & Berman, A. S. (2002). The interactive effects of infant activity level and fear on growth trajectories of early childhood behavior problems. *Development and Psychopathology*, *14*, 1–23.

Corso, P. S., Mercy, J. A., Simon, T. R., Finkelstein, E. A., & Miller, T. R. (2007). Medical costs and productivity losses due to interpersonal and self-directed violence in the United States. *American Journal of Preventative Medicine*, *32*, 474–482.

Eaves, L., Silberg, J. L., Meyer, J. M., Maes, H. H., Simonoff, E., Pickles, A., *et al.* (1997). Genetics and developmental psychopathology: 2. the main effects of genes and environment on behavioral problems in the Virginia Twin Study of Adolescent Behavioral Development. *Journal of Child Psychology & Psychiatry*, *38*, 965–980.

Eisenberger, N. I., Way, B. M., Taylor, S. E., Welch, W. T., & Lieberman, M. D. (2007). Understanding genetic risk for aggression: clues from the brain's response to social exclusion. *Biological Psychiatry*, *61*, 1100–1108.

Eisner, M. (2004). Violence and the rise of modern society. *Criminology in Europe: Newsletter of the European Society of Criminology*, *3*, 14–16.

Elliott, D. S., Pampel, F. C., & Huizinga, D. (2005). Youth violence: continuity and desistance: a supplemental report to youth violence: a report of the Surgeon General. Washington, DC: Substance Abuse and Mental Health Services Administration.

Fabio, A., Loeber, R., Balasurbramani, G. K., Roth, J., & Farrington, D. P. (2006). Why some generations are more violent than others: assessment of age, period, and cohort effects. *American Journal of Epidemiology*, *164*, 151–160.

Farrington, D. P. (1986). Age and crime. In M. Tonry & N. Morris (eds), *Crime and Justice: An Annual Review of Research* (pp. 189–250). Chicago, IL: University of Chicago Press.

Farrington, D. P. (1997). Early prediction of violent and non-violent youthful offending. *European Journal on Criminal Policy and Research*, *5*, 51–66.

Farrington, D. P., & Jolliffe, D. (2005). Cross-national comparisons of crime rates in four countries, 1981–1999. In M. Tonry & D. P. Farrington (eds), *Crime and Punishment in Western Countries, 1980–1999* (pp. 377–397). Chicago, IL: University of Chicago Press.

Fishbein, D. H. (ed) (2000). *The Science, Treatment, and Prevention of Antisocial Behavior. Application to the Criminal Justice System*. Kingston, NJ: Civic Research Institute.

Flor, H., Birbaumer, N., Hermann, C., Ziegler, S., & Patrick, C. (2002). Aversive Pavlovian conditioning is psychopaths: peripheral and central correlates. *Psychophysiology*, *39*, 505–518.

Frick, P. J., & Morris, A. S. (2004). Temperament and developmental pathways to conduct problems. *Journal of Clinical Child and Adolescent Psychology*, *33*, 54–68.

Giancola, P. R., Roth, R. M., & Dominic, J. P. (2006). The mediating role of executive functioning in the relation between difficult temperament and physical aggression. *Journal of Psychopathology and Behavioral Assessment*, *28*, 211–221.

Gjone, H., & Stevenson, J. (1997). The association between internalizing and externalizing behavior in childhood and early adolescence: genetic of environmental common influences? *Journal of Abnormal Childhood Psychology*, *25*, 277–286.

Gogtay, N., Giedd, J. N., Lusk, L., Hayashi, K. M., Greenstein, D., Vaituzis, A. C., *et al.* (2004). Dynamic mapping of human cortical development during childhood through early adulthood. *Proceedings of the National Academy of Sciences of the United States of America*, *101*, 8174–8179.

Gorman-Smith, D., & Loeber, R. (2005). Are developmental pathways in disruptive behavior the same for girls and boys? *Journal of Child and Family Studies*, *14*, 15–27.

Guerin, D. W., Gottfried, A. W., & Thomas, C. W. (1997). Difficult temperament and behavioral problems: a longitudinal study from 1.5 to 12 years. *International Journal of Behavioral Development*, *21*, 71–90.

Hawkins, J. D., Herrenkohl, T., Farrington, D. P., Brewer, D., Catalano, R. F., & Harachi, T. W. (1998). A review of predictors of youth violence. In R. Loeber & D. P. Farrington (eds), *Serious and Violent Juvenile Offenders: Risk Factors and Successful Interventions* (pp. 106–146). Thousand Oaks, CA: Sage Publications.

Henry, D., Caspi, A., Moffitt, T. E., & Silva, P. A. (1996). Temperamental and familial predictors of violence and non-violent criminal convictions: age 3 to age 18. *Developmental Psychology*, *32*, 614–623.

Henry, B., & Moffitt, T. E. (1997). Neuropsychological and neuroimaging studies of juvenile delinquency and adult criminal behavior. In D. M. Stoff & J. Breiling (eds), *Handbook of Antisocial Behavior* (pp. 280–288). New York: Wiley.

Horn, N. R., Dolan, M., Elliott, R., Deakin, J. F. W., & Woodruff, P. W. R. (2003). Response inhibition and impulsivity: an fMRI study. *Neuropsychologia*, *41*, 1959–1966.

Jacobson, K. C., Prescott, C. A., Neale, M. C., & Kendler, K. S. (2000). Cohort differences in genetic and environmental influences on retrospective reports of conduct disorder among adult male twins. *Psychological Medicine*, *30*, 775–787.

Kiehl, K. A., Smith, A. M., Hare, R. D., Mendrek, A., Forster, B. B., Brink, J., *et al.* (2001). Limbic abnormalities in affective processing by criminal psychopaths as revealed by functional magnetic resonance imaging. *Biological Psychiatry*, *50*, 677–684.

Kingston, L. M., & Prior, M. (1995). The development of patterns of stable, transient, and school-age onset aggressive behavior in young children. *American Academy of Child & Adolescent Psychiatry*, *34*, 348–358.

Koot, H. M., Oosterlaan, J., Jansen, L. M., Neumann, A., Luman, M., & van Lier, P. A. C. (in press). Individual factors. In R. Loeber, N. W. Slot, P. H. van der Laan, & M. Hoeve (eds), *Tomorrow's Criminals: The Development of Child Delinquency and Effective Interventions*. Aldershot: Ashgate.

Kumari, V., Aasen, I., Taylor, P., Ffytche, D. H., Das, M., & Barkataki, I. (2006). Neural dysfunction and violence in schizophrenia: an fMRI investigation. *Schizophrenia Research*, *84*, 144–164.

Lacourse, E., Nagin, D., Tremblay, R. E., Vitaro, F., & Claes, M. (2003). Developmental trajectories of boys' delinquent group membership and facilitation of violent behaviors during adolescence. *Development and Psychopathology*, *15*, 183–197.

Lahey, B. B., Loeber, R., Burke, J., & Rathouz, P. J. (2002). Adolescent outcomes of childhood conduct disorder among clinic-referred boys: predictors of improvement. *Journal of Abnormal Child Psychology*, *30*, 333–348.

Lahey, B. B., Loeber, R., Hart, E. L., Frick, P. J., Applegate, B., Zhang, Q., *et al.* (1995). Four-year longitudinal study of conduct disorder in boys: patterns and predictors of persistence. *Journal of Abnormal Psychology*, *104*, 83–93.

Lahey, B. B., & Waldman, I. D. (2003). A developmental propensity model of the origins of conduct problems during childhood and adolescence. In B. B. Lahey, T. E. Moffitt, & A. Caspi (eds), *The Causes of Conduct Disorder and Serious Juvenile Delinquency* (pp. 76–117). New York: Guilford Press.

Laub, J. H., & Sampson, R. J. (2003). *Shared Beginnings, Divergent Lives: Delinquent Boys up to Age 70*. Cambridge, MA: Harvard University Press.

Lemery, K. S., Essex, M. J., & Smider, N. A. (2002). Revealing the relation between temperament and behavior problem symptoms by eliminating measurement confounding: expert ratings and factor analyses. *Child Development*, *73*, 867–882.

Levenston, G. K., Patrick, C. J., Bradley, M. M., & Lang, P. J. (2000). The psychopath as observer: emotion and attention in picture processing. *Journal of Abnormal Psychology*, *109*, 373–385.

Lipsey, M. W., & Derzon, J. H. (1998). Predictors of violent or serious delinquency in adolescence and early adulthood: a synthesis of longitudinal research. In R. Loeber, & D. P. Farrington (eds), *Serious and Violent Juvenile Offenders: Risk Factors and Successful Interventions* (pp. 86–105). Thousands Oaks, CA: Sage.

Loeber, R., & Farrington, D. F. (1998). *Serious and Violent Juvenile Offenders: Risk Factors and Successful Interventions*. Thousand Oaks, CA: Sage.

Loeber, R., & Farrington, D. P. (2001). *Child delinquents: Development, Intervention and Service Needs*. Thousand Oaks, CA: Sage.

Loeber, R., Farrington, D. P., Stouthamer-Loeber, M., Moffitt, T. E., & Caspi, A. (1998). The development of male offending: key findings from the first decade of the Pittsburgh Youth Study. *Studies in Crime and Crime Prevention*, *7*, 141–172.

Loeber, R., Farrington, D. P., Stouthamer-Loeber, M., & White, H. R. (2008). *Violence and Serious Theft: Development and Prediction from Childhood to Adulthood*. New York: Routledge.

Loeber, R., Keenan, K., & Zhang, Q. (1997). Boys' experimentation and persistence in developmental pathways toward serious delinquency. *Journal of Child and Family Studies, 6*, 321–357.

Loeber, R., Pardini, D. A., Homish, D. L., Wei, E. H., Crawford, A. M., Farrington, D. P., *et al.* (2005). The prediction of violence and homicide in young men. *Journal of Consulting and Clinical Psychology, 73*, 1074–1088.

Loeber, R., Pardini, D. A., Stouthamer-Loeber, M., & Raine, A. (2007). Do cognitive, physiological and psycho-social risk and promotive factors predict desistance from delinquency in males? *Development and Psychopathology, 19*, 867–887.

Loeber, R., Wei, E., Stouthamer-Loeber, M., Huizinga, D., & Thornberry, T. (1999). Behavioral antecedents to serious and violent juvenile offending: joint analyses from the Denver Youth Survey, Pittsburgh Youth Study, and the Rochester Development Study. *Studies in Crime and Crime Prevention, 8*, 245–263.

Loeber, R., Wung, P., Keenan, K., Giroux, B., Stouthamer-Loeber, M., van Kammen, W.B., *et al.* (1993). Developmental pathways in disruptive child behavior. *Development and Psychopathology, 5*, 101–132.

Lynam, D. R. (1996). Early identification of chronic offenders: who is the fledgling psychopath? *Psychological Bulletin, 120*, 209–234.

McBurnett, K., Pfiffner, L. J., Capasso, L., Lahey, B. B., & Loeber, R. (1997). Children's aggression and DSM-II-R symptoms predicted by parent psychopathy, parenting practices, cortisol, and SES. In A. Raine, P. A. Brennan, D. P. Farrington, & S. A. Mednick (eds), *Biosocial Bases of Violence* (pp. 345–348). New York: Plenum.

Moffitt, T. E. (1993). Adolescence-limited and life-course-persistent antisocial behavior: a developmental taxonomy. *Psychological Review, 100*, 674–701.

Moffitt, T. E. (2005). The new look of behavioral genetics in developmental psychopathology: gene-environment interplay in antisocial behaviors. *Psychological Bulletin, 131*, 533–554.

Morgan, A. B., & Lilienfeld, S. O. (2000). A meta-analytic review of the relation between antisocial behavior and neuropsychological measures of executive function. *Clinical Psychology Review, 20*, 113–136.

Nagin, D. S., & Tremblay, R. E. (2001). Analyzing developmental trajectories of distinct but related behaviors: a group-based method. *Psychological Methods, 6*, 18–34.

Nagin, D., & Tremblay, R. E. (2005). What has been learned from group-based trajectory modeling? Examples from physical aggression and other problem behaviors. *Annals of the American Academy of Political and Social Science, 602*, 82–117.

Newburn, T. (2007). 'Tough on crime': penal policy in England and Wales. In M. Tonry (ed), *Crime, Punishment, and Politics in Comparative Perspective. Crime and Justice, vol. 36* (pp. 425–470). Chicago: Chicago University Press.

NICHD Early Child Care Research Network (2004). Trajectories of physical aggression from toddlerhood to middle childhood. *SRCD Monographs, 69*, 1–146.

Nigg, J. T., & Huang-Pollack, C. L. (2003). An early onset model of the role of executive functions and intelligence in conduct disorder/delinquency. In B. B. Lahey, T. E. Moffitt, & A. Caspi (eds), *Causes of Conduct Disorder and Juvenile Delinquency* (pp. 227–253). New York: Guilford.

Oldehinkel, A. J., Hartman, C. A., de Winter, A. F., Veenstra, R., & Ormel, J. (2004). Temperament profiles associated with internalizing and externalizing problems in preadolescence. *Development and Psychopathology, 16*, 421–440.

Olson, S. L., Bates, J. E., Sandy, J. M., & Lanthier, R. (2000). Early developmental precursors of externalizing behavior in middle childhood and adolescence. *Journal of Abnormal Child Psychology, 28*, 119–133.

Olweus, D. (1979). Stability of aggressive reaction patterns in males: a review. *Psychological Bulletin, 86*, 852–875.

Orobio de Castro, B., Veerman, J. W., Koops, W., Bosch, J. D., & Monshouwer, H. J. (2002). Personality and social development hostile attribution of intent and aggressive behavior: a meta-analysis. *Child Development, 73*, 916–934.

Owens, E. B., & Shaw, D. S. (2003). Predicting growth curves of externalizing behavior across the preschool years. *Journal of Abnormal Child Psychology, 31*, 575–590.

Pardini, D. (2006). The callousness pathway to severe violent delinquency. *Aggressive Behavior*, *32*, 590–598.

Piquero, A. R. (in press). Taking stock of developmental trajectories of criminal activity over the life course. In A. Liberman (ed), *The Yield of Recent Longitudinal Research on Crime and Delinquency*. New York: Springer.

Prinzie, P., Onghena, P., Hellinckx, W., Grietens, H., Ghesquière, P., & Colpin, H. (2005). Direct and indirect relationships between parental personality and externalising behaviour: the role of negative parenting. *Psychologica Belgica*, *45*, 123–145.

Raine, A. (1993). *The Psychopathology of Crime. Criminal Behavior as a Clinical Disorder*. San Diego, CA: Academic Press.

Raine, A. (2002). Annotation: the role of prefrontal deficits, low autonomic arousal, and early health factors in the development of antisocial and aggressive behavior in children. *Journal of Child Psychology and Psychiatry*, *43*, 417–434.

Raine, A., Moffitt, T. E., Caspi, A., Loeber, R., Stouthamer-Loeber, M., & Lynam, D. (2005). Neurocognitive impairments in boys on the life-course persistent antisocial path. *Journal of Abnormal Psychology*, *114*, 38–49.

Rapee, R. M. (2002). The development and modification of temperamental risk for anxiety disorders: prevention of a lifetime of anxiety? *Biological Psychiatry*, *52*, 947–957.

Rosenfeld, R. (2004). Firearms research and the crime drop. *Criminology and Public Policy*, *4*, 799–806.

Rothbart, M. K. (2004). Commentary: differentiated measures of temperament and multiple pathways to childhood disorders. *Journal of Clinical Child and Adolescent Psychology*, *33*, 82–87.

Rothbart, M. K., Ahadi, S. A., & Hershey, K. L. (1994). Temperament and social behavior in childhood. *Merrill-Palmer Quarterly*, *40*, 21–39.

Rowe, D. C. (2002). *Biology and Crime*. Los Angeles, CA: Roxbury.

Séguin, J. R., Boulerice, B., Harden, P. W., Tremblay, R. E., & Pihl, R. O. (1999). Executive functions and physical aggression after controlling for attention deficit hyperactivity disorder, general memory, and IQ. *Journal of Child Psychology and Psychiatry*, *40*, 1197–1208.

Séguin, J. R., Nagin, D., Assaad, J. M., & Tremblay, R. E. (2004). Cognitive-neuropsychological function in chronic physical aggression and hyperactivity. *Journal of Abnormal Psychology*, *113*, 603–613.

Shaw, D. S., Gilliom, M., Ingoldsby, E. M., & Nagin, D. S. (2003). Trajectories leading to school-age conduct problems. *Developmental Psychology*, *39*, 189–200.

Sterzer, P., Stadler, C., Krebs, A., Kleinschmidt, A., & Poustka, F. (2005). Abnormal neural responses to emotional visual stimuli in adolescents with conduct disorder. *Biological Psychiatry*, *57*, 7–15.

Taylor, A., & Kim-Cohen, J. (2007). Meta-analysis of gene-environment interactions in developmental psychopathology. *Development and Psychopathology*, *19*, 1029–1037.

Tolan, P. H., & Gorman-Smith, D. (1998). Development of serious and violent offending careers. In R. Loeber, & D. P. Farrington (eds), *Serious and Violent Juvenile Offenders: Risk Factors and Successful Interventions*. (pp. 68–85). Thousand Oaks, CA: Sage.

Tolan, P. H., Gorman-Smith, D., & Loeber, R. (2000). Developmental timing of onsets of disruptive behaviors and later delinquency of inner-city youth. *Journal of Child and Family Studies*, *9*, 203–230.

Tremblay, R. E., & Nagin, D. S. (2005). The developmental origins of physical aggression in humans. In R. E. Tremblay, & W. W. Hartup (eds), *Developmental Origins of Aggression* (pp. 85–106). New York: Guilford Press.

Tremblay, R. E., Nagin, D. S., Séguin, J. R., Zoccolillo, M., Zelazo, P. D., Boivin, M., *et al.* (2004). Physical aggression during early childhood: trajectories and predictors. *Pediatrics*, *114*, e43–e50.

Tremblay, R. E., Pihl, R. O., Vitaro, F., & Dobkin, P. L. (1994). Predicting early onset of male antisocial behavior from preschool behavior. *Archives of General Psychiatry*, *51*, 732–739.

Vitale, J. E., Newman, J. P., Bates, J. E., Goodnight, J., Dodge, K. A., & Pettit, G. S. (2005). Deficient behavioral inhibition and anomalous selective attention in a community sample of adolescents with psychopathic traits and low-anxiety traits. *Journal of Abnormal Child Psychology*, *33*, 461–470.

Wallace, J. F., Schmitt, W. A., Vitale, J. E., & Newman, J. P. (2000). Experimental investigations of information processing deficiencies in psychopaths: implications for diagnosis and treatment. In C. B. Gacono (ed), *The Clinical and Forensic Assessment of Psychopathy: A Practitioner's Guide* (pp. 87–109). Mahwah, NJ: Erlbaum.

Waschbusch, D. A. (2002). A meta-analytic examination of comorbid hyperactive-impulsive-attention problems and conduct problems. *Psychological Bulletin, 128,* 118–150.

Welsh, B. C., Loeber, R., Stouthamer-Loeber, M., Cohen, M. A., Farrington, F. P., & Stevens, B. R. (in press). The cost of juvenile crime in urban areas: a longitudinal perspective. *Youth Violence and Juvenile Justice.*

2

The life-course persistent pathway of antisocial behaviour: Risks for violence and poor physical health

Candice L. Odgers

Introduction

Violence is one of the leading causes of death worldwide for individuals aged 15–44 years (World Health Organization, 2002). For example, in the United States, it is estimated that each year violence causes over 2.5 million injuries and approximately 50 000 deaths (Corso *et al.*, 2007). In the end, the costs of violence, including interpersonal, self-inflicted, and collective forms of violence, translate into billions of dollars in health-care-related expenses (World Health Organization, 2007). The recognition that violence is one of the most important public health problems facing the international community has prompted researchers, clinicians, and policymakers alike to search for new strategies for reducing and preventing violence. One strategy for responding to serious and violent offending has been to focus on a subgroup of high-risk individuals who are believed to be responsible for a disproportionate amount crime and violence. This targeted approach has its origins in classic criminological observations that a small subgroup of individuals (e.g., 5-6%) are responsible for more than 50% of known crimes (Farrington *et al.*, 1986), with more recent findings demonstrating that individuals following a *life-course persistent* (LCP) pathway of antisocial behaviour (ASB) are responsible for 50–70% of officially sanctioned *violent crime* (Hodgins, 1994; Moffitt *et al.*, 2002; Odgers *et al.*, 2007).

Understanding the origins and consequences of persistent antisocial behaviour has emerged as a top research priority. Decades of longitudinal research has also repeatedly demonstrated that early onset and persistent antisocial behaviour – a pathway believed to have origins in neurodevelopmental deficits that begin very early in life – predicts a wide range of adult outcomes, including depression, substance use disorders, relationship difficulties, self-harm behaviours, poor educational outcomes, and dependence on social welfare systems (Kratzer & Hodgins, 1997; Moffitt *et al.*, 2002; Kim-Cohen *et al.*, 2003; Fergusson *et al.*, 2005; Wiesner *et al.*, 2005). More recently, a prospective link has been documented between early onset and persistent antisocial behaviour and poor adult *physical* health (Odgers *et al.*, 2007; Piquero *et al.*, 2007), including injury, sexually transmitted diseases, cardiovascular risk, immune function, and dental disease. Thus, while individuals on the LCP pathway are consuming far more than their share of criminal justice and mental health services, new evidence is showing that these individuals may also be responsible for a larger share of medical costs than previously thought.

This chapter reviews what is known about the health-related costs of early onset and persistent antisocial behaviour (most commonly referred to as the *life-course persistent* pathway of antisocial behaviour). Two types of health-related costs are considered. First, harm and injury to self and others is considered by reviewing rates of violence perpetration by males and females on the LCP pathway. Second, the physical health burden attributed to those on this pathway is summarized, with an emphasis on the importance of including both self-reported and objective assessments of physical health status in future research. Finally, the potential mechanisms underlying the association between poor physical health and antisocial behaviour are examined and directions for future research are outlined.

The LCP pathway of antisocial behaviour

The developmental origins, predicted course, and consequences for children on the LCP pathway were articulated over a decade ago in Moffitt's (1993) developmental taxonomy of antisocial behaviour. The LCP subgroup is of particular interest to those interested in the neurodevelopmental origins of violence, as the original taxonomy stated that the roots of this pathway may begin very early in life, perhaps with a causal chain that is present before or soon after birth. For example, the 'aetiological chain', although hypothesized to involve a myriad of social, familial, *and* individual factors, may originate with factors capable of producing individual differences in the neuropsychological functions of the infant nervous system, including minor physical anomalies, prenatal exposure to toxins, brain insult due to birth complications, or perhaps heritable variation in neuropsychological health (see Moffitt, 1993 for a full discussion). Indeed, there is a wealth of evidence supporting the fact that children who follow a persistently antisocial pathway suffer from deficits in neuropsychological abilities (Moffitt & Henry, 1991; Moffitt & Caspi, 2001). In fact, it has even been suggested that the age of onset per se may not be the causal influence for persistent antisocial behaviour, but instead may heightened vulnerability for mark neurodevelopmental risk in childhood (Rutter *et al.*, 2006).

Over the last 15 years, children on the LCP pathway have been intensively studied. As a result, we have learned a great deal about the origins, developmental course, and adult outcomes of this group (for a review, see Moffitt, 2006). In a nutshell, the original developmental taxonomy of antisocial behaviour proposed that at least two prototypical subtypes underlie the observed age-by-crime distribution (Moffitt, 1993): an LCP pathway characterized by social, familial, and neurodevelopmental deficits, which onsets in early childhood and distinguishes a relatively small yet persistent and pathological subgroup of individuals; and an *adolescence-limited* (AL) pathway hypothesized to be more common, relatively transient, and near normative. Adolescence-limited involvement in antisocial behaviour is believed to emerge alongside puberty as a relatively normative response to the role-less years between biological maturation and access to mature privileges and responsibilities, a period of time labelled as the 'maturity gap'. Although those on the LCP pathway are expected to experience multiple problems in adulthood, adolescence-limited individuals, given the normative nature of their pre-teen development, are hypothesized to be more successful in their transition to adulthood, provided they do not encounter snares, such as substance dependency or a criminal record.

Early onset and persistent antisocial behaviour predicts future violence

It is well established that early onset antisocial behaviour is one of the most robust predictors of later involvement in serious and violent offending (Farrington, 1995b; Kratzer & Hodgins, 1997; Caspi, 2000). Individuals on the LCP pathway have been found to display antisocial behaviour, antisocial traits, and violent behaviour well into young adulthood. Early involvement in antisocial behaviour predicts a longer duration of a crime career

(Farrington *et al.*, 2006) and has been linked to a variety of different types of violence, including serious violent offences and weapon involvement (McCluskey *et al.*, 2006), robbery, assault, domestic violence, and violence against children (Moffitt *et al.*, 2002; Woodward *et al.*, 2002), as well as juvenile and adult arrests (Schaeffer *et al.*, 2003).

Research has also demonstrated that males on the LCP pathway are at increased risk of physical violence in adulthood. For example, research from the Dunedin Multidisciplinary Health and Development Study, a 32-year longitudinal study of a birth cohort of 1000 New Zealanders, found that 26-year-old males on the LCP pathway engaged in a wide range of violent activities (Moffitt *et al.*, 2002). For example, LCP men accounted for five times their share of the cohort's violent convictions (43% of the cohort's officially sanctioned violent crime). They were also elevated on self-reported and official measures of abuse towards women, including physical abuse (e.g., beating her up, throwing her bodily) and controlling abuse (e.g., stalking her, restricting her access to her friends and family). LCP men were also the most likely to report that they had hit a child in anger (not in the course of normal discipline). Six years later, at age 32, such men continued to engage in violence towards themselves and others (Odgers *et al.*, 2007). Although many of the LCP men had been incarcerated since age 26, 33% of these men (versus 0.4% of the cohort norm and 10.2% of adolescent-onset individuals) had received a new conviction *for violence* since age 26. LCP men were also more likely to engage in controlling forms of abuse with partners and in self-reported violence (compared to the cohort norm). In total, 59% of the LCP men had engaged in at least one act of physical violence in the 6 months prior to their interview. They were also more likely to engage in violence towards themselves: 10% of the LCP men (compared to 0.4% of the cohort norm and 3% of adolescent-onset men) attempted suicide between the ages of 26 and 32. Despite the fact that the Dunedin sample was more than 10 years past the peak age for violent offending, violence among LCP men remained high.

Similar findings have been reported by other representative longitudinal studies. For example, in the Christchurch Study, another prospective cohort study following approximately 900 New Zealanders from childhood into adulthood, it has been reported that individuals with serious childhood-onset conduct problems, compared with children without conduct problems, engaged in ten times more violent crime by age 25 (Fergusson *et al.*, 2005). Young adults with childhood-onset antisocial behaviour in this cohort also engaged in significantly more violence against partners than did those with adolescent-onset antisocial behaviour (Woodward *et al.*, 2002).

It is not uncommon for divergent findings to emerge across high-risk versus normative samples. However, information from both types of populations is important to consider because representative cohort studies are best situated to inform questions of prevalence, aetiology, and prognosis, whereas high-risk studies provide a valuable source of information regarding the subgroup of high-risk individuals that many clinicians and policymakers are most interested in. Among the high-risk samples in the United States, longitudinal cohort studies have also studied subgroups of individuals with a chronic pattern of antisocial behaviour. For example, Schaeffer and colleagues (2006) followed a group of 300 inner-city boys from age 6 to age 20, and reported that boys with chronically high trajectories of antisocial behaviour are at increased risk of Conduct Disorder, juvenile and adult arrest, and antisocial personality disorder in young adulthood. Moving further across the lifespan, the Cambridge Study in Delinquent Development has reported criminal career outcomes for 400 high-risk boys followed prospectively from childhood to age 50 (Farrington *et al.*, 2006). Based on official conviction data, males with an early onset of offending (defined here as the first conviction between the ages 10–13) had the greatest number of lifetime official convictions and, when combined with those who began offending prior to age 15 (many of whom had childhood behavioural problems), had the longest criminal careers. Again, a small fraction of the males in this study (7%) accounted for over half (52%) of all officially recorded offences. Notably, official convictions peaked for these early offending groups in their mid to late 20s, and by age 50 relatively few of the men were still receiving official convictions; between age 40 and 50, there were approximately 2 officially recorded offences per 100 men. A similar population-level decline in official offending has been documented by Sampson and Laub (2003, 2005) in their follow-up of 500 men from the Glueck Study to age 70.

In the Oregon Youth Study, a sample of 200 males followed from age 12 to age 24, the chronic offending subgroup (defined using self-reported data) demonstrated higher levels of antisocial behaviour and related problems in young adulthood when compared with low-level offending subgroups (Wiesner & Capaldi, 2003; Wiesner *et al.*, 2005). However, similar trajectories of antisocial behaviour were not identified when official offending data were used (Wiesner *et al.*, 2007). The discrepancy between the use of self-reported versus official offending data to identify individuals following an early onset and persistent course is currently cause for debate, with some questioning whether an LCP pathway of criminal offending exists (Sampson & Laub, 2003). However, it has long been recognized that a reliance on official convictions may not provide a complete picture of what is happening in the lives of individuals exhibiting an early onset and persistent course of antisocial behaviour. Indeed, the original developmental taxonomy acknowledged that a population-wide process of aging out of crime would occur. That is, it was not expected that an LCP pathway of antisocial behaviour would be marked by *crime* in old age; instead, it referred to the persistence of antisocial personality characteristics or antisocial behaviours within the family (see Moffitt, 1993, p. 680). It is also important to note that trajectory-based models have their limitations (Bauer, 2007). These limitations are especially relevant when applied within high-risk samples and in the absence of evidence of measurement invariance across ages. As such, it will be important to continue to (1) utilize a wide range of methods that ensure all forms of continuing violence and/or antisocial behaviour are captured *and* (2) ensure that the limitations of analytic strategies, such as trajectory modeling, are recognized in future work.

In sum, there is a large body of research demonstrating that LCP involvement in antisocial behaviour is related to a wide spectrum of problems in adulthood, with a particularly salient link to violence during young adulthood. Three cautionary notes are required when examining the linkage between LCP involvement in antisocial behaviour and future violence. First, as researchers continue to follow cohorts across adulthood, it will be important to gather information via a range of sources (e.g., informant-reported, self-reported, observational) to test whether violent behaviours persist across the lifespan for those on the LCP pathway and the extent to which these violent behaviours are linked to antisocial personality characteristics and other antisocial behaviours.

Second, it is important to acknowledge that most children with behavioural disorders do not become serious violent offenders. Indeed, most children who exhibit antisocial behaviour problems desist before they reach adolescence or young adulthood, and many obtain relatively good outcomes (Robins, 1978; Rutter *et al.*, 2006). In other words, without evidence of persistence, such childhood conduct problems are not sufficient to signal poor outcomes in adulthood (Tremblay, 2000; Moffitt *et al.*, 2001) and, in particular, there is *little* evidence that a 'childhood-*limited*' course of antisocial behaviour is linked with adult violence (Odgers *et al.*, 2007). Questions remain, however, regarding whether aggressive behaviour in childhood-versus antisocial behaviour in general-is the key ingredient with respect to persistence. Moreover, the existence of a childhood-limited group, which does not go on to engage in higher rates of violence, raises important questions for the study of the stability of antisocial behaviour and traits overtime.

Third, the majority of the research to date has focused on the developmental course of antisocial behaviour in males. However, the reliance on male-only samples has been changing. As a result, an evidence base regarding the course and consequences of girls' antisocial behaviour is emerging; this body of research is summarized in the following.

Early onset and persistent antisocial behaviour among females *predicts future involvement in violence*

Prospective cohort studies have identified a childhood-onset and persistent subtype of females who, although fewer in number, are very similar to LCP males in terms of childhood risk factors, including neurodevelopmental risk (Odgers *et al.*, 2008), and who also experience poor prognosis in adolescence and adulthood (Kratzer & Hodgins, 1999; Coté *et al.*, 2001; Fergusson & Horwood, 2002; Broidy *et al.*, 2003; Bongers *et al.*, 2004; White & Piquero, 2004; Lahey *et al.*, 2006; Schaeffer *et al.*, 2006; Odgers *et al.*, 2008). Although research focused on the LCP pathway among females is relatively new, predictions for this pathway among females are not. The original statement of the taxonomy was intended to apply to females as well as males (Moffitt, 1994; Moffitt *et al.*, 2001). Within the developmental taxonomy, much of the gender difference in levels of antisocial behaviour is attributed to sex differences in the individual risk factors of persistent antisocial behaviour. For example, research has consistently shown that girls have lower rates of symptoms of nervous system dysfunction, difficult temperament, hyperactivity, reading failure, and learning disabilities than boys (Gorman-Smith & Loeber, 2005; Lahey *et al.*, 2006; Messer *et al.*, 2006). Thus, the consequent processes of cumulative continuity ensue for fewer girls than boys, resulting in a smaller number of girls following the LCP pathway. However, the childhood correlates of the LCP subtype are assumed to be similar across gender (Moffitt *et al.*, 2001).

Virtually all epidemiological studies testing for gender-specific pathways of antisocial behaviour have identified a 'childhood-onset' or 'early starter' pathway among females (Coté *et al.*, 2002; Fergusson & Horwood, 2002; Broidy *et al.*, 2003; Bongers *et al.*, 2004; Lahey *et al.*, 2006; Schaeffer *et al.*, 2006). For example, Coté and colleagues (2001), in a representative study of 820 Canadian girls, found that approximately 11% of the girls followed a medium-high to high trajectory of persistent disruptive behaviours between the ages of 6 and 12 and were at increased risk of juvenile Conduct Disorder. Continued follow-up of this sample to age 21 indicated that females with early and persistent behaviour problems (particularly those who were chronically high on both hyperactivity and aggression) were at increased risk of physical and psychological aggression towards their romantic partners, although they were not more likely to engage in *non-violent* criminal behaviours (Fontaine *et al.*, 2008). In a nationally representative US sample, Lahey and colleagues (2006) reported that 3.5–6.9% of the females followed an LCP pathway between the ages of 4 and 17. Schaeffer and colleagues (2006) also identified an early starter and persistent subgroup of females (9% of a cohort) among 665 girls from a representative US inner-city sample; this group went on to have the highest levels of antisocial behaviour in adulthood, including increased risk of arrests for violent offences.

Recent findings from the Dunedin Study also revealed a small group of females (7.5% of the cohort) who exhibited conduct problem symptoms in childhood and who persisted in their involvement in antisocial behaviour into young adulthood. At age 32, women on this early onset and persistent pathway were at increased risk of violence towards their partners and their children (Odgers *et al.*, 2008). At age 32, 75% of these women had engaged in at least one form of physical violence over the past 6 months (e.g., physical violence towards partners, children, or others). For example, approximately half of the women on the LCP pathway had engaged in physical violence towards partners (44.8%) or their children (41.7%) within the past 6 months. Although there was very little evidence of officially detected violence (based on official records), the majority of the LCP women were engaging in physical violence behind closed doors (according to self and informant reports). In sum, the emerging research supports the existence of a small, yet significant, subgroup of early onset and persistent females who are at risk of poor prognosis in adulthood, including violence towards partners and children.

Although the link between the LCP pathway and violence is now well documented, less is known about the physical health costs associated with early onset and persistent antisocial behaviour. However, new research is providing insights into how childhood and adolescent-onset antisocial behaviour is linked to physical health problems among both males and females; this research is reviewed in the following section.

Early onset and persistent antisocial behaviour predicts poor physical health for males and females

A recognition of the link between antisocial behaviour and medical problems is not new. Indeed, the ability of childhood Conduct Disorder to predict poor health was reported in the 1960s (Robins & Rutter, 1990), with a number of studies since that time documenting an association between antisocial behaviour and *self-reported* health problems (Farrington, 1995a; Bardone *et al.*, 1998; Shepherd & Farrington, 2003; Serbin *et al.*, 2004; Pajer *et al.*, 2006; Piquero *et al.*, 2007). We are now beginning to learn more about the relationship between antisocial behaviour and objective physical health indices and markers, including physiological reactivity, genetic vulnerabilities, biomarkers, and disease endpoints (Moffitt *et al.*, 2008). With respect to individuals on the LCP pathway, Moffitt (2006, p. 57) has articulated a new hypothesis that is now being tested, namely that 'the life-course persistent antisocial individual will be at high risk in midlife for poor physical [and mental] health, cardiovascular disease, and early disease morbidity and mortality'.

Studies that have relied on self-reported measures of physical health provide support for a linkage between childhood histories of antisocial behaviour and poor health. For example, using data from the National Collaborative Perinatal Project, a longitudinal study of approximately 2700 individuals followed from birth to ages 27 and 33, Piquero and colleagues (2007) reported that individuals on the LCP pathway versus the *adolescence-limited* pathway were more likely to report experiencing at least one of the following poor physical health outcomes: asthma, heart trouble, hypertension, kidney problems, diabetes, or ulcers. Interesting, there were no reported differences between those on the *adolescence-limited* versus *non-offending* pathways on adverse physical health outcomes.

Antisocial behaviour has also been identified as a particularly important risk factor of poor health among girls (Pajer, 1998). For example, young women who engage in antisocial behaviour are at higher risk of early and multiple pregnancies, as well as sexually transmitted disease and infection. As such, physical health complications may present a unique challenge for this subgroup of young women and their children. In one study, 93 adolescent girls (41 controls versus 52 girls with Conduct Disorder) were recruited from the community and followed for 3 years. At the three-year follow-up, adolescent girls with Conduct Disorder versus controls self-reported poorer overall health, more discomfort, more health risk behaviours as young adults, and earlier onset of adult reproductive behaviours, even when controlling for demographic factors and pre-existing health history (Pajer *et al.*, 2007). Similar results were reported in a representative sample of 1218 mothers of boys randomly selected from urban public schools in the United States. Women with versus without a history of antisocial behaviour in this study reported higher rates of long-term physical health problems even after controlling for socio-demographic factors (Pajer *et al.*, 2006).

Although self-reported and archival assessments of physical health have provided important clues regarding the relationship between antisocial behaviour and poor physical health, what is needed are studies that integrate objective biomarkers of health problems alongside well-validated and prospective assessments of antisocial behaviour. Recent findings from the Dunedin Study report both prospectively gathered assessments of antisocial behaviour from childhood to adulthood as well as objective assessments of physical health status. Here, physical health status at age 32 was assessed via medical examinations, including the collection of blood samples (to assess sexually transmitted disease and inflammation), tests of vital lung capacity via a computerized spirometer and body plethysmograph (to assess lung function), and dental examinations (to assess gum disease and decay). Self-reported measures were also collected to evaluate overall health, smoking, chronic bronchitis, injuries, and medical service usage.

Findings from the Dunedin Study support a prospective link between antisocial subtypes and adult physical health across the first 32 years of life. Here, men on the LCP pathway demonstrated the worst physical health outcomes, including higher rates of sexually transmitted diseases, dental disease, cardiovascular risk factors, inflammatory measures of immune dysfunction, injuries requiring medical treatment, and respiratory lung dysfunctions (Odgers *et al.*, 2007). For example, 27.1% of the men on the LCP pathway versus 11.5% of the men on the *no-conduct problem* pathway were above the clinical cut-off for C-reactive protein, an index of inflammation recently endorsed as an adjunct to traditional risk factor screening for cardiovascular risk by the Centers for Disease Control and Prevention (CDC) and the American Heart Association (AHA). Similarly, over 40% of the LCP men versus less than 20% of the cohort norm had symptoms of chronic bronchitis and gum disease.

Women on the LCP pathway from the Dunedin Study were also experiencing the worst physical health outcomes at age 32. Here, women on the LCP versus the *no-conduct problem* pathway were faring worse on 6 of the 11 physical health outcomes, including type 2 herpes, smoking, nicotine dependence, chronic bronchitis symptoms, gum disease, and decayed tooth surfaces (Odgers *et al.*, 2008). For example, 41.9% of the women on the LCP pathway versus 19.7% of the women on the *no-conduct problem* pathway tested positive for the herpes virus at age 32. Similarly, 40.0% of the LCP women versus less than 14.8% of the cohort norm had symptoms of chronic bronchitis.

It is also important to note that individuals who began engaging in antisocial behaviour in *adolescence* may also be at an elevated risk of poor health. In the Dunedin Study, overall comparisons of physical health problems between those on the *adolescent-onset* versus the *no-conduct problem* pathway revealed medium effect sizes for women (Cohen's $d = 0.43$) and medium-to-large effect sizes for men (Cohen's $d = 0.67$). *Adolescent-onset* men and women were not, however, experiencing the same level of physical health problems as their LCP counterparts: comparisons between the LCP versus the *adolescent-onset* subgroup on the summary index of physical health problems revealed a medium effect size for women (Cohen's $d = 0.51$) and a medium-to-large effect size for men (Cohen's $d = 0.65$) (Odgers *et al.*, 2008).

Thus, although the health of the adolescent-onset class is not as compromised as that of the LCP's, the greater size of the adolescent-onset class makes it account for an appreciable fraction of health burden.

Why is antisocial behaviour linked to poor physical health?

The possibility that antisocial behaviour is an early marker or causal factor in poor physical health is intriguing. This type of developmental perspective regarding the underlying causes of physical health problems raises the exciting possibility that primary prevention programmes could influence both antisocial behaviour and health across the lifespan. Targeted prevention efforts would be ideal, as the untreated consequences of both antisocial behaviour and poor physical health are costly. Unfortunately, research focused on the relationship between antisocial behaviour and physical health, thus far, have not been able to identify the mechanisms through which antisocial behaviour may 'get under the skin' and translate into compromised physical health. A review of related research converges on at least four possible explanations for the documented link between a persistent pattern of antisocial behaviour and poor physical health.

Antisocial individuals may engage in more health risk behaviours

One of the most widely accepted explanations for the relationship between antisocial behaviour and poor health is that individuals who engage in antisocial behaviour are also more likely to engage in more health risk behaviours (e.g., high rates of risk taking, substance abuse, reckless driving) and may be less likely to engage in health-promoting behaviours (e.g., failure to attend regular check-ups, poor diet). For example, children who engage in antisocial and disruptive behaviour are at higher risk of accidents and unintentional injuries (Schwebel *et al.*, 2002; Brehaut *et al.*, 2003) including traumatic dental injury (Sabuncuoglu, 2007) and major and minor head injuries (Lalloo & Sheiham, 2003). The link between antisocial behaviour and poor health seems particularly strong when early behavioural problems include aggression and/or attention deficit/hyperactivity disorder (ADHD) symptoms. Children with ADHD are significantly more likely to be injured while riding a bike, to receive head injuries, be hospitalized for accidental poisoning, and utilize medical services across multiple delivery settings (DiScala *et al.*; 1998, Leibson *et al.*, 2001). With respect to early physical aggression, Tremblay (2002) found that boys who engaged in physical aggression from early childhood to late adolescence were at the highest risk of causing injuries to others and to themselves. The author concluded that, because of their risky style of behaviour, these highly aggressive boys were at risk of other medical conditions such as cardiovascular problems, cancer, and brain damage. Based on this evidence, Tremblay argued that the socialization of aggressive behaviour during the preschool years should also prevent injuries throughout the lifespan. Similar findings were reported in the Cambridge Study of Delinquent Development, where injuries at ages 16–18 and 27–32 were concentrated among males with a history of antisocial behaviour and violence (Shepherd *et al.*, 2002, 2004).

The increased risk of injury and medical service use among children and adolescents with early behaviour problems is not inconsequential, as unintentional injury is the leading cause of death of children and young persons. Such findings suggest that intervention efforts with at-risk children may have the potential to *both* reduce violence and alleviate related medical problems. In an effort to test this idea, Borowsky and colleagues (2004) conducted a randomized controlled trial to evaluate the effects of a physician-administered intervention on children's violent behaviours and violence-related injuries ($N = 224$). At the nine-month follow-up, children in the intervention versus the control group exhibited lower rates of aggression and attention problems, as well as fewer fight-related injuries requiring medical care (Borowsky et al., 2004). These results provide proof of principle that efforts to reduce childhood aggression and violence may also reduce violence-related injuries and health costs among children.

The contribution of social and behavioural factors-especially during adolescence when many lifestyle habits are forming-to chronic disease and premature death has been widely recognized (Millstein et al., 1993). As children move into adolescence, there is a general increase in risk-taking behaviours. Moreover, during adolescence, young teens begin to operate in social contexts where their still-developing moral reasoning and perspective-taking skills may put them at risk (Cauffman & Steinberg, 2000). These deficits in psychosocial maturity may have unique consequences for young teens with a history of antisocial behaviour. That is, antisocial teens are more likely to engage in a range of risk-taking and health-compromising behaviours, including early exposure to substances, dangerous driving, and risky sexual behaviours (Ramrakha et al., 2007; Toumbourou et al., 2007; Odgers et al., 2008). For example, a nine-year follow-up of 625 Canadian boys found that boys high on disruptive behaviour at age 6 were significantly more likely to engage in risky health behaviours in adolescence, including alcohol abuse, tobacco use, problems with drugs, and unsafe sex (Dobkin et al., 1997). Thus, for teens with a developmental history of antisocial behaviour, the 'normative' increase in risk taking that accompanies adolescence may be amplified. Moreover, adolescents whose behaviour is severe enough to place them in a correctional facility are often left growing up within contexts that do not meet the basic prerequisites for healthy development, including a lack of proper nutrition, exercise, and medical care (Woolard et al., 2005), although some argue that prison environments may actually bolster health for disadvantaged youth by providing medical attention that has often been absent from their lives. In adulthood, these well-developed patterns of health risk behaviour, including substance use, poor self-care, and general lifestyle choices that damage health, may become heavily entrenched and resistant to change, resulting in cumulative and prolonged exposure to many causes of injury, compromised health, and disease.

In sum, the absence of health-promoting behaviours and the increased risk of health-compromising behaviours among this population is reason for concern regarding both present and future health status (Elliot, 1993). Specific strategies for targeting adolescent health are now being developed, with a specific call for an increased spotlight on adolescent health and the development of youth-friendly health services worldwide (Shribman, 2007).

LCP antisocial behaviour is related to early adversity and childhood maltreatment, which independently predict poor health outcomes

Stressful life events have been linked to a number of poor health outcomes, with exposure to early stressors believed to uniquely influence children's health and development (Gunnar & Quevedo, 2007). Early experiences for children on the LCP pathway are often characterized by high levels of family adversity, parental conflict, and increased risk of childhood maltreatment (Moffitt, 2006). In this situation, a vulnerable child is left growing up and interacting with a high-risk home and social environment. These children are being exposed to a cascade of risk that may contribute to *both* early behaviour problems and poor health outcomes.

Repetti *et al.*'s (2002) Risky Families Model describes how these types of high-risk familial contexts may 'get under the skin' and compromise present and future health. Within this model, 'risky families' are characterized by conflict and aggression and by relationships that are cold, unsupportive, and neglectful. This type of exposure is hypothesized to create vulnerabilities in children or interact with genetically based predispositions to disrupt psychosocial functioning. In doing so, risky families are believed to produce disruptions in the stress-response system (e.g., the hypothalamic-pituitary-adrenal [HPA] axis), impede psychosocial development, and encourage poor health behaviours. Dysregulation, or over-activation of the stress-response system, has been implicated in problems such as immune dysfunction, visceral obesity, or atrophy of brain structures (McEwen 2007). There is also a growing body of biological research documenting a pattern of psychophysiological, neurotransmitter, and endocrine hypoarousal in individuals at risk of antisocial behaviour and in established offenders (for a review, see Susman, 2006). Such emerging research supports the development of a pattern of persistent antisocial behaviour via a bidirectional interplay between early (and ongoing) stressors and disruptions to the neuroendocrine system. In sum, this profile of risk is hypothesized to lead to the accumulation of risk of not only mental disorders but also of major chronic diseases and early mortality. In this sense, the early home environment and early adversity is given primacy in understanding the origins and course of physical and mental health problems across the lifespan (Repetti *et al.*, 2002).

Indeed, research has demonstrated that children reared in 'risky families' have increased rates of physical symptoms and medical diagnoses. For example, the Adverse Childhood Experience Study, a large retrospective study of the childhood experiences of approximately 9500 individuals who received a standardized medical examination, documented a robust relationship between childhood exposure to abuse or household dysfunction and a number of adult diseases, including cancer, chronic lung disease, heart disease, skeletal fractures, and liver disease (Felitti *et al.*, 1998). Prospective studies have also documented a robust relationship between childhood maltreatment and objective markers of immune function and allostatic load in young adults (Danese *et al.*, 2007). The interplay between individual-level factors and early stressors, such as child maltreatment, likely involve complex interactions between individuals and their social and physical environments. Gene-environment studies are shedding new light on how early stressors may influence the course of antisocial behaviour for some children and not others. For example, seminal work in this area by Caspi and colleagues (2002) demonstrated that children with a low-activity variant of the monoamine oxidase A (MAOA) genotype were more likely to exhibit violence only if they had been exposed to maltreatment. In this study, neither the gene variant nor the environment alone was enough to confer vulnerability: both were required (Caspi *et al.*, 2002). Future studies may help us to understand how genetic variants interact with environmental exposures to confer vulnerability for both antisocial behaviour and associated health outcomes.

Relationship stress and interpersonal conflict across the lifespan have also been linked to compromised physical health (Wickrama *et al.*, 2001; de Vogli *et al.*, 2007). These findings are important because individuals with a history of antisocial behaviour often experience high levels of interpersonal conflict, including conflict with parents, teachers, peers, and in extreme cases, with the criminal justice system. Given the high levels of interpersonal conflict in the lives of individuals with a pervasive developmental history of antisocial behaviour, health risks that are conferred through the stress of interpersonal conflict may be particularly strong. Moreover, antisocial individuals may lack the types of social support networks that have been shown to buffer many of the ill-health consequences associated with exposure to stressful life events (Cohen, 2004). That is, individuals on the LCP pathway may be less likely to have intact social support networks, they are more likely to have alienated many friends and family, and are often less likely to have positive romantic relationships (Moffitt *et al.*, 2002).

In sum, individuals with an early onset and persistent history of antisocial behaviour (1) are more likely to experience early stress and adversity, (2) often experience relationships and interactions characterized by conflict, and (3) are often less likely to have intact social support networks and positive relationships to buffer the effects of these exposures. Stressful life events are often cumulative. Thus, repeated adaptations to these types of stressors for individuals on the LCP pathway may increase the likelihood of a myriad of health problems.

Antisocial individuals are likely to be high on personality traits, such as hostility and negative affect, associated with physiological vulnerability

Antisocial and violent individuals are often high on personality traits associated with physiological vulnerability. For example, antisocial children are characterized by undercontrolled temperament, irritability, temper tantrums, and impulsivity. In adolescence and young adulthood, antisocial individuals are more likely to exhibit hostility and anger and are at elevated risk of both negative affect and depressive symptoms. Many of these personality traits have themselves been linked to poor health outcomes. With respect to co-morbid conditions, males and females on the LCP pathway are more likely to meet the diagnostic criteria for depression in adulthood, which has been linked to cardiovascular disease, obesity, and related problems (Simon *et al.*, 2006; Whooley, 2006). Therefore, it is possible that the ill-health consequences associated with antisocial behaviour are the result of co-morbid conditions (e.g., depression, negative affect). Thus, research is needed that tests whether antisocial behaviour predicts specific health outcomes in the presence and/or absence of co-morbid conditions.

With respect to closely associated traits of antisocial behaviour, hostility has been independently related to a number of adverse health outcomes, including cardiovascular disease (CVD), elevated glucose levels, and diabetes (Knox *et al.*, 2004; Raikkonen *et al.*, 2004). For example, a meta-analytic review of 45 studies concluded that hostility was an independent risk factor of coronary heart disease (Miller *et al.*, 1996), with an ongoing debate regarding whether the association between hostility and heart disease is due to a direct physiological response to hostility or the increased likelihood of engaging in health-compromising behaviours. Pajer (2007) argues that the relationship between negative emotions and heart disease may onset earlier than previously thought. She makes the case that negative emotions in adolescence may facilitate the progression of early atherosclerotic lesions (proximal cause of the most common types of CVD) and, moreover, that an earlier onset of negative emotions may be important as the length of time exposed to negative emotions is a positive predictor of CVD in adults. More broadly, she argues that negative emotions in adolescents may be risk factors for the development of cardiovascular disease via dysregulation of the stress-response system (Pajer, 2007). Among the limited research available on children and adolescents, anger and aggression have been found to predict increases in triglycerides, body mass index (BMI), and blood pressure reactivity (Ravaja *et al.*, 1996; Gump *et al.*, 1999), with one study reporting that hostility among adolescents predicted the development of metabolic syndrome characteristics three years later (Raikkonen *et al.*, 2003).

In sum, closely associated traits and co-morbid conditions of antisocial behaviour may help to explain the association between antisocial behaviour and poor physical health.

Although more research is required to identify the independent contributions of antisocial behaviour, above co-morbid disorders such as depression, there is a general acceptance that many of the personality traits that go hand in hand with antisocial behaviour (e.g., hostility) also independently contribute to increased physiological vulnerability.

Social inequalities may underlie involvement in both antisocial behaviour and poor health

Disease and poor health conditions are concentrated in economically and socially marginalized segments of the population. As such, it is likely that low socio-economic status and related risk factors (e.g., low parental education, poor housing conditions, food insecurity, limited access to medical care) underlie life-course trajectories of *both* poor physical health and antisocial behaviour. It is well documented that children growing up in deprivation go on to experience poor adult health, including cardiovascular disease, obesity, and related problems (Poulton *et al.*, 2002; Galobardes *et al.*, 2006; Lawlor *et al.*, 2006; Melchior *et al.*, 2007), as well as more rapid deterioration of physical health across the lifespan (Chandola *et al.*, 2007). Indeed, socio-economic status is one of the most robust predictors of mortality and overall well-being. Therefore, it makes sense that socio-economic status will account for at least some of the relationship between antisocial behaviour and poor health, either by directly restricting access to quality health care and/or by marking a cluster of causal risk factors embedded within families and communities at the lower end of the socio-economic continuum.

Adopting this type of common risk factor approach challenges the claim that antisocial behaviour leads to poor health, or vice versa, and instead raises the possibility that both antisocial behaviour and poor health are caused by a set of common predictors. Recent findings from the Dunedin Study inform this debate through an examination of *what* factors contribute to poor adult health among children who experience socio-economic disadvantage. The study concluded that low childhood socio-economic status (SES) contributed to adult substance dependency and poor health, *but* other risk factors also made a contribution, including familial liability to mental and physical disorders, childhood/adolescent health characteristics, low childhood IQ, exposure to childhood maltreatment, and low adult socio-economic status. Together, the risk factors accounted for 55–67% of the poor health outcomes among adults exposed to low socio-economic status as children, with no single risk factor emerging as the prime explanation (Melchior *et al.*, 2007). With respect to common risk factors of antisocial behaviour and physical illness, the Cambridge Study of Delinquent Development documented an overlap between childhood predictors of antisocial behaviour and predictors of injury and cardiovascular illness at age 32 (Shepherd *et al.*, 2004). This same study also documented a relationship between offending and poor health in early adulthood, which *held* after controlling for an underlying antisocial personality disorder and childhood predictors of both offending and poor health (Farrington, 1995a). Taken together, these studies suggest that the processes mediating the link between low socio-economic status in childhood and health outcomes are multifactorial and, importantly, that antisocial behaviour may be a prime candidate for understanding variation in health outcomes both between and within socio-economic strata.

In sum, antisocial behaviour in childhood or adolescence may be related to health via a number of mechanisms, including (1) increased risk-taking and decreased health-promoting behaviours; (2) exposure to early adversity and ongoing stressful life events; (3) associated personality traits and co-morbid conditions, such as hostility and depression, that are linked to physiological vulnerability; and/or (4) a common set of risk factors, namely those that are embedded in social inequalities and also predict disparities in physical health across the lifespan. It is unlikely that any of these influences on physical health are mutually exclusive. Rather, the association between antisocial behaviour and physical health is likely to result from a dynamic interplay between many of the mechanisms reviewed here; therefore, additional research is required.

What research is needed?

This review emphasizes the need for a joint consideration of antisocial behaviour and physical health across development and raises a number of questions for future research. For example, *when does the association between antisocial behaviour and poor health begin? Do neurodevelopmental deficits and physical health problems among individuals on the LCP pathway stem from the same underlying vulnerabilities? How can recent advancements in neuroscience and related disciplines be leveraged to better understand the interplay between persistent antisocial behaviour and poor health?* The following subsection suggests research priorities for the next generation of research focused on the interplay between antisocial behaviour and health.

First, large-scale studies that combine repeated assessments of children's mental and physical health are needed. Such studies will have the ability to test the direction of the relationship between childhood physical health problems and mental disorders. Ideally, these studies will integrate state-of-the-art assessments of mental health alongside physical and/or laboratory examinations, including assessments of neurodevelopmental risk and biomarkers of health status beginning in early childhood. Newly designed studies will soon be in a position to meet these objectives (Landrigan *et al.*, 2006). In the meantime, it will be beneficial to integrate findings across established cohorts, where disease endpoints can be assessed, versus newer cohorts, which have the advantage of leveraging new technologies such as neuroimaging and biomarker assessments early in life.

Second, neuroscience is increasingly being used to study the underlying causes of both mental disorder and medical illness. With respect to mental disorder, it has been suggested that a 'joining of forces' between neuroscience, psychiatry, and allied disciplines may help us to 'solve the biggest mystery of human psychopathology': that is, 'How does an environmental factor … get inside the nervous system and alter its elements to generate the symptoms of a disordered mind?' (Caspi & Moffitt, 2006, p. 583). Similarly, there has been a 'call to action' generated by medical researchers for neuroscientists to join their efforts in isolating the causes of medical illness. For example, the research team of the large-scale Cardiovascular Health Study (CHS) recently issued an invitation to neuroscientists to help maximize the use of magnetic resonance (MR) imaging data gathered from CHS participants, in which links have already been reported between MR imaging abnormalities and CVD (Yousem *et al.*, 2004). Given the widely recognized interdependence between neurological, immune, emotional, and related systems, it is difficult to view the development of psychiatric and medical conditions in isolation. Thus, the type of multidisciplinary collaboration advocated here is viewed by many as a prerequisite for understanding the interplay between mental and physical health problems across the lifespan.

Third, the majority of the young people are relatively healthy. However, advocates argue that the trend of ignoring specific health risks that accompany adolescence must end as 'for the first time, there is now a danger of a substantial drop in life expectancy with chronic diseases, such as diabetes and early signs of cardiovascular disease, appearing in teenagers and young adults' (Schribman, 2007, p. 1057). Indeed, new types of physical health problems are emerging among young people and causing alarm among parents, teachers, and paediatricians. For example, childhood obesity rates are increasing dramatically and early initiation of substance use is believed to pose significant health risks to many young teens (US Department of Health and Human Services, 2007). Unfortunately, the role of persistent antisocial behaviour and related neurodevelopmental vulnerabilities in moderating such prevention efforts has yet to be fully considered. In particular, there is a need to understand how the relationship between antisocial behaviour and health is manifested among key subgroups of children, such as children who present with callous and unemotional traits (Hodgins, 2007; Viding *et al.*, 2007).

In sum, innovative and cross disciplinary approaches-that cut across psychology, criminology, neuroscience, biology, and medicine-are required to advance our understanding of the developmental course of both antisocial behaviour and physical health problems. Findings to date suggest that the prevention of early behavioural problems may provide an opportunity to reduce not only future crime and violence, but may also lessen the overall adult health burden. Cost-benefit analyses are required to assess the potential benefits of such prevention strategies, taking into account medical and related expenses across the life course. The challenge for researchers and practitioners is to translate emerging knowledge across these seemingly diverse disciplines into innovative research and intervention alternatives for high-risk individuals and their families.

References

Bardone, A. M., Moffitt, T. E., Caspi, A., Dickson, N., Stanton, W. R., & Silva, P. A. (1998). Adult physical health outcomes of adolescent girls with conduct disorder, depression, and anxiety. *Journal of the American Academy of Child and Adolescent Psychiatry, 37*, 594–601.

Bauer, D. J. (2007). Observations on the use of growth mixture models in psychological research. *Multivariate Behavioral Research, 42*, 757–786.

Bongers, I. L., Koot, H. M., van Der Ende, J., & Verhulst, F. C. (2004). Developmental trajectories of externalizing behaviors in childhood and adolescence. *Child Development, 75*, 1523–1537.

Borowsky, I. W., Mozayeny, S., Stuenkel, K., & Ireland, M. (2004). Effects of a primary care-based intervention on violent behavior and injury in children. *Pediatrics, 114*, E392–E399.

Brehaut, J. C., Miller, A., Raina, P., & McGrail, K. M. (2003). Childhood behavior disorders and injuries among children and youth: a population-based study. *Pediatrics, 111*, 262–269.

Broidy, L. M., Nagin, D. S., Tremblay, R. E., Bates, J. E., Brame, B., Dodge, K. A., *et al.* (2003). Developmental trajectories of childhood disruptive behaviors and adolescent delinquency: a six-site, cross-national study. *Developmental Psychology, 39*, 222–245.

Caspi, A. (2000). The child is father of the man: personality continuities from childhood to adulthood. *Journal of Personality and Social Psychology, 78*, 158–172.

Caspi, A., McClay, J., Moffitt, T. E., Mill, J., Martin, J., Craig, I. W., *et al.* (2002). Role of genotype in the cycle of violence in maltreated children. *Science, 297*, 851–854.

Caspi, A., & Moffitt, T. E. (2006). Opinion—Gene-environment interactions in psychiatry: joining forces with neuroscience. *Nature Reviews Neuroscience, 7*, 583–590.

Cauffman, E., & Steinberg, L. (2000). (Im)maturity of judgment in adolescence: why adolescents may be less culpable than adults. *Behavioral Sciences & the Law, 18*, 741–760.

Chandola, T., Ferrie, J., Sacker, A., & Marmot, M. (2007). Social inequalities in self-reported health in early old age: follow-up of prospective cohort study. *British Medical Journal, 334*, 990–993B.

Cohen, S. (2004). Social relationships and health. *American Psychologist, 59*, 676–684.

Corso, P. S., Mercy, J. A., Simon, T. R., Finkelstein, E. A., & Miller, T. R. (2007). Medical costs and productivity losses due to interpersonal violence and self- directed violence. *American Journal of Preventive Medicine, 32*, 474–482.

Coté, S., Tremblay, R. E., Nagin, D. S., Zoccolillo, M., & Vitaro, F. (2002). Childhood behavioral profiles leading to adolescent conduct disorder: risk trajectories for boys and girls. *Journal of the American Academy of Child and Adolescent Psychiatry*, *41*, 1086–1094.

Coté, S., Zoccolillo, M., Tremblay, R. E., Nagin, D., & Vitaro, F. (2001). Predicting girls' conduct disorder in adolescence from childhood trajectories of disruptive behaviors. *Journal of the American Academy of Child and Adolescent Psychiatry*, *40*, 678–684.

Danese, A., Pariante, C. M., Caspi, A., Taylor, A., & Poulton, R. (2007). Childhood maltreatment predicts adult inflammation in a life-course study. *Proceedings of the National Academy of Sciences of the United States of America*, *104*, 1319–1324.

De Vogli, R., Chandola, T., & Marmot, M. G. (2007). Negative aspects of close relationships and heart disease. *Archives of Internal Medicine*, *167*, 1951–1957.

DiScala, C., Lescohier, I., Barthel, M., & Li, G. H. (1998). Injuries to children with attention deficit hyperactivity disorder. *Pediatrics*, *102*, 1415–1421.

Dobkin, P. L., Tremblay, R. E., & McDuff, P. (1997). Can childhood behavioural characteristics predict adolescent boys' health? A nine-year longitudinal study. *Journal of Health Psychology*, *2*, 445.

Elliot, D. S. (1993). Health-enhancing and health-compromising lifestyles. In S. G. Millstein, A. C. Petersen, & E. O. Nightingale (eds), *Promoting the Health of Adolescents: New Directions for the Twenty-First Century*. New York: Oxford University Press.

Farrington, D., Ohlin, L., & Wilson, J. Q. (1986). *Understanding and Controlling Crime*. New York: Springer-Verlag.

Farrington, D. P. (1995a). Crime and physical health: illnesses, injuries, accidents and offending in the Cambridge Study. *Criminal Behaviour and Mental Health*, *5*, 261–278.

Farrington, D. P. (1995b). The development of offending and antisocial behaviour from childhood: key findings from the Cambridge Study in Delinquent Development. *Journal of Child Psychology and Psychiatry*, *36*, 929–964.

Farrington, D. P., Coid, J. W., Harnett, L., Jolliffe, D., Soteriou, N., Turner, R., et al., (2006). *Criminal Careers up to Age 50 and Life Success up to Age 48: New Findings from the Cambridge Study in Delinquent Development*. London: Home Office.

Felitti, V. J., Anda, R. F., Nordenberg, D., Williamson, D. F., Spitz, A. M., Edwards, V., et al. (1998). Relationship of childhood abuse and household dysfunction to many of the leading causes of death in adults—the Adverse Childhood Experiences (ACE) study. *American Journal of Preventive Medicine*, *14*, 245–258.

Fergusson, D. M., & Horwood, J. L. (2002). Male and female offending trajectories. *Development and Psychopathology*, *14*, 159–177.

Fergusson, D. M., Horwood, J. L., & Ridder, E. M. (2005). Show me the child at seven: the consequences of conduct problems in childhood for psychosocial functioning in adulthood. *Journal of Child Psychology and Psychiatry*, *46*, 837–849.

Fontaine, N., Carbonneau, R., Barker, E., Vitaro, F., Hébert, M., Côté, S. M., et al. (2008). Girls' hyperactivity and physical aggression during childhood predict adjustment in early adulthood: a 15-year longitudinal study. *Archives of General Psychiatry*, *65*, 320–328.

Galobardes, B., Smith, G. D., & Lynch, J. W. (2006). Systematic review of the influence of childhood socioeconomic circumstances on risk for cardiovascular disease in adulthood. *Annals of Epidemiology*, *16*, 91–104.

Gorman-Smith, D., & Loeber, R. (2005). Are developmental pathways in disruptive behaviors the same for girls and boys? *Journal of Child and Family Studies*, *14*, 15–27.

Gump, B. B., Matthews, K. A., & Raikkonen, K. (1999). Modeling relationships among socioeconomic status, hostility, cardiovascular reactivity, and left ventricular mass in African American and White children. *Health Psychology*, *18*, 140–150.

Gunnar, M., & Quevedo, K. (2007). The neurobiology of stress and development. *Annual Review of Psychology*, *58*, 145–173.

Hodgins, S. (1994). Status at age 30 of children with conduct problems. *Studies of Crime and Crime Prevention*, *3*, 41–62.

Hodgins, S. (2007). Persistent violent offending: what do we know? *British Journal of Psychiatry*, *190*, S12–S14.

Kim-Cohen, J., Caspi, A., Moffitt, T. E., Harrington, H., Milne, B. J., & Poulton, R. (2003). Prior juvenile diagnoses in adults with mental disorder—developmental follow-back of a prospective-longitudinal cohort. *Archives of General Psychiatry*, *60*, 709–717.

Knox, S. S., Weidner, G., Adelman, A., Stoney, C. M., & Ellison, C. (2004). Hostility and physiological risk in the National Heart, Lung, and Blood Institute Family Heart Study. *Archives of Internal Medicine*, *164*, 2442–2448.

Kratzer, L., & Hodgins, S. (1997). Adult outcomes of child conduct problems: a cohort study. *Journal of Abnormal Child Psychology*, *25*, 65–81.

Kratzer, L., & Hodgins, S. (1999). A typology of offenders: a test of Moffitt's theory among males and females from childhood to age 30. *Criminal Behaviour and Mental Health*, *9*, 57–73.

Lahey, B. B., van Hulle, C. A., Waldman, I. D., Rodgers, J. L., D'onofrio, B. M., Pedlow, S., *et al.* (2006). Testing descriptive hypotheses regarding sex differences in the development of conduct problems and delinquency. *Journal of Abnormal Child Psychology*, *34*, 737–755.

Lalloo, R., & Sheiham, A. (2003). Risk factors for childhood major and minor head and other injuries in a nationally representative sample. *Injury—International Journal of the Care of the Injured*, *34*, 261–266.

Landrigan, P. J., Trasande, L., Thorpe, L. E., Gwynn, C., Lioy, P. J., D'alton, M. E., *et al.* (2006). The National Children's Study: a 21-year prospective study of 100 000 American children. *Pediatrics*, *118*, 2173–2186.

Lawlor, D. A., Ronalds, G., Macintyre, S., Clark, H., & Leon, D. A. (2006). Family socioeconomic position at birth and future cardiovascular disease risk: findings from the Aberdeen children of the 1950s cohort study. *American Journal of Public Health*, *96*, 1271–1277.

Leibson, C. L., Katusic, S. K., Barbaresi, W. J., Ransom, J., & O'brien, P. C. (2001). Use and costs of medical care for children and adolescents with and without attention-deficit/hyperactivity disorder. *Journal of the American Medical Association*, *285*, 60–66.

McCluskey, C. P., McCluskey, J. D., & Bynum, T. S. (2006). Early onset offending and later violent and gun outcomes in a contemporary youth cohort. *Journal of Criminal Justice*, *34*, 531–541.

McEwen, B. S. (2007). Physiological and neurobiology of stress and adaptation: Central role of the brain. *Physiological Review*, *87*, 873–903.

Melchior, M., Moffitt, T. E., Milne, B. J., Poulton, R., & Caspi, A. (2007). Why do children from socioeconomically disadvantaged families suffer from poor health when they reach adulthood? a life-course study. *American Journal of Epidemiology*, *166*, 966–974.

Messer, J., Goodman, R., Rowe, R., Meltzer, H., & Maughan, B. (2006). Preadolescent conduct problems in girls and boys. *Journal of the American Academy of Child and Adolescent Psychiatry*, *45*, 184–191.

Miller, T. Q., Smith, T. W., Turner, C. W., Guijarro, M. L., & Hallet, A. J. (1996). A meta-analytic review of research on hostility and physical health. *Psychological Bulletin*, *119*, 322–348.

Millstein, S. G., Petersen, A. C., & Nightingale, E. O. (eds) (1993). *Promoting the Health of Adolescents: New Directions for the Twenty-First Century*. New York: Oxford University Press.

Moffitt, T. E. (1993). Adolescence-limited and life-course-persistent antisocial behavior: a developmental taxonomy. *Psychological Review*, *100*, 674–701.

Moffitt, T. E. (1994). Natural histories of delinquency. In E. Wietekamp, & H. J. Kerner (eds) *Cross-National Longitudinal Research on Human Development and Criminal Behaviour*. Dordrecht, the Netherlands: Kluwer Academic Press.

Moffitt, T. E. (2006). Life-course-persistent and adolescent-limited antisocial behavior. In D. Cicchetti, & D. J. Cohen (eds), *Developmental Psychopathology, Vol. 3: Risk, Disorder, and Adaptation*, 2 edn. New York: John Wiley & Sons.

Moffitt, T. E., Arseneault, L., Jaffee, S. R., Kim-Cohen, J., Koenen, K. C., Odgers, C. L., *et al.* (2008). Research review: DSM-V conduct disorder: research needs for an evidence base. *Journal of Child Psychology and Psychiatry and Allied Disciplines*, *49*, 3–33.

Moffitt, T. E., & Caspi, A. (2001). Childhood predictors differentiate life-course persistent and adolescence-limited antisocial pathways among males and females. *Development and Psychopathology*, *13*, 355–375.

Moffitt, T. E., Caspi, A., Harrington, H., & Milne, B. J. (2002). Males on the life-course-persistent and adolescence-limited antisocial pathways: follow-up at age 26 years. *Development and Psychopathology*, *14*, 179–207.

Moffitt, T. E., Caspi, A., Rutter, M., & Silva, P. A. (2001). *Sex Differences in Antisocial Behaviour: Conduct Disorder, Delinquency, and Violence in the Dunedin Longitudinal Study*. New York: Cambridge University Press.

Moffitt, T. E., & Henry, B. (1991). Neuropsychological studies of juvenile delinquency and violence: a review. In J. Milner (ed), *The Neuropsychology of Aggression*. Norwell, MA: Kluwer Academic.

Odgers, C. L., Caspi, A., Broadbent, J. M., Dickson, N. P., Hancox, R., Harrington, H., *et al.* (2007). Conduct problem subtypes in males predict differential health burden. *Archives of General Psychiatry*, *64*, 476–484.

Odgers, C. L., Caspi, A., Nagin, D., Piquero, A. R., Slutske, W. S., Milne, B., *et al.* (2008). Is it important to prevent early exposure to drugs and alcohol among adolescents? *Psychological Science*, *19*, 1037–1044.

Odgers, C. L., Moffitt, T. E., Caspi, A., Broadbent, J. M., Dickson, N. P., Hancox, R., *et al.* (2008). Female and male antisocial trajectories: from childhood origins to adult outcomes. *Development and Psychopathology*, *20*, 673–716.

Pajer, K., Stouthamer-Loeber, M., Gardner, W., & Loeber, R. (2006). Women with antisocial behaviour: long-term health disability and help-seeking for emotional problems. *Criminal Behaviour and Mental Health*, *16*, 29.

Pajer, K. A. (1998). What happens to 'bad' girls? A review of the adult outcomes of antisocial adolescent girls. *American Journal of Psychiatry*, *155*, 862.

Pajer, K. A. (2007). Cardiovascular disease risk factors in adolescents: do negative emotions and hypothalamic-pituitary-adrenal axis function play a role? *Current Opinion in Pediatrics*, *19*, 559–564.

Pajer, K. A., Kazmi, A., Gardner, W. P., & Wang, Y. (2007). Female conduct disorder: health status in young adulthood. *Journal of Adolescent Health*, *40*, 84.e.1–84.e.7.

Piquero, A. R., Gibson, C. L., Daigle, L., Piquero, N., & Tibbetts, S. G. (2007). Are life-course persistent offenders at risk for adverse health outcomes? *Journal of Research in Crime and Delinquency*, *44*, 185–207.

Poulton, R., Caspi, A., Milne, B. J., Thomson, W. M., Taylor, A., Sears, M. R., *et al.* (2002). Association between children's experience of socioeconomic disadvantage and adult health: a life-course study. *Lancet*, *360*, 1640–1645.

Raikkonen, K., Matthews, K. A., & Salomon, K. (2003). Hostility predicts metabolic syndrome risk factors in children and adolescents. *Health Psychology*, *22*, 279–286.

Raikkonen, K., Matthews, K. A., Sutton-Tyrrell, K., & Kuller, L. H. (2004). Trait anger and the metabolic syndrome predict progression of carotid atherosclerosis in healthy middle-aged women. *Psychosomatic Medicine*, *66*, 903–908.

Ramrakha, S., Bell, M. L., Paul, C., Dickson, N., Moffitt, T. E., & Caspi, A. (2007). Childhood behavior problems linked to sexual risk taking in young adulthood: a birth cohort study. *Journal of the American Academy of Child and Adolescent Psychiatry*, *46*, 1272–1279.

Ravaja, N., Keltikangasjarvinen, L., & Keskivaara, P. (1996). Type A factors as predictors of changes in the metabolic syndrome precursors in adolescents and young adults—a 3-year follow-up study. *Health Psychology*, *15*, 18–29.

Repetti, R. L., Taylor, S. E., & Seeman, T. E. (2002). Risky families: family social environments and the mental and physical health of offspring. *Psychological Bulletin*, *128*, 330–366.

Robins, L. & Rutter, M. (eds) (1990). *Straight and Deviant Pathways from Childhood to Adulthood*. New York: Cambridge University Press.

Robins, L. N. (1978). Sturdy childhood predictors of adult antisocial behavior—replications from longitudinal-studies. *Psychological Medicine*, *8*, 611–622.

Rutter, M., Kim-Cohen, J., & Maughan, B. (2006). Continuities and discontinuities in psychopathology between childhood and adult life. *Journal of Child Psychology and Psychiatry*, *47*, 276–295.

Sabuncuoglu, O. (2007). Traumatic dental injuries and attention-deficit/hyperactivity disorder: is there a link? *Dental Traumatology*, *23*, 137–142.

Sampson, R. J., & Laub, J. H. (2003). Life-course desisters? trajectories of crime among delinquent boys followed to age 70. *Criminology*, *41*, 555–592.

Sampson, R. J., & Laub, J. H. (2005). A life-course view of the development of crime. *Annals of the American Academy of Political and Social Science*, *602*, 12–45.

Schaeffer, C. M., Petras, H., Ialongo, N., Masyn, K. E., Hubbard, S., Poduska, J., *et al.* (2006). A comparison of girls' and boys' aggressive-disruptive behavior trajectories across elementary school: prediction to young adult antisocial outcomes. *Journal of Consulting and Clinical Psychology*, *74*, 500–510.

Schaeffer, C. M., Petras, H., Ialongo, N., Poduska, J., & Kellam, S. (2003). Modeling growth in boys' aggressive behavior across elementary school: links to later criminal involvement, conduct disorder, and antisocial personality disorder. *Developmental Psychology*, *39*, 1020–1035.

Schwebel, D. C., Speltz, M. L., Jones, K., & Bardina, P. (2002). Unintentional injury in preschool boys with and without early onset of disruptive behavior. *Journal of Pediatric Psychology*, *27*, 727–737.

Serbin, L. A., Stack, D. M., de Genna, N., Grunzeweig, N., Temcheff, C. E., Schwartzman, A. E., *et al.* (2004). When aggressive girls become mothers: problems in parenting, health, and development across two generations. *Aggression, Antisocial Behavior, and Violence among Girls: A Developmental Perspective*. New York: Guilford Publications, Inc.

Shepherd, J., & Farrington, D. (2003). The impact of antisocial lifestyle on health—family, school, and police interventions can reduce health risks. *British Medical Journal*, *326*, 834–835.

Shepherd, J., Farrington, D., & Potts, J. (2002). Relations between offending, injury and illness. *Journal of the Royal Society of Medicine*, *95*, 539–544.

Shepherd, J., Farrington, D., & Potts, J. (2004). Impact of antisocial lifestyle on health. *Journal of Public Health*, *26*, 347–352.

Shribman, S. (2007). Adolescent health: an opportunity not to be missed. *Lancet*, *369*, 1788–1789.

Simon, G. E., von Korff, M., Saunders, K., Miglioretti, D. L., Crane, P. K., van Belle, G., *et al.* (2006). Association between obesity and psychiatric disorders in the US adult population. *Archives of General Psychiatry*, *63*, 824–830.

Susman, E. J. (2006). Psychobiology of persistent antisocial behavior: Stress, early vulnerabilities and the attenuation hypothesis. *Neuroscience and Biobehavioral Reviews*, *30*, 376–89.

Toumbourou, J. W., Stockwell, T., Neighbors, C., Marlatt, G. A., Sturge, J., & Rehm, J. (2007). Adolescent health 4—interventions to reduce harm associated with adolescent substance use. *Lancet*, *369*, 1391–1401.

Tremblay, R. E. (2000). The development of aggressive behavior during childhood: what have we learned in the past century? *International Journal of Behavioral Development*, *24*, 129–141.

Tremblay, R. E. (2002). Prevention of injury by early socialization of aggressive behavior. *Injury Prevention*, *8*, IV17–IV21.

US Department of Health and Human Services (2007). The Surgeon General's call to action to prevent and reduce underage drinking. US Department of Health and Human Services, Office of the Surgeon General.

Viding, E., Frick, P. J., & Plomin, R. (2007). Aetiology of the relationship between callous-unemotional traits and conduct problems in childhood. *British Journal of Psychiatry*, *190*, S33–S38.

White, N. A., & Piquero, A. R. (2004). A preliminary empirical test of Silverthorn and Frick's delayed-onset pathway in girls using an urban, African-American, US-based sample. *Criminal Behaviour and Mental Health*, *14*, 291–309.

Whooley, M. A. (2006). Depression and cardiovascular disease: healing the broken-hearted. *Journal of the American Medical Association*, *295*, 2874–2881.

Wickrama, K. A. S., Lorenz, F. O., Wallace, L. E., Peiris, L., Conger, R. D., & Elder, G. H. (2001). Family influence on physical health during the middle years: the case of onset of hypertension. *Journal of Marriage and the Family*, *63*, 527–539.

Wiesner, M., & Capaldi, D. M. (2003). Relations of childhood and adolescent factors to offending trajectories of young men. *Journal of Research in Crime and Delinquency*, *40*, 231–262.

Wiesner, M., Capaldi, D. M., & Kim, H. K. (2007). Arrest trajectories across a 17-year span for young men: relation to dual taxonomies and self-reported offense trajectories. *Criminology*, *45*, 835–863.

Wiesner, M., Kim, H. K., & Capaldi, D. M. (2005). Developmental trajectories of offending: validation and prediction to young adult alcohol use, drug use, and depressive symptoms. *Development
and Psychopathology*, *17*, 251–270.

Woodward, L. J., Fergusson, D. M., & Horwood, L. J. (2002). Romantic relationships of young people
with childhood and adolescent onset antisocial behavior problems. *Journal of Abnormal Child
Psychology*, *30*, 231–243.

Woolard, J. L., Odgers, C., Lanza-Kaduce, L., & Daglis, H. (2005). Juveniles within adult correctional
settings: legal pathways and developmental considerations. *International Journal of Forensic Mental
Health*, *4*, 1–18.

World Health Organization (2002). World report on violence and health. Geneva, Switzerland: WHO
Press.

World Health Organization (2007). Third milestones of a Global Campaign for Violence Prevention
report, 2007: scaling up. Geneva, Switzerland: WHO Press.

Yousem, D. M., Bryan, R. N., Beauchamp Jr., N. J., & Arnold, A. M. (2004). A national neuroimaging
database: a call to action. *American Journal of Neuroradiology*, *25*, 908–909.

3

Violent behaviour among people with schizophrenia: A framework for investigations of causes, effective treatment, and prevention

Sheilagh Hodgins

Violent criminal offending among persons with schizophrenia

There is now robust evidence demonstrating that both men and women with schizophrenia[1] are at elevated risk compared to the general population to be convicted of non-violent criminal offences, at higher risk to be convicted of violent criminal offences, and at even higher risk to be convicted of homicide (Wallace *et al.*, 2004). For example, we examined a birth cohort composed of all the 358 180 persons born in Denmark from 1944 through 1947 who were followed until their mid-forties. We excluded those who had died or emigrated before the end of the follow-up period. The official criminal records of cohort members who had been admitted to a psychiatric ward at least once with a discharge diagnosis of schizophrenia were compared with those who had not had psychiatric admissions: the risk of a violent crime was elevated 4.6 (3.8–5.6) times among the men and 23.2 (14.4–37.4) times among the women with schizophrenia versus those with no admissions to a psychiatric ward (Brennan *et al.*, 2000). Similar elevations in risk have been documented among persons with schizophrenia identified in other birth and populations cohorts (Hodgins, 1992; Tiihonen *et al.*, 1997; Arseneault *et al.*, 2000; Wallace *et al.*, 2004). Although fewer women than men, both with and without schizophrenia, are convicted of crimes, schizophrenia confers a greater risk of offending among women than among men.

This association between schizophrenia and violent offending is robust; it has been observed by different research teams who recruited samples from countries with different cultures and health and justice systems, and who measured the association of schizophrenia and offending using different experimental designs including longitudinal investigations of birth and population cohorts, comparisons of people with schizophrenia and their neighbours, and diagnostic studies of random samples of convicted offenders. There is no evidence to suggest that the elevated rates of violent offending among persons with schizophrenia compared to the general population result from discrimination on the part of the criminal justice systems in the countries where these investigations were conducted (for a discussion, see Hodgins & Janson, 2002). It is important to note that these convictions resulted from crimes that were committed in the community and not in psychiatric wards, where aggressive behaviour towards others rarely, if ever, leads to criminal prosecution.

Results of the epidemiological investigations are consistent in showing that the proportions of persons with schizophrenia who commit crimes vary from one study to another, although the elevations in risk among those with schizophrenia compared to the general

---

[1] The term schizophrenia is used to refer to both schizophrenia and schizoaffective disorder.

population are similar (Hodgins, 1998). In countries with high rates of violent crime, proportionately more individuals with schizophrenia have convictions for violent crime than in a country with lower rates of violent crime. This observation suggests that at least some of the factors that contribute to violent crime in the general population also influence violent crime among persons with schizophrenia. The proportions of persons with schizophrenia who acquire convictions for violent crime also vary by time period, reflecting differences in policies regarding diversion of mentally ill persons accused of crimes from the justice system to the health system (for further discussion, see Hodgins & Janson, 2002). Most violent offences committed by persons with schizophrenia are assaults. Although homicides attract much attention from the media, they are rare. In some countries, all persons accused of homicide undergo thorough psychiatric evaluations prior to trial. These evaluations have been used to estimate the proportion of homicides that are committed by individuals with schizophrenia and estimates vary from 6% to 28%, indicating substantial variation between and within countries by time period (Erb et al., 2001). Because the number of homicides varies greatly from one country to another while the prevalence of schizophrenia is relatively stable at just less than 1%, the numbers of persons with schizophrenia who commit homicides differs across countries. Thus, the proportion of persons with schizophrenia who engage in violence varies by place and time period, but evidence shows that it always remains higher than the proportion of offenders in the general population.

Why does it matter?

The findings reported in the preceding reflect a huge amount of human suffering, on the part of the victims and their families and on the part of the perpetrators. Schizophrenia is a devastating illness that, in most cases, limits most aspects of functioning through adult life (Mueser & McGurk, 2004). The evidence now shows that some of those stricken with this brain disorder present a propensity for engaging in aggressive behaviour towards others that leads to further negative consequences. In addition, individuals with schizophrenia are more likely than the general population to be the victims of crime (Teplin et al., 2005), particularly of assaults, and one of the strongest predictors of physical victimization is their own aggressive behaviour (Walsh et al., 2003; Silver et al., 2005; Hodgins et al., 2007). Violent crimes committed by persons with schizophrenia also matter because of the associated financial burden they place on society. Studying violence[2] among persons with schizophrenia will inform the development of treatments and prevention programmes aimed at reducing such behaviours and, perhaps, further understanding of the brain mechanisms involved in aggressive behaviour.

People with schizophrenia are commonly perceived as unpredictable and dangerous (Crisp et al., 2005), with public fears outweighing the actual risk of being injured by an individual with severe mental illness (Steadman et al., 1998). Public perceptions of dangerousness, regardless of their accuracy, play a central role in fostering stigma (Link et al., 1987). Consequently, violence committed by some individuals with severe mental illness promotes stigmatization and rejection of all persons with severe mental illness. Stigmatization may affect diagnostic decision making and treatment (Walsh & Fahy, 2002; Clark & Rowe, 2006), pose barriers to recovery and integration in the community, and compromise quality of life (Link & Pelham, 2006).

---

[2] The term violence is used to refer to physical aggression towards another person that may or may not lead to criminal prosecution. The terms violence and aggressive behaviour are used interchangeably.

Implications of violent offending among persons with schizophrenia

Treatment of persons with schizophrenia that successfully reduced aggressive behaviour would contribute to lowering rates of violent criminality. As noted in the preceding, it would reduce the homicide rate, but also the rate of other forms of violence. For example, in the Danish cohort described earlier, 2.2% of the men had severe mental illness and committed 8.4% of the physically aggressive sex offences, 9.0% of the non-physically aggressive sex offences, and in all comprised 8.1% of the sex offenders (Alden *et al.*, 2007).

Given the numbers of persons with schizophrenia who engage in violent criminal offending, there are important consequences for both the health and criminal justice systems. Adult mental health services provide care for a subgroup of individuals with schizophrenia who present high levels of violent behaviour. For example, we recently assessed a sample of 205 inpatients with severe mental illness from a UK inner-city mental health trust, most of who suffered from schizophrenia. The patients were, on average, in their late thirties and more than 80% had previously required inpatient care. Official criminal records indicated that 46.7% of the men and 16.5% of the women had at least one conviction for a violent crime, and on average, the violent offenders had each been convicted of more than two crimes. The 82 men with criminal records had committed 1792 crimes and the 23 female offenders had committed 458 crimes (Hodgins *et al.*, 2007). The risks of conviction in this sample of patients compared to the general UK population were similar to those observed in comparisons of severely mentally ill inpatient and general population samples in Sweden and Denmark. This subgroup of patients with a history of violence presents a challenge to general mental health services. Some of these patients are transferred to forensic inpatient services, which have dramatically increased in capacity, not only in the UK but also in several other European countries (Priebe *et al.*, 2005). Most forensic beds are occupied by men with schizophrenia (Hodgins & Müller-Isberner, 2004).

Many persons with schizophrenia are incarcerated (Davies, 2004a, 2004b, 2004c). Rates vary from one country to another, and within countries from one time period to another, depending on policies designed to divert the mentally ill accused or convicted of crimes from the justice system to the health system. In studies of inmate populations, rates of schizophrenia are much higher than rates for age- and sex-matched general population samples (Fazel & Danesh, 2002). Within correctional facilities, people with schizophrenia fail to obtain adequate and appropriate treatment for their illness and are frequently physically abused (Wolff *et al.*, 2007).

Also consistent with the epidemiological evidence on the elevated rates of violent offending among persons with schizophrenia is emerging evidence that antisocial behaviour in adolescence is a precursor to schizophrenia. Robins (1966) was the first to note that a disproportionate number of adolescent delinquents subsequently developed schizophrenia. A recent study in Denmark examined a cohort composed of all the offenders aged 15–19 years old in 1992. Of the 780 who were still alive in Denmark in 2001, 3.3% had developed schizophrenia compared with the expected 0.7%. The odds of developing schizophrenia among those with a history of violent criminal offending (versus those with only non-violent offending) were 4.59 (1.54–13.74) (Gosden *et al.*, 2005). We compared a sample of all the 1992 individuals who as teenagers contacted a clinic for substance misuse in a large metropolitan area of Sweden in the years 1968–72 with a randomly selected general population sample matched for sex, age, and birthplace. By age 50, four times more males and eight times more females in the clinic than the general population sample had been hospitalized with schizophrenia (Hodgins *et al.*, in preparation). These results are consistent with the epidemiological investigations that identified antisocial behaviour prior to illness onset among a subgroup of offenders with schizophrenia (Hodgins, 1992; Wallace *et al.*, 2004).

Thus, individuals who develop schizophrenia contribute disproportionately to violent crime rates. Presently, general adult mental health services fail to assess and manage their risk of violence or to provide them with treatments designed to reduce violent behaviour. More and more of these individuals are being transferred to costly forensic inpatient services (Hodgins & Müller-Isberner, 2004) and are being incarcerated. Among adolescents engaging in antisocial and criminal behaviours, a disproportionate number develop schizophrenia.

Schizophrenia is also associated with elevated rates of aggressive behaviour towards others

An interview protocol that combines information from patients and collateral informants has been developed specifically to assess aggressive behaviour and victimization among persons with mental disorders (Steadman *et al.*, 1998); studies have shown that severely mentally ill patients report aggressive incidents at only a slightly lower rate than do collaterals (Steadman *et al.*, 1998). In our study of the UK inpatients with severe mental illness, 41.7% of the men and 21.2% of the women reported having engaged in at least one serious assault sometime in their life, 49.2% of the men and 38.8% of the women reported having engaged in at least one act of physical aggression against another person in the previous six months, and 21.7% of the men and 18.8% of the women reported engaging in a life-threatening act of violence against another person in the previous six months. A study of a large sample of outpatients with psychosis found that one in five had assaulted another person over a two-year period (Walsh *et al.*, 2001). Similarly, other studies of samples of outpatients with schizophrenia report rates of any physically aggressive behaviour towards others ranging from 8% to 77% during the previous six months and rates of life-threatening violence towards others ranging from 0 to 40% (Hodgins *et al.*, 2007). As noted previously, rates of convictions for violent crimes are lower among woman than men with schizophrenia, but several studies suggest that the prevalence of aggressive behaviour is similar (Walsh *et al.*, 2001; Dean *et al.*, 2006; Hodgins *et al.*, 2007). Importantly, the correlates of violent offending and of physically aggressive behaviour towards others when patients are living in the community are similar.

Psychotic symptoms and violence

Recent studies of large population samples indicate that psychotic symptoms are more common than previously thought (Stefanis *et al.*, 2002). One US study revealed that 5.1% of 38 132 adults reported psychotic-like experiences. The presence of psychotic-like experiences was associated with a fivefold increase in the risk of assaulting another person (Mojtabai, 2006). Yet, the results of studies on the association of positive symptoms of psychosis and violent behaviour among persons with schizophrenia are contradictory (Appelbaum *et al.*, 2000; Bjørkly, 2002a, 2002b). The lack of consistency in the evidence results primarily from methodological features of studies including retrospective assessment of symptoms and failure to take account of other factors such as previous violence, childhood behaviour problems, and intoxication, which are known to be associated with violence (Appelbaum *et al.*, 2000; Bjørkly, 2002a, 2002b; Hodgins *et al.*, 2003). There is some evidence that when positive symptoms are accompanied by depression or distress, the risk of aggressive behaviour is elevated, even after controlling for a previous history of antisocial behaviour[3] and current and past substance misuse (Hodgins *et al.*, 2003; Crocker *et al.*, 2005).

The evidence is consistent, however, in showing that the correlates of violent behaviour during acute episodes of psychosis among patients hospitalized in a psychiatric ward differ from the correlates of violent behaviour that occurs in the community. Many acutely psychotic patients who are in most cases admitted involuntarily to psychiatric wards behave aggressively. The aggressive behaviour declines rapidly in the days following admission. Aggressive incidents in an acute psychiatric ward are as common among women as men, and unlike aggressive behaviour that occurs in the community, they are strongly associated with confusion and thought disorder (Steinert, 2002; Krakowski & Czobor, 2004).

Among people with schizophrenia, the lack of association between aggressive behaviour and positive symptoms of psychosis is not surprising if considered in light of evidence that psychosocial functioning generally is not associated with positive symptoms. Aggressive behaviour reflects a lack of interpersonal skills, or simply one aspect of psychosocial functioning. Interpersonal skills, community activities, and work skills are most strongly associated with performance on neuropsychological tests, negative symptoms, and depression, and not with positive symptoms (Bowie *et al.*, 2006). We assessed psychosocial functioning among 248 men with schizophrenia living in the community who had been recruited from forensic and general psychiatric services. Psychosocial functioning was defined to include measures of independent living, occupational functioning, social and leisure activities, and the absence of aggressive behaviour, substance misuse, and self-harm. We found that psychosocial functioning was associated with two static predictors—level of education and past diagnoses of substance misuse disorders—and three current predictors—depression, noncompliance with antipsychotic medication, and experiences of physical victimization (Hodgins *et al.*, in press). The results of this study confirmed findings of previous investigations showing that factors other than positive symptoms are most strongly associated with real-life functioning among persons with schizophrenia.

Our study, however, did not include a measure of cognitive impairment. Not only is the level of cognitive impairment a major determinant of psychosocial functioning, it is also a core feature of schizophrenia. Deficits in cognitive performance characterize children and adolescents developing the illness, are present at onset of illness, remain stable over time, and are largely explained by genetic factors (Cannon & Clarke, 2005; Green *et al.*, 2005; Toulopoulou *et al.*, 2007; McCabe *et al.*, 2008). Although individuals developing schizophrenia and those already affected perform more poorly than age-matched healthy persons on all measures of cognitive functioning, there is wide variation in levels of cognitive performance among persons with schizophrenia. Thus, if aggressive behaviour is viewed as one aspect of psychosocial functioning, then similar to other aspects of psychosocial functioning it too is not strongly, nor consistently, associated with positive symptoms of psychosis.

A typology of offenders with schizophrenia

Another reason for the inconsistent results concerning the association of psychotic symptoms and violence is that studies have compared offenders having schizophrenia with non-offenders

---

[3] The term antisocial behaviour is used to refer to a wide array of behaviours that break social norms, rules, and laws, and that by definition includes substance misuse.

having schizophrenia, thereby assuming that the offenders constitute a homogeneous group. The evidence, however, does not support this presumption. Among offenders who are not mentally ill, findings have been accumulated indicating that there are subtypes defined by age at onset and persistence of antisocial behaviour that differ as to aetiology and response to treatment (Moffitt & Caspi, 2001). Among offenders with schizophrenia, subtypes defined by age of onset and persistence of antisocial behaviour are also apparent. Consequently, studies that compare violent and non-violent offenders obscure features that distinguish subtypes of violent offenders with schizophrenia such that findings are difficult to interpret.

We have been conducting a programme of research based on the hypothesis that there are three types of offenders who differ as to age of onset and persistence of antisocial behaviour. The early starters display a pattern of antisocial behaviour that onsets in childhood or early adolescence and remains stable across the lifespan. They are usually convicted of crimes prior to illness onset. By contrast, a large group of violent offenders with schizophrenia show no antisocial behaviour prior to onset of the prodrome or illness and then repeatedly engage in aggressive behaviour towards others. A small group of individuals who display a chronic course of schizophrenia show no aggressive behaviour prior to their late thirties or early forties and then engage in serious violence, often killing those who care for them.

Early start offenders with schizophrenia

Early start offenders with schizophrenia have been defined in different ways: those with a conviction for violence prior to illness onset, those with a history of childhood conduct problems, and those who met the criteria for Conduct Disorder (CD) prior to age 15. Compared to other offenders with schizophrenia, those with a childhood history of conduct problems, defined in any of these ways, are convicted for more non-violent and violent crimes (Fulwiler & Ruthazer, 1999; Crocker *et al.*, 2005; Mueser *et al.*, 2006), commit a more diverse array of crimes (Hodgins, 2004), and have criminal histories similar to those of offenders who are not mentally ill who also have a childhood history of conduct problems (Hodgins & Côté, 1993; Schug *et al.*, 2007). In addition, almost all display a pattern of substance misuse going back to early adolescence (Fulwiler *et al.*, 1997; Mueser *et al.*, 1999; Tengström *et al.*, 2001; Moran & Hodgins, 2004).

For reasons currently not understood, CD and conduct problems are precursors of schizophrenia. For example, a prospective, longitudinal investigation of a large Dutch population sample observed that aggressive behaviour in childhood is associated with thought disorder in adulthood (Ferdinand & Verhulst, 1995). Similarly, a prospective investigation of a US population cohort observed that aggressive behaviour in early adolescence is associated with personality disorders that are genetically linked to schizophrenia (Bernstein *et al.*, 1996). The prospective studies of children at risk of schizophrenia by virtue of having a close relative with the disorder, usually the mother, observed that a proportion of the males who developed schizophrenia had displayed conduct problems through childhood. The most direct and robust evidence that CD is a precursor of schizophrenia comes from a prospective investigation that followed a New Zealand birth cohort to age 26. Forty per cent of the cohort members who developed schizophreniform disorders had displayed CD prior to age 15 (Kim-Cohen *et al.*, 2003). In clinical samples of adults with schizophrenia, the prevalence of CD is lower. The CD modules of the Structured Clinical Interview for DSM-III-R and IV were designed to retrospectively diagnose CD prior to age 15. We have used this interview protocol, in some studies supplemented by information from family members, school, and social service and justice files, to diagnose CD among adults with schizophrenia. In most samples, the prevalence is approximately 20% among both women and men (Hodgins *et al.*, 1998), but in the UK sample of inpatients described earlier, for example, CD prior to age 15 characterized 42.0% of the men and 22.4% of the women (Hodgins *et al.*, 2008). Although these samples of patients with schizophrenia were recruited in general psychiatric services, the prevalence of CD is higher among patients in forensic services, and it is further elevated among those incarcerated (Hodgins *et al.*, 1998).

CD and conduct problems are not only precursors of schizophrenia but are also more common among people who develop schizophrenia than in the general population. Recent estimates of the prevalence of CD prior to age 15 range from 7.5% among boys and 3.9% among girls in a large UK cohort (Green *et al.*, 2004) to 12.0% among boys and 7.1% among girls in a US sample (Nock *et al.*, 2006). These prevalence rates are much lower than that observed prospectively in the Dunedin Study among the cohort members who developed schizophreniform disorders or among clinical samples of adults with schizophrenia. This more recent evidence is consistent with older findings from a US investigation of a population sample of 20 000 adults, in which higher rates of CD were observed among persons with than without schizophrenia (Robins *et al.*, 1991) and the number of CD symptoms present prior to age 15 was found to be positively and linearly associated with the likelihood of developing schizophrenia (Robins, 1993). Then, the accumulated evidence indicates that the prevalence of CD is higher among people who develop schizophrenia than in the general population and that the gender difference is less. Thus, not only is the proportion of offenders greater in the population of persons who develop schizophrenia than in the general population, so also is the proportion of offenders who display an early onset and stable pattern of antisocial behaviour.

We conducted an investigation to examine the association of CD prior to age 15 and crime and aggressive behaviour among a sample of 248 men with schizophrenia who were, on average, aged 39.8 years at the time of the study (Hodgins *et al.*, 2005). They were assessed in the two weeks prior to discharge from hospital using multiple sources of information including complete criminal records. Fifty-two (21%) of these men met the criteria for CD prior to age 15. Incident rate ratios (IRRs) were calculated to estimate the association between CD and the number of convictions for violent crimes. CD diagnosis was associated with an increase of 2.29 (1.31–4.03) in the number of convictions for violent crimes after controlling for lifetime diagnoses of alcohol abuse, drug abuse, and/or dependence. Each CD symptom present before the age of 15 was associated with a 1.15 (1.06–1.25) increase in the number of convictions for violent crime, again after controlling for diagnoses of substance misuse disorders. CD and CD symptoms were also associated with the number of convictions for non-violent crimes, as depicted in Fig. 3.1.

We replicated these results in the sample of UK inpatients with severe mental illness described previously (Hodgins *et al.*, 2007). In this study, after controlling for sex, age, current alcohol and drug use, CD prior to age 15 was associated with a twofold (odds ratio 2.5, 1.17–5.36) increase in the number of convictions for violent crimes. Again, after controlling for sex, age, and substance misuse, each CD symptom present before age 15 was associated with a slight increase in the number of violent crimes (odds ratio 1.16, 1.01–1.35). Both CD diagnosis and the number of CD symptoms were also associated with the number of convictions for non-violent crimes. No sex differences in the association of CD and later offending were detected. The results of these two studies indicate that among individuals who develop schizophrenia, as among those who do not, CD in childhood is a precursor of criminal offending in adulthood. They concur with results from other studies that used

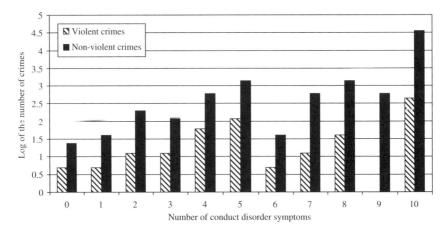

Fig. 3.1 Number of non-violent and violent crimes as a function of the number of Conduct Disorder symptoms among men with schizophrenia.

different definitions of childhood conduct problems (Rice & Harris, 1995; Fulwiler & Ruthazer, 1999; Tengström *et al.*, 2004).

Both in the general population (Moffitt & Caspi, 2001) and among people with schizophrenia, not surprisingly, CD is a precursor of aggressive behaviour, as well as violent crime. The same instrument (Steadman *et al.*, 1998) has been used in three studies to assess aggressive behaviour among people with schizophrenia and its association with CD. In the UK sample of severely ill men and women in their late thirties, we found that after controlling for age, sex, and current substance misuse, CD diagnosis prior to age 15 was associated with increased odds of aggressive behaviour towards others in the previous six months (odds ratio 2.66, 1.24–5.68), as was each CD symptom (odds ratio 1.29, 1.11–1.50) (Hodgins *et al.*, 2008).

The 248 men with schizophrenia described earlier were studied for 24 months following discharge from hospital (Hodgins *et al.*, 2005). They and an informant were interviewed at 6-month intervals to document aggressive behaviour. CD was associated with increased risk of aggressive behaviour (odds ratio 2.39, 1.18–4.83) that remained after controlling for current substance misuse and lifetime diagnoses of alcohol abuse and/or dependence, but fell below significant after controlling for lifetime drug abuse and/or dependence diagnoses. Each CD symptom present prior to age 15 was associated with an increase in the risk of engaging in aggressive behaviour towards others after controlling for current and past substance misuse (odds ratio 1.23, 1.09–1.40). We also undertook analyses with this sample to further investigate the role of psychotic symptoms in four 6-month periods when patients were living in the community. Symptoms were measured at the beginning of each 6-month period, and at the end of the period, both collateral informants and patients reported on aggressive behaviour that had occurred in the previous 6 months. We assessed positive and negative symptoms of psychosis, three paranoid symptoms, as well as depression and anxiety, and changes in levels of these symptoms. In regression models, we first entered the presence or absence of Antisocial Personality Disorder (APD; the adult diagnosis that requires the presence of CD prior to age 15), then current substance misuse measured both by self-reports and hair and urine analyses, and then the symptoms and changes in symptoms. In the final model, the risk of aggressive behaviour was increased 6 times by a diagnosis of APD and 1.5 times by the number of clinically relevant positive symptoms, by the change in the level of positive symptoms, and by the presence of anxiety (Hodgins, 2008).

Similar findings emerged from analyses of baseline data collected for a large trial of medications in the United States. Although this study used the same instrument to assess aggressive behaviour as did our studies, unlike the study mentioned in the preceding, symptoms were not measured prospectively but at the same time as the aggressive behaviour. More than two CD symptoms were found to be associated with aggressive behaviour in the previous 6 months after controlling for numerous confounders, and as in our studies, there was no association with substance misuse after taking account of childhood conduct problems. Whereas positive symptoms and depression were positively associated with life-threatening violence, negative symptoms were protective. A combination of above median scores for positive symptoms and below median scores for negative symptoms was associated with a threefold increase in risk of life-threatening violence (Swanson *et al.*, 2006).

Thus, the accumulated evidence indicates that CD is a precursor of schizophrenia in a minority of cases, it is more common among individuals who develop schizophrenia than in the general population, and among adults with schizophrenia, a diagnosis of CD and the number of CD symptoms present prior to age 15 are associated with violent behaviour through adulthood. Although some studies do show that positive symptoms are associated with aggressive behaviour even after taking account of CD, the existing evidence indicates that those with CD are not distinguished from other patients with schizophrenia by symptom profiles (Moran & Hodgins, 2004). Based on a comparison of the results of a small number of studies, the strength of the association between CD in childhood and violence in adulthood appears to be similar among individuals who develop schizophrenia (Hodgins *et al.*, 2005; Swanson *et al.*, 2006; Hodgins *et al.*, 2008) as it is among those who do not (Siminoff *et al.*, 2004; Loeber *et al.*, 2005). In addition, the number of CD symptoms prior to age 15 is linearly associated with the development of APD in adulthood among persons with schizophrenia, as it is in the general population (Robins *et al.*, 1991).

There is little prospective research on individuals who present conduct problems in childhood and who subsequently develop schizophrenia. The lack of prospectively collected data is not surprising given the challenge of identifying the very small number of individuals with conduct problems many years before they develop schizophrenia. An important finding has emerged from the prospective longitudinal investigation of a birth cohort in Dunedin, New Zealand. As previously noted, and consistent with other epidemiological evidence, the risk of violence was elevated among cohort members who developed schizophreniform disorder by age 26. This association was partially explained by the presence of both aggressive behaviour at ages 7, 9, and 11 and psychotic-like experiences at age 11 (Arseneault *et al.*, 2003). Most other relevant findings on the childhood characteristics of individuals with conduct problems who develop schizophrenia are derived from studies of clinical samples of adults in which data on childhood is collected retrospectively from multiple sources, some objective—school, social service, and juvenile justice records—and some subjective—reports from patients, parents, and older siblings. For example, in our sample of 248 men with schizophrenia, we compared those with and without CD prior to age 15. More of those with, than without, CD obtained lower than average marks in elementary school, failed to graduate from secondary school, and prior to age 18 abused substances, experienced physical abuse, and were institutionalized (Hodgins *et al.*, 2005). The results of other similar studies concur (Schanda *et al.*, 1992; Fulwiler *et al.*, 1997; Tengström *et al.*, 2001).

Several studies have reported that rates of mental illness among first-degree relatives did not differ for those with and without CD, whereas rates of criminality and substance misuse were elevated among fathers and brothers (Mueser *et al.*, 1999; Tengström *et al.*, 2001; Hodgins *et al.*, 2005; Hodgins *et al.*, 2008). Older studies had observed higher rates of criminality among the relatives of persons with schizophrenia compared with the general population. We had hypothesized that those with CD prior to illness onset had relatives who engaged in crime (Hodgins, Toupin, & Côté, 1996). Subsequent studies have shown that although greater proportions of parents and siblings of those with than without CD prior to illness onset acquired criminal convictions, the differences between the two groups are not always statistically significant. As there are no studies that compare individuals with childhood CD who do and do not develop schizophrenia, it is not possible to compare family liability in the two groups. It is known, however, that among children with CD those who go on to become persistent offenders are distinguished from the others by having more relatives who present externalizing disorders (Odgers *et al.*, 2007).

We and others (Joyal *et al.*, 2003; Stirling *et al.*, 2005) have proposed that among men with schizophrenia, those with early onset persistent antisocial behaviour display fewer brain abnormalities than those without a history of antisocial behaviour. This proposition is based on evidence from studies that compare violent and non-violent patients with schizophrenia, only a few of which distinguish early starters (for a review, see Naudts & Hodgins, 2006), and from studies that compare patients having schizophrenia with and without co-occurring substance misuse disorders (for a review, see Potvin *et al.*, 2008). Results suggest that among patients with schizophrenia, those who present an early onset stable pattern of antisocial behaviour perform better on tests tapping specific executive functions (Wisconsin Card-Sorting Test, Trail-Making Test, Wechsler Adult Intelligence Scale [WAIS], Trigram Test, Control Oral Word Association Test), more poorly on assessments of orbitofrontal functions, show fewer neurological soft signs, display larger reductions in volume of the amygdala, more structural abnormalities in the orbitofrontal system, and more abnormalities of white matter in the amygdala-orbitofrontal system, and smaller reductions of the hippocampus. Thus, early start offenders with schizophrenia may be distinguished by better executive functioning, higher verbal skills, and greater impulsivity than other men with schizophrenia. This evidence is, however, derived from studies that examined small, poorly characterized samples and that used definitions of violence and measures of brain function and structure that varied markedly. There is only one functional magnetic resonance imaging (fMRI) study that has examined men with schizophrenia and compared those with and without CD (Joyal *et al.*, 2007). The results of this investigation concur with the conclusions of the literature review in showing dysfunction in the orbital prefrontal cortex among those with prior CD. Dysfunction in this brain region has been associated with antisocial behaviour, and specifically with impaired inhibition, attention, and lower-order executive functions (Damasio, 2000). Thus, cognitive impairment—a core feature of schizophrenia that strongly impacts on psychosocial functioning—may distinguish individuals who display an early onset and stable pattern of antisocial behaviour from others with the illness.

We speculate that individuals with CD who are developing schizophrenia may be characterized by lower levels of anxiety, heart rate, and cortisol, similar to other children and adolescents with CD (Lorber, 2004; Susman, 2006; van Goozen *et al.*, 2007). Consequently, changes in brain function and structure resulting from the toxic effects of chronically elevated levels of cortisol and an overactive hypothalamic-pituitary-adrenal (HPA) axis would be less among those with, than without, CD. Consistent with this notion, one study recently reported that individuals with both schizophrenia spectrum disorders and APD (which requires CD prior to age 15) showed lower skin conductance orienting and arousal than individuals with only APD or only a schizophrenia spectrum disorder (Schug *et al.*, 2007).

Implications for the aetiology of schizophrenia and CD

The accumulated evidence suggests that among persons with schizophrenia, CD is directly associated with criminal offending and substance abuse that begins in adolescence and persists across the lifespan but not with the presentation of the illness. These findings may be interpreted to suggest that among persons with schizophrenia, CD is a distinct co-morbid disorder and not a consequence of abnormalities associated with the developing schizophrenia. Elevated rates of criminality and substance misuse among first-degree relatives would possibly suggest a distinct aetiology for CD. However, the robust finding that the prevalence of CD is higher among people who develop schizophrenia than in the general population indicates that there is a link between the two disorders.

Heritability estimates for schizophrenia are high, usually over 80% (Gottesman, 1993). Presently, it is thought that this brain disorder develops as a result of many genes, each of which confers vulnerability that is further enhanced by untoward events occurring during pregnancy, at birth, in early childhood, and at adolescence (Mueser & McGurk, 2004). We have developed hypotheses to guide future research aimed at furthering understanding of the aetiological processes leading to the development of individuals with CD in childhood and adolescence and schizophrenia in adulthood.

Hypothesis I: individuals at genetic risk of schizophrenia are at increased risk of exposure to environmental factors known to contribute to an early onset and stable pattern of antisocial behaviour

There is robust evidence showing that an early onset and stable pattern of antisocial behaviour is also hereditary, with estimates of heritability at about 50% (Kruger *et al.*, 2002; Moffitt, 2005). Behavioural-genetic studies concur in showing that both shared and non-shared environments contribute to antisocial behaviour, particularly in childhood (Kruger *et al.*, 2002; Moffitt, 2005). The non-genetic factors, both those that characterize families and parents and those that characterize children, associated with the development of persistent antisocial behaviour may be more common among children at genetic risk of schizophrenia and in their families than in the general population. Consider the first factors that are active during pregnancy and at birth. There is considerable evidence indicating that among people who develop schizophrenia, foetal neural development is disrupted in the first trimester, at the end of the second trimester, and at birth (Takei *et al.*, 1995; Lane *et al.*, 1997; Ismail *et al.*, 2000; Buka *et al.*, 2001; Cannon, Jones *et al.*, 2002). In studies of general population samples, obstetrical complications coupled with family problems (Hodgins *et al.*, 2001) and maternal smoking (Räsänen *et al.*, 1999; Maughan *et al.*, 2004) and drinking (d'Onofrio *et al.*, 2007) during pregnancy have been associated with conduct problems among the offspring. All of these factors are more common among people with schizophrenia than in the general population. Only one study, to our knowledge, has assessed the association between obstetrical complications and an early onset pattern of antisocial behaviour and violence among persons with schizophrenia. In a large birth cohort, complications in the neonatal period were found to be associated with an increased risk (odds ratio 2.79, 1.71–4.56) of violent criminal offending (Hodgins *et al.*, 2002).

Many studies have identified characteristics of families and parents that contribute to the initiation and maintenance of antisocial behaviour. These include socio-economic status of the family, mother's age, level of education and mental health, parenting practices, physical abuse of the child, family conflict, and changes in caregiver (Moffitt & Caspi, 2001); all of these have been associated with the development of schizophrenia (Jones *et al.*, 1994;

Tienari *et al.*, 1994; Cannon, Caspi *et al.*, 2002; Walker *et al.*, 2004; Read *et al.*, 2005; Morgan *et al.*, 2007). Further, studies have shown that both mothers and fathers who themselves display antisocial behaviour engage in parenting practices that contribute to conduct problems among their offspring (Lahey *et al.*, 1988; Frick *et al.*, 1992; Caspi *et al.*, 2004; Jaffee *et al.*, 2004). Largely because of the difficulty in identifying children who will later develop schizophrenia, there are almost no studies of parenting practices in this population. Thus, although highly speculative at this stage, we propose that individuals with CD prior to the onset of schizophrenia would experience insults in the prenatal and perinatal periods, resulting from maternal behaviour, poor attachment to parents, and poor parenting, especially inadequate and inappropriate supervision, harsh and inconsistent discipline, and a lack of appropriate models for coping with stress.

Hypothesis II: brain and neuroendocrine abnormalities present among children who are developing schizophrenia render them vulnerable for antisocial and aggressive behaviour

Adults with schizophrenia display both structural and functional brain abnormalities (Miyamoto *et al.*, 2003; Mueser & McGurk, 2004), some of which are observed at illness onset prior to the use of antipsychotic medication (Pantelis *et al.*, 2005). Post-mortem studies of brains of individuals with schizophrenia, studies of obstetrical complications, studies of the consequences of disturbances in utero such as minor physical anomalies, and neurocognitive assessments in childhood of individuals who subsequently developed schizophrenia suggest that brain abnormalities are present before illness onset (Rapoport *et al.*, 2005). In addition, recent evidence shows that the increase in symptoms of anxiety that precedes onset, in most cases, is reflected in an overreactive HPA axis as indicated by levels of cortisol and increased pituitary volumes (Garner *et al.*, 2005; Pariante *et al.*, 2005).

Individuals who present an early onset and stable pattern of antisocial behaviour are characterized by deficits in performance in neuropsychological tests and specific features of temperament and behaviour that are observed as early as 3 years of age (Moffitt & Caspi, 2001), and lower than average heart rate and cortisol levels (Moffitt & Caspi, 2001; Lorber, 2004; Loney *et al.*, 2006; Susman, 2006; van Goozen *et al.*, 2007). Children with conduct problems also present marked abnormalities in the recognition of emotions in the faces of others. For example, in one study, they reported neutral faces to be hostile, consistent with their behaviour that suggests they constantly feel threatened by others (Dadds *et al.*, 2006; Frick & Marsee, 2006). The small subgroup of children with CD who also present callous-unemotional traits fail to recognize fear in the faces and voices of others (Blair *et al.*, 2006).

In a sample of treatment-resistant patients with schizophrenia, a history of arrest was found to be associated with poor recognition of emotions, most particularly fearful faces, after adjusting for age, education, duration of illness, and symptom severity. The number of arrests for violent crimes was associated with the misinterpretation of faces as fear or sadness, whereas aggressive behaviour was associated with misinterpreting faces as angry (Weiss *et al.*, 2006). Adults with schizophrenia display deficits in the recognition of emotions in the faces of others (Schneider *et al.*, 2006), which are present at illness onset and in the prodromal phase (Addington *et al.*, 2008). Studies have also shown that the deficit characterizes many of their healthy siblings leading to the suggestion that it may signal the presence of one or more susceptibility genes for schizophrenia (Bediou *et al.*, 2007). If such a deficit were present in childhood, it might contribute to conduct problems. For example, the failure to recognize anger in the face of adults would deprive the child of information that their behaviour was inappropriate, the failure to recognize fear in others would be associated with a lack of empathy and understanding of others (Blair *et al.*, 2006), and a general failure to recognize emotions would be associated with problems with peers (d'Acremont & van der Linden, 2007).

Longitudinal prospective investigations suggest that children vulnerable for schizophrenia display motor delays, neurological signs, receptive language deficits, and lower than average IQ scores (Cannon, Caspi *et al.*, 2002; Cannon & Clarke, 2005; Laurens *et al.*, 2007). These characteristics may limit learning how not to be aggressive that occurs from toddlerhood through middle childhood (Broidy *et al.*, 2003).

Next steps

We hypothesize that there are two distinct developmental trajectories leading to schizophrenia. The most common pathway is characterized by emotional problems, usually anxiety, and a growing sensitivity to stress through adolescence. The second, less common, pathway is characterized by conduct problems and a reduced sensitivity to stress. In order to test this hypothesis, we wanted to identify children at risk of schizophrenia. Historically, this has always been done by identifying children with an affected relative, usually the parent. Such a strategy, however, is limited in that the majority of adults with schizophrenia do not have an affected relative (Gottesman, 1993). Consequently, we have attempted to develop a procedure for identifying at-risk children in the community. Based on a detailed review of the prospective investigations of children with an affected relative and of population cohorts that have identified the childhood characteristics of individuals who developed schizophrenia, we established a list of antecedents that had been replicated. We added to this list psychotic-like experiences that had been found by one prospective study to characterize 11-year-old children who subsequently developed schizophreniform disorder (Poulton *et al.*, 2000). We defined a triad of antecedents of schizophrenia to include (1) a caregiver report of motor and/or speech delay or abnormality, (2) a child report in the clinical range for internalizing problems on the Strengths and Difficulties Questionnaire (SDQ) or a caregiver report in the clinical range for externalizing and peer problems on the SDQ, and (3) a child report of at least one 'certain' psychotic-like experience.

Based on analyses of the first 548 children and caregivers screened, we found that 9.2% of the boys and 4.1% of the girls met the criteria for the triad of antecedents (Laurens *et al.*, 2007). Further, just as the prevalence of schizophrenia is elevated among persons of African-Caribbean heritage living in the UK, we found that the prevalence of the triad of antecedents was also significantly elevated among children of African-Caribbean heritage (Laurens *et al.*, 2008). Among the children who presented the triad of antecedents, there are distinct groups. Among the boys, 27.3% obtained scores within the clinical range of the SDQ for emotional problems but not for conduct problems, 36.4% obtained scores within the clinical range of the SDQ for conduct problems but not for emotional problems, 2.3% obtained scores within the clinical range of the SDQ for both emotional and conduct problems, and 34.1% obtained scores within the clinical range of the SDQ on another subscale, most commonly that assessing problems with peers; the comparable figures for the girls are 54.5%, 18.2%, 12.1%, and 15.2%, respectively. Until these children pass through the age of risk of schizophrenia, we will not know how many develop the illness.

We have now screened more than 4000 9-to-11 year olds, and the prevalence of the triad of antecedents remains stable. Presently, we are examining a sample of children who present the triad of antecedents, some of whom also have an affected relative and some who do not, children with an affected relative, and children who have neither the antecedents of schizophrenia nor an affected relative. The children and their caregivers complete a diagnostic interview, the caregiver provides information about the family and all caregivers, and the children complete neuropsychological tests, structural and functional brain imaging, and a session to measure Event-Related Potentials.

In addition, we are conducting further studies of adults with schizophrenia who have a history of CD in order to refine our understanding of their distinguishing features, including neurological soft signs, performance on neuropsychological tests, structural brain abnormalities, and response to antipsychotic medication.

Type II offenders with schizophrenia

Type II offenders with schizophrenia present no history of antisocial or aggressive behaviour prior to illness onset. Thereafter, they repeatedly engage in aggressive behaviour towards others. Such a pattern of aggressive behaviour that onsets in adulthood is very rare, as almost all persistently violent offenders have a long history of antisocial and aggressive behaviour stretching back into childhood (Loeber et al., 2005; Moffitt, 2006). When a pattern of aggressive behaviour onsets in adulthood, it is usually associated with some form of brain disorder (see for example, Hodgins et al., 1996). In the sample of 248 men with schizophrenia we recruited from forensic and general psychiatric hospitals, we compared the offenders who did not have a childhood history of antisocial behaviour—that is, our Types II and III—with those who did—our Type I. Those without antisocial behaviour prior to illness onset, compared with those with prior CD, included similar proportions with at least one conviction for a violent crime, but on average had acquired fewer convictions for violent crimes and fewer convictions for non-violent crimes. Importantly, however, a greater proportion of patients without antisocial behaviour prior to illness onset had been convicted for a homicide (23.9%) compared with patients with prior CD (10.4%) (X^2[N = 186] = 3.99, p = 0.046). As would be expected, patients with no history of antisocial behaviour prior to illness onset were significantly older at first conviction for a violent crime than were those with prior CD.

There are few studies of patients with schizophrenia, having no history of antisocial behaviour prior to illness onset, who repeatedly engage in aggressive behaviour towards others. Some evidence (Mueser et al., 1999, 2006) suggests that they may be particularly vulnerable to illicit drug use and that drug use may be directly associated with their violent behaviour. In the study described in the preceding, we found no differences in the prevalence of lifetime diagnoses of alcohol abuse and/or dependence or drug abuse and/or dependence among patients with and without antisocial behaviour prior to illness onset. Similarly, in our study of the UK inpatient sample, we found no difference in levels of substance misuse between those with and without CD prior to age 15; although half of the patients in this study presented a substance misuse problem, in the subsequent two years, only 3% of the men and 5% of the women received a treatment targeting this problem. Yet, there are effective treatments for substance misuse among persons with schizophrenia (Green et al., 2007). Drug use by patients with schizophrenia puts them at risk of violence in several different ways. With impaired social cognition, such patients make contact with antisocial offenders who congregate in high-crime areas with high levels of violence in order to purchase illicit drugs and use up their limited financial resources, which may subsequently impact on nutrition. The use of either alcohol or illicit drugs further contributes to limiting their psychosocial functioning generally and to increasing their cognitive impairments. It usually also limits their engagement with services and their compliance with medication. Further, the consequences of different substances on an already malfunctioning brain, and most specifically on the fragile dopaminergic and serotonergic systems, may lower the threshold for engaging in aggressive behaviour. Understanding of the links between substance misuse and violence among persons with schizophrenia with no history of antisocial behaviour prior to illness onset is a priority for future research.

Although substance use by persons with schizophrenia has attracted a great deal of attention, no studies to our knowledge have examined the links between the progressive brain changes that characterize the illness and aggressive behaviour. Further, studies have not been undertaken to understand if individual reactions to these brain changes, and/or to illness onset, are linked to violence. Patients with schizophrenia who repeatedly engage in aggressive behaviour in the absence of a prior history of such behaviour represent a distinct subgroup. Further research is needed to identify the processes leading to the aggressive behaviour and treatments to end it.

Type III Offenders with Schizophrenia
These are men in their late thirties with chronic schizophrenia and no history of antisocial or aggressive behaviour who kill, or try to kill, someone, often a caregiver. Among men with schizophrenia, the number of convictions for violent offences decreases with the age at first conviction (Hodgins, 2004). But, this is not true of homicide. Homicides are often committed by patients with schizophrenia who have no history of violence or antisocial behaviour (Beaudoin *et al.*, 1993; Erb *et al.*, 2001). We know of only one study that has examined this type of offender. It was based on the large amount of research showing that callousness is associated with aggressive behaviour. Using our sample of 248 men with schizophrenia, we found that clinical ratings of Deficient Affective Experience (shallow affect, callousness, lack of remorse, a failure to accept responsibility for one's own actions) were associated with violent offending and negative symptoms, but not with CD or substance misuse (Sunak, 2006). Similarly, in a study of persistently aggressive inpatients, three distinct groups were identified, one of which was characterized by a lack of remorse (Nolan *et al.*, 2003). We hypothesize that among patients with schizophrenia, Deficient Affective Experience may be a state that fluctuates as do psychotic symptoms and that when present increases the vulnerability for aggressive behaviour towards others.

Conclusion

The available evidence indicates that schizophrenia is associated with an increased risk of non-violent and violent crime and of aggressive behaviour towards others. Offenders with schizophrenia constitute a heterogeneous population. Developing a typology of offenders with schizophrenia that is relevant to aetiology and to treatment will provide a framework for investigating causal mechanisms and for studies of the effectiveness of treatment packages that address the characteristics of each type of offender.

Acknowledgements

The author would like to thank many collaborators from around the world who contributed to the studies reported in this chapter, and M. Rutter and J. Veverra who commented on earlier versions of the same, as well as the patients and families who gave generously of their time to provide the data.

The author acknowledges financial support from the European Union; agencies in Canada, Finland, Germany, and Sweden; the Trustees and R&D funds of the South London and Maudsley NHS Foundation Trust; and the Department of Health via the National Institute for Health Research (NIHR) Specialist Biomedical Research Centre for the Mental Health Award to South London and Maudsley NHS Foundation Trust (SLaM) and the Institute of Psychiatry at King's College London.

References

Addington, J., Penn, D., Woods, S. W., Addington, D., & Perkins, D. O. (2008). Facial affect recognition in individuals at clinical high risk for psychosis. *British Journal of Psychiatry, 192,* 67–68.

Alden, A., Brennan, P., Hodgins, S., & Mednick, S. (2007). Psychotic disorders and sex offending in a Danish birth cohort. *Archives of General Psychiatry, 64*(11), 1251–1258.

Appelbaum, P. S., Robbins, P. C., & Monahan, J. (2000). Violence and delusions: data from the MacArthur Violence Risk Assessment Study. *American Journal of Psychiatry, 157,* 566–572.

Arseneault, L., Cannon, M., Murray, R. Poulton, R., Caspi, A., & Moffitt, T. E. (2003). Childhood origins of violent behaviour in adults with schizophreniform disorder. *British Journal of Psychiatry, 183,* 520–525.

Arseneault, L., Moffitt, T. E., Caspi, A., Taylor, P. J., & Silva, P. A. (2000). Mental disorders and violence in a total birth cohort: results from the Dunedin Study. *Archives of General Psychiatry, 57*(10), 979–986.

Beaudoin, M. N., Hodgins, S., & Lavoie, F. (1993). Homicide, schizophrenia, and substance abuse or dependency. *Canadian Journal of Psychiatry, 38,* 541–546.

Bediou, B., Asri, F., Brunelin, J., Krolak-Salmon, P., D'amato, T., Saoud, M., *et al.* (2007). Emotion recognition and genetic vulnerability to schizophrenia. *British Journal of Psychiatry, 191,* 126–130.

Bernstein, D. P., Cohen, P., Skodol, A., Bezirganian, S., & Brook, J. S. (1996). Childhood antecedents of adolescent personality disorders. *American Journal of Psychiatry, 153,* 907–913.

Bjørkly, S. (2002a). Psychotic symptoms and violence towards others—a literature review of some preliminary findings: Part 1. *Delusions. Aggression and Violent Behavior, 7,* 617–631.

Bjørkly, S. (2002b). Psychotic symptoms and violence towards others—a literature review of some preliminary findings: Part 2. *Hallucinations. Aggression and Violent Behavior, 7,* 605–615.

Blair, R. J. R., Peschardt, K. S., Budhani, S., Mitchell, D. G. V., & Pine, D. S. (2006). The development of psychopathy. *Journal of Child Psychology and Psychiatry, 47*(3/4), 262–275.

Bowie, C. R., Reichenberg, A., Patterson, T. L., Heaton, R. K., & Harvey, P. D. (2006). Determinants of real-world functional performance in schizophrenia subjects: correlations with cognition, functional capacity, and symptoms. *American Journal of Psychiatry, 163*(3), 418–425.

Brennan, P., Mednick, S. A., & Hodgins, S. (2000). Major mental disorders and criminal violence in a Danish birth cohort. *Archives of General Psychiatry, 57,* 494–500.

Broidy, L. M., Tremblay, R. E., Brame, B., Fergusson, D., Horwood, J. L., Moffitt, T. E., *et al.* (2003). Developmental trajectories of childhood disruptive behaviors and adolescent delinquency: a six-site, cross-national study. *Developmental Psychology, 39*(2), 222–245.

Buka, S. L., Tsuang, M. T., Torrey, E. F., Klebanoff, M. A., Bernstein, D., & Yolken, R. H. (2001). Maternal infections and subsequent psychosis among offspring. *Archives of General Psychiatry, 58,* 1032–1037.

Cannon, M., Caspi, A., Moffitt, T. E., Harrington, H., Taylor, A., Murray, R. M., *et al.* (2002). Evidence for early-childhood, pan-developmental impairment: specific to Schizophreniform Disorder. *Archives of General Psychiatry, 59,* 449–456.

Cannon, M., & Clarke, M. C. (2005). Risk for schizophrenia—broadening the concepts, pushing back the boundaries. *Schizophrenia Research, 79*(1), 5–13.

Cannon, M., Jones, P. B., & Murray, R. M. (2002). Obstetric complications and schizophrenia: historical and meta-analytic review. *American Journal of Psychiatry, 159*(7), 1080–1092.

Caspi, A., Moffitt, T. E., Morgan, J., Rutter, M., Taylor, A., Arsenault, L., *et al.* (2004). Maternal expressed emotion predicts children's anti-social behaviour problems: using monozygotic-twin differences to identify environmental effects on behavioural development. *Developmental Psychology*, 40(2), 149–161.

Clark, T., & Rowe, R. (2006). Violence, stigma and psychiatric diagnosis: the effects of a history of violence on psychiatric diagnosis. *Psychiatric Bulletin*, 30, 254–256.

Crisp, A., Gelder, M., Goddard, E., & Meltzer, H. (2005). Stigmatisation of people with mental illnesses: a follow-up study wihtin the Changing Minds Campaign of the Royal college of Psychiatrists. *World Psychiatry*, 4(2), 106–113.

Crocker, A. G., Mueser, K. T., Drake, R. E., Clark, R. E., McHugo, G. J., Ackerson, T. H., *et al.* (2005). Antisocial personality, psychopathy, and violence in persons with dual disorders. *Criminal Justice and Behavior*, 32(4), 452–476.

D'Acremont, M., & van der Linden, M. (2007). Memory for angry faces, impulsivity, and problematic behavior in adolescence. *Journal of Abnormal Child Psychology*, 35(2), 313–324.

D'Onofrio, B. M., van Hulle, C. A., Waldman, I. D., Rodgers, J. L., Rathouz, P. J., & Lahey, B. B. (2007). Casual inferences regarding prenatal alcohol exposure and childhood externalizing problems. *Archives of General Psychiatry*, 64(III), 1296–1304.

Dadds, M. R., Perry, Y., Hawes, D. J., Merz, S., Riddell, A. C., Haines, D. J., *et al.* (2006). Attention to the eyes reverses fear-recognition deficits in child psychopathy. *British Journal of Psychiatry*, 189, 280–281.

Damasio, A. R. (2000). A neural basis for sociopathy. *Archives of General Psychiatry*, 57(2), 128–129.

Davies, N. (2004a). Scandal of society's misfits dumped in jail. *The Guardian*, 6 Dec.

Davies, N. (2004b). Trapped in a cycle of self-harm and despair for want of a psychiatric bed. *The Guardian*, 7 Dec.

Davies, N. (2004c). Wasted lives of the young let down by jail system. *The Guardian*, 8 Dec.

Dean, K., Walsh, E., Moran, P., Tyler, P., Creed, F., Byford, S., *et al.* (2006). Violence in women with psychosis in the community: prospective study. *British Journal of Psychiatry*, 188, 264–270.

Erb, M., Hodgins, S., Freese, R., Müller-Isberner, R., & Jöckel, D. (2001). Homicide and schizophrenia: maybe treatment does have a preventive effect. *Criminal Behaviour and Mental Health*, 11(1), 6–26.

Fazel, S., & Danesh, J. (2002). Serious mental disorder in 23000 prisoners: a systematic review of 62 surveys. *Lancet*, 259, 545–550.

Ferdinand, R. F., & Verhulst, F. C. (1995). Psychopathology from adolescence into young adulthood: an 8-year follow- up study *American Journal of Psychiatry*, 152, 1586–1594.

Frick, P. J., Lahey, B. B., Loeber, R., Stouthamer-Loeber, M., Christ, M. A. G., & Hanson, K. (1992). Familial risk factors to oppositional defiant disorder and conduct disorder: parental psychopathology and maternal parenting. *Journal of Consulting and Clinical Psychology*, 60(1), 49–55.

Frick, P. J., & Marsee, M. A. (2006). Psychopathy and developmental pathways to antisocial behavior in youth. In C. J. Patrick (ed), *Handbook of Psychopathy* (pp. 353–374). New York: Guilford Press.

Fulwiler, C., Grossman, H., Forbes, C., & Ruthazer, R. (1997). Early-onset substance abuse and community violence by outpatients with chronic mental illness. *Psychiatric Services*, 48, 1181–1185.

Fulwiler, C., & Ruthazer, R. (1999). Premorbid risk factors for violence in adult mental illness. *Comprehensive Psychiatry*, 40(2), 96–100.

Garner, B., Pariante, C. M., Wood, S. J., Velakoulis, D., Philips, L., Soulsby, B., *et al.* (2005). Pituitary volume predicts future transition to psychosis in individuals at ultra-high risk of developing psychosis. *Biological Psychiatry*, 58, 417–423.

Gosden, N. P., Kramp, P., Gabrielsen, G., Andersen, T. F., & Sestoft, D (2005). Violence of young criminals predicts schizophrenia: a 9-year register-based follow-up of 15- to 19-year-old criminals. *Schizophrenia Bulletin*, 31(3), 759–768.

Gottesman, I. I. (1993). Origins of schizophrenia: past as prologue. In R. Plomin, & G. E. McClean (eds), *Nature, Nuture and Psychology* (pp. 231–244). Washington, DC: American Psychological Association.

Green, A. I., Drake, R. E., Brunette, M. F., & Noordsy, D. L. (2007) Schizophrenia and co-occurring substance use disorder. *American Journal of Psychiatry*, 164, 402–408.

Green, E. K., Raybould, R., MacGregor, S., Gordon-Smith, K., Heron, J., Hyde, S., *et al.* (2005). Operation of the schizophrenia susceptibility gene, neuregulin 1, across traditional diagnostic boundaries to increase risk for bipolar disorder. *Archives of General Psychiatry, 62*, 642–648.

Green, H., McGinnity, A., Meltzer, H., Ford, T., & Goodman, R. (2004). Mental health of children and young people in Great Britain 2004. London: Office for National Statistics.

Hodgins, S. (1992). Mental disorder, intellectual deficiency and crime: evidence from a birth cohort. *Archives of General Psychiatry, 49*, 476–483.

Hodgins, S. (1998). Epidemiological investigations of the associations between major mental disorders and crime: methodological limitations and validity of the conclusions. *Social Psychiatry and Psychiatric Epidemiology, 33*(1), 9–37.

Hodgins, S. (2004). Criminal and antisocial behaviours and schizophrenia: a neglected topic. In W. F. Gattaz, & H. Häfner (eds), *Search for the Causes of Schizophrenia, Vol V* (pp. 315–341). Darmstadt, Germany: Steinkopff Verlag.

Hodgins, S. (2008). Criminality among persons with severe mental illness. In K. Soothill, M. Dolan, & P. Rogers (eds), *Handbook of Forensic Mental Health (chapter 16)*. Devon, UK: Willan Publishing.

Hodgins, S., Alderton, J., Cree, A., Aboud, A., & Mak, T. (2007). Aggressive behaviour, victimisation, and crime among severely mentally ill patients requiring hospitalisation. *British Journal of Psychiatry, 191*, 343–350.

Hodgins, S., & Côté, G. (1993). Major mental disorder and APD: a criminal combination. *Bulletin of the American Academy of Psychiatry and the Law, 21*, 155–160.

Hodgins, S., Côté, G., & Toupin, J. (1998). Major mental disorders and crime: an etiological hypothesis. In D. Cooke, A. Forth, & R. D. Hare (eds), *Psychopathy: Theory, Research and Implications for Society* (pp. 231–256). Dordrecht, the Netherlands: Kluwer Academic Publishers.

Hodgins, S., Cree, A., Alderton, J., & Mak, T. (2008). From conduct disorder to severe mental illness: associations with aggressive behaviour, crime and victimization. *Psychological Medicine, 38*, 975–987.

Hodgins, S., Hiscoke, U. L., & Freese, R. (2003). The antecedents of aggressive behavior among men with schizophrenia: a prospective investigation of patients in community treatment. *Behavioral Sciences and the Law, 21*, 523–546.

Hodgins, S., & Janson, C. G. (2002). *Criminality and Violence among the Mentally Disordered: The Stockholm Metropolitan Project*. Cambridge University Press.

Hodgins, S., Kratzer, L., & McNeil, T. D. (2001). Obstetric complications, parenting, and risk of criminal behavior. *Archives of General Psychiatry, 58*, 746–752.

Hodgins, S., Kratzer, L., & McNeil, T. F. (2002). Obstetrical complications, parenting practices and risk of criminal behavior among persons who develop major mental disorders. *Acta Psychiatrica Scandinavica, 105*, 179–188.

Hodgins, S., Larsson, G., & Larm, P. (in preparation). Developing schizophrenia among adolescents with substance misuse problems.

Hodgins, S., Lincoln, T., & Mak, T. (in press). Functional outcome in schizophrenia: a novel definition and predictors. *Social Psychiatry and Psychiatric Epidemiology*.

Hodgins, S., Mednick, S. A., Brennan, P., Schulsinger, F., & Engberg, M. (1996). Mental disorder and crime: evidence from a Danish birth cohort. *Archives of General Psychiatry, 53*, 489–496.

Hodgins, S., & Müller-Isberner, R. (2004). Preventing crime by people with schizophrenic disorders: the role of psychiatric services. *British Journal of Psychiatry, 185*, 245–250.

Hodgins, S., Tiihonen, J., & Ross, D. (2005). The consequences of Conduct Disorder for males who develop schizophrenia: associations with criminality, aggressive behavior, substance use, and psychiatric services. *Schizophrenia Research, 78*, 323–335.

Hodgins, S., Toupin, J., & Côté, G. (1996). Schizophrenia and antisocial personality disorder: a criminal combination. In L. B. Schlesinger (ed), *Explorations in Criminal Psychopathology* (pp. 217–237). Springfield, IL: Charles C. Thomas Publisher.

Ismail, B., Cantor-Graae, E., & McNeil, T. (2000). Minor physical anomalies in schizophrenia: cognitive, neurological, and other clinical correlates. *Journal of Psychiatric Research, 34*, 45–56.

Jaffee, S. R., Caspi, A., Moffitt, T. E., & Taylor, A. (2004). Physical maltreatment victim to antisocial child: evidence of an environmentally mediated process. *Journal of Abnormal Psychology, 113*(1), 44–55.

Jones, P., Rodgers, B., Murray, R., & Marmot, M. (1994). Child developmental risk factors for adult schizophrenia in the British 1946 birth cohort. *Lancet, 344,* 1398–1401.

Joyal, C., Hallé, P., Hodgins, S., & Lapierre, D. (2003). Letter to the Editor: drug abuse and/or dependence and better neuropsychological performance in patients with schizophrenia. *Schizophrenia Research, 63*(3), 297–299.

Joyal, C. C., Putkonen, A., Mancini-Marïe, A., Hodgins, S., Kononen, M., Boulay, L., *et al.* (2007). Violent persons with schizophrenia and comorbid disorders: a functional magnetic resonance imaging study. *Schizophrenia Research, 91,* 97–102.

Kim-Cohen, J., Caspi, A., Moffitt, T. E., Harrington, H. L., Milne, B. J., & Poulton, R. (2003) Prior juvenile diagnoses in adults with mental disorder: developmental follow-back of a prospective longitudinal cohort. *Archives of General Psychiatry, 60,* 709–717.

Krakowski, M., & Czobor, P. (2004). Gender differences in violent behaviours: relationship to clinical symptoms and psychosocial factors. *American Journal of Psychiatry, 161*(3), 459–465.

Kruger, R. F., Hicks, B. M., Patrick, C. J., Carlson, S. R., Iacono, W. G., & McGue, M. (2002). Etiologic connections among substance dependence, antisocial behavior, and personality: modeling the externalizing spectrum. *Journal of Abnormal Psychology, 111*(3), 411–424.

Lahey, B. B., Piacentini, J. C., McBurnett, K., Stone, P., Hartidagen, S., & Hynd, G. (1988). Psychopathology in the parents of children with conduct disorder and hyperactivity. *American Academy of Child and Adolescent Psychiatry, 27*(2), 163–170.

Lane, A., Kinsella, A., Murphy, P., Byrne, M., Keenan, J., Colgan, K., *et al.* (1997). The anthropometric assessment of dysmorphic features in schizophrenia as an index of its developmental origins. *Psychological Medicine, 27*(5), 1155–1164.

Laurens, K. R., Hodgins, S., Maughan, B., Murray, R. M., Rutter, M. L., & Taylor, E. A. (2007). Community screening for psychotic-like experiences and other putative antecedents of schizophrenia in children aged 9–12 years. *Schizophrenia Research, 90,* 130–146.

Laurens, K. R., West, S. A., Murray, R. M., & Hodgins, S. (2008). Psychotic-like experiences and other antecedents of schizophrenia in children aged 9-12 years: a comparison of ethnic and migrant groups in the United Kingdom. *Psychological Medicine, 38*(8), 1103–1111.

Link, B. G., Cullen, F. T., Frank, J., & Wozniak, J. F. (1987). The social rejection of former mental patients: Understanding why labels matter. *American Journal of Sociology, 92,* 1461–1500.

Link, B. G., & Pelham, J. C. (2006). Stigma and its public health implications. *Lancet, 367*(9509), 528–529.

Loeber, R., Pardini, D., Homish, D., Wei, E., Crawford, A., Farrington, D., *et al.* (2005). The prediction of violence and homicide in young men. *Journal of Consulting and Clinical Psychology, 73* (6), 1074–1088.

Loney, B. R., Butler, M. A., Lima, E. N., Counts, C. A., & Eckel, L.A. (2006). The relation between salivary cortisol, callous-unemotional traits, and conduct problems in an adolescent non-referred sample. *Journal of Child Psychology and Psychiatry, 47*(1), 30–36.

Lorber, M. F. (2004). Psychophysiology of aggression, psychopathy, and conduct problems: a meta-analysis. *Psychological Bulletin, 130*(4), 531–552.

Maughan, B., Taylor, A., Caspi, A., & Moffitt, T. E. (2004). Parental smoking and early childhood conduct problems: testing genetic and environmental explanations of the association. *Archives of General Psychiatry, 61,* 836–843.

McCabe, J. H., Lambe, M. P., Cnattingius, S., Torrång, A., Björk, C., Sham, P. C., etal. (2008). Scholastic achievement at age 16 and risk of schizophrenia and other psychoses: a national cohort study. *Psychological Medicine, 38*(8), 1133–1140.

Miyamoto, S., LaMantia, A. S., Duncan, G. E., Sullivan, P., Gilmore, J. H., & Lieberman, J. A. (2003). Recent advances in the neurobiology of schizophrenia. *Molecular Interventions, 3,* 27–39.

Moffitt, T. E. (2005). Genetic and environmental influences on antisocial behaviors: evidence from behavioral-genetic research. *Advances in Genetics, 55,* 41–104.

Moffitt, T. E. (2006). Life-course-persistent versus adolescence-limited antisocial behaviour. In D. Cicchetti, & D. Cohen (eds), *Developmental Psychopathology, Vol 3: Risk, Disorder, and Adaptation*, 2nd edn (pp. 570–598). Hoboken, NJ: John Wiley & Sons, Inc.

Moffitt, T. E., & Caspi, A. (2001). Childhood predictors differentiate life-course persistent and adolescence-limited antisocial pathways among males and females. *Development and Psychopathology, 13*(2), 355–375.

Mojtabai, R. (2006). Psychotic-like experiences and interpersonal violence in the general population. *Social Psychiatry and Psychiatric Epidemiology, 40,* 1–8.

Moran, P., & Hodgins, S. (2004). The correlates of co-morbid antisocial personality disorder in schizophrenia. *Schizophrenia Bulletin, 30*(4), 791–802.

Morgan, C., Kirkbride, J., Leff, J., Craig, T., Hutchinson, G., McKenzie, K., *et al.* (2007). Parental separation, loss and psychosis in different ethnic groups: a case-control study. *Psychological Medicine, 37,* 495–503.

Mueser, K. T., & McGurk, S. R. (2004). Schizophrenia. *Lancet, 363,* 2063–2072.

Mueser, K. T., Crocker, A. G., Frisman, L. B., Drake, R. E., Covell, N. H., & Essock, S.M. (2006). Conduct disorder and antisocial personality disorder in persons with severe psychiatric and substance use disorders. *Schizophrenia Bulletin, 32*(4), 626–636.

Mueser, K. T., Rosenberg, S. D., Drake, R. E., Miles, K. M., Wolford, G., Vidaver, R., *et al.* (1999). Conduct disorder, antisocial personality disorder and substance use disorders in schizophrenia and major affective disorders. *Journal of Studies on Alcohol, 60,* 278–284.

Naudts, K. H., & Hodgins, S. (2006). Schizophrenia and violence. *A search for neurobiological correlates. Current Opinion in Psychiatry, 19,* 533–538.

Nock, M. K., Kazdin, A. E., Hiripi, E., & Kessler, R. C. (2006). Prevalence, subtypes, and correlates of DSM-IV conduct disorder in the National Comorbidity Survey Replication. *Psychological Medicine, 36*(5), 699–710.

Nolan, K. A., Czobor, P., Roy, B. B., Platt, M. M., Shope, C. B., Citrome, L. L., *et al.* (2003). Characteristics of assaultive behavior among psychiatric inpatients. *Psychiatric Services, 54*(7), 1012–1016.

Odgers, C. L., Milne, B. J., Caspi, A., Crump, R., Poulton, R., & Moffitt, T. E. (2007). Predicting prognosis for the conduct-problem boy: can family history help? *Journal of the American Academy of Child and Adolescent Psychiatry, 46*(10), 1240–1249.

Pantelis, C., Yücel, M., Wood, S. J., Velakoulis, D., Sun, D., Berger, G., *et al.* (2005). Structural brain imaging evidence for multiple pathological processes at different stages of brain development in schizophrenia. *Schizophrenia Bulletin, 31*(3), 672–696.

Pariante, C. M., Dazzan, P., Danese, A., Morgan, K. D., Brudagli, F., Morgan, C., *et al.* (2005). Increased pituitary volume in antipsychotic-free and antipsychotic-treated patients of the AESOP First-Onset Psychosis Study. *Neuropsychopharmacology, 30,* 1923–1931.

Potvin, S., Joyal, C. C., Pelletier, J., & Stip, E. (2008). Contradictory cognitive capacities among substance-abusing patients with schizophrenia: a meta-analysis. *Schizophrenia Research, 100,* 242–251.

Poulton, R., Caspi, A., Moffitt, T. E., Cannon, M., Murray, R., & Harrington, H. L. (2000). Children's self-reported psychotic symptoms and adult schizophreniform disorder: a 15-year longitudinal study. *Archives of General Psychiatry, 57*(11), 1053–1058.

Priebe, S., Badesconyi, A., Fioritti, A., Hansson, L., Kilian, R., Torres-Gonzales, F., *et al.* (2005). Reinstitutionalisation in mental health care: comparison of data on service provision from six European countries. *British Medical Journal, 330,* 123–126.

Rapoport, J. C., Addington, A. M., & Frangou, S. (2005). The neurodevelopmental model of schizophrenia: update 2005. *Molecular Psychiatry, 10,* 439–449.

Räsänen, P., Hakko, H., Isohanni, M., Hodgins, S., Järvelin, M-R., & Tiihonen, J. (1999). Maternal smoking during pregnancy and risk of criminal behavior in the Northern Finland 1966 birth cohort. *American Journal of Psychiatry, 156*(6), 857–862.

Read, J., van Os, J., Morrison, A. P., & Ross, C. A. (2005). Childhood trauma, psychosis and schizophrenia: a literature review with theoretical and clinical implications. *Acta Psychiatrica Scandinavica, 112,* 330–350.

Rice, M. E., & Harris, G. T. (1995). Psychopathy, schizophrenia, alcohol abuse, and violent recidivism. *International Journal of Law and Psychiatry*, *18*, 333–342.

Robins, L. (1966). *Deviant Children Grown Up*. Baltimore, MD: Williams and Wilkins.

Robins, L. N. (1993). Childhood conduct problems, adult psychopathology, and crime. In S. Hodgins (ed), *Mental Disorder and Crime* (pp. 173–207). Newbury Park, CA: Sage Publications, Inc.

Robins, L. N., Tipp, J., & Przybeck, T. (1991). Antisocial personality. In L. N. Robins, & D. Regier (eds), *Psychiatric disorders in America: The Epidemiologic Catchment Area Study* (pp. 258–290). New York: Macmillan/Free Press.

Schanda, H., Fs, P., Topitz, A., Fliedl, R., & Knecht, G. (1992). Premorbid adjustment of schizophrenic criminal offenders. *Acta Psychiatrica Scandinavica*, *86*, 121–126.

Schneider, F., Gur, R. C., Koch, K., Backes, V., Amunts, K., Shah, J., *et al.* (2006). Impairment in the specificity of emotion processing in schizophrenia. *American Journal of Psychiatry*, *163*, 442–447.

Schug, R. A., Raine, A., & Wilcox, R. R. (2007). Psychophysiological and behavioural characteristics of individuals comorbid for antisocial personality disorder and schizophrenia-spectrum personality disorder. *British Journal of Psychiatry*, *191*, 408–414.

Silver, E., Arseneault, L., Langley, J., Caspi, A., & Moffitt, T. E. (2005). Mental disorder and violent victimization in a total birth cohort. *American Journal of Public Health*, *95*, 2015–2021.

Siminoff, E., Elander, J., Holmshaw, J., Pickles, A., Murray, R., & Rutter, M. (2004). Predictors of antisocial personality. *Continuities from childhood to adult life*. *British Journal of Psychiatry*, *184*, 118–127.

Steadman, H. J., Mulvey, E. P., Monahan, J., Robbins, P. C., Applebaum, P. S., Grisso, T., *et al.* (1998). Violence by people discharged from acute psychiatric inpatient facilities and by others in the same neighborhoods. *Archives of General Psychiatry*, *55*, 393–401.

Stefanis, N. C., Hanssen, M., Smirnis, N. K., Avramopoulos, D. A., Evdokimidis, I. K., Stefanis, C. N., *et al.* (2002). Evidence that three dimensions of psychosis have a distribution in the general population. *Psychological Medicine*, *32*, 347–358.

Steinert, T. (2002). Prediction of inpatient violence. *Acta Psychiatrica Scandinavica*, *106*, 133–141.

Stirling, J., Lewis, S., Hopkins, R., & White, C. (2005). Cannabis use prior to first onset psychosis predicts spared neurocognition at 10-year follow-up. *Schizophrenia Research*, *75*, 135–137.

Sunak, S. (2006). Deficient effective experience and violence in schizophrenia. M.Sc. thesis, Department of Forensic Mental Health Science, Institute of Psychiatry, King's College London.

Susman, E. J. (2006). Psychobiology of persistent antisocial behavior: stress, early vulnerabilities and the attenuation hypothesis. *Neuroscience and Biobehavioral Review*, *30*, 376–389.

Swanson, J. W., Swartz, M. S., van Dorn, R. A., Elbogen, E. B., Wagner, H. R., Rosenbeck, R. A., *et al.* (2006). A national study of violent behavior in persons with schizophrenia. *Archives of General Psychiatry*, *63*(5), 490–499.

Takei, N., Sham, P. C., O'Callaghan, E. O., Glover, G., & Murray, R. M. (1995). Early risk factors in schizophrenia: place and season of birth. *European Psychiatry*, *10*, 165–170.

Tengström, A., Hodgins, S., Grann, M., Långström, N., & Kullgren, G. (2004). Schizophrenia and criminal offending: the role of psychopathy and substance misuse. *Criminal Justice and Behavior*, *31*(4), 1–25.

Tengström, A., Hodgins, S., & Kullgren, G. (2001). Men with schizophrenia who behave violently: the usefulness of an early versus late starters typology. *Schizophrenia Bulletin*, *27*, 205–218.

Teplin, L., McClelland, G. M., Abram, K. M., & Weiner, D. A. (2005). Crime victimization in adults with severe mental illness: comparison with the National Crime Victimization Survey. *Archives of General Psychiatry*, *62*, 911–921.

Tienari, P., Wynne, L. C., Moring, J., Lahti, I., Naarala, M., Sorri, A., *et al.* (1994). The Finnish adoptive family study of schizophrenia. *Implications for family research. British Journal of Psychiatry*, *164*(suppl 23), 20–26.

Tiihonen, J., Isohanni, M., Rasanen, P., Koiranen, M., & Moring, J. (1997). Specific major mental disorders and criminality: a 26-year prospective study of the 1996 Northern Finland birth cohort. *American Journal of Psychiatry*, *154*(6), 840–845.

Toulopoulou, T., Picchioni, M., Rijsdijk, F., Hua-Hall, M., Ettinger, U., Sham, P., et al. (2007). Substantial genetic overlap between neurocognition and schizophrenia: genetic modeling in twin samples. *Archives of General Psychiatry, 64*, 1348–1355.

Van Goozen, S. J. M., Fairchild, G., Snoek, H., & Harold, G. T. (2007). The evidence for a neurobiological model of childhood antisocial behaviour. *Psychological Bulletin, 133*(1), 149–182.

Walker, E., Kestler, L., Bollini, A., & Hochman, K. M. (2004). Schizophrenia: etiology and course. *Annual Review of Psychology, 55*, 401–430.

Wallace, C., Mullen, P. E., & Burgess, P. (2004). Criminal offending in schizophrenia over a 25-year period marked by deinstitutionalization and increasing prevalence of comorbid substance use disorders. *American Journal of Psychiatry, 161*(4), 716–727.

Walsh, E., & Fahy, T. (2002). Violence in society. *British Medical Journal, 325*, 507–508.

Walsh, E., Gilvarry, C., Samele, C., Harvey, K., Manley, C., Tyrer, P., et al. (2001). Reducing violence in severe mental illness: randomized controlled trial of intensive case management compared with standard care. *British Medical Journal, 323*(10), 1093–1097.

Walsh, E., Moran, P., Scott, C., McKenzie, K., Burns, T., Creed, F., et al. (2003). UK700 Group. Prevalence of violent victimisation in severe mental illness. *British Journal of Psychiatry, 183*, 233–238.

Weiss, E. M., Kohler, C. G., Nolan, K. A., Czobor, P., Volavka, J., Platt, M. M., et al. (2006). The relationship between history of violent and criminal behavior and recognition of facial expression of emotions in men with schizophrenia and schizoaffective disorder. *Aggressive Behaviour, 32*, 187–194.

Wolff, N., Litz, C., & Shi, J. (2007). Rates of sexual victimization in prison for inmates with and without mental disorders. *Psychiatric Services, 58*, 1087–1094.

4

The use of callous-unemotional traits to define important subtypes of antisocial and violent youth

Paul J. Frick and Amelie Petitclerc

Introduction

Research has consistently indicated that serious and violent adult offenders often show histories of antisocial and aggressive behaviour dating back to early childhood (Marshall & Cooke, 1999). Similarly, within juvenile samples, serious and violent offenders often show a history of conduct problems that pre-date their illegal acts (Vermeiren, 2003). Thus, understanding serious and violent offending is intertwined with understanding broader patterns of antisocial and aggressive behaviour in children and adolescents. Given their link to violence, it is not surprising that there is rather extensive research literature investigating the development, assessment, prevention, and treatment of serious of conduct problems in youth (Loeber & Farrington, 2000; Raine, 2002; Dodge & Pettit, 2003; Vermeiren, 2003; Frick, 2006).

This research has resulted in a long list of factors that can place a child at risk of acting in an antisocial and aggressive manner. They include dispositional risk factors such as neurochemical (e.g., low serotonin) and autonomic (e.g., low resting heart rate) irregularities, neurocognitive deficits (e.g., deficits in executive functioning), deficits in the processing of social information (e.g., a hostile attributional bias), temperamental vulnerabilities (e.g., poor emotional regulation), and personality predispositions (e.g., impulsivity). In addition, there are at least as many contextual risks including factors in the child's prenatal (e.g., exposure to toxins), early child care (e.g., poor quality child care), family (e.g., ineffective discipline), peer (e.g., association with deviant peers), and neighbourhood (e.g., high levels of exposure to violence) environments.

Although research has been very successful in documenting these many and diverse risk factors, it has led to great debate over the best way to integrate these factors into comprehensive causal models to explain the development of antisocial behaviour. There are a few points of agreement, however. First, it is clear that for any model to explain the development of aggressive and antisocial behaviour, it must consider the potential role of multiple risk factors. For example, Stouthamer-Loeber *et al.* (2002) reported that, in a high-risk sample of urban youth, the number of risk factors showed a linear association with risk of serious and persistent delinquency. Second, it is now generally accepted that causal models must consider the possibility that subgroups of antisocial youth may have very different patterns of behavioural problems and distinct causal mechanisms underlying their antisocial and aggressive behaviours (Moffitt, 2003; Frick, 2006). Third, it is becoming increasingly clear that causal models need to integrate research on the development of antisocial and aggressive behaviour with research on normally developing youth. For example, research has suggested that the ability to adequately regulate emotion and behaviour and the ability to feel empathy and guilt towards others seem to play a role in the development of severe conduct problems in youth (Frick & Morris, 2004). As a result, understanding the processes involved in the normal development of these abilities can also be critical for understanding how they may go awry in some youth and place them at risk of acting in an aggressive or antisocial manner. Such an approach, which underlies the developmental psychopathology perspective (Rutter & Sroufe, 2000), could also be critical for advancing interventions focusing on preventing antisocial behaviour by enhancing child development prior to the onset of behavioural problems.

One notable example of a causal model that has integrated these important considerations is the distinction that has been made between a childhood and an adolescence onset to severe conduct problems. A number of reviews have summarized research supporting the distinction between children who begin showing severe conduct problems in childhood versus those whose onset of severe antisocial behaviour coincides with the onset of puberty (Patterson, 1996; Moffitt, 2003). In addition to the different patterns of onset, the childhood-onset group is more likely to show aggressive behaviours in childhood and adolescence and is also more likely to continue to show antisocial and criminal behaviour into adulthood (Moffitt et al., 2002). Further, this group seems to show greater levels of both dispositional (e.g., temperamental risk, low intelligence) and contextual (e.g., family dysfunction, poverty) risk compared to the adolescent-onset group. The adolescence-onset group seems to be deviant largely by showing more affiliation with delinquent peers and higher levels of rebelliousness and authority conflict (Moffitt, 2003).

Based on these findings, there have been several theories offered as to how these groups may differ on the developmental mechanisms underlying their behavioural disturbance. For example, Moffitt (1993, 2003) proposed that children in the childhood-onset group develop their problem behaviour through a transactional process involving a difficult and vulnerable child (e.g., impulsive, with verbal deficits) who experiences an inadequate rearing environment (e.g., poor parental supervision, poor-quality schools). This dysfunctional transactional process disrupts the child's socialization leading to poor social relations with persons both inside (e.g., parents and siblings) and outside the family (e.g., peers and teachers). These disruptions lead to enduring vulnerabilities that can negatively affect the child's psychosocial adjustment across multiple developmental stages. In contrast, children in the adolescence-onset group are viewed as engaging in antisocial and delinquent behaviours as a misguided attempt to obtain a subjective sense of maturity and adult status in a way that is maladaptive (e.g., breaking societal norms) but encouraged by an antisocial peer group. Given that their behaviour is viewed as an exaggeration of a process specific to adolescence, and not due to an enduring vulnerability, their antisocial behaviour is less likely to persist beyond adolescence. However, they may still have impairments that persist into adulthood due to the consequences of their adolescent antisocial behaviour (e.g., a criminal record, dropping out of school, substance abuse).

Although the distinction between childhood-onset and adolescence-onset trajectories has been very useful for explaining two separate pathways through which children may develop severe aggressive and antisocial behaviour, it is important to note that clear differences in risk factors between the two groups have not always been found (Lahey et al., 2000), and the applicability of this model to girls requires further testing (Silverthorn & Frick, 1999). More importantly, research has begun extending this conceptualization by exploring whether additional distinctions could be made. There is growing evidence to suggest that an important distinction can be made within the childhood-onset group, based on the presence of a callous and unemotional (CU) affective style. This distinction is similar to the distinction made within samples of antisocial adults using the construct of psychopathy (Patrick, 2006).

CU traits and developmental models of psychopathy

Lacking empathy, an absence of guilt, and a callous use of others for one's own gain have been prominent in most conceptualizations of psychopathy (Cleckley, 1976; Hare, 1993). There is still substantial debate about exactly how many dimensions best capture the construct of psychopathy in adults (see Cooke *et al.*, 2006 for a discussion). However, at least three correlated dimensions consistently emerge in samples of both adults (Cooke *et al.*, 2006) and youth (Frick & White, 2008). One dimension includes these CU traits and has been variously labelled as 'deficient affective experience' (Cooke *et al.*, 2006) or the 'affective factor' (Hare, 2003). The other two dimensions involve narcissistic traits and an impulsive and/or irresponsible behavioural style.

In addition to the disagreement as to how many dimensions best represent the construct of psychopathy, there has also been great debate as to what dimension may be most important for defining the construct or whether methods that combine across these dimensions may be most appropriate (Cooke *et al.*, 2006). For example, Lynam's (1996) conceptualization of the 'fledgling psychopath' in youth focused on the combination of impulsivity and severe conduct problems. In support of this conceptualization, Lynam noted that children with a diagnosis of both Attention Deficit Hyperactivity Disorder (ADHD) and Conduct Disorder typically showed the most severe and chronic patterns of antisocial behaviour. Similarly, a number of studies have reported that the impulsivity and irresponsibility dimension from many measures of psychopathy often shows the strongest and most consistent correlations with measures of conduct problems, delinquency, and other antisocial indices (Lynam, 1998; Kotler & McMahon, 2005; Frick & White, 2008).

However, for a construct to be important for subtyping within antisocial individuals, it also needs to show important areas of independence from general measures of antisocial behaviour: that is, if a dimension accounts for the same variance as general antisocial behaviour in predicting important external criteria (e.g., risk of future aggression and violence), the incremental utility of this dimension is limited and it is unlikely to designate a distinct group *within* antisocial individuals. In adult samples, it is the CU dimension that seems to be most specific to individuals high on psychopathic traits compared to other antisocial individuals (Cooke & Michie, 1997). There is also some evidence that the same may be true for youth: that is, a large proportion of youth with childhood-onset conduct problems show high rates of impulsivity, but it seems to be the subgroup with CU traits who show characteristics often associated with psychopathy (Barry *et al.*, 2000).

Therefore, in this chapter, we focus on a theoretical model that uses the CU dimension of psychopathy to differentiate important subgroups of childhood-onset antisocial and violent youth. One limitation in taking this approach is that most measures of psychopathy that have been used in past research with youth typically include only a limited number of items specifically assessing this dimension, often with as few as 4 (Forth *et al.*, 2003) or 6 (Frick & Hare, 2001) items. As a result, many existing measures of CU traits have often had some significant psychometric limitations, such as displaying poor internal consistency in detained samples of adolescents (Poythress *et al.*, 2006). In an attempt to overcome these limitations, a more extended assessment of these traits (24 items) has been tested in a large (n = 1443) community sample of German adolescents of ages 12–18 (Essau *et al.*, 2006) and a moderate-sized (n = 248) sample of juvenile offenders of ages 12–20 in the United States (Kimonis *et al.*, 2008). In both samples, a similar factor structure emerged with three factors (e.g., Uncaring, Callousness, Unemotional) loading on a higher-order CU dimension providing the best fit in both samples (see Table 4.1 for items). Importantly, the total scores proved to be internally consistent in both samples (α: 0.77–0.81) and these scores were related to antisocial behaviour, aggression, delinquency, and other measures of emotional functioning in ways consistent with past research on psychopathy.

Another important issue for using CU traits as a method for differentiating a subgroup of antisocial youth is whether the behaviours that define these traits are stable enough in children or adolescents to warrant the designation of 'traits' that implies some level of stability across development (Edens *et al.*, 2001; Seagrave & Grisso, 2002). There are now a number of studies showing that these traits are relatively stable from late childhood to early adolescence when assessed by both self-report (Munoz & Frick, 2007) or parent report (Frick, Kimonis *et al.*, 2003; Obradovic *et al.*, 2007). Further, there is evidence of fairly strong measurement invariance in scales assessing these traits, such that the items used show a relatively stable structure from ages 8 through 16 (Obradovic *et al.*, 2007). Importantly, this level of stability does not imply that these traits are unchangeable. That is, Frick, Kimonis *et al.* (2003) reported that, despite the high level of stability in these traits in a sample that started with an average age of 12, there were a significant number of youth who decreased in their level of CU traits over the four-year study (see also Lynam *et al.*, 2007 for a similar pattern of change over a longer period of development). Further, youth who decreased in their level of CU traits showed lower levels of conduct problems, came from homes of higher socio-economic status, and experienced more effective parenting. Thus, CU traits do appear to be at least somewhat malleable and their change is related to factors in the child's psychosocial environment.

Table 4.1 Dimensions of callous-unemotional traits

Unemotional	Uncaring	Callousness
I do not show my emotions to others.	I work hard on everything I do. (**I**)	I do not care about doing things well.
I express my feelings openly. (**I**)	I always try my best. (**I**)	I do not like to put the time into doing things well.
I hide my feelings from others.	I care about how well I do at school or work. (**I**)	I do not feel remorseful when I do something wrong.
It is easy for others to tell how I am feeling. (**I**)	I do things to make others feel good. (**I**)	I do not care about being on time.
I am very expressive and emotional. (**I**)	I apologize to persons I hurt. (**I**)	I do not care if I get into trouble.
	I feel bad or guilty when I do something wrong. (**I**)	I seem very cold and uncaring to others.
	I easily admit to being wrong. (**I**)	The feelings of others are unimportant to me
	I try not to hurt others' feelings. (**I**)	I do not care who I hurt to get what I want.
		I am concerned about the feelings of others. (**I**)
		What I think is right and wrong is different from what other people think.

Note: These three dimensions emerged from factor analyses in non-referred German adolescents (Essau *et al.*, 2006) and detained adolescents in the United States (Kimonis *et al.*, in press). **I**, items that are reversed.

It is also important to note that these studies on the stability of CU traits have largely focused on the developmental period from later childhood to early adolescence. However, Dadds *et al.* (2005) found moderate one-year stability estimates for parent-reported CU traits ($r = 0.55$) in a community sample of Australian children who were 4–9 years of age. Further, several studies have now shown that measures of CU traits in childhood and adolescence are predictive of measures of psychopathy in adulthood (Blonigen *et al.*, 2006; Burke *et al.*, 2007; Lynam *et al.*, 2007).

CU traits, aggression, and delinquency

Thus, research clearly suggests that some antisocial youth or youth with conduct problems show high levels of CU traits and these traits can be assessed reliably in samples with children as young as age 3 (Kimonis *et al.*, 2006) and 4 (Dadds *et al.*, 2005). Further, this research suggests that these traits are relatively stable across extended periods of development. However, as noted previously, a key issue is whether the presence or absence of CU traits designates important subgroups within antisocial or violent youth.

One of the most important and useful aspects of the construct of psychopathy in adult samples has been its ability to designate a particularly violent and chronic subgroup of antisocial individuals (Douglas *et al.*, 2006). There is now a fairly substantial body of research to suggest that this may also be the case in samples of youth. Edens *et al.* (2007) conducted a meta-analysis of 21 studies, all of which used the same measure to assess CU traits, with non-overlapping samples of juvenile offenders. They reported an overall effect size of $r = 0.24$ and $r = 0.25$ for measures of CU traits in predicting general and violent offending, respectively. Similarly, two qualitative reviews that focused only on published studies but included studies with non-offending samples and multiple measures of CU traits found 33 published studies using child or adolescent samples in which CU traits were associated with more severe conduct problems, delinquency, or aggression (Frick & Dickens 2006; Frick & White, 2008). Eighteen of these studies were cross-sectional studies demonstrating contemporaneous associations between CU traits and antisocial behaviour and 15 were longitudinal studies demonstrating predictive relations between these two constructs. Further, these reviews documented 5 published studies showing an association between CU traits and poor treatment outcome.

These reviews provide compelling evidence that antisocial youth with CU traits tend to show more severe and stable conduct problems, aggression, and delinquency. However, there is evidence to suggest that this group of youth is also distinct in the type of conduct problems and aggression they exhibit. Specifically, antisocial youth with CU traits, whether studied in a community sample (Frick, Cornell, Barry *et al.*, 2003), in clinic-referred samples (Stafford & Cornell, 2003; Enebrink *et al.*, 2005), or in detained samples (Murrie *et al.*, 2004; Kruh *et al.*, 2005), show more severe aggression overall than youth without these traits. However, their aggression is also more likely to be premeditated (i.e., with planning and forethought) and more likely to be for instrumental gain (i.e., to obtain money, goods, or dominance). In contrast, antisocial youth without high levels of CU traits tend to show less severe aggression overall and their aggression seems to be limited to impulsive or reactive aggression, which is in response to real or perceived provocation (Frick, Cornell, Barry *et al.*, 2003; Kruh *et al.*, 2005). This association between CU traits and more severe and proactive aggression has been found as early as in the preschool years (Kimonis *et al.*, 2006).

One critical issue in research on the association between CU traits and aggression is whether the association is found for both boys and girls. Several studies have found that CU traits are highly associated with aggression in girls (Marsee *et al.*, 2005; Odgers *et al.*, 2005; Marsee & Frick, 2007). However, Edens *et al.*'s (2007) meta-analysis of offending samples of adolescents found that the effect size of CU traits predicting violent offending was lower for girls than for boys, although the effects sizes for predicting general offending were comparable across sex. One possible reason for these conflicting results could be the low base rate of violent offending in samples of girls that could attenuate the effect size estimates (Edens *et al.*, 2007). However, it is also possible that aggression may be expressed differently in girls and boys (Crick & Grotpeter, 1995), and most studies have not assessed the type of aggression that is most often displayed by girls. In support of this latter possibility, Marsee and Frick (2007) studied both physical and relational aggression in a sample of detained adolescent girls. Relational aggression focused on attempts to harm others by hurting their social relationships, such by gossiping about them, lying about them, or excluding them from groups. Marsee and Frick (2007) reported that CU traits were associated with both physical aggression and relational aggression, but (a) this association was somewhat stronger for relational aggression ($r = 0.47, p < 0.001$) than for physical aggression ($r = 0.34, p < 0.05$) and (b) the association with relational aggression remained strong even after controlling for physical aggression ($\beta = 0.44, p < 0.001$).

CU traits, and emotional and social-cognitive functioning

In line with their different patterns of aggressive behaviour, antisocial youth with and without CU traits also differ on several emotional and social-cognitive characteristics (see Frick & White, 2008 for a review). First, several studies of non-referred (Frick, Cornell, Bodin, *et al.*, 2003) and clinic-referred (Frick *et al.*, 1999) children and non-referred (Essau *et al.*, 2006) and detained (Pardini, 2006) adolescents have reported that youth with CU traits display higher levels of thrill and adventure seeking or fearlessness. Second, youth with CU traits show lower levels of anxiety than other youth with conduct problems, controlling for their level of impulsivity and conduct problems. Specifically, there is evidence for a suppression effect between CU traits on one hand and impulsivity and conduct problems on the other in their association with anxiety symptoms. Although impulsivity and conduct problems are positively associated with anxiety symptoms, CU traits are negatively related to anxiety symptoms, and these specific relationships are stronger when the other variable is controlled. This suppressor effect has been found in samples of clinic-referred school-aged children (Frick *et al.*, 1999) and non-referred school-aged girls (Hipwell *et al.*, 2007), as well as in samples of adults (Frick *et al.*, 2000; Hicks & Patrick, 2006). A negative association between CU traits and anxiety symptoms was also found in male adolescent offenders screened for anxiety disorders (Dolan & Rennie, 2007).

In addition to lower expressions of fear and anxiety, youth with CU traits evidence different processing of emotional stimuli when compared with other youth with conduct problems (Frick & White, 2008). For instance, a study of antisocial adolescents showed that, whereas impulsivity and conduct problems are associated with facilitated processing of negative emotional words, CU traits are associated with slower processing of these stimuli (Loney *et al.*, 2003). Further, children with psychopathic tendencies show weaker electrodermal responses to others' distress (Blair, 1999). When asked to identify others' emotions, children and adolescents with CU traits have difficulty discriminating negative emotional expressions (Stevens *et al.*, 2001). This finding was replicated in a non-clinical sample of 7-year-old twins, and this relationship was found to be explained by genetic factors common to both poor emotional discrimination and CU traits (Petitclerc *et al.*, 2007).

These emotional characteristics of youth with CU traits may influence their moral development and could be important for explaining their aggressive behaviour. Youth with high CU traits, for instance, are more likely than their peers to think that it is acceptable to commit a moral transgression (i.e., impairing others' physical or material well-being) if there are no rules against it, and they are less likely to make reference to others' welfare to justify not transgressing (Blair, 1997; Fisher & Blair, 1998; Blair *et al.*, 2001; Rogers *et al.*, 2006). This impaired moral reasoning, along with their poorer recognition of and lower autonomic reactions to others' distress, may explain why CU traits are associated with more frequent use of aggression in general, and more frequent use of instrumental aggression in particular (Frick, Cornell, Barry *et al.*, 2003; Kruh *et al.*, 2005).

In contrast, for youth with conduct problems but without elevated CU traits, higher levels of negative emotions and increased responsiveness to emotional stimuli may explain their predominant use of reactive, rather than instrumental, aggression (Frick, Cornell, Barry *et al.*, 2003). Also, children with conduct problems but without CU traits are more likely to interpret neutral facial expressions as anger (Dadds *et al.*, 2006). Similarly, in social situations, children without CU traits are more likely to show a hostile attribution bias in social situations (i.e., more likely to attribute a hostile intent to others) (Frick, Cornell, Bodin, *et al.*, 2003) and have more difficulty in coming up with prosocial responses to provocation (Waschbusch, Walsh, *et al.*, 2007), both of which could increase the likelihood of reactive aggressive behaviour.

Common characteristics in antisocial youth with and without CU traits

Despite their distinct behavioural, emotional, and social-cognitive characteristics, antisocial youth with and without CU traits share some important characteristics. For example, both subtypes are likely to present non-compliance and physical aggression starting in early childhood (Waschbusch, Carrey *et al.*, 2007). In addition, evidence from studies of early externalizing behaviour problems suggests that the vast majority of youth with childhood-onset conduct problems show high levels of impulsivity and hyperactivity. Indeed, impulsivity and hyperactivity in early childhood are among the best early predictors of childhood antisocial behaviour (Richman *et al.*, 1982; Tremblay *et al.*, 1994) and of a childhood-onset pattern of antisocial behaviour in particular (Moffitt & Caspi, 2001). Although they may have distinct underlying neurocognitive vulnerabilities (Blair *et al.*, 2005), high levels of impulsive and hyperactive symptoms have been documented in antisocial youth both with and without CU traits (Christian *et al.*, 1997; Colledge & Blair, 2001; Frick, Cornell, Bodin, *et al.*, 2003; Mathias *et al.*, 2007).

These behavioural features common to antisocial youth with and without CU traits have been associated with the temperament dimension of effortful inhibitory control. According to Rothbart and Bates (1998), effortful inhibitory control is the ability to inhibit a dominant response to initiate a subdominant response. It is an active inhibitory system that involves attentional skills and serves to modulate approach behaviour according to situational and/or parental demands (Rothbart & Ahadi, 1994), and to modulate more reactive aspects of temperament such as anger and fear (Rothbart, Derryberry *et al.*, 1994). Effortful inhibitory control starts to develop in the second year of life and continues to evolve, mostly during the preschool years (Rothbart *et al.*, 2006). Individual differences in effortful inhibitory control show moderate stability during early childhood (Kochanska *et al.*, 2000).

Several studies support the association between low effortful inhibitory control and impulsivity/hyperactivity and with early antisocial behaviour more generally. In 3-year-old boys, effortful inhibitory control is associated with externalizing behaviour problems, and especially their impulsive/inattentive component (Olson *et al.*, 2005). It is also associated concurrently with impulsivity and externalizing problems in childhood (Eisenberg *et al.*, 2004) and pre-adolescence (Oldehinkel *et al.*, 2004), and is associated prospectively with externalizing problems during childhood (Eisenberg *et al.*, 2004) and adolescence (Eisenberg *et al.*, 2005).

Rothbart and her colleagues (Rothbart, Ahadi *et al.*, 1994) have suggested two mechanisms involving effortful inhibitory control that may help to inhibit aggressive behaviour. First, effortful inhibitory control allows a child to redirect his or her attention from immediate personal gratification to the possible consequences of his or her behaviour. Second, it can allow individuals to attend to others' distress and other social cues rather than focusing on their own sympathetic distress (Rothbart *et al.*, 2006). Thus, poor effortful inhibitory control could add to the risk of aggressive behaviour conferred by the different patterns of emotional functioning found in antisocial youth with and without CU traits. Specifically, for children who experience weaker emotional reactions to others' distress (i.e., those with CU traits), poor effortful inhibitory control could further impair their ability to recognize when their goal-directed behaviour is potentially harmful to others and to inhibit such behaviour. For children who are highly emotionally reactive, and are at risk of more reactive forms of aggression (i.e., those children with conduct problems but low on CU traits), poor effortful inhibitory control could increase their difficulty to regulate their high arousal and interfere with their ability to interpret distress and other social cues in others.

Developmental pathway for antisocial youth with high CU traits

This discussion of effortful control and its role in the development of aggression in youth both high and low on CU traits illustrates the importance of integrating research on normal early development with research on samples of youth with conduct problems. Using this same approach, it is important to consider some of the distinct developmental mechanisms that may be operating for youth with and without CU traits.

As noted previously, low levels of emotional reactivity to negative stimuli, especially distress in others, and low proneness to fear seem to be specific to youth with CU traits. Fear develops late in the first year of life and serves as a reactive inhibitory control system (Rothbart & Bates, 1998). Lower proneness to fear may lead to the development of CU traits by interfering with the experience of affective discomfort following misbehaviour, a discomfort that normally differentiates into feelings of guilt, as the child develops (Kochanska, 1993). Fowles (1980, 1984) expressed similar ideas, emphasizing the role of fear in learning (or conditioning) in the context of punishment cues: fearless individuals, because of a lower sensitivity to punishment cues, would fail to learn to inhibit behaviours usually associated with punishment, including antisocial and violent behaviour. Thus, lower proneness to fear could lead to the development of CU traits and more generally impair internalization of rules, which would then place the child at risk of engaging in aggressive and other antisocial behaviour.

In support of this model, fear observed in infancy was associated with lower aggression, higher empathy, and higher guilt as reported by mothers at ages 6–7 years (Rothbart *et al.*, 1994).

Similarly, fearlessness assessed at age 2 predicted higher levels of externalizing behaviour problems at age 5 (Calkins *et al.*, 2007) and predicted more stable trajectories of externalizing behaviour problems between ages 2 and 8 (Shaw *et al.*, 2003). In an older sample that explicitly tested the mediational role of CU traits, Pardini (2006) reported that the association between fearlessness and violent delinquency was mediated by the presence of CU traits in a sample of adjudicated adolescents.

Based on the previous discussion, children with both fearlessness and poor effortful inhibitory control would be at the most risk of the development of CU traits. Indeed, according to Kochanska's (1993) theory of the development of conscience (which refers to internalization of rules, cooperation in discipline contexts, guilt, empathy), early fear would be necessary for the emergence of the affective component of conscience (guilt, empathy), whereas early effortful inhibitory control would be necessary for its behavioural component (inhibition in the context of rules). Although no studies have yet tested the role of these two temperamental dimensions in the development of CU traits specifically, there is empirical evidence for them as independent predictors of persistent pre-adolescent antisocial behaviour (Tremblay *et al.*, 1994) and adult psychopathic personality (Glenn *et al.*, 2007).

Besides their direct association with children's conscience development, early fear levels could also act as a moderator in the relationship between parenting and children's conscience. For toddlers who are relatively fearful, parents' use of low-power assertion predicts higher conscience three years later, whereas for their relatively fearless peers, parental power assertion is unrelated to conscience development (Kochanska, 1991; Kochanska *et al.*, 2007). In contrast, a positive mother-child relationship is associated with later conscience development in relatively fearless toddlers, whereas no such relationship can be found for relatively fearful children (Kochanska *et al.*, 2007). Similarly, in the pre-adolescent years, parental use of corporal punishment and the child's perception of lower parental warmth and/or involvement predict increases in CU traits over a one-year period. However, the relationship involving low parental warmth and/or involvement appears to be stronger for children who are low in anxiety (Pardini *et al.*, 2007). This suggests that children's family experiences may not have direct effects on the development of CU traits; rather, the role of the family environment may be moderated by the child's dispositional characteristics.

The issue of the relative importance of genetic and environmental factors in the aetiology of CU traits has been investigated more directly in two studies of twins at school entry. Twin studies are useful to estimate the relative contribution of genetic factors and two types of environmental factors (either shared or not shared by twins of the same family) to explain individual differences in a given trait (Neale & Cardon, 1992). The twin design relies on the fact that monozygotic twins have 100% of their genes in common, whereas dizygotic twins share on average 50% of their genes. There is evidence of an influence of genetic factors when monozygotic twins are more similar on a trait than dizygotic twins are. The remaining intra-familial resemblance is attributed to what is called the 'shared environment', whereas the proportion of variance unique to each twin of monozygotic pairs is attributed to non-shared environmental factors, and includes measurement error (Neale & Cardon, 1992).

In the Quebec Newborn Twins Study (QNTS), additive genetic factors and non-shared environmental factors were about equally important in explaining individual differences in teacher-rated CU traits, whereas there was no significant influence of shared environmental factors (Petitclerc *et al.*, 2007). In the Twins Early Development Study (TEDS) sample, however, the relative contribution of genetic and shared and non-shared environmental factors in teacher-rated CU traits varied as a function of gender (Viding *et al.*, 2007). In boys, genetic factors accounted for about two thirds of the variance in CU traits, whereas non-shared environmental factors accounted for the remaining variance, with no significant effect of shared environmental factors. In girls, genetic factors explained approximately half of the variance in CU traits, and there was a modest but significant (0.20) contribution of shared environmental factors, with the remaining variance explained by non-shared environmental factors (Viding *et al.*, 2007).

The results of these twin studies, showing limited or no influence of shared environmental factors to explain individual differences in children's CU traits, must be interpreted in light of what 'shared environment' means in quantitative genetic analyses of twin data. Shared environmental factors are non-genetic influences that make the twin siblings more similar to each other (Turkheimer & Waldron, 2000). They are not equivalent to familial factors. Hence, if two children from the same family are affected differently by the same environmental factor (e.g., family events, parenting behaviours), because of some genetically or environmentally driven child characteristic, this would not be part of 'shared environmental' influences. Therefore, the results of studies on the genetic-environmental aetiology of CU traits in children are consistent with findings reviewed earlier showing that parenting effects on the development of children's conscience or CU traits may not be main effects but effects that are moderated by child factors, such as temperamental differences in the child's emotional reactivity and fearlessness (Kochanska, 1991; Kochanska *et al.*, 2007; Pardini *et al.*, 2007).

Genetically informative studies are also useful to explain the aetiology of the relationship between CU traits and conduct problems. Results of Viding *et al.*'s (2007) study indicated that most of the association between CU traits and conduct problems in 7-year-old children is explained by common genetic influences on both types of behaviours. Similarly, a common genetic factor was found for self-reported CU traits and antisocial behaviour in a sample of Swedish adolescents (Larsson *et al.*, 2007). These results suggest that both types of behaviours share a genetically based vulnerability (Larsson *et al.*, 2007).

Besides their genetic correlation with conduct problems, CU traits in middle childhood may moderate the relationship between parenting and conduct problems. This moderation effect is analogous to the moderation effect reviewed earlier, in which children's fearlessness attenuated the relationship between power-assertive parenting and the development of CU traits. Whereas a parenting style characterized by lack of involvement, low positive reinforcement, low supervision, and inconsistent and coercive parenting behaviour is associated with higher conduct problems in children with low CU traits, such a relationship is not found in children with high CU traits (Wootton *et al.*, 1997; Oxford *et al.*, 2003; Hipwell *et al.*, 2007). One characteristic of children with CU traits may help understand these findings: children with CU traits tend to perceive adults as less capable of imposing limits and of prevailing when conflicts arise (Schneider *et al.*, 2003). In children with such a lower 'sense of containment', there is no relationship between ineffective parenting and externalizing child behaviour, contrary to the positive relationship observed in children who perceive their parents as more able to 'contain' their behaviour (Schneider *et al.*, 2003).

Developmental pathway for antisocial youth with low CU traits

Although there are no epidemiological data, it appears that only a minority of youth with childhood-onset conduct problems show high rates of CU traits (Christian *et al.*, 1997). Further, although their aggression seems to be less severe and more reactive in nature, children with childhood-onset conduct problems without CU traits still show significant levels of aggression (Frick, Cornell, Bodin, *et al.*, 2003) and appear to be at risk of delinquency in adolescence (Frick *et al.*, 2005). Thus, it is also important to have models to explain the development of conduct problems in youth without CU traits.

Many theories have focused on problems regulating negative emotions for this group (Frick & Morris, 2004; Frick, 2006). Poor emotional regulation is characterized by both high negative emotionality (including fear, anxiety, and anger) and poor effortful control of these emotions (Calkins & Fox, 2002). In support of the importance of these two dimensions as correlates of conduct problems, high levels of anger have been associated with more aggression in childhood (Eisenberg *et al.*, 2004; Schultz *et al.*, 2004), and this relationship is strongest when children also have poor effortful inhibitory control (Eisenberg *et al.*, 2004). Measures of poor emotional regulation have been related to aggressive behaviour in the preschool years (Chang *et al.*, 2003) and to externalizing behaviour problems in the pre-adolescent years (Pardini *et al.*, 2006).

The association between problems in emotional regulation and a child's propensity to display conduct problems and aggressive behaviour can be both direct and indirect (Robison *et al.*, 2005). For example, a child who tends to react with strong angry and hostile emotions may act aggressively within the context of these strong emotions without thinking of the potential consequences of these acts (Shields & Cicchetti, 1998; Hubbard, *et al.*, 2002). In contrast, poor emotional regulation could lead to aggression indirectly by impairing social cognitive skills that allow a child to effectively process and respond to information in social situations (Dodge & Frame, 1982; Dodge & Pettit, 2003). Research on aggressive children who show strong emotional reactions has indicated that these children tend to selectively attend to hostile cues in peer interactions (Dodge *et al.*, 1986), they make hostile attributions to the intent of peer behaviours when the intent is not readily apparent (Dodge *et al.*, 1997), and they more readily access aggressive responses to peer provocations (Asarnow & Callan, 1985). In addition, a child who lacks the ability to competently regulate emotional arousal is more likely to be rejected by his or her peers (Rubin *et al.*, 1998). Such peer rejection can lead a child to miss out on important socializing experiences that take place within the peer group, such as learning appropriate and effective social skills (Renshaw & Asher, 1982; Dodge *et al.*, 2003).

Poor emotional regulation can also influence how a child responds to socialization attempts by parents, making them more sensitive to the quality of parenting. As noted previously, in contrast to children with high CU traits, ineffective parenting practices seem to be highly associated with conduct problems in youth low on CU traits (Wootton *et al.*, 1997; Oxford *et al.*, 2003; Hipwell *et al.*, 2007). This finding is consistent with other research showing that, in middle childhood, the positive relationship between parental use of harsh discipline and boys' externalizing behaviour problems is strongest in boys with higher fear levels (Colder *et al.*, 1997). Prospective studies have also shown that parenting quality is more strongly associated with externalizing problems at age 3 (Belsky *et al.*, 1998) and in middle childhood (Kochanska, 1991) for children who had higher negative emotionality (higher fear and distress to limitation) as toddlers.

Further supporting evidence of the role of parenting among highly reactive children comes from research on young children described as having a 'difficult temperament', which refers to the child being easily upset, showing intense emotional reactions, being difficult to soothe, and showing irregularity in biological functions (Thomas & Chess, 1977). In a study of young children, a difficult temperament was associated with more externalizing problems and this temperament moderated the relationship between parenting and externalizing problems (van Zeijl *et al.*, 2007). Both low-positive and high-negative discipline strategies were more strongly related with young children's externalizing problems among children with a difficult temperament than among those with an easy temperament (van Zeijl *et al.*, 2007). Thus, children with poor effortful inhibitory control and higher levels of negative emotions may be at risk of conduct problems especially when parents resort to coercive behaviour.

Conclusions

In conclusion, the available research suggests that there are a number of distinct causal pathways that can lead children to act in a severely antisocial and aggressive manner. Two such pathways, both involving children with a childhood onset to their conduct problems, were the primary focus of this chapter because they appear to account for a large proportion of violent offenders in adolescence and adulthood (Moffitt *et al.*, 2002). Both trajectories involve impulsive and poorly regulated behaviour. However, the first pathway seems to involve a temperament characterized by a low level of emotional reactivity that can lead to problems in a child's development of empathy, guilt, and other aspects of conscience. These CU traits can place a child at risk of showing severe conduct problems and instrumental aggression. In contrast, the second pathway appears to involve high levels of emotional reactivity that can make it difficult for a child to develop regulatory strategies to control his or her emotions and behaviour resulting in impulsive conduct problems and reactive aggression. This second pathway is also strongly related to problematic parenting strategies.

In defining these distinct causal pathways, we have tried to integrate research on normal development with research on children and adolescents who show conduct problems and aggression. This developmental psychopathological approach is important for theoretical models of aggressive and violent behaviour for several reasons. First, it can provide a framework for integrating the many risk factors that have been associated with conduct problems and aggression (e.g., impulsivity, problematic parenting, poor emotional regulation) into comprehensive causal models that clearly define the key causal mechanisms through which the risk factors influence the developing child. Second, the developmental psychopathological approach outlined in this chapter recognizes that a child's membership in these pathways is not unchangeable. For example, we have outlined several temperamental vulnerabilities that can place a child at risk of developing conduct problems and aggression. However, this approach recognizes that there are likely to be many children who show the temperamental vulnerabilities but who nevertheless do not develop significant behavioural problems. Identifying protective factors that can foster more optimal development, even in the context of either temperamental or environmental risk, could be critical for developing more effective interventions for youth with severe conduct problems.

Thus, in addition to the implications for causal theories, this research has important implications for improving our interventions designed to prevent or reduce the level of aggression and violence in youth. Given that a large proportion of violent and aggressive adolescents have a history of childhood conduct problems, it is important to intervene early in the developmental trajectory of problem behaviour. In support of this approach, there is consistent evidence that the effectiveness of treatments for conduct problems decrease with age (Kazdin, 1995; Brestan & Eyberg, 1998; Frick, 1998). However, most existing preventive programmes target children who have started to show significant conduct problems at an early age (e.g., Webster-Stratton *et al.*, 2004). By focusing on the early developmental processes that can precede even these early conduct problems, it opens the possibility of prevention programmes that promote optimal development in children with certain risk factors (e.g., a fearless temperament, poor emotional regulation) even before the behavioural problems emerge.

In addition to intervening early, the current developmental model could help in tailoring interventions to the needs of youth in the different pathways. Specifically, some of the most effective interventions for antisocial and violent youth are approaches that do not provide a single type of intervention to all youth. Instead, they provide a system for assessing the unique needs of individual youth and designing an individualized approach to treatment to meet those needs (e.g., Henggeler *et al.*, 1998). Research on the distinct developmental processes leading to conduct problems across the different subgroups of antisocial and aggressive youth could help to highlight some factors that may be important to target for most youth with serious conduct problems (e.g., problems of impulse control, development of effortful control strategies) and others that may be important to target for only certain subgroups of youth (e.g., empathy development, anger control).

Unfortunately, there have been few studies to date that have directly tested whether youth in the various developmental pathways respond differentially to treatment. In one notable exception, Hawes and Dadds (2005) reported that clinic-referred boys (ages 4–9) with conduct problems and CU traits were less responsive to a parenting intervention than boys with conduct problems who were low on CU traits. However, this differential effectiveness was not consistently found across all phases of the treatment. That is, children with and without CU traits seemed to respond equally well to the first part of the intervention that focused on teaching parents methods of using positive reinforcement to encourage prosocial behaviour. In contrast, only the group without CU traits showed added improvement with the second part of the intervention that focused on teaching parents more effective discipline strategies. In another study of the differential response to treatment of youth with CU traits, Waschbusch, Carrey *et al.* (2007) reported that children (ages 7–12) with conduct problems and CU traits responded less well to behaviour therapy alone than children with conduct problems without CU traits. However, these differences largely disappeared when stimulant medication was added to the behaviour therapy, although the children with CU traits were still less likely to score in the normative range than those without these traits.

Clearly, much more research is needed on the response to treatment of children with CU traits. However, these two studies provide strong motivation for such research. Both studies suggest that children with CU traits may be more difficult to treat but are not unresponsive to treatment. They do respond to certain types of interventions. Research on the unique developmental mechanisms underlying their antisocial behaviour could provide important clues as to what types of interventions may be the most effective for this group of youth who seem to be at particularly high risk of violent behaviour in adolescence (Frick, 2006). Thus, there is some cause for at least cautious optimism that this research on CU traits could guide more effective interventions for a subgroup of youth who operate at a high cost to society because of their chronic and serious delinquent and aggressive acts.

References

Asarnow, J. R., & Callan, J. W. (1985). Boys with peer adjustment problems: social cognitive processes. *Journal of Consulting and Clinical Psychology*, *53*, 80–87.

Barry, C. T., Frick, P. J., DeShazo, T. M., McCoy, M. G., Ellis, M., & Loney, B. R. (2000). The importance of callous-unemotional traits for extending the concept of psychopathy to children. *Journal of Abnormal Psychology*, *109*, 335–340.

Belsky, J., Hsieh, K-H., & Crnic, K. (1998). Mothering, fathering, and infant negativity as antecedents of boys' externalizing problems and inhibition at age 3 years: differential susceptibility to rearing experience? *Development and Psychopathology*, *10*, 301–319.

Blair, R. J. R. (1997). Moral reasoning and the child with psychopathic tendencies. *Personality and Individual Differences*, *22*, 731–739.

Blair, R. J. R. (1999). Responsiveness to distress cues in the child with psychopathic tendencies. *Personality and Individual Differences*, *27*, 135–145.

Blair, R. J. R., Mitchell, D., & Blair, K. (2005). *The Psychopath: Emotion and the Brain*. Malden, MA: Blackwell.

Blair, R. J. R., Monson, J., & Frederickson, N. (2001). Moral reasoning and conduct problems in children with emotional and behavioural difficulties. *Personality and Individual Differences, 31,* 799–811.

Blonigen, D. M., Hicks, B. M., Krueger, R. F., Patrick, C. J., & Iacono, W. G. (2006). Continuity and change in psychopathic traits as measured via normal-range personality: a longitudinal-biometric study. *Journal of Abnormal Psychology, 115,* 85–95.

Brestan, E. V., & Eyberg, S. M. (1998). Effective psychosocial treatments of conduct-disordered children and adolescents: 29 years, 82 studies, and 5,272 kids. *Journal of Clinical Child Psychology Special Issue: Empirically Supported Psychosocial Interventions for Children, 27,* 180–189.

Burke, J. D., Loeber, R., & Lahey, B. B. (2007). Adolescent conduct disorder and interpersonal callousness as predictors of psychopathy in young adults. *Journal of Clinical Child and Adolescent Psychology, 36,* 334–346.

Calkins, S. D., Blandon, A. Y., Williford, A. P., & Keane, S. P. (2007). Biological, behavioral, and relational levels of resilience in the context of risk for early childhood behavior problems. *Development and Psychopathology, 19,* 675–700.

Calkins, S. D., & Fox, N. A. (2002). Self-regulatory processes in early personality development: a multilevel approach to the study of childhood social withdrawal and aggression. *Development and Psychopathology, 14,* 477–498.

Chang, L., Schwartz, D., Dodge, K. A., & McBride-Chang, C. (2003). Harsh parenting in relation to child emotion regulation and aggression. *Journal of Family Psychology, 17,* 598–606.

Christian, R. E., Frick, P. J., Hill, N. L., Tyler, L., & Frazer, D. R. (1997). Psychopathy and conduct problems in children: II. Implications for subtyping children with conduct problems. *Journal of the American Academy of Child and Adolescent Psychiatry, 36,* 233–241.

Cleckley, H. (1976). *The Mask of Sanity,* 5th edn. St. Louis, MO: Mosby.

Colder, C. R., Lochman, J. E., & Wells, K. C. (1997). The moderating effects of children's fear and activity level on relations between parenting practices and childhood symptomatology. *Journal of Abnormal Child Psychology, 25,* 251–263.

Colledge, E., & Blair, R. J. R. (2001). The relationship in children between the inattention and impulsivity component of attention deficit and hyperactivity disorder and psychopathic tendencies. *Personality and Individual Differences, 30,* 1175–1187.

Cooke, D. J., & Michie, C. (1997). An item response theory analysis of the Hare Psychopathy Checklist-Revised. *Psychological Assessment, 9,* 3–14.

Cooke, D. J., Michie, C., & Hart, S. D. (2006). Facets of clinical psychopathy: toward clearer measurement. In C. J. Patrick (ed), *Handbook of Psychopathy* (pp. 91–106). New York: Guilford Press.

Crick, N. R., & Grotpeter, J. K. (1995). Relational aggression, gender, and social-psychological adjustment. *Child Development, 66,* 710–722.

Dadds, M. R., Fraser, J., Frost, A., & Hawes, D. J. (2005). Disentangling the underlying dimensions of psychopathy and conduct problems in childhood: a community study. *Journal of Consulting and Clinical Psychology, 73,* 400–410.

Dadds, M. R., Perry, Y., Hawes, D. J., Merz, S., Riddell, A. C., Haines, D. J., *et al.* (2006). Attention to eyes and fear-recognition deficits in child psychopathy. *British Journal of Psychiatry, 189,* 280–281.

Dodge, K. A., & Frame, C. L. (1982). Social cognitive biases and deficits in aggressive boys. *Child Development, 53,* 620–635.

Dodge, K. A., Lansford, J., Burks, V. S., Bates, J. E., Pettit, G. S., Fontaine, R., *et al.* (2003). Peer rejection and social information processing factors in the development of aggressive behaviour problems in children. *Child Development, 74,* 374–393.

Dodge, K. A., Lochman, J. E., Harnish, J. D., Bates, J. E., & Pettit, G. S. (1997). Reactive and proactive aggression in school children and psychiatrically impaired chronically assaultive youth. *Journal of Abnormal Psychology, 106,* 37–51.

Dodge, K. A., & Pettit, G. S. (2003). A biopsychosocial model of the development of chronic conduct problems in adolescence. *Developmental Psychology Special Issue: Violent Children, 39,* 349–371.

Dodge, K. A., Pettit, G. S., McClaskey, C. L., & Brown, M. (1986). Social competence in children. *Monographs of the Society for Research in Child Development, 51*(213), 1–85.

Dolan, M. C., & Rennie, C. E. (2007). Is juvenile psychopathy associated with low anxiety and fear in conduct-disordered male offenders? *Journal of Anxiety Disorders, 21,* 1028–1038.

Douglas, K. S., Vincent, G. M., & Edens, J. F. (2006). Risk for criminal recidivism: the role of psychopathy. In C. J. Patrick (ed), *Handbook of Psychopathy* (pp. 533–554). New York: Guilford Press.

Edens, J. F., Campbell, J. S., & Weir, J. M. (2007). Youth psychopathy and criminal recidivism: a meta-analysis of the psychopathy checklist measures. *Law and Human Behavior, 31,* 53–75.

Edens, J. F., Skeem, J. L., Cruise, K. R., & Cauffman, E. (2001). Assessment of 'juvenile psychopathy' and its association with violence: a critical review. *Behavioral Sciences and the Law, Special Issue: Youth Violence, 19,* 53–80.

Eisenberg, N., Spinrad, T. L., Fabes, R. A., Reiger, M., Cumberland, A., Shepart, S. A., *et al.* (2004). The relations of effortful control and impulsivity to children's resiliency and adjustment. *Child Development, 75,* 25–46.

Eisenberg, N., Zhou, Q., Spinrad, T. L., Valiente, C., Fabes, R. A., & Liew, J. (2005). Relations among positive parenting, children's effortful control, and externalizing problems: a three-wave longitudinal study. *Child Development, 76,* 1055–1071.

Enebrink, P., Andershed, H., & Långström, N. (2005). Callous-unemotional traits are associated with clinical severity in referred boys with conduct problems. *Nordic Journal of Psychiatry, 59,* 431–440.

Essau, C. A., Sasagawa, S., & Frick, P. J. (2006). Callous-unemotional traits in a community sample of adolescents. *Assessment, 13,* 454–469.

Fisher, L., & Blair, R. J. R. (1998). Cognitive impairment and its relationship to psychopathic tendencies in children with emotional and behavioural difficulties. *Journal of Abnormal Child Psychology, 26,* 511–519.

Forth, A. E., Kosson, D., & Hare, R. D. (2003). *The Hare PCL: Youth Version.* Toronto, ON: Multi-Health Systems.

Fowles, D. C. (1980). The three arousal model: implications of Gray's two-factor learning theory for heart rate, electrodermal activity, and psychopathy. *Psychophysiology, 17,* 87–104.

Fowles, D. C. (1984). Biological variables in psychopathology: a psychobiological perspective. In E. Adams, & P. B. Sutker (eds), *Comprehensive Handbook of Psychopathology* (pp. 77–110). New York: Plenum.

Frick, P. J., (1998). *Conduct Disorders and Severe Antisocial Behavior.* New York: Plenum Press.

Frick, P. J. (2006). Developmental pathways to conduct disorder. *Child and Adolescent Psychiatric Clinics of North America, 15,* 311–331.

Frick, P. J., Cornell, A. H., Barry, C. T., Bodin, S. D., & Dane, H. E. (2003). Callous-unemotional traits and conduct problems in the prediction of conduct problem severity, aggression and self-report of delinquency. *Journal of Abnormal Child Psychology, 31,* 457–470.

Frick, P. J., Cornell, A. H., Bodin, S. D., Dane, H. E., Barry, C. T., & Loney, B. R. (2003). Callous-unemotional traits and developmental pathways to severe conduct problems. *Developmental Psychology Special Issue: Violent Children, 39,* 246–260.

Frick, P. J., & Dickens, C. (2006). Current perspectives on conduct disorder. *Current Psychiatry Reports, 8,* 59–72.

Frick, P. J., & Hare, R. D. (2001). *The Antisocial Process Screening Device.* Toronto, ON: Multi-Health Systems.

Frick, P. J., Kimonis, E. R., Dandreaux, D. M., & Farell, J. M. (2003). The 4-year stability of psychopathic traits in non-referred youth. *Behavioral Sciences and the Law, 21,* 713–736.

Frick, P. J., Lilienfeld, S. O., Edens, J. F., Poythress, N. G., & McBurnett, K. (2000). The association between anxiety and antisocial behaviour. *Primary Psychiatry, 7,* 52–57.

Frick, P. J., Lilienfeld, S. O., Ellis, M., Loney, B. R., & Silverthorn, P. (1999). The association between anxiety and psychopathy dimensions in children. *Journal of Abnormal Child Psychology, 27,* 383–392.

Frick, P. J., & Morris, A. S. (2004). Temperament and developmental pathways to conduct problems. *Journal of Clinical Child and Adolescent Psychology, 33,* 54–68.

Frick, P. J., Stickle, T. R., Dandreaux, D. M., Farrell, J. M., & Kimonis, E. R. (2005). Callous-unemotional traits in predicting the severity and stability of conduct problems and delinquency. *Journal of Abnormal Child Psychology*, *33*, 471–487.

Frick, P. J., & White, S.F. (2008). The importance of callous-unemotional traits for the development of aggressive and antisocial behavior. *Journal of Child Psychology and Psychiatry*, *49*, 359–375.

Glenn, A. L., Raine, A., Venables, P. H., & Mednick, S. A. (2007). Early temperamental and psychophysiological precursors of adult psychopathic personality. *Journal of Abnormal Psychology*, *116*, 508–518.

Hare, H. D. (1993). *Without Conscience: The Disturbing World of Psychopaths among Us*. New York: Simon & Schuster (Pocket Books).

Hare, R. D. (2003). *The Hare Psychopathy Checklist-Revised* (2nd edn). Toronto, ON: Multi-Health Systems.

Hawes, D. J., & Dadds, M. R. (2005). The treatment of conduct problems in children with callous-unemotional traits. *Journal of Consulting and Clinical Psychology*, *73*, 737–741.

Henggeler, S. W., Schoenwald, S. K., Borduin, C. M., Rowland, M. D., & Cunningham, P. B. (1998). *Multisystemic Treatment of Antisocial Behavior in Children and Adolescents*. New York: Guilford.

Hicks, B. M., & Patrick, C. J. (2006). Psychopathy and negative emotionality: analyses of suppressor effects reveal distinct relations with emotional distress, fearfulness, and anger-hostility. *Journal of Abnormal Psychology*, *115*, 276–287.

Hipwell, A. E., Pardini, D. A., Loeber, R., Sembower, M., Keenan, K., & Stouthamer-Loeber, M. (2007). Callous-unemotional behaviors in young girls: shared and unique effects relative to conduct problems. *Journal of Clinical Child and Adolescent Psychology*, *36*, 293–304.

Hubbard, J. A., Smithmyer, C. M., Ramsden, S. R., Parker, E. H., Flanagan, K. D., Dearing, K. F., *et al.* (2002). Observational, physiological, and self-report measures of children's anger: relations to reactive versus proactive aggression. *Child Development*, *73*, 1101–1118.

Kazdin, A. E. (1995). *Conduct Disorders in Childhood and Adolescence* (2nd edn). Thousand Oaks, CA: Sage Publications, Inc.

Kimonis, E. R., Frick, P. J., Boris, N. W., Smyke, A. T., Cornell, A. H., Farrell, J. M., *et al.* (2006). Callous-unemotional features, behavioral inhibition, and parenting: independent predictors of aggression in a high-risk preschool sample. *Journal of Child and Family Studies*, *15*, 741–752.

Kimonis, E. R., Frick, P. J., Skeem, J., Marsee, M. A., Cruise, K., Munoz, L. C., *et al.* (2008). Assessing callous-unemotional traits in adolescent offenders: validation of the inventory of callous-unemotional traits. *International Journal of Law and Psychiatry*, *31*, 241–252.

Kochanska, G. (1991). Socialization and temperament in the development of guilt and conscience. *Child Development*, *62*, 1379–1392.

Kochanska, G. (1993). Toward a synthesis of parental socialization and child temperament in early development of conscience. *Child Development*, *64*, 325–347.

Kochanska, G., Aksan, N., & Joy, M. E. (2007). Children's fearfulness as a moderator of parenting in early socialization: two longitudinal studies. *Developmental Psychology*, *43*, 222–237.

Kochanska, G., Murray, K. T., & Harlan, E. T. (2000). Effortful control in early childhood: continuity and change, antecedents, and implications for social development. *Developmental Psychology*, *36*, 220–232.

Kotler, J. S., & McMahon, R. J. (2005). Child psychopathy: theories, measurement, and relations with the development and persistence of conduct problems. *Clinical Child and Family Psychology Review*, *8*, 291–325.

Kruh, I. P., Frick, P. J., & Clements, C. B. (2005). Historical and personality correlates to the violence patterns of juveniles tried as adults. *Criminal Justice and Behavior*, *32*, 69–96.

Lahey, B. B., Miller, T. L., Schwab-Stone, M., Goodman, S. H., Waldman, I. D., Canino, G., *et al.* (2000). Age and gender differences in oppositional behavior and conduct problems: a cross-sectional household study of middle childhood and adolescence. *Journal of Abnormal Psychology*, *109*, 488–503.

Larsson, H., Tuvblad, C., Rijsdijk, F. V., Andershed, H., Grann, M., & Lichtenstein, P. (2007). A common genetic factor explains the association between psychopathic personality and antisocial behavior. *Psychological Medicine*, *37*, 15–26.

Loeber, R., & Farrington, D. P. (2000). Young children who commit crime: epidemiology, developmental origins, risk factors, early interventions, and policy implications. *Development and Psychopathology*, *12*, 737–762.

Loney, B. R., Frick, P. J., Clements, C. B., Ellis, M. L., & Kerlin, K. (2003). Callous-unemotional traits, impulsivity, and emotional processing in adolescents with antisocial behavior problems. *Journal of Clinical Child and Adolescent Psychology*, *32*, 66–80.

Lynam, D. R. (1996). Early identification of chronic offenders: Who is the fledgling psychopath? *Psychological Bulletin*, *120*, 209–234.

Lynam, D. R. (1998). Early identification of the fledgling psychopath: locating the psychopathic child in the current nomenclature. *Journal of Abnormal Psychology*, *107*, 566–575.

Lynam, D. R., Caspi, A., Moffitt, T. E., Loeber, R., & Stouthamer-Loeber, M. (2007). Longitudinal evidence that psychopathy scores in early adolescence predict adult psychopathy. *Journal of Abnormal Psychology*, *116*, 155–165.

Marsee, M. A., & Frick, P. J. (2007). Exploring the cognitive and emotional correlates to proactive and reactive aggression in a sample of detained girls. *Journal of Abnormal Child Psychology*, *35*, 969–981.

Marsee, M. A., Silverthorn, P., & Frick, P. J. (2005). The association of psychopathic traits with aggression and delinquency in non-referred boys and girls. *Behavioral Sciences and the Law*, *23*, 803–817.

Marshall, L. A., & Cooke, D. J. (1999). The childhood experiences of psychopaths: a retrospective study of familial and societal factors. *Journal of Personality Disorders*, *13*, 211–225.

Mathias, C. W., Furr, R. M., Daniel, S. S., Marsh, D. M., Shannon, E. E., & Dougherty, D. M. (2007). The relationship of inattentiveness, hyperactivity, and psychopathy among adolescents. *Personality and Individual Differences*, *43*, 1333–1343.

Moffitt, T. E. (1993). Adolescence-limited and life-course-persistent antisocial behavior: a developmental taxonomy. *Psychological Review*, *100*, 674–701.

Moffitt, T. E. (2003). Life-course-persistent and adolescence-limited antisocial behavior: a 10-year research review and a research agenda. In B. B. Lahey, T. E. Moffitt, & A. Caspi (eds), *Causes of Conduct Disorder and Juvenile Delinquency* (pp. 49–75). New York: Guilford Press.

Moffitt, T. E., & Caspi, A. (2001). Childhood predictors differentiate life-course persistent and adolescence-limited antisocial pathways among males and females. *Development and Psychopathology*, *13*, 355–375.

Moffitt, T. E., Caspi, A., Harrington, H., & Milne, B. J. (2002). Males on the life-course-persistent and adolescence-limited antisocial pathways: follow-up at age 26 years. *Development and Psychopathology*, *14*, 179–207.

Muñoz, L. C., & Frick, P. J. (2007). The reliability, stability, and predictive utility of the self-report version of the antisocial process screening device. *Scandinavian Journal of Psychology*, *48*, 299–312.

Murrie, D. C., Cornell, D. G., Kaplan, S., McConville, D., & Levy-Elkon, A. (2004). Psychopathy scores and violence among juvenile offenders: a multi-measure study. *Behavioral Sciences and the Law*, *22*, 49–67.

Neale, M. C., & Cardon, L. R. (1992). *Methodology for Genetic Studies of Twins and Families*. Dordrecht, the Netherlands: Kluwer Academic Publications.

Obradovic, J., Pardini, D. A., Long, J. D., & Loeber, R. (2007). Measuring interpersonal callousness in boys from childhood to adolescence: an examination of longitudinal invariance and temporal stability. *Journal of Clinical Child and Adolescent Psychology*, *36*, 276–292.

Odgers, C. L., Reppucci, N. D., & Moretti, M. M. (2005). Nipping psychopathy in the bud: an examination of the convergent, predictive, and theoretical utility of the PCL-YV among adolescent girls. *Behavioral Sciences and the Law*, *23*, 743–763.

Oldehinkel, A. J., Hartman, C. A., De Winter, A. F., Veenstra, R., & Ormel, J. (2004). Temperament profiles associated with internalizing and externalizing problems in preadolescence. *Development and Psychopathology*, *16*, 421–440.

Olson, S. L., Sameroff, A. J., Kerr, D. C. R., Lopez, N. L., & Wellman, H. M. (2005). Developmental foundations of externalizing problems in young children: the role of effortful control. *Development and Psychopathology*, *17*, 25–45.

Oxford, M., Cavell, T. A., & Hughes, J. N. (2003). Callous/unemotional traits moderate the relation between ineffective parenting and child externalizing problems: a partial replication and extension. *Journal of Clinical Child and Adolescent Psychology*, *32*, 577–585.

Pardini, D. A. (2006). The callousness pathway to severe violent delinquency. *Aggressive Behavior*, *32*, 590–598.

Pardini, D. A., Barry, T. D., Barth, J. M., Lochman, J. E., & Wells, K. C. (2006). Self-perceived social acceptance and peer social standing in children with aggressive-disruptive behaviors. *Social Development*, *15*, 46–64.

Pardini, D. A., Lochman, J. E., & Powell, N. (2007). The development of callous-unemotional traits and antisocial behavior in children: Are there shared and/or unique predictors? *Journal of Clinical Child and Adolescent Psychology*, *36*, 319–333.

Patrick, C. J. (2006). Back to the future: Cleckley as a guide to the next generation of psychopathy research. In C. J. Patrick (ed), *Handbook of Psychopathy* (pp. 605–613). New York: Guilford Press.

Patterson, G. R. (1996). Some characteristics of a developmental theory for early-onset delinquency. In M. F. Lenzenweger, & J. J. Haugaard (eds), *Frontiers of Developmental Psychopathology* (pp. 81–124). New York: Oxford University Press.

Petitclerc, A., Boivin, M., Dionne, G., Vitaro, F., Brendgen, M., Tremblay, R. E., *et al.* (2007 Mar). Poor emotion discrimination and reward dominance in 7-year-old twins with callous-noncompliant behavior. Poster presented at the Society for Research in Child Development (SRCD) Biennial Meeting, Boston, MA.

Poythress, N. G., Douglas, K. S., Falkenbach, D., Cruise, K., Lee, Z., Murrie, D. G., *et al.* (2006). Internal consistency reliability of the self-report antisocial process screening device. *Assessment*, *13*, 107–113.

Raine, A. (2002). Biosocial studies of antisocial and violent behavior in children and adults: a review. *Journal of Abnormal Child Psychology*, *30*, 311–326.

Renshaw, P. D., & Asher, S. R. (1982). Social competence and peer status: the distinction between goals and strategies. In K. H. Rubin, & H. S. Ross (eds), *Peer Relationships and Social Skills in Childhood* (pp. 375–395). New York: Springer-Verlag.

Richman, N., Stevenson, J., & Graham, P. J. (1982). *Preschool to School: A Behavioural Study*. London: Academic Press.

Robison, S. D., Frick, P. J., & Morris, A. S. (2005). Temperament and parenting: implications for understanding developmental pathways to conduct disorder. *Minerva Pediatrics*, *57*, 373–388.

Rogers, J., Viding, E., Blair, R. J. R., Frith, U., & Happé, F. (2006). Autism spectrum disorder and psychopathy: shared cognitive underpinnings or double hit? *Psychological Medicine*, *36*, 1789–1798.

Rothbart, M. K., & Ahadi, S. (1994). Temperament and the development of personality. *Jounral of Abnormal Psychology*, *103*, 55–66.

Rothbart, M. K., Ahadi, S., & Hershey, K. L. (1994). Temperament and social behavior in children. *Merrill-Palmer Quarterly*, *40*, 21–39.

Rothbart, M. K., & Bates, J. E. (1998). Temperament. In W. Damon, & N. Eisenberg (eds), *Handbook of Child Psychology, Vol 3: Social, Emotional, and Personality Development*, 5th edn (pp. 105–176). Hoboken, NJ: John Wiley & Sons Inc.

Rothbart, M. K., Derryberry, D., & Posner, M. I. (1994). A psychobiological approach to the development of temperament. In J. E. Bates, & T. D. Wachs (eds), *Temperament: Individual Differences at the Interface of Biology and Behavior* (pp. 83–116). Washington, DC: American Psychological Association.

Rothbart, M. K., Posner, M. I., & Kieras, J. (2006). Temperament, attention, and the development of self-regulation. In K. McCartney, & D. Phillips (eds), *Blackwell Handbook of Early Childhood Development* (pp. 338–357). Malden, MA: Blackwell Publishing.

Rubin, K. H., Bukowski, W., & Parker, J. G. (1998). Peer interactions, relationships, and groups. In W. Damon (ed), *Handbook of Child Psychology: Vol. 3. Social, Emotional, and Personality Development* (pp. 619–700). New York: Wiley.

Rutter, M., & Sroufe, L. A. (2000). Developmental psychopathology: concepts and challenges. *Development and Psychopathology Special Issue: Reflecting on the Past and Planning for the Future of Developmental Psychopathology*, *12*, 265–296.

Schneider, W. J., Cavell, T. A., & Hughes, J. N. (2003). A sense of containment: potential moderator of the relation between parenting practices and children's externalizing behaviors. *Development and Psychopathology*, *15*, 96–117.

Schultz, D., Izard, C. E., & Bear, G. (2004). Children's emotion processing: relations to emotionality and aggression. *Development and Psychopathology*, *16*, 371–387.

Seagrave, D., & Grisso, T. (2002). Adolescent development and the measurement of juvenile psychopathy. *Law and Human Behavior*, *26*, 219–239.

Shaw, D. S., Gilliom, M., Ingoldsby, E. M., & Nagin, D. S. (2003). Trajectories leading to school-age conduct problems. *Developmental Psychology*, *39*, 189–200.

Shields, A., & Cicchetti, D. (1998). Reactive aggression among maltreated children: the contributions of attention and emotion dysregulation. *Journal of Clinical Child Psychology*, *27*, 381–395.

Silverthorn, P., & Frick, P. J. (1999). Developmental pathways to antisocial behavior: the delayed-onset pathway in girls. *Development and Psychopathology*, *11*, 101–126.

Stafford, E., & Cornell, D. G. (2003). Psychopathy scores predict adolescent inpatient aggression. *Assessment*, *10*, 102–112.

Stevens, D., Charman, T., & Blair, R. J. R. (2001). Recognition of emotion in facial expressions and vocal tones in children with psychopathic tendencies. *The Journal of Genetic Psychology*, *162*, 201–211.

Stouthamer-Loeber, M., Loeber, R., Wei, E., Farrington, D. P., & Wikström, P. H. (2002). Risk and promotive effects in the explanation of persistent serious delinquency in boys. *Journal of Consulting and Clinical Psychology*, *70*, 111–123.

Thomas, A., & Chess, S. (1977). *Temperament and Development*. New York: University Press.

Tremblay, R. E., Pihl, R. O., Vitaro, F., & Dobkin, P. L. (1994). Predicting early onset of male antisocial behavior from preschool behavior. *Archives of General Psychiatry*, *51*, 732–739.

Turkheimer, E., & Waldron, M. (2000). Nonshared environment: a theoretical, methodological, and quantitative review. *Psychological Bulletin*, *126*, 78–108.

Van Zeijl, J., Mesman, J., Stolk, M. W., Alink, L. R. A., van IJzendoorn, M. H., Bakermans-Krunenburg, M. J., *et al.* (2007). Differential susceptibility to discipline: the moderating effect of child temperament on the association between maternal discipline and early childhood externalizing problems. *Journal of Family Psychology*, *21*, 626–636.

Vermeiren, R. (2003). Psychopathology and delinquency in adolescents: a descriptive and developmental perspective. *Clinical Psychology Review*, *23*, 277–318.

Viding, E., Frick, P. J., & Plomin, R. (2007). Aetiology of the relationship between callous-unemotional traits and conduct problems in childhood. *British Journal of Psychiatry*, *190*(suppl 49), s33–s38.

Waschbusch, D. A., Carrey, N. J., Willoughby, M. T., King, S., & Andrade, B. F. (2007). Effects of methylphenidate and behavior modification on the social and academic behavior of children with disruptive behavior disorders: the moderating role of callous/unemotional traits. *Journal of Clinical Child and Adolescent Psychology*, *36*, 629–644.

Waschbusch, D. A., Walsh, T. M., Andrade, B. F., King, S., & Carrey, N. J. (2007). Social problem-solving, conduct problems, and callous-unemotional traits in children. *Child Psychiatry and Human Development*, *37*, 293–305.

Webster-Stratton, C., Reid, M. J., & Hammond, M. (2004). Treating children with early-onset conduct problems: intervention outcomes for parent, child, and teacher training. *Journal of Clinical Child and Adolescent Psychology*, *33*, 105–124.

Wootton, J. M., Frick, P. J., Shelton, K. K., & Silverthorn, P. (1997). Ineffective parenting and childhood conduct problems: the moderating role of callous-unemotional traits. *Journal of Consulting and Clinical Psychology*, *65*, 301–308.

5

Aggression in young children with concurrent callous-unemotional traits: Can the neurosciences inform progress and innovation in treatment approaches?

Mark R. Dadds and Tracy Rhodes

Introduction

Violence and antisocial behaviour (VAB) are a consistent and central feature of human history. Approaches to understanding their causes, manifestations, and remediation cover all aspects of human endeavour: religious, sociological, medical, legal, and ethological. The focus of this chapter is the use of the emerging tools of neuroscience and psychology to present a speculative discussion of one particular type of VAB: the individualistic type that characterizes the life histories of a small but significant number of people, usually males, in all societies. By this, we mean a chronic pattern of self-interested behaviour that offends the rights of and thus causes harm to other people, and society in general.

The natural history of this behavioural pattern is quite well known (Loeber & Farrington, 2000): it usually begins early in life as repetitive oppositional behaviour, impulsivity, and aggression in the child, with his environments typified by violence and instability. Across the years, he progresses through a series of predictable milestones such as school failure, drug use, and criminal involvement, developing a pattern that once established is largely intractable to the efforts of our juvenile justice and psychiatric systems. Thanks to decades of research, we also know a lot about how to best identify and manage these problems, as a lot is known about how, when, and why interventions work and do not work. The first subsection will briefly review evidence for the effectiveness of current interventions. As will be shown, there are well-characterized and evaluated interventions that can successfully remediate and prevent early pathways into VAB. We also have a wealth of information about when these interventions fail to produce change. This will lead us to a discussion, necessarily speculative, about whether the rapid progress being made in the neurobiology of VAB can help inform the development of new approaches to help us when the traditional interventions fail.

First to the successful treatments; put simply, parenting is the 'clean water' of mental health and parenting interventions are the 'clean water' of child psychiatry. Early identification of VAB (i.e., roughly before adolescence) that leads to effective engagement of the families, of such children, into best-practice services, can and does lead to positive change in a large proportion of cases (Serketich & Dumas, 1996). There is little point in reviewing the literature in support of this claim here, as decades of research have lead to several review papers and a number of meta-analyses. Overall, this literature shows that parenting interventions focused on teaching parents how to positively engage with their child and promote prosocial behaviour, and effectively reduce aggression and antisocial behaviour using non-violent, sensitive discipline strategies, are the treatment of choice for the early emergence of VAB.

The science of these parenting interventions began in the 1960s when pioneers such as Gerry Patterson, John Reid, Robert Wahler, and Rex Forehand applied the operant learning theory to understand how parents' and children's behaviour shapes and maintains each other's aggressive versus prosocial behaviour. The idea of 'coercive family process' in which aggressive loops become self-sustaining (Patterson, 1982) is arguably one of the great ideas of the 20th century in the behavioural sciences. Importantly, these researchers showed empirically that programmed changes in parental responding led to reliable and clinically significant changes in child behaviour. From the 1980s onwards, treatments were packaged into readily disseminated modules that have spread all over the world and have considerable empirical support in efficacy and effectiveness trials-for example, the Incredible Years (Webster-Stratton, 1998), Triple P (Sanders & Turner, 2005), and Multisystemic Therapy (Henggeler, 1999), just to name a few. It is difficult to overstate the conclusion, coming from research across all major continents of the world, that these interventions represent one of the major achievements of the mental health sciences.

There are three important riders to this conclusion. First is the issue of 'reach'. Many children and their families do not access these best-practice services (Turner & Sanders, 2006). The reasons for this are many, including unavailability of local services and expertise, family alienation from the health-care system, and chaotic families that are not consistent in attendance and tend to drop out. Consequently, an important focus of current clinical research and service development is to maximize the extent to which high-risk children are afforded effective services. To date, there are several lineages of such research. Of particular note is the creative application of public health models of service delivery to these parenting interventions (Prinz & Sanders, 2007). At the other extreme, even simple solutions such as telephoning parents to prompt their attendance at appointments can improve engagement rates in parents of VAB children (Watt *et al.*, 2007).

The second rider is that families of children showing early signs of VAB are often beset with a range of other mental health and social problems. Reviews, such as by Miller and Prinz (1990), have documented the common co-occurrence of interparental violence and discord, depression, substance abuse problems, social isolation, and poverty that pose direct threats to our ability to engage and produce change in parent-child processes and outcomes. The main challenge, and one that the behavioural sciences has not shied from, is to integrate the parenting interventions into broader clinical approaches. The primary aim of these interventions is to address the multiple problems of many of these families without producing cluttered, cumbersome interventions that are impossible to implement except by the most skilled and motivated clinicians. Again, there are many examples of empirically supported programmes that specifically provide clinical strategies for managing complex systems of family problems associated with VAB in young children (e.g., Henggeler & Borduin, 1990; Sanders & Turner, 2005; Dadds & Hawes, 2006).

The third rider is one that has received relatively little attention and thus will be the main focus of this chapter. Although much effort is underway to parse the heterogeneous population of aggressive children into more sensible subgroupings, they are still treated as a unity with respect to best possible treatments. Given that parent training literature arose from within a social learning perspective, it is not surprising that the traits of the children themselves attracted little attention. Recent evidence suggests, however, that child factors are predictive of outcomes; further, there appears to a small proportion of children who do not appear to benefit from the receipt of our best available services.

For example, Hawes and Dadds (2005) recently showed that young oppositional boys with a 'cold' temperamental form of aggression (callous-unemotional traits, CU) did not benefit from improvements in parenting relative to their 'hot' peers. In this study, a sample of boys from 3 to 8 years of age were treated using a standardized parenting intervention and measures were taken before, after, and at 6 months follow-up. As a group, the parents and their sons showed a typical no-diagnosis rate of about 60% at the completion of treatment. Having high CU traits was a unique predictor of poor response to treatment even after controlling for parenting and family characteristics, socio-economic status, parents' implementation of the programme, and other characteristics of the child. Direct observations of the parent-child interactions in the home showed that the only variable differentiating the high-CU group were their responsiveness to the 'time-out' procedure. When removed from ongoing interactions and placed in a quiet area due to aggression or antisocial behaviour, these children showed little emotion and their parents rated this particular procedure as less effective than the parents' of low-CU children.

This observation squares well with literature showing that high-CU children are generally less emotional, less influenced by parenting, and more likely to have a genetic basis to both the CU traits and their aggressive/antisocial behaviour (see Chapter 4). More generally, it exemplifies that there are specific traits that characterize and differentiate children's problems into groups that may have very different aetiologies and thus require different treatment approaches. There can be no doubt that the future will see increasing differentiation of VAB children into meaningful subgroups, but at present the dichotomy of VAB children into high- versus low-CU traits is receiving considerable support for its predictive validity and will be used throughout the rest of this chapter. Given the high genetic loading for VAB in the high-CU subgroup (Viding et al., 2005), it is likely that neurobiological markers may be more evident. In what follows, we will first ask what is it about high-CU traits that make them more immune to parenting. This will take us into the fascinating area of emotion processing. We will also review animal models of early bioparenting interactions, and we will speculate about how specific patterns of disturbance might be targeted using combined or synergistic biological and behavioural procedures. Two examples of emerging work will be drawn upon to illustrate this potential: oxytocin (OT) in attachment processes and cycloserine in fear learning.

Emotion processing and CU traits in children

Analysing how people respond to emotional faces has become a major tool in the neurosciences: the emotional face is a 'superstimulus' (e.g., Tinbergen, 1951) that automatically sets off specific neural systems that are central to our emotional and interpersonal lives. There is increasing evidence that neural and behavioural responses to emotional stimuli, specifically emotional faces, differ between healthy people and those with various forms of psychopathology. There is also some evidence that specific responses to particular emotions (e.g., fear versus anger versus happiness) can differentiate between various forms of psychopathology such as bipolar disorder, depression, anxiety, and aggression (e.g., Guyer et al., 2007; Leist & Dadds, in press).

Of particular interest to us is that adult psychopaths, those with 'cold' forms of VAB, and even children with psychopathic tendencies are hyporesponsive to emotional faces, particularly those displaying fear (see Blair, 2003 for a review): that is, they show deficits in recognizing fear on other's faces, as well as diminished behavioural and visceral responses to these stimuli. Recent studies with adult psychopaths have shown diminished responses in the amygdala to such stimuli by using functional magnetic resonance imaging (fMRI) mapping (Deeley *et al.*, 2006). Systems within the amygdala modulate attention and responsiveness to emotionally salient stimuli, and form links between cues and salient outcomes. One of the most reliable ways of eliciting a response in the amygdala is to present a fearful face. Although the amygdala is responsive to any emotionally salient cue, it is highly reactive to the configuration of widened eyes with the whites enlarged as seen in fear (Fox & Damjanovic, 2006).

Why would psychopathy and indeed children with CU traits be associated with deficits in recognizing fear? Can this finding help inform how best to help these children? Adolphs and colleagues (2005) have conducted extensive work on the neural bases of fear blindness. In particular, they showed that fear blindness in an amygdala-damaged patient is due to neglect of the eye region: unlike healthy people, the patient fails to naturally attend to the most emotionally salient aspects of the environment, in this case the eyes of other people. Interestingly, he also showed that this deficit could be overcome by asking the subject to look at the eyes of the target face: there was no problem recognizing fear once the relevant data were accessed.

Could fear recognition deficits in children with high psychopathy traits also be due to attentional problems? A recent study found that adolescent high-CU males showed the expected deficits in fear recognition, but that these disappeared when the participants were asked specifically to 'look at the eyes' of the stimulus faces (Dadds *et al.*, 2006). When asked to 'look at the mouth' of the stimulus faces, their deficits in fear recognition returned. These findings suggest that children with high-CU traits have problems with the allocation of attention to critically salient aspects of the environment similar to those with fear blindness due to amygdala damage.

In a follow-up study, Dadds *et al.* (2008), used computerized eye tracking to measure gaze characteristics of young males while viewing a series of emotional faces. The results showed the CU traits were associated with deficits in the attention given to salient emotional aspects of the environment, in this case other people's eyes. This deficit is one of the reasons that people with high psychopathy have trouble recognizing fear, the emotion that is uniquely associated with communication via the eyes. The study also shows that the deficit is present at least as early as adolescence.

The eyes of course can be regarded as 'superstimuli' (Tinbergen, 1951) to humans and in healthy people sets off various automatic processes, perhaps the most basic of which is immediate attention. This automatic attention to the eyes of other people occurs very early in the newborn child and is intricately involved in attachment processes and the development of many human qualities such as the development of empathy and theory of mind (e.g., see Skuse, 2003). What happens when a child lacks the automatic tendency to focus on the eyes of others? The answer to this is not fully known but there are good reasons to believe that the deficit will interfere with parent-child bonding, depriving the child of the building blocks for the development of empathic concern, and specifically, all but only the most superficial information about the consequences of his or her behaviour on other people.

Blair (2003) has presented a number of models of how deficits in fear recognition may signal a failure of violence-inhibition mechanisms. That is, mammals will generally inhibit aggression once a conspecific demonstrates submission. If one cannot recognize submission or distress, it is likely that the aggression will arise and continue unmodulated. We feel that the explanatory strength of this model will increase when couched in a developmentally precise context. That is, as well as representing a failure to inhibit aggression, failure to attend to critical emotional cues will compromise the development of more complex human systems that require emotion recognition as a building block. Typical examples of this would be the development of attachment bonds, empathy, moral conscience, and theory of mind. Most of these building blocks are laid down in infancy.

Our knowledge of early attentional processes, neural function, and parent-child interactions is quite limited for the human; however, there is a lot to be learned by some of the exciting work currently being done using animal models. Specifically, these models show that there are critical periods, very early in life, in which the interactions between parenting and biological processes in the young animal are synergistic and productive of lifelong changes in the biological and behavioural propensities of the mammal. To fully appreciate this work, we need to first introduce two neurobiological systems that are known to play a role in VAB. As we will see, there is emerging evidence that the cortisol and serotonergic systems may function differently in emotionally reactive versus high-CU children with VAB.

HPA axis function differentiates subtypes of VAB and is responsive to early parenting

Information about the role of the hypothalamic-pituitary-adrenal (HPA) axis in mental health is primitive yet promising, and there is clear evidence that the system plays a role in the development and expression of VAB (van Goozen et al., 2007) Further, its role is intimately linked with the history and quality of parenting the child has received, and its specific patterns of disturbance may help us understand the 'hot' versus 'cold' expressions of VAB in young children. The following focuses on two key aspects of HPA functioning: the cortisol and serotinergic systems and their relationship to early parenting experiences.

Cortisol is a hormone involved in stress response modulation and is a rough marker of stress reactivity in humans and rats (as corticosteroids). In people who have suffered acute stress (trauma sufferers) and those who are highly reactive to challenges (high-anxious people), cortisol levels are generally elevated. Of interest, low cortisol is a marker of people with high and chronic levels of VAB, especially the 'cold' or high-CU traits subset. This has been found in adult perpetrators of violent crimes and 'psychopaths' (see van Goozen et al., 2007), and children with 'psychopathic' traits (Loney et al., 2006). This finding is typically interpreted within a broad understanding that psychopaths are fearless and not perturbed by the outcomes of their behaviour and effects on other people. Recent animal models, however, indicate that there is a lot more to be learned about cortisol in early learning and about threat and the interpersonal attachment systems in which this learning occurs.

The first example comes from the innovative work of Sullivan and colleagues (e.g., Moriceau & Sullivan, 2005). All young mammals will naturally seek out and remain centred around the nest and the mother. Pairing the smells of the mother and/or nest with an aversive stimulus produces radically different effects depending on the age of the pup. After approximately 9–12 days of age, a pup that associates the nest with discomfort will show avoidance; before that time, the opposite occurs. Strong associations between the nest odours and discomfort will ironically lead to increased preference for the nest. Around this time, the amygdala of the pup undergoes rapid growth and this change is dependent on the activation of corticosterone (or cortisol in humans) in the system at that time. Thus, with sufficient cortisol, amygdala functioning emerges and is associated with learning to recognize and avoid aversive stimuli in the environment. Dysfunction of the cortisol systems associated with hypoamygdala responsiveness leads to an organism that exhibits diminished registration and avoidance of aversive stimuli. Taken together, this shows remarkable parallels to the characteristics of the low-CU or psychopathy subset of VAB.

Other work has shown more directly the important role of serotonin (5-HTT [5-hydroxy-tryptamine]) and cortisol in the development of normal versus 'cold' aggression. Haller *et al.* (2005) found that, in rats, there is an inverse relationship between activation of serotonergic systems (5-HTT neurons in the dorsal raphe nucleus) and attacks on non-vulnerable targets (offensive or normal aggression), which is consistent with an inhibitory influence of 5-HTT on aggression. In contrast, these systems appear unrelated to attacks on vulnerable targets (abnormal predatory aggression). Similarly, lesions of various serotonergic systems modulate offensive but not predatory aggression (de Bruin *et al.*, 1983). In humans, it is well known that serotonergic medication can be used to reduce 'emotional' or 'hot' aggression in certain personality disorders but has little or no effect on aggression in chronic offenders. Haller *et al.* (2005) suggested that the reduced influence of the serotonergic system in cold aggression could be due to the overriding effects of central amygdala activation or changes in prefrontal cortical functioning. Alternatively, it is possible that low glucocorticoid secretion impairs the functioning of the 5-HTT system, which explains the low efficacy of this system in controlling aggression under these circumstances.

Various authors have argued that 5-HTT stabilizes information processing in various neural systems, resulting in controlled behavioural, affective, and cognitive output. Spoont (1992) argues that high levels of 5-HTT lead to excessive restraint, cognitive inflexibility, and anxiety whereas low levels lead to disinhibition and distractibility. Coccaro *et al.* (1997) proposed that the threshold for aggressive reactions is modulated by overall serotonergic system function: low function may disinhibit aggression (to self and others) by lowering thresholds to stimuli that elicit irritation and aggression and blunting sensitivity to cues that signal punishment (Spoont, 1992).

Of particular interest to this chapter is that there is emerging data to show that 5-HTT manipulations may directly influence facial emotion processing. As noted, it is well known that serotonergic agents can stabilize mood and thus reduce irritable aggression in people with various forms of mood and personality problems. Merens *et al.* (2007) reviewed empirical evidence that the effects of 5-HTT on mood are mediated by specific changes in emotional information processing. They present clear evidence that even short-term manipulations of 5-HTT levels produce reliable changes in responses to emotional faces, including recognition skills, and that these are particularly evident for fear faces. The specific direction of change was predicted by the pre-existing levels of psychopathology in the subjects, their baseline skills in emotion recognition, and whether the 5-HTT effects were measured immediately or over longer courses of treatment. This work is important in showing that common mood stabilizers might in part work by changing basic emotion recognition processes. Although provocative, the review reported no such research with children and no focus on aggression.

Although the exact determinants of various forms of aggression are likely to involve multiple interacting biological and behavioural systems, the preceding examples show that differentiating cold versus hot aggression by serotonergic versus cortisol systems has support across multiple research methods and species. The main advantage of Sullivan *et al.*'s (see Moriceau & Sullivan, 2005) and Haller *et al.*'s (2005) animal models is that they show that experimentally induced changes in these systems lead directly to the changes in stimulus preferences and aggression, respectively. Therefore, these changes are more than just correlational artefacts of an overwhelmingly complex system. In natural development, complex interactions of various systems are likely to be the rule. For example, serotonergic function interacts with testosterone through puberty. Keleta *et al.* (2007) assessed the interactive effects of chronic anabolic androgenic steroid (T) exposure and brain 5-HTT depletion on aggression in pubertal male rats. The 5-HTT depletion resulted in significantly decreased locomotor activity and increased irritability but had no effect on sexual behaviour, partner preference, or aggression. T alone had no effect on locomotion, irritability, or sexual behaviour but increased partner preference and aggression. The most striking effect of combining T and depletion was a significant increase in attack frequency as well as a significant decrease in the latency to attack, particularly following physical provocation. Similarly, in humans, Popma *et al.* (2007) showed that cortisol moderates the relationship between testosterone and aggression in VAB boys such that low cortisol amplifies the relationship of testosterone to vert aggression through this critical period.

So, can these models be related back to parenting and the young child at risk of VAB? Baby rhesus monkeys suffering high rates of maternal rejection and abuse in their first month of life often produce less 5-HTT and these effects can come to characterize families through generations. In a study conducted by Maestripieri *et al.* (2006), the effects of maternal behaviour on brain 5-HTT in the offspring were observed in both infants that were reared by their genetic mothers and infants reared by foster mothers. Infants who became abusive as adults had about 10–20% less 5-HTT than did infants who did not become abusive as parents or infants who were not exposed to maternal abuse.

It is interesting that in most of the animal models, the age at which the effects are brought about is critical; however, once established, the effects remain remarkably constant throughout adulthood (e.g., Maestripieri *et al.*, 2006; Kaffman & Meaney, 2007). Through childhood, however, variations in the system of interest may be the rule. Given that out treatments are generally aimed at preventing the problem from becoming a permanent feature, understanding its early course is a priority. In one of the few longitudinal studies of serotonergic function, Auerbach *et al.* (1999) categorized children according to their polymorphisms of the 5-HTT transporter promoter gene (*5-HTTLPR*) and assessed emotional reactivity through the first year of life. At 2 months of age, infants possessing the short/short (s/s) alleles of *5-HTTLPR* (low 5-HTT) received higher scores on the negative emotionality and distress to limitations scales than those infants possessing the short/long (s/l) or long/long (l/l) alleles. At 12 months, the association reversed: infants with the s/s alleles did not show more negative emotionality and actually scored significantly lower on measured behaviours such as intensity of facial fear, intensity of escape behaviour, and active escape manoeuvres. The authors speculate that these changes are likely due to complex bioenvironmental interactions in which early emotionality may elicit more concern and attention from their caregivers, which in turn helped these infants to become able to best regulate their own behavioural arousal or distress.

Although this is speculative, it is consistent with the finding of developmental change in behavioural characteristics associated with high vagal tone. High vagal tone in early infancy is related to higher distress and negative reactivity, whereas by 14 months, high vagal tone can reverse and be associated with positive outcomes of sociability and ease of approach (Calkins & Fox, 1992). Similarly, Sullivan's (see Moriceau & Sullivan, 2005) demonstration of critical period reversal in cortisol-dependent associative learning in the rat pup again alerts us that timing is crucial in understanding the important interactions between biological development and the parenting environment.

One of the dramatic demonstrations of the effects of parenting on lifelong changes in biological vulnerability comes from Meany's work on the nurturance and epigenetics of brain development (e.g., see Kaffman & Meaney, 2007). His initial work showed that natural variations in the degree to which mother rats lick and groom their offspring produce important changes in the behaviour of pups. Over the years, his impressive body of literature has expanded to where we now know that environmental adversity results in chained patterns of parent-offspring interactions, and low levels of nurturance (licking and grooming) increase stress reactivity in the pup through sustained effects on gene expression in brain regions known to regulate behavioural, endocrine, and autonomic responses to stress. Although such effects might be adaptive, the associated cost involves an increased risk of stress-related illness (see Parent *et al.*, 2005 for a review).

In conclusion, we have seen in this subsection that the neurobiology of VAB varies according to the type of aggression: the distinction between hot and cold (or callous-unemotional in humans?) maps nicely onto distinctions between serotonergic- and cortisol-dependent functions. Put simply, in both humans and animals, there is clear evidence that serotonergic dysregulation appears to be related to decreased thresholds for explosive violence, whereas low cortisol appears to be associated with colder more predatory violence associated with low capacity for fear, aversive conditioning (or punishment insensitivity; see Dadds & Salmon, 2004), and probably associated with diminished amygdala involvement in attention and responsiveness to emotionally salient stimuli. These relationships are unlikely to be linear; rather, complex interrelationships between hormonal and neurobiological agents (e.g., testosterone and 5-HTT) that occur at critical and sensitive periods of critical epigenetic and neural transcription (e.g., early nurturance and epigenetic changes to hippocampal development, testosterone and 5-HTT at puberty, cortisol and amygdala development in aversive attachment conditioning during days 6–12 in rat pups) will be the rule.

By way of linking this subsection on the biological underpinnings of hot versus cold aggression back to the earlier subsection on emotion recognition, recent research has linked genetics, serotonergic function, and emotion recognition using fMRI methods. As noted, adults with psychopathy show reduced amygdala activation when presented with fear faces and this is consistent with most theories of psychopathy as involving a core deficit in emotional responsiveness. Although not 'psychopathic', men who have suffered early childhood abuse and violence and have the short polymorphisms of the monoamine oxidase A (MAOA) gene associated with low serotonergic function are at risk of chronic antisocial behaviour (Caspi *et al.*, 2002). However, these men show hyperresponsiveness of the amygdala to fear faces in fMRI studies (see Meyer-Lindenberg & Zink, 2007). These findings bring current findings about the genetics of VAB into the equation relating to responsiveness of the amygdala as a marker of 'cold' and 'hot' forms of VAB.

It should be noted that the preceding discussion does not lead us to the obvious corollary that interventions that directly modify serotonergic and cortisol function may help with VAB. Unfortunately, medications for diminished serotonergic and cortisol function are intensive and intrusive in that they require long-term daily use and are characterized by variable side effects, and there is little evidence to suggest that they reduce aggressive behaviour in antisocial populations. Although serotonergic drugs are used in adolescents and sometimes children, primarily for depression and behavioural problems related to mood instability, they offer little in the way of a general intervention for the early development of VAB except for extreme cases of explosive aggression. More potential might be realized, however, should we learn more about the conditions, both behavioural and biological, that are associated with healthy serotonergic and cortisol function.

Implications for the development of innovative interventions

The preceding discussion leads us back to the question of whether interventions can produce positive changes in children's attention to and understanding of the emotional environment directly through the HPA and neural systems that support these functions, and the environment that shapes their expression. There are several promising indications.

In terms of behavioural interventions, it has been shown that simply directing people's attention to emotionally significant stimuli does alter their registration and understanding of these stimuli (Dadds *et al.*, 2006); it is unlikely, however, that this could lead to any long-term gains without some other powerful changes in place. When adults with autism are trained to attend to and interpret emotional faces, their accuracy levels increase and compensatory changes in neural activity, measured via fMRI, are observed (Bölte *et al.*, 2006). Thus, in the short term at least, there is evidence that targeted training in reading emotions does lead to change.

With children, it is likely that such changes would have the best impact if timed to coincide with relevant developmental changes and placed in the context of ongoing parent-child interactions. Recent work on emotion talk between children and their attachment figures has shown that children's understanding of the emotional world and their own emotions can be enhanced by training parents to regularly engage their offspring in conversational reviews of day-to-day emotional events. The impact of these interventions have so far been demonstrated in healthy (Reese & Newcombe, 2007) and clinically referred children (Salmon *et al.*, submitted), but data on the impact of the interventions on mental health are yet to be gathered.

Emotional attention and understanding can also be altered biochemically. Animal research has shown that the neuropeptide oxytocin (OT) enhances social recognition and approach behaviour, while decreasing social avoidance and aggression (Lim & Young, 2006). These findings have led some (Bartz & Hollander, 2006) to suggest that OT may have a role in the enhancement and treatment of relationships (i.e., parent-child bonds, couple distress), and the amelioration of disorders characterized by social deficits (i.e., autism, schizophrenia). Emerging research with humans has shown that OT nasal administration (24–27 IU) enhances trust (Kosfeld *et al.*, 2005), identification of emotions in the eyes of others (Domes *et al.*, 2007), the benefits of social support during social stress tasks (Heinrichs *et al.*, 2003), and reduced responsiveness to social threat stimuli (Kirsch *et al.*, 2005). For example, in the study by Domes *et al.* (2007), 30 males received OT (24 IU) or a placebo before tests of one's ability to read subtle facial cues of internal emotion states. OT participants were better able to infer the emotional state of the actors and effects were stronger for faces rated difficult to read. The authors argued that one possible mechanism underlying this effect was OT enhancement of eye gaze during face perception. Of relevance is that face perception is a basic process in interpersonal communication (Haxby *et al.*, 2002). Critical information is taken from the eyes, and to a lesser extent the mouth, where individuals assess the degree of interest, threat, and emotion of another (Haxby *et al.*, 2000, 2002; Domes *et al.*, 2007). In fact, amount of eye gaze has been found to be predictive of one's ability to interpret the intentions of others and the meaning of social situations (Klin *et al.*, 2002; Garrett *et al.*, 2004; Spezio *et al.*, 2007).

A recent study suggests eye-gaze enhancement is one mechanism that may be associated with improved face perception and interpersonal communication from OT administration. Guastella, Mitchell and Dadds (2008) showed that a single dose of nasal spray OT increased eye gaze to the eye region of other people's faces. Disorders characterized by deficits in communication and emotion perception, such as autism (Baron-Cohen *et al.*, 2001;

Klin *et al.*, 2002; Dalton *et al.*, 2005), schizophrenia (Loughland *et al.*, 2002), and fragile X syndrome (Garrett *et al.*, 2004), and of particular interest, psychopathic traits in young people (Dadds *et al.*, 2006) are associated with deficits in face perception and eye gaze. OT may have therapeutic value in the treatment of these disorders. Interestingly, the direction to focus attention towards the eyes in disordered populations ameliorates some emotion-perception deficits (Dadds *et al.*, 2006). Clearly, OT has the potential to be used in interventions that aim to alleviate social attachment and communication deficits.

The missing part of this research is the consideration of possible synergies between biochemical and behavioural interventions. Emotional training improves attention to and understanding of the emotional world, as does OT administration. What would result from carefully targeted interactions between the two? If OT improves some aspects of autism, what would happen if it was administered during training on emotion-recognition tasks or better, during intensive interactions with a loving caregiver, or during training on emotion-recognition tasks? We argue that a key direction of this research should be to explore how such interventions can be integrated into caregiving relationships at sensitive developmental periods for children with specified deficits in emotion processing, such as the aforementioned children with CU traits and VAB.

There are precious few examples of the targeted use of bioagents to enhance specific psychological experiences. We are unaware of any synergistic biobehavioural interventions currently available for VAB in young people. Thus, we will draw an example from another area: one of the more exciting developments of recent years has been the potential of biobehavioural synergy as exemplified by the use of D-cycloserine (DCS) in fear learning. Although we are not claiming this has direct relevance to the treatment of VAB, we finish by putting this forward as a positive example of this emerging line of thinking.

Interacting biological and behavioural systems: the example of DCS
Pavlovian conditioning studies have shown that the partial N-methyl-D-aspartate (NMDA) agonist DCS facilitates the extinction of learned fear in animals when administered immediately before or even shortly after extinction training (Richardson, Ledgerwood, Cranney, 2004). It appears that DCS strengthens extinction memories so they may be more easily retrieved during subsequent exposures to fear-relevant cues. When DCS is administered chronically to patients over weeks and months, it has no effect on symptoms of anxiety (Heresco-Levy *et al.*, 2002). When administered acutely in combination with psychological extinction-based procedures, however, it may enhance treatment outcome in height phobic (Ressler *et al.*, 2004), social phobic (Hofmann *et al.*, 2006; Guastella, Dadds *et al.*, 2008), and obsessive compulsive (Kushner *et al.*, 2007) patients (cf: two negative results with non-clinic subjects; Guastella, Dadds *et al.*, 2007; Guastella, Lovibond *et al.*, 2007).

Overall, this research supports a radical new approach to the treatment of psychological disorders that enhances the adaptive learning that occurs in therapy via medication. That is, DCS has effects that are specific to emotionally significant learning experiences. This represents one of the first demonstrations of targeted biological-behavioural interactions in the remediation of behavioural disorders. It is not a huge leap to imagine that the future will see the development of more of these synergistic interventions: that is, medications are used in short bursts during prescribed psychological experiences. What would happen if OT was administered to children who then experienced a targeted period of intense love and attachment with a responsive caregiver? How might the acute normalization of cortisol functioning affect a child who was undergoing a prescribed series of positive experiences with emotionally significant scenarios?

These imagined interventions raise many questions, not the least of which are aesthetic and ethical, as do all fruitful innovations in science. For instance, how could we work to improve attachment bonds with parents that are absent, emotionally disturbed, or abusive? How palatable is it to society, let alone the specific parents and children, to be directly modifying the mechanics of attachment? Ultimately, the value of these will probably lie in the psychological context in which they are applied. That is, the use of medications for directly stopping VAB is ethically odious, even forgetting its low acceptability and, thus, low impact value. It is a different matter, however, if medications could be applied acutely to enhance experiences that we know instinctively and scientifically to be 'good'-that is, psychologically healthy. Examples of this are facing and overcoming fears, communicating affection and understanding with loved ones and trusted caregivers, and learning to understand and care about the emotions of other people.

Implications for specific parenting strategies
We would like to end by discussing the preceding with reference to the specific parenting strategies that are the centrepiece of available parenting interventions for early signs of VAB. As noted, these interventions fall into two broad categories: positive parent-child engagement and reward strategies in which parents are helped to establish positive engagement with their child and deliberately reward prosocial behaviour, and a non-violent discipline strategy for responding to instances of child VAB. The most common strategy used for the latter is 'time-out' in child instances of VAB, resulting in the child being temporarily removed from any reward for the aggression. Traditionally, these techniques were developed and continue to be interpreted within the operant theory: that is, rewards are used to increase prosocial behaviour and time-out to reduce problem behaviour. The operant aspects of these procedures, however, are only the tip of the iceberg and many writers now invoke ideas from attachment and self-regulation theories to better characterize their implementation (e.g., Dadds & Hawes, 2006). Clearly, any move to better understand the specific nature of the patterns of disturbance seen for problem children can lead to a rethinking of how these strategies can be best employed.

In this regard, we have been particularly interested in how these strategies work with 'hot' versus 'cold' variants of VAB. Our research has shown first that reward strategies are rated as effective with both variants (Hawes & Dadds, 2005). Time-out, however, appears to be less effective with 'cold' children (Hawes *et al.*, 2005; see also Dadds & Salmon, 2004 for a review of the idea of 'punishment insensitivity'). As noted, these children are insensitive to emotional stimuli and tend to be less outwardly perturbed by time-out (Hawes & Dadds, 2005). On the other hand, 'hot' children become outwardly quite emotional during discipline.

Our clinical work and the findings referred to here lead us to propose the following corollaries for the use of the time-out technique. Hot children may be particularly sensitive to threat cues, and the reason for implementing time-out is often interpersonal in nature (an argument); allowing the emotion to escalate before implementing time-out is problematic. More specifically, during the instructions for the child to go to time-out, close and direct eye contact from the parent can lead to acutely elevated stress responses and result in escalation and aggression from the child. We are careful with these children to advise parents to avoid 'getting in the child's face' too much, and especially to avoid aggressive facial emotion and eye contact.

On the other hand, 'cold' children are more likely to come into conflict due to inappropriate reward seeking behaviour, and are unlikely to attend to the salient emotional aspects of the time-out procedure. Taken together, this literature indicates that increasing emotional salience and indeed close eye contact should increase the chances of a positive outcome for these children. We find that getting very close to the child and calmly attempting to make direct eye contact actually has the positive and opposite effect of focusing the 'cold' child on what should be the salient aspect of the situation, rather than the inappropriate reward they are so often seeking at the expense of others.

This is one simple example of how more precise delineation of the child's pattern of disturbance can lead to new ways of thinking about even our most well-established strategies. We expect that the next several years will see increasing precision brought to the specific strategies that can be used to help children and parents learn alternatives to aggression.

In summary, this chapter started with the empirically supported idea that parenting interventions offer the best clinical and public health solution to early onset aggression and antisocial behaviour in children. Unfortunately, there are systemic-, family-, and child-level factors that are associated with poorer outcomes for these children. We focused on the least well researched of these: characteristics of children that predict chronic antisocial behaviour and poor treatment responses. We argued that rapid progress is being made in the developmental neurosiences of aggression, and we reviewed a number of examples of human and animal models that help us think more precisely about the development of aggression and its treatment. Hopefully, this chapter may help inspire growth in the cross-fertilization between bourgeoning neurosciences of VAB and the clinical sciences responsible for working with these children.

Acknowledgements

The authors thank John Brennan, David Hawes, Subodha Wimalaweera, and Ana Lopes for their comments on a oratory presentation of this chapter, and collaboration in general. They also thank the Australian Research Council and the National Health and Medical Research Council of Australia for funding support.

References

Adolphs, R., Gosselin, F., Buchanan, T. W., Tranel, D., Schyns, P., & Damasio, A. (2005). A mechanism for impaired fear recognition after amygdala damage. *Nature*, *433*, 68–72.

Auerbach, J., Geller, V., Lezer, S., Shinwell, E., Belmaker, R. H., Levine, J., *et al.* (1999). Dopamine D4 receptor (*D4DR*) and serotonin transporter promoter (*5-HTTLPR*) polymorphisms in the determination of temperamental 2-month-old infants. *Molecular Psychiatry*, *4*, 369–373.

Baron-Cohen, S., Wheelwright, S., Hill, J., Raste, Y., & Plumb, I. (2001). The 'Reading the Mind in the Eyes' test, revised version: a study with normal adults, and adults with Asperger syndrome or high-functioning autism. *Journal of Child Psychology and Psychiatry*, *42*, 241–251.

Bartz, J. A., & Hollander, E. (2006). The neuroscience of affiliation: forging links between basic and clinical research on neuropeptides and social behavior. *Hormones and Behavior*, *50*(4), 518–528.

Blair, R. J. (2003). Neurobiological basis of psychopathy. *British Journal of Psychiatry*, *182*, 5–7.

Bölte, S., Hubl, D., Feineis-Matthews, S., Prvulovic, D., Dierks, T., & Poustka, F. (2006). Facial affect recognition training in autism: Can we animate the fusiform gyrus? *Behavioral Neuroscience*, *120*, 211–216.

Calkins, S., & Fox, N. (1992). The relations among infant temperament, security of attachment, and behavioral inhibition at twenty-four months. *Child Development*, *63*, 1456–1472.

Caspi, A., McClay, J., Moffitt, T. E., Mill, J., Martin, J., Craig, I. W., *et al.* (2002). Role of genotype in the cycle of violence in maltreated children. *Science*, *297*, 851–854.

Coccaro, E. F., Kavoussi, R. J., Trestman, R. L., Gabriel, S. M., Cooper, T. B., & Siever, L. J. (1997). 5-HTT function in human subjects: intercorrelations among central serotonin indices and aggressiveness. *Psychiatry Research, 73*, 1–14.

Dadds, M. R., El Masry, Y., Wimalaweera, S., & Guastella, A. J. (2008). Reduced eye gaze explains fear recognition deficits in psychopathy. *Journal of the American Academy of Child and Adolescent Psychiatry, 47*, 455–463.

Dadds, M. R., & Hawes, D. (2006). Integrated Family Intervention for Child Conduct Problems: *A Behaviour-Attachment-Systems Intervention for Parents*. Brisbane: Australian Academic Press.

Dadds, M. R., Perry, Y., Hawes, D. J., Merz, S., Riddell, A. C., Haines, D. J., et al. (2006). Look at the eyes: fear recognition in child psychopathy. *British Journal of Psychiatry, 189*, 180–181.

Dadds, M. R., & Salmon, K. (2003). Learning and temperament as alternate pathways to punishment insensitivity in antisocial children. *Clinical Child and Family Psychology Review, 6*, 69–86.

Dalton, K. M., Nacewicz, B. M., Johnstone, T., Schaefer, H. S., Gernsbacher, M. A., Goldsmith, H. H., et al. (2005). Gaze fixation and the neural circuitry of face processing in autism. *Nature Neuroscience, 8*(4), 519–526.

De Bruin, J. P., van Oyen, H. G., & van de Poll, N. (1983). Behavioural changes following lesions of the orbital prefrontal cortex in male rats. *Behavioral Brain Research, 10*(2/3), 209–232.

Deeley, Q., Daly, E., Surguladze, S., Tunstall, N., Mezey, G., Beer, D., et al. (2006). Facial emotion processing in criminal psychopathy: preliminary functional magnetic resonance imaging study. *British Journal of Psychiatry, 189*, 533–539.

Domes, G., Heinrichs, M., Michel, A., Berger, C., & Herpertz, S. (2007). Oxytocin improves 'mind reading' in humans. *Biological Psychiatry, 61*(5), 731–733.

Fox, E., & Damjanovic, L. (2006). The eyes are sufficient to produce a threat superiority effect. *Emotion, 6*, 534–539.

Garrett, A. S., Menon, V., MacKenzie, K., & Reiss, A. L. (2004). Here's looking at you, kid: neural systems underlying face and gaze processing in fragile X syndrome. *Archives of General Psychiatry, 61*, 281–288.

Guastella, A., Mitchell, P. B., & Dadds, M. R. (2008). Oxytocin increases gaze to the eye region of human faces. *Biological Psychiatry, 63*, 3–5.

Guastella, A. J., Dadds, M. R., Lovibond, P. F., Mitchell, P., & Richardson, R. (2007). A randomized controlled trial of the effect of D-Cycloserine on exposure therapy for spider fears. *Journal of Psychiatric Research, 41*, 466–471.

Guastella, A. J., Dadds, M. R., Richardson, R., Rapee, R. M., Gaston, J. E., Mitchell, P., et al. (2008). A randomised controlled trial of D-Cycloserine enhancement of CBT for social phobia. *Biological Psychiatry, 63*, 544–549.

Guastella, A. J., Lovibond, P. F., Dadds, M. R., Mitchell, P., & Richardson, R. (2007). A randomized controlled trial for the effect of D-Cycloserine on conditioning and extinction in humans. *Behaviour Research and Therapy, 45*(4), 663–672.

Guyer, E. A., McClure, B. E., Adler, D. A., Brotman, A. M., Rich, A. B., Kimes, S. A., et al. (2007). Specificity of facial expression labeling deficits in childhood psychopathology. *Journal of Child Psychology and Psychiatry and Allied Disciplines, 48*(9), 863–871.

Haller, J., Mikics, E., Halasz, J., & Toth, M. (2005). Mechanisms differentiating normal from abnormal aggression: glucocorticoids and serotonin. *European Journal of Pharmacology, 526*, 89–100.

Hawes, D. M., & Dadds, M. R. (2005). Callous-unemotional traits are a risk factor for poor treatment response in young conduct problem children. *Journal of Consulting and Clinical Psychology, 73*, 737–741.

Haxby, J. V., Hoffman, E. A., & Gobbini, M. I. (2000). The distributed human neural system for face perception. *Trends in Cognitive Science, 4*, 223–233.

Haxby, J. V., Hoffman, E. A., & Gobbini, M. I. (2002). Human neural systems for face recognition and social communication. *Biological Psychiatry, 51*, 59–67.

Heinrichs, M., Baumgartner, T., Kirschbaum, C., & Ehlert, U. (2003). Social support and oxytocin interact to suppress cortisol and subjective responses to psychosocial stress. *Biological Psychiatry, 54*(12), 1389–1398.

Henggeler, S. (1999). Multisystemic therapy: an overview of clinical procedures, outcomes and policy implications. *Child Psychology and Psychiatry Review, 4*(1), 2–10.

Henggeler, S., & Borduin, C. (1990). *Family Therapy and Beyond: A Multisystemic Approach to Treating the Behaviour Problems of Children and Adolescents.* Pacific Grove, CA: Brooks Cole.

Heresco-Levy, U., Kremer, I., Javitt, D. C., Goichman, R., Reshef, A., Blanaru, M., *et al.* (2002). Pilot-controlled trial of D-cycloserine for the treatment of post-traumatic stress disorder. *The International Journal of Neuropsychopharmacology, 5*(4), 301–307.

Hofmann, S. G., Meuret, A. E., Smits, J. A., Simon, N. M., Pollack, M. H., Eisenmenger, K., *et al.* (2006). Augmentation of exposure therapy for social anxiety disorder with D-Cycloserine. *Archives of General Psychiatry, 63,* 298–304.

Kaffman, A., & Meaney, M. (2007). Neurodevelopmental sequelae of postnatal maternal care in rodents: clinical and research implications of molecular insights. *Journal of Child Psychology and Psychiatry, 48,* 224–244.

Keleta, Y. B., Lumia, A. R., Anderson, G. M., & McGinnis, M. Y. (2007) Behavioral effects of pubertal anabolic androgenic steroid exposure in male rats with low serotonin. *Brain Research, 1132,* 129–138.

Kirsch, P., Esslinger, C., Chen, Q., Mier, D., Lis, S., Siddhanti, S., *et al.* (2005). Oxytocin modulates neural circuitry for social cognition and fear in humans. *The Journal of Neuroscience, 25*(49), 11489–11493.

Klin, A., Jones, W., Schultz, R., Volkmar, F., & Cohen, D. (2002). Visual fixation patterns during viewing of naturalistic social situations as predictors of social competence in individuals with autism. *Archives of General Psychiatry, 59,* 809–816.

Kosfeld, M., Heinrichs, M., Zak, P.J., Fischbacher, U., & Fehr, E. (2005). Oxytocin increases trust in humans. *Nature, 435*(7042), 673–676.

Kushner, M. G., Kimb, S.W., Donahuea, C., Thurasa, P., Adsona, D., Kotlyara, M., *et al.* (2007). D-Cycloserine augmented exposure therapy for Obsessive-Compulsive Disorder. *Biological Psychiatry, 62,* 835–838.

Leist, T., & Dadds, M. R. (in press). Emotion recognition and psychopathology: disentangling the contributions of child traits and early maltreatment. Clinical Child Psychology and Psychiatry.

Lim, M. M., & Young, L. (2006). Neuropeptidergic regulation of affiliative behavior and social bonding in animals. *Hormones and Behaviour, 50*(4), 506–517.

Loeber, R., & Farrington, D. P. (2000). Young children who commit crime: epidemiology, developmental origins, risk factors, early interventions, and policy implications. *Development and Psychopathology, 12,* 737–762.

Loney, B. R., Butler, M. A., Lima, E. N., Counts, C. A., & Eckel, L. A. (2006). The relation between salivary cortisol, callous-unemotional traits, and conduct problems in an adolescent non-referred sample. *Journal of Child Psychology and Psychiatry, 47,* 30–36.

Loughland, C. M., Williams, L. M., & Gordon, E. (2002). Schizophrenia and affective disorder show different visual scanning behavior for faces: a trait versus state-based distinction? *Biological Psychiatry, 52*(4), 338–348.

Maestripieri, D., Higley, J. D., Lindell, S. G., Newman, T. K., McCormack, K. M., & Sanchez, M. M., (2006). Early maternal rejection affects the development of monoaminergic systems and adult abusive parenting in rhesus macaques (*Macaca mulatta*). *Behavioral Neuroscience, 120*(5), 1017–1024.

Merens, W., Willem van der Does, A. J., & Spinhoven, P. (2007). The effects of serotonin manipulations on emotional information processing and mood. *Journal of Affective Disorders, 103*(1–3), 43–62.

Meyer-Lindenberg, A., & Zink, C. F. (2007). Imaging genetics for neuropsychiatric disorders. *Child and Adolescent Psychiatric Clinics of North America, 16,* 581–597.

Miller, G. E., & Prinz, R. J. (1990). Enhancement of social learning family interventions for childhood Conduct Disorder. *Psychological Bulletin, 108*(2), 291–307.

Moriceau, S., & Sullivan, R. M. (2005). Neurobiology of infant attachment. *Developmental Psychobiology, 47,* 230–242.

Parent, C., Zhang, T. Y., Caldji, C., Bagot, R., Champagne, F. A., Pruessner, J., *et al.* (2005). Maternal care and individual differences in defensive responses. *Current Directions in Psychological Science, 14*(5), 229–233.

Patterson, G. R., (1982). Coercive Family Process. Eugene, OR: Castalia Publishing Co.

Popma, A., Vermeiren, C., Geluk, T., Rinne, T., van den Brink, W., Knol, D., *et al.* (2007). Cortisol moderates the relationship between testosterone and aggression in delinquent male adolescents. *Biological Psychiatry*, *61*, 405–411.

Prinz, R. J., & Sanders, M. R. (2007). Adopting a population-level approach to parenting and family support interventions. *Clinical Psychology Review*, *27*(6), 739–749.

Reese, E., & Newcombe, R. (2007). Training mothers in elaborative reminiscing enhances children's autobiographical memory and narrative. *Child Development*, *78*, 1153–1170.

Ressler, K. J., Rothbaum, B. O., Tannenbaum, L., Anderson, P., Graap, K., Zimand, E., *et al.* (2004). Cognitive enhancers as adjuncts to psychotherapy: use of D-cycloserine in phobic individuals to facilitate extinction of fear. *Archives of General Psychiatry*, *61*(11), 1136–1144.

Richardson, R., Ledgerwood, L., & Cranney, J. (2004). Facilitation of fear extinction by D-Cycloserine: theoretical and clinical implications. *Learning and Memory*, *11*, 510–516.

Salmon, K., Dadds, M. R., Hawes, D., & Allen, J. (submitted). Can emotional language skills be taught during parent training for conduct problem children?

Sanders, M. R., & Turner, K. M. (2005). Reflections on the challenges of effective dissemination of behavioural family intervention: our experience with the triple P—Positive Parenting Program. *Child and Adolescent Mental Health*, *10*(4), 158–169.

Serketich, W. J., & Dumas, J. (1996). The effectiveness of behavioral parent training to modify antisocial behavior in children: a meta-analysis. *Behavior Therapy*, *27*, 171–186.

Skuse, D. (2003). Fear recognition and the neural basis of social cognition. *Child and Adolescent Mental Health*, *8*, 50–60.

Spezio, M. L., Huang, P. S., Castelli, F., & Adolphs, R. (2007). Amygdala damage impairs eye contact during conversations with real people. *The Journal of Neuroscience*, *27*(15), 3994–3997.

Spoont, M. R. (1992). Modulatory role of serotonin in neural information processing: implications for human psychopathology. *Psychological Bulletin*, *112*, 330–350.

Tinbergen, N., (1951). *The Study of Instinct*. Oxford: Oxford University Press.

Turner, K. M., & Sanders, M. R. (2006). Dissemination of evidence-based parenting and family support strategies: learning from the triple P—Positive Parenting Program system approach. *Aggression and Violent Behavior*, *11*(2), 176–193.

Van Goozen, S., Fairchild, G., Snoek, H., & Harold, G. T. (2007). The evidence for a neurobiological model of antisocial behavior. *Psychological Bulletin*, *133*, 149–182.

Viding, E., Blair, R. J., Moffitt, T. E., & Plomin, R. (2005). Evidence of substantial genetic risk for psychopathy in 7-year-olds. *Journal of Child Psychology and Psychiatry*, *46*, 592–597.

Watt, B. D., Hoyland, M., Best, D., & Dadds, M. D. (2007). Treatment participation among children with conduct problems and the role of telephone reminders. *Journal of Child Family Studies*, *16*, 522–530.

Webster-Stratton, C. (1998). Preventing conduct problems in Head Start children. *Journal of Consulting and Clinical Psychology*, *66*, 715–730.

6

The dynamics of threat, fear, and intentionality in the conduct disorders: Longitudinal findings in the children of women with post-natal depression

Jonathan Hill, Lynne Murray, Vicki Leidecker, and Helen Sharp

Introduction

Conduct disorders among young children are common in the general population (prevalence 5-10% depending on the threshold). They are disabling, often leading to antisocial behaviours and multiple mental health and personality problems in later life (Moffitt *et al.*, 2002). The causes involve an interplay between inherited characteristics such as emotional expression and regulation, and family and wider social influences (Hill, 2002). Commonly, conduct disorder symptoms develop in association with high levels of environmental threat in the form of parental hostility, physical abuse, and marital discord and violence. This is probably accounted for in part by correlated parental and child risks, but is also likely to reflect a direct causal relationship (Jaffee, Moffitt, Caspi, Taylor, & Arseneault, 2002; Jaffee *et al.*, 2005). The implications of high levels of chronic threat for social information processing and emotion regulation were addressed by Dodge and colleagues in their hypotheses linking physical abuse to hostile attributional biases, anger, and reactive aggression (Orobio *et al.*, 2002). However, studies of other social information processes, and the role of fear, in the conduct disorders have been conducted largely independently of consideration of the role of environmental threat. Deficits in emotion recognition (Denham *et al.*, 2002), pragmatic language use (Gilmour *et al.*, 2004), and social fear processing (Blair *et al.*, 2006) have been conceptualized as risk factors for the conduct disorders without substantial environmental contributions. Two pathways to conduct disorders have thus been hypothesized: one involving anger and reactive aggression with a substantial threat contribution and the other characterized by limitations in social and emotional processing, arising without substantial environmental influences leading to callous-unemotional traits and proactive aggression. Studies of the neurobiology of aggression and conduct disorders have focused mainly on the second pathway implicating impaired social emotion processing arising without substantial environmental contributions.

In this chapter, we consider possible mechanisms whereby high environmental threat may lead to modifications in the activity of key brain structures, in particular the amygdala, and hence to aggression and conduct disorders. We present the case that under conditions of threat children may learn coping strategies that reduce amygdala activation and fear, which in turn increases vulnerability to aggression and conduct disorders. Children with high emotional reactivity reared in threatening or unsupportive environments and who make use of such coping strategies may be particularly vulnerable to conduct disorders. We then go on to describe findings from a longitudinal study in which we examined whether insecure attachment in infancy predicted threat-related social cognitions at age 5 years of the kind that we hypothesize will be associated with reduced amygdala activation. We also report associations between these threat-related social cognitions and conduct disorder symptoms in the children of women with post-natal depression (PND).

Amygdala function, threat, and the conduct disorders

Normally, the amygdala contributes to social learning and social responsiveness through its roles in the establishment of stimulus-punishment associations and in fear processing. Psychopathy in adults and callous-unemotional traits in children are thought to arise from a reduced ability to form the stimulus-punishment associations necessary for successful social-ization, coupled with a lack of responsiveness to expressions of fear in others. As a result, individuals with psychopathy do not learn to avoid actions that will harm others (Blair, 2006). Amygdala dysfunction has been identified as a causal factor of adult psychopathy, on the basis that deficits seen in psychopathic disorder are similar to those found following amygdala lesions, and adult psychopaths show reduced amygdala activation in functional imaging studies (Blair *et al.*, 2006) . Psychopathic disorder and callous-unemotional traits in children are thought to stem from amygdala dysfunction without significant contribution from environmental factors (Viding *et al.*, 2005; Blair *et al.*, 2006).

On the other hand, studies of the role of parenting in relation to callous-unemotional traits do not conform to this general view. Cornell and Frick (2007) investigated the interplay between temperament and guilt and empathy in a middle-class sample of 3 to 5-year-olds. Children nominated by their peers as being behaviourally inhibited were rated by their parents as showing more guilt and empathy than uninhibited children. This is consistent with a link between temperamental fearlessness, likely to have a substantial genetic contribution, and dimensions of callous-unemotional traits. However, in the uninhibited subgroup of chil-dren, guilt and empathy were lower among those experiencing greater parent-reported incon-sistent parenting (Cornell & Frick, 2007). Thus, the biological risk of callous-unemotional traits is modified by the quality of the parental environment. Parenting characteristics were also related to outcome in a study of 120 aggressive 11-year-olds followed for one year (Pardini *et al.*, 2007). Callous-unemotional traits displayed moderate temporal stability and predicted increases in antisocial behaviour. However, children exposed to lower levels of physical punishment showed decreases in such traits, and those experiencing higher levels of parental warmth and involvement had decreases in both callous-unemotional traits and antisocial behaviour. Lower levels of anxiety were associated with increasing callous-unemotional traits only in children who described their primary caregiver as exhibiting low warmth and involvement. These findings do not necessarily apply to children with severe callous-unemotional traits; however, they do point to the need to include possible environ-mental mechanisms in neurobiological hypotheses for these traits.

The amygdala subserves a much broader set of functions than those thought to be relevant to psychopathy, some of which may increase vulnerability in unfavourable environments. In particular, it enables preferential processing of stimuli that are emotional and potentially threatening, and it is implicated in the effect of arousal on memory whereby information associated with strong emotions is better remembered (Phelps & LeDoux, 2005). Thus, the child living in an environment of chronic threat may experience repeated negative emotions underpinned by these amygdala-mediated processes. This may result in anger-driven reactive aggression, or in attempts to resolve the fearful state. Given that parents are commonly the source of the threat, they are also unlikely to be able to help the child in reducing their fear by providing comfort.

Derryberry and Rothbart (1997) eloquently outlined the potential consequences for the child of attempting to manage threat without support: where the child is unable to find comfort or protection from caregivers when threatened, he 'may come to rely upon primarily avoidant strategies, disengaging attention from the threatening situation without attending to sources of relief and available coping options' (p. 647). They outline two major possible consequences of this strategy with implications for disruptive behaviour problems. Firstly, it is likely to reduce the child's capacity to attend to the details of the threatening information, and hence reduce the appropriateness and effectiveness of his responses. The child who is less able to cope with challenging social situations is more likely to find maladaptive, for example, coercive, ways of dealing with them. Secondly, 'if this strategy were used too extensively, the child may fail to benefit from the more positive effects of felt anxiety ... in impulse control, empathy, and conscience' (Derryberry & Rothbart 1997). Although evidence is not available regarding children's ability to reduce amygdala activation using avoidant strategies, adults can be taught avoidant strategies in the form of reappraisal of standard negative stimuli, and this has been shown to reduce amygdala activation in response to those stimuli (Ochsner *et al.*, 2002). If children were able to reduce amygdala activity via analogous mechanisms, this would provide a means of adapting to high environmental threat, simultaneously increasing vulnerability to the conduct disorders as a result of impaired social learning and emotion processing.

Threat, emotion regulation, and social information processing in the conduct disorders

Several kinds of avoidant strategy can be envisaged, such as withdrawing attention from the source of threat or denial that there is a threat. Within interpersonal exchanges, perceived threat can also be varied depending on the interpretation that is put on others' behaviours. What others' behaviours are 'about', otherwise referred to as their intentionality (Searle, 1983), can be construed in terms of their motives, attitudes, emotions, or plans. This is what Dennett (1987) refers to as 'adopting the intentional stance' although 'responding in' might be more appropriate to children because it is not implied that they make a choice. The alternative is to respond in the 'physical stance', whereby social behaviours do not have intentionality with respect to mental states and instead are viewed as no more than sounds or movements (Dennett, 1987; Bolton & Hill, 2004). Thus, the raised voice of a caregiver, which according to the intentional stance is angry and threatening, becomes simply a louder sound when interpreted using the physical stance, and similarly, the threatening gesture of a peer is only an arm raised.

Intentionality is similar to mentalization but is more restricted in its scope, as mentalization refers not only to responding using the intentional stance but also to the range of competences required in implementing it effectively (Fonagy & Target, 2006). Intentionality also differs from 'theory of mind' as currently conceived (Carpendale & Lewis, 2004). Theory of mind refers to the ability to take the perspective of another accurately, whereas intentionality refers to a mode of interpreting and responding irrespective of whether the interpretations are correct or the responding appropriate. Theory of mind is generally tested under emotionally neutral conditions and is thought of as a general capability, whereas intentionality may be examined in relation to varying emotional demands and the same individual may show marked variations depending on those demands.

In the study reported here, the extent to which the child responded in the intentional or physical stance was assessed using a doll play challenge (Murray, Woolgar *et al.*, 1999). Children were asked to show what happens in their families at bedtime (low threat), in a bad and nasty time (high threat), and in a happy and best time (low threat), and their accounts were rated on an intentionality scale. Responding using the intentional stance in a doll play task has two elements, making use of the plastic objects to represent people and their surroundings, and showing the interpersonal reasons for the doll play characters' behaviours. Higher intentionality scores were assigned where both elements were clearly present and lower scores where one or both were to some degree lacking. Details of the scoring and are provided in the 'Method' section.

The role of attachment processes

Links between emotion regulation and intentionality are likely to be influenced by attachment processes. Fonagy and Target (1997) argued that secure attachment provides the psychosocial basis for acquiring an understanding of others' minds. The child is likely to maintain the intentional stance if expressions of fear or distress in the face of threat elicit comfort from a caregiver, but may otherwise drop to the physical stance, simultaneously alleviating the negative emotions and reducing opportunities to further understand the caregiver's mind. Thus, we expect insecure attachment to be associated with responding using the physical stance under conditions of threat.

Whether a child responds using the intentional stance is also likely to be influenced by factors other than attachment security. For example, theory-of-mind capabilities are likely to enhance the use of the intentional stance when responding to social challenges (Fonagy, 2006). However, we predict that this general capability does not equip the child to maintain this stance in the face of threat and so will only be associated with intentionality in response to low-threat social challenges. The quality of family conversations about mental states and feelings has also been found to be related to mentalizing abilities (Dunn & Brown, 2001), and may be expected to be associated with making use of the intentional stance. We predict that the context of family conversations is crucial to the context in which it promotes intentionality. The quality of family interactions while responding to and regulating anger or distress is likely to be related to the child's capacity to maintain the intentional stance in the face of threat. By contrast, family interactional patterns where negative emotions are not aroused will be associated with the child's ability to maintain the intentional stance in low-threat contexts. In this study, theory of mind and the quality of mother-child conversations in a non-threatening context were assessed at age 5, so that these predictions could be tested.

Implications of lower intentionality for conduct problems

If a child responds habitually to threat with reduced intentionality, he may come to this avoidant strategy more generally in regulating fear or anxiety, along the lines outlined by Derryberry and Rothbart (1997). However, the child who drops to the physical stance to deal with fear or anxiety may become vulnerable to antisocial behaviours in at least four ways: firstly, he reduces his capacity to process the details of the social situation and hence his ability to respond appropriately; secondly, he is deprived of the regulatory function of anxiety or fear to inhibit impulsive actions; thirdly, the emotional responsiveness associated with empathy and conscience is reduced; and fourth, by turning away from the mental state of the other, he becomes indifferent to the damaging consequences of his actions.

In a previous study, we tested our hypothesis that conduct disordered children are prone to using an avoidant strategy to deal with fear through lowering intentionality by comparing boys referred with conduct disorder symptoms and community controls using story stem challenges (Hill *et al.*, 2007). The key contrast was between challenges that involved fear and distress (a child is frightened by a dog, a child is distressed after being scalded) and those with conflict (a fight between two children, an argument between parents). There was a significant interaction term between the conduct disordered versus control groups, and fear and/or distress versus conflict stories, because conduct disordered boys had lower intentionality scores than controls but only in response to story stem challenges involving fear and distress .

Attachment and conduct problems

Associations between attachment and conduct problems have been demonstrated in cross-sectional and prospective studies (Lyons-Ruth *et al.*, 1997; Speltz *et al.*, 1999; Belsky & Fearon, 2002; Burgess *et al.*, 2003; Keller *et al.*, 2005; Guttmann-Steinmetz & Crowell, 2006; Moss *et al.*, 2006). However, there have been variations in the type of insecure attachment associated with conduct disorder symptoms and in whether or not attachment security is associated with symptoms only in interaction with other factors such as fearlessness or social risk (Belsky & Fearon 2002). Current concepts and models of the way that attachment security may be relevant to the conduct disorders also vary substantially. One line of argument suggests that attachment security contributes to conduct disorders only inasmuch as it affects the child's capacity to solicit emotional support in dealing with the vulnerabilities that directly lead to aggressive and disruptive behaviours (Greenberg *et al.*, 2001; Keller *et al.*, 2005). This is in contrast to proposals that envisage direct links between attachment status and conduct disorders (Moss *et al.*, 2006). For example, aggressive behaviours may be seen as a manifestation of attempts to cope with the consequences of disorganised attachment.

Attachment insecurity or disorganization is not, however, the only influence on emotion regulation, and it may be that the mechanisms in the conduct disorders involve interplay between attachment and other emotion regulatory processes. For example, Burgess *et al.* (2003) hypothesized that risk for externalizing behaviour problems might arise from both the low temperamental fearfulness and down-regulation of fear associated with avoidant attachment. They found that the combination of fearlessness assessed at 24 months and avoidant attachment assessed at 14 months predicted externalizing behaviour problems at 4 years. Thus, the available evidence is consistent with there being effects of attachment on conduct disorders only in the presence of other risks, as evidenced in statistical interactions, and with conduct disorder symptoms as direct manifestations of attachment processes and thus main effects

Gender, social information processing, and the conduct disorders

Males have higher rates of conduct disorders in childhood than females (Moffitt *et al.*, 2001). This is mainly because males are exposed to more risk factors than females rather than because males are more vulnerable. Gender differences in peer relationships were identified as a key factor in the elevated rates of conduct disorders in the Dunedin Health and Development Study. Some of these differences may be relevant to the development of intentionality in social interactions. Boys tend to engage in physical competitive activities and to develop relationships that emphasize dominance and status, whereas girls' groups are commonly oriented towards verbal and emotional intimacy (Maccoby, 2002). Girls are therefore more likely to be experienced in tracking interpersonal processes using the intentional stance than boys.

The role of parental depression

Associations between maternal depression and behaviour problems in children are well documented (Hay *et al.*, 2003). These do not establish that maternal depression is the key risk because it is associated with other psychiatric disorders and psychosocial risks. For example, many women with depression have a history of conduct problems and marked interpersonal difficulties in adult life (Jaffee, Moffitt, Caspi, Fombonne, *et al.*, 2002; Hill *et al.*, 2004). Rates of conduct disorders among the children of mothers with depression and antisocial personality disorder are higher than among those with depression only (Kim-Cohen, Caspi, Rutter *et al.*, 2006). In turn, the adverse parenting environment may arise from psychosocial risks associated with maternal personality disorder, such as elevated rates of physical maltreatment and exposure to domestic violence (Kim-Cohen, Caspi, Rutter *et al.*, 2006). Where it can be shown that maternal depression is the key risk, a critical issue in the investigation of possible mechanisms concerns the timing of the maternal disorder.

Post-natal depression (PND) has been of interest both because of possible effects on early mother-infant interactions (Murray, Fiori-Cowley *et al.*, 1996) and evidence from animal studies that early perturbations of maternal care may affect gene expression and neurodevelopment (Szyf *et al.*, 2007). Establishing the specific contribution of PND to psychopathology requires measurement of depression outside of the post-partum period because there are strong associations between antenatal depression and PND, and between PND and subsequent persistence or recurrence of depression (Hay *et al.*, 2003). Hay *et al.* addressed this issue by assessing not only PND but also antenatal depression and maternal depression when children were age 1, 4, and 11 years, in an urban community sample. PND predicted violence reported by parents and teachers at age 11, after accounting for depression assessed at other time points. The biological father's history of arrests made an independent contribution to violence at age 11, together with PND. Previous findings from the study described in this chapter have also indicated that there may be a persistent effect on child psychological adjustment of PND not accounted for by subsequent episodes of depression, nor by associated psychosocial factors (Murray, Sinclair *et al.*, 1999). There is, therefore, some evidence of a persistent effect of PND, with two major caveats. Firstly, statistical power to examine the contrast between depression confined to the post-partum period and later depression is generally limited by the strong association between the two. For example, in the study of Hay *et al.*, of the 26 mothers with PND, only 7 did not have a recorded recurrence of major depression. Secondly, there is some evidence of familial aggregation of PND (Forty *et al.*, 2006; Murphy-Eberenz *et al.*, 2006), so the association may be accounted for by common genetic effects on PND and child psychopathology.

There is increasing evidence that risks interact in the development of the conduct disorders. For example, the association between child maltreatment and antisocial behaviour problems is higher among individuals with a functional polymorphism conferring low levels of expression of the gene encoding the neurotransmitter-metabolizing enzyme monoamine oxidase A (MAOA; Caspi *et al.*, 2002; Kim-Cohen, Caspi, Taylor *et al.*, 2006). The way in which reduced MAOA may contribute to risk of conduct problems in the presence of maltreatment is not known; however, animal studies point to the possibility of a link between altered monoamine levels and hyperreactivity to stress (Ward *et al.*, 1998). In rats, MAO (A and B) inhibition during brain development results in increased aggression in response to social threat (Mejia *et al.*, 2002). Animal studies also find that maternal behaviour during the first days of the post-partum period has long-term effects on reactivity to threat (Menard & Hakvoort, 2007). Thus, genetic and early environmental vulnerabilities to conduct disorders may arise from emotional reactivity, in interaction with subsequent environmental threats (Frick & Morris, 2004). We have previously reported that boys referred with conduct problems show both dysregulated aggression and reduced intentionality in response to distress portrayed in doll play scenarios (Hill *et al.*, 2007). Thus, if PND is associated with elevated emotional reactivity, we expect that there will be an interaction between it and reduced intentionality to threat in relation to conduct problems in children.

We set out to test the following hypotheses:

1. Insecure attachment in infancy will be associated with lower intentionality, specifically in response to a high threat doll play challenge, at 5 years.
2. Theory of mind and quality of observed mother-child conversations will be associated with intentionality scores in tasks where no threat is posed, but will not be associated with lower intentionality in response to threat.
3. Lower intentionality, specifically in response to threat, at 5 years will be associated with conduct disorder symptoms in interaction with maternal PND.
4. Insecure attachment in infancy will be associated with elevated conduct disorder problems at 5 years, mediated by intentionality in response to threat.
5. Male gender will be associated with lower intentionality, which will mediate the association between gender and conduct disorder symptoms in the children of women with PND.

Participants

All participants provided written informed consent prior to taking part in this Cambridgeshire Local Ethics Committee-approved study. The sample comprised 82 children participating in a prospective longitudinal study of the impact of PND on child development (Murray, 1992). There were 47 children of mothers with PND (mean age = 60.5 months, SD = 1.0), and 35 control children (mean age = 60.3, SD = 0.9). The gender and social class distributions in each of the PND and control groups were very similar (Table 6.1). The distribution of attachment categories assessed using the Strange Situation Test at age 18 months was as follows: secure, 43; avoidant, 34; ambivalent, 2; and disorganized, 3. So only secure (N = 43) and insecure (N = 39) groups were contrasted in the data analyses. Children of mothers with PND had elevated levels of insecure attachment compared with children of control mothers (Table 6.1).

The original sample comprised 100 mother-infant dyads, recruited at approximately 8 weeks post-partum. Initial recruitment was through screening a community sample of 702 primiparous mothers of healthy, full-term infants for PND, by administering the Edinburgh Postnatal Depression Scale (EPDS; Cox *et al.*, 1987) at 6 weeks post-partum. Women scoring over 12 on the EPDS were interviewed: 61 women who met the Research Diagnostic Criteria (Spitzer *et al.*, 1978) for depressive disorder were identified, 58 of whom were recruited for the study. Forty-two non-depressed mothers randomly selected from the same post-natal population were also recruited. All the mothers were white, their mean age was 28 years (SD = 4), 64% were in the upper- to middle-class households (UK Standard Occupation Classification: I, II, or III non-manual), and 49% had been in full-time educa-

Table 6.1 Descriptive statistics for the control and post-natal depression (PND) groups.

	Control (N = 35)	PND (N = 47)	P
Mean age in months	60.5 (1.0)	60.3 (0.9)	0.34
Proportion of males	49%	47%	0.87
Proportion of social class I, II, III non-manual	69%	64%	0.65
Proportion of insecure attachment at 18 months	26%	64%	0.001
Proportion of maternal depression at 18 months–5 years	17%	51%	0.002
Proportion of child involvement in marital discord	14%	40%	0.01
Proportion who did not pass the false belief task	12%	20%	0.36
Mean McCarthy General Cognitive Index	111.1 (10.3)	111.2 (12.8)	0.96
Mean McCarthy Verbal Subscale	57.1 (10.3)	58.3 (10.6)	0.61
Mean maternal–child-focused speech	1.21 (1.1)	1.14 (0.9)	0.75
Mean intentionality–bedtime	7.40 (2.28)	7.28 (2.95)	0.86
Mean intentionality–bad and nasty time	6.06 (3.65)	6.02 (3.41)	0.96
Mean intentionality–happy and best time	4.91 (3.38)	5.06 (3.27)	0.84

Values of P were derived from two-sided independent groups t-tests and chi-square tests.

Values in parentheses are the standard deviation.

tion for at least 12 years. Of the original sample of 100 assessed in infancy, 94 (50 PND, 44 controls) were assessed at age 5 years and videotaped assessments of the children in a doll play procedure were available for 82 children[1].

Measures

Assessment at age 18 months

Infant attachment
The quality of infant attachment to the mother at 18 months was assessed using the Strange Situation procedure (Ainsworth & Wittig, 1969). Attachment was classified from videotapes following the procedures described by Ainsworth *et al.* (1978) and by Main and Solomon (1990). Cohen's kappa coefficient for the secure, avoidant, ambivalent, and disorganized attachment classifications of the two research groups who independently scored 63 randomly selected videotapes of the Strange Situation was 0.94 (see Murray, Fiori-Cowley *et al.*, 1996).

Assessments at age 5 years

Recent maternal depression
Mothers were interviewed using the Schedule for Affective Disorders and Schizophrenia, Lifetime Version (SADS-L; Endicott & Spitzer, 1978). Episodes of DSM Major Depressive Disorder occurring between the time the child was 18 months old and the present were recorded along with timing of onset and remission.

---

[1] Technical problems, such as poor sound quality, meant that tapes could not be rated for 12 children.

Chronic difficulties and child involvement in parental discord
The Life Events and Difficulties Schedule (LEDS; Brown & Harris, 1978) was used to assess current chronic difficulties. In addition to the usual LEDS probes, a number were introduced to elicit information about the degree to which the child had been actively exposed to, or was the focus of, any marital conflict, over the past 12 months.

Cognitive development
The McCarthy Scales of Children's Development were administered (McCarthy, 1972). These scales have been widely used in research and are a valid and reliable measure of children's cognitive development. Two scales were used: the General Cognitive Index (GCI) and the Verbal Subscale.

Theory of mind
The procedure of Wimmer and Perner (1983) was used: the child was presented with a narrative involving two characters and containers. The protagonist puts some chocolate into one of the containers and then leaves the scene; in his absence, his mother moves the chocolate to one of the other containers. On returning, the protagonist wants the chocolate. The child is asked where the character will look, having first established that the child knows the correct location. Success was scored where the child both remembered the correct location and represented the protagonist's false belief. Of the 82 children, 4 were unable to locate the chocolate correctly, so the sample size for analyses of theory of mind was 78. Of these children, 13 (16%) failed the false belief item.

Maternal communication with the child during a snack: maternal sensitivity
The mother and child were shown into a comfortably furnished room and were provided with some light refreshments, including fruit juice, oranges, and a cake. These items were, in part, selected to elicit the mother's involvement in helping the child, and possible control over what and how much the child ate. The quality of the mother's communication with the child was coded from a transcript of the 10-minute snack interaction. Ratings were designed to provide a parallel to the analysis of mothers' speech to their infants when they were 2 months old. They reflected positive comments, genuine questions, and expansions and extensions relevant to the child or to a common focus of interest. Inter-rater reliability and associations with family adversity were reported previously (Murray, Sinclair, *et al.*, 1999).

Conduct disorder symptoms
Teachers completed the Preschool Behaviour Checklist, which consists of 22 items covering externalizing and internalizing behaviours (McGuire & Richman, 1988). The six conduct disorder items—fights, destructive, difficult to manage, interferes with other children, has tantrums, and teases other children—were summed to create the scale used in this study.

Dolls' house assessment
The dolls' house procedure has been described in previous publications of this study (Murray, **Woolgar** *et al.*, 1999). The child was shown a doll house that was furnished but had no doll characters in it. The back of the house was removed so that the child's play could be video-recorded through the observation window. The researcher explained to the child that they were going to pretend that this was the child's own house and asked him or her to choose

figures to represent the people in the child's family. The researcher then asked the child to show what happened in the family during four scenes: a meal time (warm-up), bedtime, bad and nasty time, and happy and best time. The researcher was not directive on the use of the play materials; however, standard probes were introduced in order to ensure that the child did respond to the demands of the scene. In the bedtime story, the questions 'Do you go straight to sleep?' or 'Does it sometimes take some time' and 'Do you wake up in the night sometimes' were always asked. In the bad and nasty time, if the child could not think of one, or said that they never occur, the administrator said, 'Let's pretend it is a bad and nasty time', and similarly for the happy and best time. Where the child told a story that was not apparently related to the demands of the scene, the administrator would respond along the lines of, 'Is that what happens when it is a (e.g., bad and nasty) time?'

The child's stories were rated using a coding scheme that was developed for use with the MacArthur Story Stem Battery (MSSB; Hill *et al.*, 2000; Emde *et al.*, 2003; Minnis *et al.*, 2006; Hill *et al.*, 2007). Some minor modifications were made of the rating rules to take account of the differences between the dolls' house play procedure and the MSSB.

The intentionality scale assesses the extent to which the reasons for the doll participants' behaviours, in terms of mental states such as needs, desires, feelings, and beliefs, are made explicit or can be readily inferred from the behaviours. This is a 12-point scale in which ratings of 10–12 require that explicit reference be made to the feelings or motives of the participants, whereas ratings in the 7–9 range are made where mental states can be readily inferred but are not referred to explicitly. For example, in the 'bad and nasty time' scenario, a sequence in which the child says, 'There is a big storm in the night and Michael is frightened and goes into his parent's room for a cuddle' would contribute to a rating in the 10–12 range. By contrast, 'There is a big storm in the night and Michael goes into his parent's room for a cuddle' would contribute to a rating in the 7–9 range. Contributions to ratings of 4–6 come from portrayed actions whose intentionality refer to physical circumstances of the doll characters, rather than their states of mind or motives: for example, 'There is a big storm in the night. Michael is mending his bike.' Ratings in the lowest range (1–3) reflect sequences where the dolls are manipulated outside of the rules of their symbolic function: for example, 'There is a big storm in the night, and Michael flies up on to the roof, and then slides down the chimney.'

All of the doll play assessments were rated blind to all of the assessments at 18 months and 5 years. Inter-rater reliability (intraclass correlation coefficient) **on** assessments from 20 children ranged between 0.72–0.85 for the scales used in this study.

Variables and Analyses

The distributions of intentionality scores were examined using histograms and were found to be appropriate for parametric analyses; however, the teacher-rated externalizing symptoms were skewed and so analyses were conducted using the log-transformed scores. Associations with earlier and concurrent measures were examined using correlation coefficients, two-sided between-group *t*-tests, and analysis of covariance (ANCOVA). Contrasts in associations with attachment security and gender across different dolls' house scenarios were examined using repeated-measures ANCOVA with appropriate covariates and testing for interactions with scenario type. Predictions of teacher-rated conduct disorder symptoms were examined in multiple linear regressions, including interaction terms to test whether effects were modified by risks such as PND. In view of the moderate correlations among them, the tolerance value of each intentionality variable in the regression analyses was used as a check for multicollinearity. Tolerance values of 0.1 and higher are generally regarded as acceptable. Mediation was examined in linear regression using the method outlined by Baron and Kenny (1986), whereby variable B may be considered as a mediator between variables A and C, if there are associations between A–B, A–C, and B–C, and the contribution of A to C becomes non-significant when considered jointly with variable B.

Results

The PND and control groups did not differ significantly in mean GCI and Verbal Subscale scores, proportions passing the false belief task, and maternal sensitivity during a snack (Table 6.1). Children of mothers with PND were more likely to have been exposed to maternal depression between 18 months and 5 years, and to be involved in marital discord as 5-year-olds. Only 4 mothers met the criteria for DSM Major Depression at the 5-years assessments, of which 3 were in the PND group. The groups did not differ in mean intentionality scores assessed in the doll play procedure at 5 years.

Intentionality scores in each of the scenarios were moderately correlated: bedtime with bad and nasty time ($r = 0.57$, $p < 0.001$), bedtime with happy and best time ($r = 0.53$, $p < 0.001$), and bad and nasty time with happy and best time ($r = 48$, $p < 0.001$). There were weak associations between GCI scores (but not the Verbal Subscale) and intentionality in the bedtime story ($r = 0.23$, $p = 0.03$), but no associations with scores in the other scenarios. There were no associations between intentionality in any of the dolls' house scales and social class, the child's age, maternal depression between 18 months and 5 years, or the child's involvement in current marital conflict. Unless otherwise stated, all analyses were conducted after controlling for GCI.

Infant attachment security and intentionality at age 5

Hypothesis 1 was examined in repeated-measures ANCOVA. Overall, mean intentionality scores were lower in the bad and nasty time story compared with the bedtime story ($p < 0.001$)

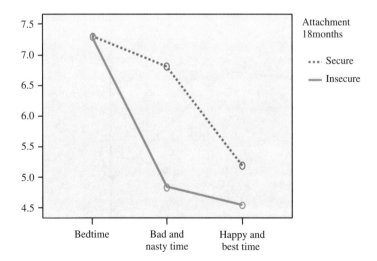

Fig. 6.1 Estimated marginal mean intentionality scores comparing children who were secure and insecure at 18 months in low- and high-threat scenarios at the age of 5 years

Table 6.2 Mean intentionality scores at age 5 years contrasting children rated secure and insecure at age 18 months.

	Secure (N = 43)	Insecure (N = 39)	Mean (95% CI)	*P*	*P* cov
Intentionality–bedtime	7.53 (3.13)	7.10 (3.05)	0.63 (−0.93–1.79)	0.53	0.59
Intentionality–nasty time	7.26 (3.59)	4.69 (2.90)	2.56 (1.12–4.00)	0.001	0.001
Intentionality–happy time	5.58 (3.35)	4.36 (3.15)	1.22 (−0.21–2.66)	0.094	0.098

The table shows unadjusted means and mean differences and their 95% confidence intervals. The *P* values are from independent groups two-sided *t*-tests and *P* cov values are from analysis of covariance, controlling for McCarthy general cognitive ability scores.

and in the happy and best time compared with the bad and nasty time ($p = 0.029$). The interaction term between insecure attachment at 18 months and doll play scenario in the prediction of intentionality at 5 years was statistically significant ($F[2,78] = 5.48$, $p = 0.006$; Fig. 6.1). Follow-up analyses revealed that infant attachment security was associated with intentionality in the high-threat, bad and nasty time, scenario but not the low-threat, bedtime and happy and best time, scenarios (Table 6.2). Infant attachment explained 13% of the variance in intentionality scores in the bad and nasty time scenario at 5 years ($\beta = -0.36$, $p = 0.001$).

Hypothesis 2 was tested in repeated-measures ANCOVA testing for interactions between passing the false belief task and doll play scenario, and maternal sensitivity and doll play scenario in the prediction of intentionality. Attachment security was retained in the models because of its association with intentionality in the bad and nasty time scenario. The interaction term between passing the false belief task and doll play scenario was statistically significant ($F[2,73] = 3.21$, $p = 0.046$; Fig. 6.2), and the interaction between maternal sensitivity and doll play scenario approached statistical significance ($F[2,77] = 2.79$, $p = 0.068$). Follow-up analyses were conducted in three separate hierarchical linear regressions, entering attachment, theory of mind, and maternal sensitivity jointly in the second step (Table 6.3). Theory of

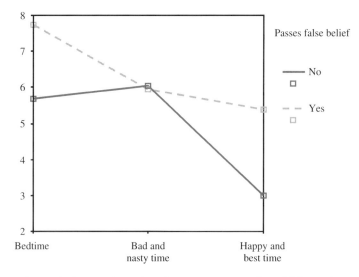

Fig. 6.2 Estimated marginal mean intentionality scores comparing children who passed and who failed the false-belief task in low- and high-threat scenarios at age 5, controlling for attachment

Table 6.3 Summary of multiple linear regression analyses predicting intentionality in low- and high-threat scenarios.

Intentionality	ΔR^2	ΔF	df	P	Variables	β	P
Bedtime	0.13	3.56	3.73	0.018	Attachment	−0.04	0.70
					Theory of mind	0.21	0.068
					Maternal sensitivity	0.26	0.021
Bad and nasty time	0.13	3.73	3.73	0.015	Attachment	−0.36	0.001
					Theory of mind	−0.01	0.92
					Maternal sensitivity	0.02	0.84
Happy and best time	0.10	2.86	3.73	0.045	Attachment	−0.17	0.14
					Theory of mind	0.26	0.035
					Maternal sensitivity	0.06	0.61

mind and maternal sensitivity were each associated with intentionality in the low-threat bedtime scenario, but neither was associated with intentionality in the high-threat bad and nasty time scenario, which was only predicted by attachment status. Only theory of mind was associated with intentionality in the happy and best scenario.

Intentionality, attachment, theory of mind, maternal sensitivity, and conduct disorder symptoms at age 5

There were no associations between the log-transformed teacher-rated conduct disorder symptoms and family social class ($t = 0.82$, $p = 0.41$), age of child ($r = -0.08$, $p = 0.49$), maternal depression between 18 months and 5 years ($t = 0.68$, $p = 0.50$), or involvement in current marital conflict ($t = 1.24$, $p = 0.22$).

In order to test Hypothesis 3, the log-transformed teacher symptom scores were first regressed on intentionality scores in the low- and high-threat scenarios, controlling for CGI scores. In tests for possible effects of collinearity among the intentionality scores, the tolerance of each variable was 0.6 or higher. None made a significant contribution to the model (Table 6.4). When groups by intentionality interaction terms were added in the third step, there was a significant interaction between maternal PND and intentionality in the bad and

Table 6.4 Summary of hierarchical regression analysis for the prediction of teacher-rated conduct disorder symptoms from intentionality ratings in low- and high-threat scenarios.

Step	ΔR^2	ΔF	df	P	Variables	β	P
1	0.02	1.37	1.80	0.25	McCarthy GCI	0.13	0.25
2	0.10	2.77	3.77	0.047	McCarthy GCI	0.18	0.10
					BTI	−0.06	0.70
					BNI	−0.24	0.07
					HBI	−0.06	0.67
3	0.18	4.52	4.73	0.003	McCarthy IQ	0.19	0.065
					BTI	−0.14	0.40
					BNI	0.18	0.30
					HBI	0.05	0.77
					Group (PND vs control)	0.14	0.17
					BTI by group	−0.17	0.39
					BNI by group	−0.65	0.001
					HBI by group	−0.04	0.82

BTI, bedtime intentionality; BNI, bad and nasty time intentionality; HBI, happy and best time intentionality, PND; post-natal depression; McCarthy GCI, McCarthy General Cognitive Index.

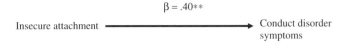

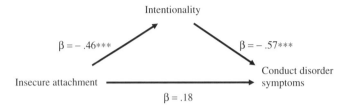

Fig. 6.3 Mediation by intentionality in the high-threat scenario (bad and nasty time) of the association between insecure attachment at 18 months and teacher-rated conduct disorder symptoms at age 5 years in the post-natal depression (PND) group (Notes: ** $p < 0.01$, *** $p < 0.001$)

nasty time scenario. In follow-up analyses, intentionality in the high-threat, bad and nasty time, scenario accounted for 31% of the variance in the teacher-rated conduct symptom scores ($\beta = -0.57$, $p < 0.001$) in the maternal PND group, but only 3% in the control group. There were no statistically significant interactions between social class ($\beta = -0.06$, $p = 0.63$), maternal depression between ages 18 months and 5 years ($\beta = 0.10$, $p = 0.49$), or involvement in marital conflict ($\beta = -0.14$, $p = 0.32$) and intentionality in predicting teacher-rated conduct problems.

In view of the interaction between intentionality in the bad and nasty time scenario and PND, we tested Hypothesis 4, which is intentionality would mediate the association between attachment and conduct disorder symptoms, only in the PND group (Fig. 6.3). In the first step, intentionality in the high-threat scenario was regressed on attachment security in the PND group. Insecure attachment explained 21% of the variance in intentionality scores ($\beta = -0.46$, $p = 0.001$). Then, teacher-rated conduct symptoms were regressed on to attachment security, which explained 16% of the variance ($\beta = 0.40$, $p = 0.006$). Finally, we examined whether the contribution of attachment security to teacher-rated conduct disorder symptoms in the PND group was altered by the introduction of intentionality. When attachment security was entered into the hierarchical regression after intentionality, the explained variance fell from 16% to 3% ($\beta = 0.18$, $p = 0.21$), and the contribution of intentionality remained significant ($\beta = -0.48$, $p = 0.001$), consistent with mediation.

Theory of mind was not associated with conduct disorder symptoms in the overall sample ($t = 1.38$, $p = 0.12$) or in the PND group ($t = 1.22$, $p = 0.23$), neither was maternal sensitivity assessed in the snack task (overall sample: $r = -0.18$, $p = 0.10$; PND group: $r = -0.16$, $p = 0.28$).

Gender, intentionality, and conduct disorder symptoms

Boys had lower intentionality scores than girls in all three scenarios, and the interaction term between gender and scenario was non-significant (Table 6.5). Of specific relevance to mediation (Hypothesis 5), in the PND group, gender explained 25% of the variance in intentionality scores in the high-threat bad and nasty time scenario ($\beta = 0.50$, $p = <0.001$), and 22% of the variance in the log-transformed teacher-rated conduct symptoms ($\beta = 0.47$, $p = 0.001$). When gender was entered into the hierarchical regression after intentionality, the

Table 6.5 Mean intentionality scores at age 5 years contrasting boys and girls.

	Female (N = 43)	Male (N = 39)	Mean difference (95% CI)	P	P cov
Intentionality–bedtime	8.51 (2.51)	6.03 (3.15)	2.49 (1.24–3.73)	<0.001	<0.001
Intentionality–nasty time	7.47 (3.18)	4.46 (3.19)	3.00 (1.60–4.40)	<0.001	<0.001
Intentionality–happy time	6.47 (3.43)	3.38 (2.24)	3.08 (1.79–4.37)	<0.001	<0.001

The table shows unadjusted means and mean differences and their 95% confidence intervals. The P values are from independent groups two-sided t-tests and P cov values are from analysis of covariance, controlling for McCarthy general cognitive ability scores.

explained variance fell from 22% to 5% ($\beta = 0.25$, $p = 0.088$). This was consistent with mediation by intentionality in the context of high threat of the association between gender and conduct disorder symptoms in the PND group.

Gender, attachment, intentionality, and conduct disorder symptoms

When gender and attachment were examined jointly in linear regression, each made contributions to intentionality in the high-threat bad and nasty time scenario, both in the overall sample ($\Delta R^2 = 0.25$; gender: $\beta = -0.36$, $p < 0.001$; attachment: $\beta = -0.28$, $p = 0.005$) and in the PND group ($\Delta R^2 = 0.34$; gender: $\beta = -0.39$, $p = 0.005$; attachment: $\beta = -0.33$, $p = 0.015$). Teacher-rated conduct symptoms were then regressed on to gender and infant attachment security jointly in the overall sample and each made independent contributions ($\Delta R^2 = 0.16$; gender: $\beta = 0.25$, $p = 0.022$; attachment: $\beta = 0.27$, $p = 0.014$; Fig. 6.4). In the PND group, gender and attachment jointly explained 28% of the variance in conduct symptoms (gender: $\beta = 0.37$, $p = 0.01$; attachment: $\beta = 0.27$, $p = 0.055$). In hierarchical linear regression with intentionality entered followed by gender and attachment, their joint contribution to the variance in conduct symptom scores fell to 6% (gender: $\beta = 0.23$, $p = 0.12$; attachment: $\beta = 0.15$, $p = 0.30$), consistent with mediation by intentionality of the links between both attachment security and gender and conduct disorder symptoms in the PND group.

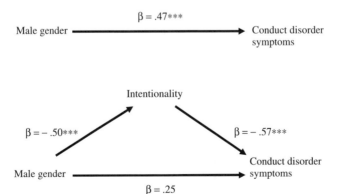

Fig. 6.4 Mediation by intentionality in the high-threat scenario (bad and nasty time) of the association between male gender and teacher-rated conduct disorder symptoms at age 5 years in the postnatal depression (PND) group (Notes: *** $p < 0.001$)

Discussion

The central ideas informing this study were that responding using the intentional stance promotes effective social action but may expose the child to fear in threatening situations, and that inhibiting the intentional stance may reduce fear but promote conduct disorder symptoms. We considered four possible influences on the use of the intentional stance: attachment security, gender, theory of mind, and maternal sensitivity assessed in a non-threatening task. Attachment security indexes how effectively the infant seeks comfort from a caregiver in the face of a threat, and therefore we expect that the secure infant is more able than the insecure one to reduce fear or anxiety while maintaining the intentional stance specifically in threatening situations. The child's fear is also reduced by understanding the situation better, and understanding enhances their strategies for resolving the problem. Girls generally engage in social interactions that require higher levels of interpersonal understanding than boys; so, they may be expected to be more adept in using the intentional stance when asked to respond to social challenges. Theory-of-mind competences are associated with the capacity to perspective-take which we predicted would promote responding using the intentional stance in low-threat scenarios. Maternal sensitivity in non-threatening contexts is also likely to promote intentional stance use, but only in low-threat situations.

We assessed the extent to which the 5-year-old child uses the intentional stance in dolls' house tasks with an intentionality scale, contrasting high- and low-threat scenarios. Children rated as securely attached with their mothers at age 18 months showed evidence, in their doll play responses, of being better able to preserve the intentional stance than insecure children in a high-threat 'bad and nasty time' scenario, but not in low-threat 'bedtime' and 'happy and best time' scenarios. Girls had higher intentionality scores than boys across all three scenarios. Theory of mind competence and maternal sensitivity were also each associated with intentionality, but the interaction terms indicated that this was confined to the low-threat scenarios. Thus, the findings were consistent with there being domain-specific processes whereby attachment, theory-of-mind competences, and maternal sensitivity contribute to the maintenance of the intentional stance via mechanisms that are threat dependent.

We also hypothesized that lower intentionality impairs the regulation of social aggression through its impact on social understanding and through fear reduction particularly when responding to actual or perceived threats. In this study, only intentionality in the high-threat scenario was associated with teacher-rated conduct disorder symptoms, and only in the children of women with PND. Furthermore, intentionality mediated the associations between attachment security and gender and conduct disorder symptoms in the PND group.

Interaction between intentionality and PND

Although intentionality emerged as central to the relationships between threat, attachment, gender, social cognition, and conduct disorder symptoms, its association with conduct symptoms was not uniform across the sample. Intentionality in the high-threat scenario explained 31% of the variance in symptoms among children exposed to PND but only 3% in the control group. Although PND was associated with subsequent maternal depression and with the likelihood of the child being involved in marital discord at age 5, only PND moderated the effect of intentionality. We could not, however, rule out the possibility of moderation by antenatal depression, or conditions co-morbid with PND such as maternal anxiety disorders.

We predicted the interaction on the basis that animal studies found associations between early perturbations of mothering and emotional reactivity, and the combination of high reactivity and lower intentionality may create the conditions for conduct disorder symptoms.

However, we did not have measures at age 5 of emotional reactivity and so could not test this hypothesis directly. Some indirect support is provided by follow-up of this sample to age 16, in which the children of mothers with PND had greater depressive symptomatology, compared with those not exposed to PND, mediated via elevated morning cortisol at age 13 (Halligan *et al.*, 2004, 2007). This pathway did not appear to be explained by depression or other psychosocial factors after the post-natal period. Alterations in hypothalamus-pituitary-adrenal (HPA) axis functioning and early exposure to maternal depression have also been associated with emotional reactivity in infants (Huot *et al.*, 2004; Davis *et al.*, 2007). Thus, the PND by intentionality interaction in predicting conduct disorder symptoms may reflect an interaction with emotional reactivity related to early parenting in the PND group.

Attachment security and intentionality

The finding of an association between infant attachment and intentionality in response to threat at 5 years is in contrast with several studies finding low stability of attachment security, and stressing the openness of attachment processes to later experience (Waters *et al.*, 2000; Thompson & Raikes, 2003). In spite of clear evidence in this sample that early psychosocial adversity (PND) was associated with later adversities (maternal depression in the preschool years and current involvement of the child in marital discord), none of these risks was associated with intentionality ratings. In a previous report from the same study (Murray, Woolgar *et al.*, 1999), recent and current family adversities were associated with a several features of children's dolls' house representations. Most of these referred to the content of the narratives, such as how much neglect was portrayed. This suggests that some aspects of children's representations of family relationships, especially their content, may be influenced by recent experiences, whereas others such as the strategy for interpersonal information processing may have its origins, or be evidenced, in early attachment security.

Strengths and limitations of the study

The study design had several strengths. The sample was representative of the local community in that it had been recruited from post-natal wards, and there was a high participation rate and retention of subjects at follow-up. There was, however, a higher representation of more advantaged families than in the United Kingdom generally. Relevant standardized assessments were conducted at 18 months and at 5 years, and ratings of the dolls' house assessments were made according to written rating rules and blind to all other information about the subjects, except gender. The sequence of scenarios in the doll's house procedure developed by Murray and colleagues was well suited to testing hypotheses regarding continuities from infant attachment status. Although bedtime may in some families be difficult or emotional, the majority of the children told everyday stories of bedtime routines, and seemed to regard it as relatively undemanding emotionally. In the bad and nasty time, most children provided accounts of conflict or threat, some of them quite severe. Where children did not portray events relevant to the theme, the administrator reminded them, so that in most cases it was clear that the child was responding to the emotional implications of the scenario.

Implications for the neurobiology of aggression

The amygdala has rightly taken centre stage in neurobiological models of aggression. In particular, reduced amygdala activation may contribute to both social and emotion regulation processes in callous-unemotional behaviours. Accounts of the causes of amygdala underactivation have generally given priority to deficits, possibly with substantial genetic contributions. We have argued in this chapter that forms of adaptation to threat in childhood may also lead to underactivation of the amygdala. We have focused on the role of avoidant mechanisms in the face of threat, and their role in generating vulnerability to the conduct disorders. The findings reported here are consistent with there being a threat-related avoidant strategy, in the form of lowered intentionality, associated with a history of insecure attachment and also with male gender, which contributes to vulnerability to conduct disorder symptoms. Whether or not children develop avoidant strategies in the face of threat, and hence reduced amygdala activation, will require prospective study of the temporal relationship between environmental insults such as physical abuse, and subsequent behavioural and neurobiological processes.

Acknowledgements

This work was supported by the Tedworth Charitable Trust. Lynne Murray was supported by a senior research fellowship from the Medical Research Council.
    The dolls' house assessments were administered by Alison Hipwell. Vicki Leidecker coded the dolls' house assessments, supervised by Jonathan Hill and Helen Sharp, as part of her research project for the Liverpool University Division of Clinical Psychology.

References

Ainsworth, M. D., Blehar, M. C., Waters, E., & Wall, S. (1978). *Patterns of Attachment: A Psychological Study of the Strange Situation*. Hillsdale, NJ: Earlbaum.
Ainsworth, M. D., & Wittig, B. A. (1969). Attachment and exploratory behaviour in 1-year olds in a Strange Situation. In B. M. Foss (ed), *Determinants of Infant Behaviour (Vol 4)*. London: Methuen.
Baron, R. M., & Kenny, D. A. (1986). The moderator-mediator variable distinction in social psychological research: conceptual, strategic, and statistical considerations. *Journal of Personality and Social Psychology*, *51*, 1173–1182.
Belsky, J., & Fearon, R. M. (2002). Infant-mother attachment security, contextual risk, and early development: a moderational analysis. *Development and Psychopathology*, *14*, 293–310.
Blair, R. J. (2006). The emergence of psychopathy: implications for the neuropsychological approach to developmental disorders. *Cognition*, *101*, 414–442.
Blair, R. J., Peschardt, K. S., Budhani, S., Mitchell, D. G., & Pine, D. S. (2006). The development of psychopathy. *Journal of Child Psychology and Psychiatry*, *47*, 262–276.
Bolton, D., & Hill, J. (2004). *Mind, Meaning and Mental Disorder*, (2nd edn). Oxford, UK: Oxford University Press
Brown, G. W., & Harris, T. (1978). *Social Origins of Depression: Study of Psychiatric Disorders in Women*. London: Tavistock.
Burgess, K. B., Marshall, P. J., Rubin, K. H., & Fox, N. A. (2003). Infant attachment and temperament as predictors of subsequent externalizing problems and cardiac physiology. *Journal of Child Psychology and Psychiatry*, *44*, 819–831.
Carpendale, J. I., & Lewis, C. (2004). Constructing an understanding of mind: the development of children's social understanding within social interaction. *The Behavioral and Brain Sciences*, *27*, 79–96.
Caspi, A., McClay, J., Moffitt, T. E., Mill, J., Martin, J., Craig, I. W., *et al.* (2002). Role of genotype in the cycle of violence in maltreated children. *Science*, *297*, 851–854.
Cornell, A. H., & Frick, P. J. (2007). The moderating effects of parenting styles in the association between behavioral inhibition and parent-reported guilt and empathy in preschool children. *Journal of Clinical Child and Adolescent Psychology*, *36*, 305–318.

Cox, J. L., Holden, J. M., & Sagovsky, R. (1987). Detection of postnatal depression. Development of the 10-item Edinburgh Postnatal Depression Scale. *British Journal of Psychiatry, 150*, 782–786.

Davis, E. P., Glynn, L. M., Schetter, C. D., Hobel, C., Chicz-DeMet, A., & Sandman, C. A. (2007). Prenatal exposure to maternal depression and cortisol influences infant temperament. *Journal of the American Academy of Child and Adolescent Psychiatry, 46*, 737–746.

Denham, S. A., Caverly, S., Schmidt, M., Blair, K., DeMulder, E., Caal, S., *et al.* (2002). Preschool understanding of emotions: contributions to classroom anger and aggression. *Journal of Child Psychology and Psychiatry, 43*, 901–916.

Dennett, D. (1987). *The Intentional Stance.* Cambridge, MA: MIT Press.

Derryberry, D., & Rothbart, M. K. (1997). Reactive and effortful processes in the organization of temperament. *Development and Psychopathology, 9*, 633-652

Dunn, J., & Brown, J. (2001). Emotion, pragmatics and developments in emotion understanding in the preschool years. In D. Bakhurst, & S. Shanker (eds), *Jerome Bruner: Language, Culture, Self.* Thousand Oaks, CA: Sage.

Emde, R. N., Wolf, D. P., & Oppenheim, D. (2003). *Revealing the Inner Worlds of Young Children. The MacArthur Story Stem Battery and Parent-Child Narratives.* New York: Oxford University Press.

Endicott, J., & Spitzer, R. L. (1978). A diagnostic interview: the schedule for affective disorders and schizophrenia. *Archives of General Psychiatry, 35*, 837–844.

Fonagy, P. (2006). The mentalization-focused approach to social development. In J. G. Allen, & P. Fonagy (eds), *Handbook of Mentalization-Based Treatment* (pp. 53–100). Chichester, UK: Wiley.

Fonagy, P., & Target, M. (1997). Attachment and reflective function: their role in self-organization. *Development and Psychopathology, 9*, 679–700.

Fonagy, P., & Target, M. (2006). The mentalization-focused approach to self pathology. *Journal of Personality Disorders, 20*, 544–576.

Forty, L., Jones, L., MacGregor, S., Caesar, S., Cooper, C., Hough, A., *et al.* (2006). Familiality of postpartum depression in unipolar disorder: results of a family study. *American Journal of Psychiatry, 163*, 1549–1553.

Frick, P. J., & Morris, A. S. (2004). Temperament and developmental pathways to conduct problems. *Journal of Clinical Child and Adolescent Psychology, 33*, 54–68.

Gilmour, J., Hill, B., Place, M., & Skuse, D. H. (2004). Social communication deficits in conduct disorder: a clinical and community survey. *Journal of Child Psychology and Psychiatry, 45*, 967–978.

Greenberg, M. T., Speltz, M. L., DeKlyen, M., & Jones, K. (2001). Correlates of clinic referral for early conduct problems: variable- and person-oriented approaches. *Development and Psychopathology, 13*, 255–276.

Guttmann-Steinmetz, S., & Crowell, J. A. (2006). Attachment and externalizing disorders: a developmental psychopathology perspective. *Journal of the American Academy of Child and Adolescent Psychiatry, 45*, 440–451.

Halligan, S. L., Herbert, J., Goodyer, I. M., & Murray, L. (2004). Exposure to postnatal depression predicts elevated cortisol in adolescent offspring. *Biological Psychiatry, 55*, 376–381.

Halligan, S. L., Herbert, J., Goodyer, I., & Murray, L. (2007). Disturbances in morning cortisol secretion in association with maternal postnatal depression predict subsequent depressive symptomatology in adolescents. *Biological Psychiatry, 62*, 40–46.

Hay, D. F., Pawlby, S., Angold, A., Harold, G. T., & Sharp, D. (2003). Pathways to violence in the children of mothers who were depressed postpartum. *Developmental Psychology, 39*, 1083–1094.

Hill, J. (2002). Biological, psychological and social processes in the conduct disorders. *Journal of Child Psychology and Psychiatry, 43*, 133–164.

Hill, J., Fonagy, P., Lancaster, G., & Broyden, N. (2007). Aggression and intentionality in narrative responses to conflict and distress story stems: an investigation of boys with disruptive behaviour problems. *Attachment and Human Development, 9*, 223–237.

Hill, J., Hoover, D., & Taliaferro, G. (2000). *Revised Manual for the MacArthur Narrative Completion Task.* Topeka, KS: Menninger Clinic.

Hill, J., Pickles, A., Rollinson, L., Davies, R., & Byatt, M. (2004). Juvenile- versus adult-onset depression: multiple differences imply different pathways. *Psychological Medicine, 34*, 1483–1493.

Huot, R. L., Brennan, P. A., Stowe, Z. N., Plotsky, P. M., & Walker, E. F. (2004). Negative affect in offspring of depressed mothers is predicted by infant cortisol levels at 6 months and maternal depression during pregnancy, but not postpartum. *Annals of the New York Academy of Science*, *1032*, 234–236.

Jaffee, S. R., Caspi, A., Moffitt, T. E., Dodge, K. A., Rutter, M., Taylor, A., *et al.* (2005). Nature × nurture: genetic vulnerabilities interact with physical maltreatment to promote conduct problems. *Developmental Psychopathology*, *17*, 67–84.

Jaffee, S. R., Moffitt, T. E., Caspi, A., Fombonne, E., Poulton, R., & Martin, J. (2002). Differences in early childhood risk factors for juvenile-onset and adult-onset depression. *Archives of General Psychiatry*, *59*, 215–222.

Jaffee, S. R., Moffitt, T. E., Caspi, A., Taylor, A., & Arseneault, L. (2002). Influence of adult domestic violence on children's internalizing and externalizing problems: an environmentally informative twin study. *Journal of the American Academy of Child and Adolescent Psychiatry*, *41*, 1095–1103.

Keller, T. E., Spieker, S. J., & Gilchrist, L. (2005). Patterns of risk and trajectories of preschool problem behaviors: a person-oriented analysis of attachment in context. *Development and Psychopathology*, *17*, 349–384.

Kim-Cohen, J., Caspi, A., Rutter, M., Tomas, M. P., & Moffitt, T. E. (2006). The caregiving environments provided to children by depressed mothers with or without an antisocial history. *American Journal of Psychiatry*, *163*, 1009–1018.

Kim-Cohen, J., Caspi, A., Taylor, A., Williams, B., Newcombe, R., Craig, I. W., *et al.* (2006). MAOA, maltreatment, and gene-environment interaction predicting children's mental health: new evidence and a meta-analysis. *Molecular Psychiatry*, *11*, 903–913.

Lyons-Ruth, K., Easterbrooks, M. A., & Cibelli, C. D. (1997). Infant attachment strategies, infant mental lag, and maternal depressive symptoms: predictors of internalizing and externalizing problems at age 7. *Developmental Psychology*, *33*, 681–692.

Maccoby, E. E. (2002). Gender and social exchange: a developmental perspective. *New Direction for Child and Adolescent Development*, *95*, 87–105.

Main, M., & Solomon, J. (1990). Procedures for identifying infants as disorganised/disoriented during the Ainsworth Strange Situation. In M. Greenberg, D. Cicchetti, & E. M. Cummings (eds), *Attachment in the Preschool Years*. Chicago, IL: University of Chicago Press.

McCarthy, D. (1972). *McCarthy Scales of Children's Abilities*. New York: Psychological Corporation.

McGuire, J., & Richman, N. (1988). *PreSchool Behaviour Checklist (PBCL) Handbook*. Windsor, UK: NFER-Nelson.

Mejia, J. M., Ervin, F. R., Baker, G. B., & Palmour, R. M. (2002). Monoamine oxidase inhibition during brain development induces pathological aggressive behavior in mice. *Biological Psychiatry*, *52*, 811–821.

Menard, J. L., & Hakvoort, R. M. (2007). Variations of maternal care alter offspring levels of behavioural defensiveness in adulthood: evidence for a threshold model. *Behavioural Brain Research*, *176*, 302–313.

Minnis, H., Millward, R., Sinclair, C., Kennedy, E., Greig, A., Towlson, K., *et al.* (2006). The computerized MacArthur Story Stem Battery—a pilot study of a novel medium for assessing children's representations of relationships. *International Journal of Methods in Psychiatric Research*, *15*, 207–214.

Moffitt, T. E., Caspi, A., Harrington, H., & Milne, B. J. (2002). Males on the life-course-persistent and adolescence-limited antisocial pathways: follow-up at age 26 years. *Developmental Psychopathology*, *14*, 179–207.

Moffitt, T. E., Caspi, A., Rutter, M., & Silva, P. (2001). *Sex Differences in Antisocial Behaviour*. Cambridge, UK: Cambridge University Press.

Moss, E., Smolla, N., Cyr, C., Dubois-Comtois, K., Mazzarello, T., & Berthiaume, C. (2006). Attachment and behavior problems in middle childhood as reported by adult and child informants. *Developmental Psychopathology*, *18*, 425–444.

Murphy-Eberenz, K., Zandi, P. P., March, D., Crowe, R. R., Scheftner, W. A., Alexander, M., *et al.* (2006). Is perinatal depression familial? *Journal of Affective Disorders*, *90*, 49–55.

Murray, L. (1992). The impact of postnatal depression on infant development. *Journal of Child Psychology and Psychiatry*, *33*, 543–561.

Murray, L., Fiori-Cowley, A., Hooper, R., & Cooper, P. (1996). The impact of postnatal depression and associated adversity on early mother-infant interactions and later infant outcome. *Child Development*, *67*, 2512–2526.

Murray, L., Sinclair, D., Cooper, P., Ducournau, P., Turner, P., & Stein, A. (1999). The socioemotional development of 5-year-old children of postnatally depressed mothers. *Journal of Child Psychology and Psychiatry*, *40*, 1259–1271.

Murray, L., Woolgar, M., Briers, S., & Hipwell, A. (1999). Children's social representations in dolls' house play and theory of mind tasks, and their relation to family adversity and child disturbance. *Social Development*, *8*, 179–200.

Ochsner, K. N., Bunge, S. A., Gross, J. J., & Gabrieli, J. D. (2002). Rethinking feelings: an fMRI study of the cognitive regulation of emotion. *Journal of Cognitive Neuroscience*, *14*, 1215–1229.

Orobio, D. C., Veerman, J. W., Koops, W., Bosch, J. D., & Monshouwer, H. J. (2002). Hostile attribution of intent and aggressive behavior: a meta-analysis. *Child Development*, *73*, 916–934.

Pardini, D. A., Lochman, J. E., & Powell, N. (2007). The development of callous-unemotional traits and antisocial behavior in children: are there shared and/or unique predictors? *Journal of Clinical Child and Adolescent Psychology*, *36*, 319–333.

Phelps, E. A., & LeDoux, J. E. (2005). Contributions of the amygdala to emotion processing: from animal models to human behavior. *Neuron*, *48*, 175–187.

Searle, J. (1983). *Intentionality*. Cambridge, UK: Cambridge University Press.

Speltz, M. L., DeKlyen, M., & Greenberg, M. T. (1999). Attachment in boys with early onset conduct problems. *Developmental Psychopathology*, *11*, 269–285.

Spitzer, R. L., Endicott, J., & Robins, E. (1978). Research diagnostic criteria: rationale and reliability. *Archives of General Psychiatry*, *35*, 773–782.

Szyf, M., McGowan, P., & Meaney, M. J. (2007). The social environment and the epigenome. *Environmental and Molecular Mutagenesis*, *49*(1), 46–60.

Thompson, R. A., & Raikes, H. A. (2003). Toward the next quarter-century: conceptual and methodological challenges for attachment theory. *Development Psychopathology*, *15*, 691–718.

Viding, E., Blair, R. J., Moffitt, T. E., & Plomin, R. (2005). Evidence for substantial genetic risk for psychopathy in 7-year-olds. *Journal of Child Psychology and Psychiatry*, *46*, 592–597.

Ward, H. E., Johnson, E. A., Goodman, I. J., Birkle, D. L., Cottrell, D. J., & Azzaro, A. J. (1998). Corticotropin-releasing factor and defensive withdrawal: inhibition of monoamine oxidase prevents habituation to chronic stress. *Pharmacology, Biochemistry and Behavior*, *60*, 209–215.

Waters, E., Weinfield, N. S., & Hamilton, C. E. (2000). The stability of attachment security from infancy to adolescence and early adulthood: general discussion. *Child Development*, *71*, 703–706.

7

The amygdala and ventromedial prefrontal cortex: Functional contributions and dysfunction in psychopathy

R. James R. Blair

Introduction

Psychopathy is a developmental disorder (Lynam *et al.*, 2007) marked by emotional dysfunction (reduced guilt and empathy) and antisocial behaviour (Harpur *et al.*, 1988; Hare, 1991; Frick, 1995). The disorder is not equivalent to the psychiatric diagnoses of Conduct Disorder (CD) or Antisocial Personality Disorder (ASPD) (DSM-IV) or Conduct Disorder and Dissocial Personality Disorder (ICD 10) (for full details on the assessment of psychopathy, see Patrick, 2006). These psychiatric diagnoses concentrate on the antisocial behaviour shown by the individual rather than any putative cause such as the emotion dysfunction seen in psychopathy. A distinctive feature of psychopathy is that it confers an increased risk of both reactive and instrumental aggression (Cornell *et al.*, 1996; Frick *et al.*, 2003). Reactive aggression is triggered by a frustrating or threatening event and involves unplanned, enraged attacks on the object perceived to be the source of the threat or frustration. This aggression type is often accompanied by anger and can be considered 'hot'. Importantly, it is initiated without regard for any potential goal. This is in direct contrast with instrumental aggression, which is *purposeful and goal directed* (e.g., to obtain the victim's possessions). Furthermore, instrumental aggression need not be accompanied by an emotional state, such as anger, and can be considered 'cold'. Many emotional disorders (e.g., childhood bipolar disorder and Post-Traumatic Stress Disorder) confer an increased risk of reactive aggression (Blair *et al.*, 2005). However, psychopathy is the only psychiatric condition to also confer an increased risk of instrumental aggression.

The goal of this review is to consider the cognitive neuroscience of psychopathy. In short, the functional contributions of two core neural systems, evidence of their dysfunction in psychopathy, and the developmental consequences of these dysfunctions will be considered. The primary causes of the disorder-that is, the contribution of genes and the environment-will not be considered in detail. However, the strong suggestion here is that there is a genetic contribution to the emotion dysfunction that is the core of psychopathy and which will be described in this chapter. Currently, there are no known environmental factors (including trauma and neglect) that can give rise to the pathophysiology seen in psychopathy (see Blair, 2007). Instead, these environmental factors are associated with increased responsiveness in the amygdala in particular (see Blair, 2007) rather than the decreased responsiveness seen in psychopathy. This, of course, does not imply that social and environmental factors have no impact on the development of the disorder. Indeed, it will be argued, in the following, that they have a significant impact on how the disorder manifests in the individual.

The two core neural systems that will be considered in this chapter are the amygdala and the ventromedial prefrontal cortex (vmPFC). The term *amygdala* was first used by

Burdach (1819–22) to describe an almond-shaped mass of grey matter in the anterior portion of the human temporal lobe. Later work subdivided the amygdala into distinct nuclei with a primary division being made between the basolateral and central nuclei (Johnston, 1923), a division that remains in the literature today. For this chapter, the vmPFC is considered to include Brodmann's areas 10 and 11 and inferior regions of the rostral anterior cingulate cortex and subgenual cingulate cortex (BA 32 and 24). Regions of the vmPFC have considerable interconnectivity with the amygdala (Price, 2003).

Functions of the amygdala and VmPFC

The amygdala

The goal here is not to provide a complete overview on the functions of the amygdala and the vmPFC but to describe those functions implicated in understanding psychopathy. The amygdala is involved in stimulus-reinforcement learning. At one stage, the general view was that the basolateral nuclei received sensory input and allowed the formation of conditioned stimulus-unconditioned stimulus associations. These associations then allowed the basolateral amygdala to control the activity of the central nucleus, which in turn allowed the control of hypothalamic and brainstem structures to orchestrate behavioural, autonomic, and neuroendocrine responses (LeDoux, 1998; Davis, 2000). However, it is now clear that the basolateral amygdala does more than control the central nucleus (Everitt et al., 2003; Schoenbaum & Roesch, 2005). In particular, it allows the transmission of stimulus-reinforcement association information (i.e., reinforcement expectancies) forward to the vmPFC for appropriate decision making (see the following subsection; Schoenbaum & Roesch, 2005).

Much work has stressed the role of the amygdala with respect to aversive conditioning (LeDoux, 1998; Buchel & Dolan, 2000; Davis, 2000). However, it is now clear that the amygdala also plays a role in appetitive conditioning (Gottfried et al., 2002; Everitt et al., 2003). Moreover, it plays a role in instructed fear, showing greater responsiveness to stimuli that subjects have been simply told will anticipate shock (Phelps et al., 2001). Presumably, the instructed fear stimulus is semantically associated with conditioned stimuli and thus comes to activate the amygdala.

Aversive and appetitive conditioning involve the interaction of the temporal cortex and the amygdala (LeDoux, 1998). Conditioned stimuli, represented within the temporal cortex, become associated with valence information represented within the amygdala. As the connections between the temporal cortex and the amygdala are reciprocal (Amaral et al., 1992), the activity of neurons representing emotional stimuli in the temporal cortex is further augmented by reciprocal feedback from the amygdala. Emotional attention can be understood in terms of this interaction (Pessoa & Ungerleider, 2004; Mitchell et al., 2006). Representations of emotional stimuli in the temporal cortex are primed by the amygdala as a function of the degree to which they activate the amygdala. As such, emotional distracters should and do cause greater interference on task performance than do neutral distracters (Erthal et al., 2005; Mitchell et al., 2006; Blair et al., 2007). Conversely, if the emotional stimulus is relevant to task performance, then there will be facilitation of performance, relative to neutral stimuli. This can be seen in emotional lexical decision paradigms where healthy volunteers are usually significantly faster or more accurate to judge that emotional letter strings (e.g., 'murder') are words rather than neutral letter strings (e.g., 'table') (Graves et al., 1981; Lorenz & Newman, 2002; Nakic et al., 2006).

Considerable data indicate that the amygdala is involved in the processing of emotional expressions (for reviews, see Adolphs, 2002; Blair, 2003). However, there are two issues that remain open to debate. The first of these concerns which expressions the amygdala responds to. There have been suggestions that the amygdala responds to all emotional expressions (Winston *et al.*, 2003; Fitzgerald *et al.*, 2006). However, a considerable number of other studies have not supported this view (Morris *et al.*, 1996; Blair *et al.*, 1999; LaBar *et al.*, 2003). Moreover, a meta-analysis of the literature strongly supported the suggestion that the amygdala is particularly responsive to fearful expressions (Murphy *et al.*, 2003).

The second, related, issue concerns the nature of the function of the amygdala's response to expression information. One influential view suggests that the 'amygdala monitors the environment for stimuli that signal an increased probability of threat' and that the 'magnitude of amygdala activation may be inversely related to the amount of information concerning the nature of the threat' (Whalen, 1998; p. 180). According to this view, fearful faces are innately specified threat stimuli that 'engage the amygdala to a greater degree than angry faces because they require more information concerning the nature of a probable threat' (Whalen, 1998; p. 180). Fearful expressions are considered more ambiguous threats than angry expressions because they provide less information regarding the source of the threat and thus lead to increased amygdala activity.

A second view suggests that fearful faces should be viewed as 'reinforcers that modulate the probability that a particular behaviour will be performed in the future' and this function as reinforcers lead to amygdala activity (Blair, 2003; p. 564). In contrast, angry expressions are considered to 'serve to inform the observer to stop the current behavioural action' and 'can be seen as triggers for response reversal' (Blair, 2003; p. 564). In line with this position, angry faces have been shown to activate regions of the inferior frontal cortex (Murphy *et al.*, 2003). This region is consistently implicated in reversal learning (Cools *et al.*, 2002; Budhani *et al.*, 2007).

A recent study by Hooker and colleagues (2006) allowed a direct contrast of these views. In this study, healthy participants were presented with images of individuals displaying fearful and happy expressions either towards novel objects (i.e., probable threats) or empty space (i.e., no information was provided regarding the nature of the threat). If amygdala activation is inversely related to the amount of information regarding the nature of the threat (i.e., related to increased ambiguity), then there should be greater activation to the fearful expression when presented alone, relative to when it was presented as a response to an object. Alternatively, if the amygdala treats particular expressions as reinforcers (i.e., cues to stimulus-reinforcement learning), then the amygdala should show greater activity when there are object stimuli to associate with the expression reinforcement. The data clearly supported the latter suggestion: there was significantly greater amygdala activity when there were object stimuli to associate with the expression reinforcement (Hooker *et al.*, 2006). In short, and as noted by Hooker and colleagues, the data indicated that the 'amygdala uses social signals to rapidly and flexibly learn threatening and rewarding associations' (p. 8915).

The VmPFC

Much of the clinical neuroscience literature stresses a role for the vmPFC in emotional regulation (Phillips *et al.*, 2003; Rauch *et al.*, 2006). Thus, animal work has shown that train stimulation of the medial prefrontal cortex in rats suppresses neuronal activity in the basolateral nucleus of the amygdala, that is otherwise seen to conditioned stimuli (Rosenkranz *et al.*, 2003). However, which regions of the vmPFC are involved in emotional regulation in

humans remains unclear. The rostral anterior cingulate cortex has frequently been implicated (Whalen *et al.*, 1998; Pezawas *et al.*, 2005; Etkin *et al.*, 2006), with the subgenual anterior cingulate cortex appearing to receive emotional information from the amygdala (Pezawas
et al., 2005; Budhani *et al.*, 2007) and the supragenual cingulated cortex acting to suppress
the amygdala (Pezawas *et al.*, 2005; Etkin *et al.*, 2006). In our own work, we have observed
activity in a slightly lateral, polar region of the vmPFC in tasks requiring the suppression of
emotional distracter information (Blair *et al.*, 2007; Mitchell *et al.*, 2007). This region has
also been typically activated for tasks in which participants are explicitly instructed to
suppress their emotional reactions (Beauregard *et al.*, 2001; Ohira *et al.*, 2006).

Although some regions of the vmPFC are involved in emotional regulation, it is important to note that the vmPFC, as articulated in the preceding, is a large area that is likely
implicated in a variety of functions. Considerable data indicate a role for the vmPFC in
encoding reinforcement outcome information (Knutson & Cooper, 2005; Schoenbaum &
Roesch, 2005; Rushworth *et al.*, 2007). Indeed, the vmPFC appears to receive reinforcement
expectation information in stimulus-reinforcement-based instrumental learning paradigms
(such as the animal go/no-go task, referred to in the human literature as the passive avoidance learning paradigm). The availability of this information is critical for appropriate decision making (Schoenbaum & Roesch, 2005; Kosson *et al.*, 2006). Moreover, vmPFC lesions
actually diminish reinforcement-expectancy activity in the basolateral nucleus of the
amygdala (Schoenbaum *et al.*, 2003); that is, suppression is not the only interaction that the
vmPFC has with the amygdala.

Considerable progress has been made on the functional contributions of the vmPFC.
Suggestions have been made that the orbitofrontal cortex normalizes the value of competing
outcomes so that the value of differing rewards such as apples and oranges can be compared
(Montague & Berns, 2002; Schoenbaum & Roesch, 2005). In line with these suggestions,
recent recording work demonstrated the existence of cells in the orbitofrontal cortex
that encode the value of offered and chosen goods. They show greater activity to smaller
amounts of a more desirable object relative to greater amounts of a less desirable object
(Padoa-Schioppa & Assad, 2006).

Interestingly, although the vmPFC is importantly involved in the representation of value
information crucial for stimulus selection, this region itself does not appear to directly select
between responses. There have been suggestions that the vmPFC is involved in the *comparison* of values and stimulus selection (Arana *et al.*, 2003; Blair, 2004; Schoenbaum & Roesch,
2005). However, such suggestions made clear predictions: if the vmPFC is involved in the
comparison of values, it should show differential responsiveness to parameters that increase
choice difficulty on the basis of value information. We examined two such parameters on
vmPFC activity: the degree of difference in reinforcement associated with the chosen and
non-chosen object (the greater the differential in value, the easier the decision making; Blair,
Marsh *et al.*, 2006), and the number of objects to choose between (the fewer objects with
different values to choose between, the easier the decision making; Marsh *et al.*, 2007). In
both the studies, vmPFC activity was seen to vary as a function of the reinforcement associated with the chosen stimulus. However, it was not influenced by either the degree of difference in reinforcement associated with the chosen and non-chosen object (Blair, Marsh *et al.*,
2006) or the number of objects to choose between (Marsh *et al.*, 2007). In short, the vmPFC
is importantly involved in the representation of value information but does not directly
select between responses.

It appears plausible that the dorsomedial prefrontal cortex may be operating on the
translation of reinforcement expectancy information into response tendencies to mediate

response selection. Considerable work has demonstrated a role for this cortex in the monitoring and resolution of response conflict (Cohen *et al.*, 2000; Botvinick *et al.*, 2004). If reinforcement expectancies are translated as approach or avoidance tendencies, then response options that are close in reinforcement value should be associated with similar strength approach or avoidance tendencies and greater response conflict (cf. Blair, Marsh *et al.*, 2006). Similarly, the greater the number of response options, the greater should be the response conflict (cf. Marsh *et al.*, 2007). Certainly, dorsal regions of the anterior cingulate cortex did show significant activity in response to both the degree of difference in reinforcement associated with the chosen and non-chosen object and the number of objects to choose between (Blair, Marsh *et al.*, 2006; Marsh *et al.*, 2007).

On a related note, the vmPFC has been consistently implicated in reversal learning in animal (Iversen & Mishkin, 1970; Dias *et al.*, 1996; Izquierdo *et al.*, 2004) and some human work (Fellows & Farah, 2003; O'Doherty *et al.*, 2003; Budhani *et al.*, 2007). During reversal learning, the vmPFC shows a significant *reduction* in activity during reversal errors (trials when a previously rewarded response is now punished; Budhani *et al.*, 2007). It is possible that this signaling in the vmPFC may be needed for the detection of contingency change and thus the initiation of reversal learning (Budhani *et al.*, 2007). Alternatively, this region may orchestrate reversal learning by representing the reinforcement associated with the two responses: the vmPFC appears to track the expectation of reinforcement associated with not only chosen but also non-chosen objects (Blair, Marsh *et al.*, 2006; Hampton *et al.*, 2006; Padoa-Schioppa & Assad, 2006). It has been argued that the vmPFC may increase the representation of reward expectancy associated with the non-chosen object if the chosen object does not elicit reward (Hampton *et al.*, 2006). By this latter account, as the old correct response becomes more frequently punished, the expectancy of reward associated with it decreases. Simultaneously, the expectancy of reward associated with the now correct response increases. When the expectancy of reward associated with the now correct response is greater than the expectancy of reward associated with the old correct response, the participant should switch their responding (cf. Hampton *et al.*, 2006).

The cognitive neuroscience of psychopathy: amygdala and vmPFC dysfunction

In the preceding section, I described the core functions of the amygdala and vmPFC that I believe are of core relevance to the understanding of psychopathy. In this next section, I will consider the data indicating amygdala and vmPFC dysfunction in psychopathy.

Amygdala dysfunction

As noted earlier, a considerable literature implicates the amygdala in stimulus-reinforcement association formation (LeDoux, 1998; Buchel & Dolan, 2000; Davis, 2000). Individuals with psychopathy show pronounced impairment on tasks reliant on the ability to form such associations. For example, some of the earliest findings in psychopathy were demonstrations of the impairment in aversive conditioning (Hare, 1970; Lykken, 1957). Moreover, recent functional magnetic resonance imaging (fMRI) work has demonstrated that individuals with psychopathy show reduced amygdala activity during aversive conditioning (Birbaumer *et al.*, 2005). Related to this function, the amygdala allows conditioned stimuli to prime brainstem threat circuits mediating the startle reflex such that a startle probe elicits greater startle after a threatening prime relative to a neutral prime (Davis, 2000). Individuals with psychopathy do not show appropriate augmentation of the startle reflex following a negative prime (Patrick *et al.*, 1993; Levenston *et al.*, 2000). The amygdala also plays a role in instructed fear, when subjects are told that a stimulus is associated with shock (Phelps *et al.*, 2001). Individuals with psychopathy show reduced autonomic responses, relative to comparison individuals, to instructed fear cues (e.g., Hare *et al.*, 1978).

Earlier, I related emotional attention to stimulus-reinforcement learning and the consequent interaction between the temporal cortex and the amygdala (Pessoa & Ungerleider, 2004; Mitchell *et al.*, 2006). If there is amygdala dysfunction in psychopathy, individuals with the disorder should show significantly less interference by emotional distracters. Two studies have directly examined this issue. Christianson *et al.* (1996) showed that emotional, relative to neutral, content in images caused significantly less interference with the recollection of non-emotional, peripheral content in individuals with psychopathy relative to comparison individuals. Mitchell *et al.* (2006) reported significantly less interference in motor responding in individuals with psychopathy from emotional distracters presented immediately before and after the very rapidly presented target stimuli. A second prediction of amygdala dysfunction in psychopathy with respect to emotional attention is that if the emotional stimulus is relevant to task performance, then individuals with the disorder should show less facilitation by emotional *targets*. In line with this prediction, individuals with psychopathy show significantly less facilitation by emotional words relative to comparison individuals on the emotional lexical decision task (Williamson *et al.*, 1991; Lorenz & Newman, 2002).

FMRI data can also reveal the priming of emotional representations in the temporal cortex by reciprocal amygdala activation (i.e., emotional attention). Thus, several studies have shown heightened fusiform and/or temporal cortex responses to emotional expressions relative to neutral ones, presumably as a consequence of reciprocal feedback of the amygdala to this region of the temporal cortex (Mitchell *et al.*, 2007). Studies examining expression processing in both adults with psychopathy (Deeley *et al.*, 2006) and children with psychopathic traits (Marsh *et al.*, under revision) have shown a reduced differential response within the fusiform cortex to fearful expressions relative to neutral expressions. These data are consistent with reduced priming of emotion-relevant representations in the temporal cortex by reciprocal amygdala activation in individuals with psychopathy (although only Marsh *et al.* under revision observed reduced amygdala activity). In addition, recent work has shown that (i) patients with amygdala lesions show reduced eye gaze to the eye region, (ii) this is related to their impairment in fearful face recognition, and (iii) attentional instructions to focus on the eye region abolish the recognition impairment (Adolphs *et al.*, 2005). Similarly, Dadds and colleagues (2006) have reported reduced eye gaze to the eye region in children with psychopathic tendencies and that attentional instructions to focus on the eye region abolish their recognition impairment. In short, children with psychopathic tendencies show similar emotional attention-related impairments as patients with amygdala lesions.

As noted, the amygdala appears particularly responsive to fearful expressions (Murphy *et al.*, 2003). Although multiple studies have shown specific impairments in fearful expression processing in individuals with psychopathic tendencies (Blair *et al.*, 2004; Montagne *et al.*, 2005; Dadds *et al.*, 2006), not all studies have reported such deficits (Kosson *et al.*, 2002; Glass & Newman, 2006). However, a recent meta-analysis of 20 studies examining expression recognition in psychopathy and other instrumentally aggressive populations demonstrated a robust link between these antisocial populations and specific deficits in recognizing fearful expressions (Marsh & Blair, 2007). Moreover, imaging work in subclinical adult populations (Gordon *et al.*, 2004) and children with psychopathic tendencies (Marsh *et al.*, in press) has shown reduced amygdala responses to fearful expressions in individuals with psychopathic tendencies.

VmPFC dysfunction

As noted in the preceding, the amygdala feeds forward reinforcement information associated with stimuli to the vmPFC, which then represents this outcome information (Schoenbaum & Roesch, 2005). Given the indications of amygdala dysfunction described earlier, it can be expected that individuals with psychopathy will show anomalous vmPFC activity in response to amygdala activation. Indeed, in their fMRI study of fearful expression processing, Marsh *et al.* (in press) report reduced functional connectivity between the amygdala and the vmPFC in the children with psychopathic tendencies relative to the comparison children. Moreover, Birbaumer *et al.* (2005) reported reduced vmPFC activity as well as reduced amygdala activity in individuals with psychopathy during aversive conditioning. Similarly, a study examining performance on the Prisoner's Dilemma in a subclinical population found reduced amygdala and vmPFC differentiation in individuals with psychopathic tendencies in Blood-oxygen-level dependent (BOLD) response when making cooperation relative to defection choices (Rilling *et al.*, 2007). In addition, a study of emotional memory reported reduced amygdala and vmPFC responses to emotional words in individuals with psychopathy (Kiehl *et al.*, 2001).

The suggestion is that reinforcement expectancy information is critical for optimal decision making (Montague & Berns, 2002; Schoenbaum & Roesch, 2005). In line with this, vmPFC lesions have been demonstrated to show impairment in decision making (Bechara *et al.*, 2000). Moreover, this impairment on the Iowa gambling task is also reliant on appropriate amygdala functioning (Bechara *et al.*, 1999)-as can be predicted given the amygdala's role in feeding forward reinforcement expectancy information to the vmPFC. Individuals with psychopathy show impairment on the Iowa gambling task (Blair *et al.*, 2001; Mitchell *et al.*, 2002) as do subclinical populations with psychopathic tendencies (van Honk *et al.*, 2002). Neuroimaging data have confirmed that other stimulus-reinforcement-based decision-making tasks such as the passive avoidance learning task (Kosson *et al.* 2006) and the differential reward-punishment task (Blair, Marsh *et al.* 2006) are also reliant on integrated amygdala-vmPFC activity. Individuals with psychopathy show impairment on both these tasks (Newman & Kosson, 1986; Blair *et al.*, 2004; Blair, Leonard *et al.*, 2006).

The role of the vmPFC in the representation of reinforcement expectancies is also crucial for behavioural extinction and reversal learning either because of its role in prediction error signaling (Budhani *et al.*, 2007) or because of its role in tracking the reinforcement associated with the non-chosen object (Hampton *et al.*, 2006). Individuals with psychopathy are impaired in both behavioural extinction (Newman *et al.*, 1987) and reversal learning (Mitchell *et al.*, 2002; Budhani & Blair, 2005; Budhani *et al.*, 2006). Moreover, neuroimaging data of children with psychopathic tendencies performing a reversal-learning paradigm have recently been obtained (Finger *et al.*, 2008). In this study, children with psychopathic tendencies and comparison children performed a probabilistic reversal-learning paradigm similar to that described by Budhani *et al.* (2007), who had demonstrated that healthy adults showed a reduced BOLD response within the vmPFC to punished incorrect reversal phases responses relative to correct responses; this is consistent with the suggestion that the vmPFC is responding to the prediction error, the failure to receive the anticipated reward. In the study by Finger *et al.* (2008), the comparison children also showed significant reductions in

BOLD responses in the vmPFC to punished incorrect reversal responses relative to correct responses. In contrast, the children with psychopathic tendencies did not.

The human neuroimaging literature has consistently implicated the inferior and dorsomedial prefrontal cortex in reversal learning: both regions show greater BOLD responses to punished reversal errors relative to rewarded correct responses (Cools et al., 2002; Kringelbach & Rolls, 2003; Budhani et al., 2007). Interestingly, although children with psychopathic tendencies did not show the appropriate reduction in BOLD response to punished incorrect reversal phases responses relative to correct responses in the vmPFC, they did show increases in BOLD response, equivalent to comparison children, in the inferior and dorsomedial prefrontal cortex to the same contrast (Finger et al., 2008). This is important because it indicates that any vmPFC detection of reinforcement contingency changes cannot be responsible for the recruitment of this cortex to effect a change in response (cf. Budhani et al., 2007). Indeed, these data suggest a degree of independence in these functional processes. Importantly, there are many cues for error detection that do not rely on a reinforcement-based prediction error signal (cf. Holroyd et al., 2004). It appears that children with psychopathic tendencies are sensitive to such cues and successfully recruit regions necessary for response change accordingly.

In this context, it is worth noting the behavioural performance of adults with psychopathy on reversal learning paradigms (Budhani et al., 2006). Following a punished incorrect response, adults with psychopathy are as likely to change their response on the subsequent trial as comparison individuals. This was not readily accounted for in the Budhani et al. (2006) study. However, the findings of Finger et al. (2008), showing appropriate recruitment of the dorsomedial and inferior frontal cortex to punished reversal errors, perhaps provide an explanation.

It can be assumed that reinforcement information, in the context of reversal learning and other paradigms, serves two functions: first, it changes the outcome expectancy associated with the stimulus, and second, if it is punishment information, it prompts an immediate change in behaviour. The first function involves the vmPFC in the representation of appetitive and aversive outcome information, and the second involves the dorsomedial and inferior frontal cortex in the orchestration of behavioural change (see the preceding paragraphs). On the basis of both Budhani et al.'s (2006) behavioural and Finger et al.'s (2008) fMRI results, the second function appears to be intact in psychopathy. Punishment information appropriately activates the dorsomedial and inferior frontal cortex (cf. Finger et al., 2008) orchestrating a shift in responding on the immediate subsequent trial (cf. Budhani et al., 2006).

In contrast, the first function, the role of the vmPFC in the representation of outcome information, appears to be dysfunctional in psychopathy (cf. Finger et al., 2008). This suggests that response selection on the basis of outcome information should be impaired. Adults with psychopathy show impairment on trials subsequent to a rewarded correct response: they are significantly more likely to revert to the previously rewarded, now no longer correct, response than comparison individuals (Budhani et al., 2006). These are trials that are likely to be particularly under the control of outcome expectancy calculations.

Conclusions: developmental consequences of amygdala and VmPFC dysfunction

I began this chapter by describing the functional contributions of the two core regions that I believe are dysfunctional in psychopathy and presented data indicating dysfunction in the functioning of these regions in individuals with the disorder. In this last section, I aim to briefly consider why this dysfunction may lead to the development of the disorder.

As noted earlier, the amygdala is crucial for stimulus-reinforcement learning and responding to emotional expressions, particularly fearful expressions that, as reinforcers, are important initiators of such learning. Moreover, the amygdala is involved in the formation of both stimulus-punishment and stimulus-reward associations. Individuals with psychopathy show impairment in stimulus-reinforcement learning (whether punishment- or reward-based) and responding to fearful and sad expressions. It is argued that this impairment drives much of the syndrome of psychopathy. Stimulus-reinforcement learning is crucial for socialization, for learning that some things are bad to do, and individuals with psychopathy fail to take advantage of standard socialization techniques (Wootton et al., 1997). As such, they are more likely to learn to use antisocial strategies to achieve their goals. The reduced amygdala responding also diminishes empathy-based learning following the witnessing of another's distress and leads to reduced empathy generally. Finally, the impairment in stimulus-reward learning may relate to the reduced attachment reported in this disorder (Hare, 2003): individuals with psychopathy may find their caregivers less rewarding stimuli and be less motivated to maintain contact with them.

The vmPFC is considered critical for the representation of reinforcement information that can then be used by other structures, such as the dorsomedial frontal cortex, to implement behaviour. Impairment in vmPFC functioning means that individuals with psychopathy will show impaired decision making. This will contribute to their disordered lifestyle and may increase the risk of drug abuse. Moreover, because the vmPFC is so important for successful decision making, its dysfunction will increase the probability that individuals with the disorder will make less than optimal decisions when attempting to achieve their goals. As such, this will increase the risk of frustration and potentially frustration-based reactive aggression.

Can the model described here explain all aspects of psychopathy? The answer is almost certainly not. There are aspects of psychopathy (e.g., the grandiose sense of self and superficial charm) that are not clear developmental consequences of the impairment described in the preceding section. It will be interesting to determine whether these relate to additional impairments or that they are consequences of how the dysfunction described interacts with the individual's social environment.

Importantly, the above suggests pharmacological treatment strategies. Whereas some pharmacological compounds such as propranolol decrease amygdala activity, others such as yohimbine increase it. Theoretically it might be possible to increase the responsiveness of the systems described such that clinically based socialization strategies (e.g., empathy induction and victim awareness) might allow the individual to form more appropriate associations regarding the distress of others and actions that harm others. In short, it is to be hoped that the increased basic understanding of this disorder may soon be translated into therapeutic strategies that will help the individuals concerned.

Acknowledgements

This research was supported by the Intramural Research Program of the National Institutes of Health and the National Institute of Mental Health (NIH:NIMH).

References

Adolphs, R. (2002). Neural systems for recognizing emotion. *Current Opinion in Neurobiology, 12,* 169–177.

Adolphs, R., Gosselin, F., Buchanan, T. W., Tranel, D., Schyns, P., & Damasio, A. R. (2005). A mechanism for impaired fear recognition after amygdala damage. *Nature, 433,* 68–72.

Amaral, D. G., Price, J. L., Pitkanen, A., & Carmichael, S. T. (1992). Anatomical organization of the primate amygdaloid complex. In J. P. Aggleton (ed), *The Amygdala: Neurobiological Aspects of Emotion, Memory, and Mental Dysfunction* (pp. 1–66). New York: Wiley.

Arana, F. S., Parkinson, J. A., Hinton, E., Holland, A. J., Owen, A. M., & Roberts, A. C. (2003). Dissociable contributions of the human amygdala and orbitofrontal cortex to incentive motivation and goal selection. *Journal of Neuroscience, 23,* 9632–9638.

Beauregard, M., Levesque, J., & Bourgouin, P. (2001). Neural correlates of conscious self-regulation of emotion. *Journal of Neuroscience, 21,* RC165.

Bechara, A., Damasio, H., Damasio, A. R., & Lee, G. P. (1999). Different contributions of the human amygdala and ventromedial prefrontal cortex to decision-making. *Journal of Neuroscience, 19,* 5473–5481.

Bechara, A., Tranel, D., & Damasio, H. (2000). Characterization of the decision-making deficit of patients with ventromedial prefrontal cortex lesions. *Brain, 123*(Pt 11), 2189–2202.

Birbaumer, N., Veit, R., Lotze, M., Erb, M., Hermann, C., Grodd, W., *et al.* (2005). Deficient fear conditioning in psychopathy: a functional magnetic resonance imaging study. *Archives of General Psychiatry, 62,* 799–805.

Blair, J. (2007). Dysfunctions of medial and lateral orbitofrontal cortex in psychopathy. *Annals of the New York Academy of Science, 1121,* 461–479.

Blair, K. S., Leonard, A., Morton, J., & Blair, R. J. R. (2006). Impaired decision making on the basis of both reward and punishment information in individuals with psychopathy. *Personality and Individual Differences, 41,* 155–165.

Blair, K. S., Marsh, A. A., Morton, J., Vythilingham, M., Jones, M., Mondillo, K., *et al.* (2006). Choosing the lesser of two evils, the better of two goods: specifying the roles of ventromedial prefrontal cortex and dorsal anterior cingulate cortex in object choice. *Journal of Neuroscience, 26,* 11379–11386.

Blair, K. S., Smith, B. W., Mitchell, D. G., Morton, J., Vythilingam, M., Pessoa, L., *et al.* (2007). Modulation of emotion by cognition and cognition by emotion. *Neuroimage, 35,* 430–440.

Blair, R. J., Colledge, E., & Mitchell, D. G. (2001). Somatic markers and response reversal: Is there orbitofrontal cortex dysfunction in boys with psychopathic tendencies? *Journal of Abnormal Child Psychology, 29,* 499–511.

Blair, R. J. R. (2003). Facial expressions, their communicatory functions and neuro-cognitive substrates. *Philosophical Transactions of the Royal Society of London: Series B Biological Sciences, 358,* 561–572.

Blair, R. J. R. (2004). The roles of orbital frontal cortex in the modulation of antisocial behavior. *Brain and Cognition, 55,* 198–208.

Blair, R. J. R., Mitchell, D. G. V., & Blair, K. S. (2005). *The Psychopath: Emotion and the Brain.* Oxford: Blackwell.

Blair, R. J. R., Mitchell, D. G. V., Leonard, A., Budhani, S., Peschardt, K. S., & Newman, C. (2004). Passive avoidance learning in individuals with psychopathy: modulation by reward but not by punishment. *Personality and Individual Differences, 37,* 1179–1192.

Blair, R. J. R., Morris, J. S., Frith, C. D., Perrett, D. I., & Dolan, R. (1999). Dissociable neural responses to facial expressions of sadness and anger. *Brain, 122,* 883–893.

Botvinick, M. M., Cohen, J. D., & Carter, C. S. (2004). Conflict monitoring and anterior cingulate cortex: an update. *Trends in Cognitive Science, 8,* 539–546.

Buchel, C., & Dolan, R. J. (2000). Classical fear conditioning in functional neuroimaging. *Current Opinions in Neurobiology, 10,* 219–223.

Budhani, S., & Blair, R. J. (2005). Response reversal and children with psychopathic tendencies: success is a function of salience of contingency change. *Journal of Child Psychology and Psychiatry, 46,* 972–981.

Budhani, S., Marsh, A. A., Pine, D. S., & Blair, R. J. (2007). Neural correlates of response reversal: considering acquisition. *Neuroimage, 34*, 1754–1765.

Budhani, S., Richell, R. A., & Blair, R. J. (2006). Impaired reversal but intact acquisition: probabilistic response reversal deficits in adult individuals with psychopathy. *Journal of Abnormal Psychology, 115*, 552–558.

Christianson, S. A., Forth, A. E., Hare, R. D., Strachan, C., Lidberg, L., & Thorell, L. H. (1996). Remembering details of emotional events: a comparison between psychopathic and nonpsychopathic offenders. *Personality and Individual Differences, 20*, 437–443.

Cohen, J. D., Botvinick, M., & Carter, C. S. (2000). Anterior cingulate and prefrontal cortex: who's in control? *Nature Neuroscience, 3*, 421–423.

Cools, R., Clark, L., Owen, A. M., & Robbins, T. W. (2002). Defining the neural mechanisms of probabilistic reversal learning using event-related functional magnetic resonance imaging. *Journal of Neuroscience, 22*, 4563–4567.

Cornell, D. G., Warren, J., Hawk, G., Stafford, E., Oram, G., & Pine, D. (1996). Psychopathy in instrumental and reactive violent offenders. *Journal of Consulting and Clinical Psychology, 64*, 783–790.

Dadds, M. R., Perry, Y., Hawes, D. J., Merz, S., Riddell, A. C., Haines, D. J., *et al.* (2006). Attention to the eyes and fear-recognition deficits in child psychopathy. *British Journal of Psychiatry, 189*, 280–281.

Davis, M. (2000). The role of the amygdala in conditioned and unconditioned fear and anxiety. In J. P. Aggleton (ed), *The Amygdala: A Functional Analysis* (pp. 289–310). Oxford: Oxford University Press.

Deeley, Q., Daly, E., Surguladze, S., Tunstall, N., Mezey, G., Beer, D., *et al.* (2006). Facial emotion processing in criminal psychopathy. *Preliminary functional magnetic resonance imaging study. British Journal of Psychiatry, 189*, 533–539.

Dias, R., Robbins, T. W., & Roberts, A. C. (1996). Dissociation in prefrontal cortex of affective and attentional shifts. *Nature, 380*, 69–72.

Erthal, F. S., de Oliveira, L., Mocaiber, I., Pereira, M. G., Machado-Pinheiro, W., Volchan, E., *et al.* (2005). Load-dependent modulation of affective picture processing. *Cognitive, Affective and Behavioral Neuroscience, 5*, 388–395.

Etkin, A., Egner, T., Peraza, D. M., Kandel, E. R., & Hirsch, J. (2006). Resolving emotional conflict: a role for the rostral anterior cingulate cortex in modulating activity in the amygdala. *Neuron, 51*, 871–882.

Everitt, B. J., Cardinal, R. N., Parkinson, J. A., & Robbins, T. W. (2003). Appetitive behavior: impact of amygdala-dependent mechanisms of emotional learning. *Annals of the New York Academy of Sciences, 985*, 233–250.

Fellows, L. K., & Farah, M. J. (2003). Ventromedial frontal cortex mediates affective shifting in humans: evidence from a reversal learning paradigm. *Brain, 126*, 1830–1837.

Finger, E. C., Marsh, A. A., Mitchell, D. G. V., Reid, M. E., Sims, C., Budhani, S., *et al.* (2008). Abnormal ventromedial prefrontal cortex function in children with psychopathic traits during reversal learning. *Archives of General Psychiatry, 65*, 586–594.

Fitzgerald, D. A., Angstadt, M., Jelsone, L. M., Nathan, P. J., & Phan, K. L. (2006). Beyond threat: amygdala reactivity across multiple expressions of facial affect. *Neuroimage, 30*, 1441–1448.

Frick, P. J. (1995). Callous-unemotional traits and conduct problems: a two-factor model of psychopathy in children. *Issues in Criminological and Legal Psychology, 24*, 47–51.

Frick, P. J., Cornell, A. H., Barry, C. T., Bodin, S. D., & Dane, H. E. (2003). Callous-unemotional traits and conduct problems in the prediction of conduct problem severity, aggression, and self-report delinquency. *Journal of Abnormal Child Psychology, 31*, 457–470.

Glass, S. J., & Newman, J. P. (2006). Recognition of facial affect in psychopathic offenders. *Journal of Abnormal Psychology, 115*, 815–820.

Gordon, H. L., Baird, A. A., & End, A. (2004). Functional differences among those high and low on a trait measure of psychopathy. *Biological Psychiatry, 56*, 516–521.

Gottfried, J. A., O'Doherty, J., & Dolan, R. J. (2002). Appetitive and aversive olfactory learning in humans studied using event-related functional magnetic resonance imaging. *Journal of Neuroscience, 22*, 10829–10837.

Graves, R., Landis, T., & Goodglass, H. (1981). Laterality and sex differences for visual recognition of emotional and non-emotional words. *Neuropsychologia, 19,* 95–102.

Hampton, A. N., Bossaerts, P., & O'Doherty, J. P. (2006). The role of the ventromedial prefrontal cortex in abstract state-based inference during decision making in humans. *Journal of Neuroscience, 26,* 8360–8367.

Hare, R. D. (1970). *Psychopathy: Theory and Research.* New York: Wiley.

Hare, R. D. (1991). *The Hare Psychopathy Checklist-Revised.* Toronto, ON: Multi-Health Systems.

Hare, R. D. (2003). *Hare Psychopathy Checklist-Revised (PCL-R),* 2nd edn. Toronto, ON: Multi-Health Systems.

Hare, R. D., Frazelle, J., & Cox, D. N. (1978). Psychopathy and physiological responses to threat of an aversive stimulus. *Psychophysiology, 15,* 165–172.

Harpur, T. J., Hakstian, A. R., & Hare, R. D. (1988). The factor structure of the Psychopathy Checklist. *Journal of Consulting and Clinical Psychology, 56,* 741–747.

Holroyd, C. B., Nieuwenhuis, S., Yeung, N., Nystrom, L., Mars, R. B., Coles, M. G., *et al.* (2004). Dorsal anterior cingulate cortex shows fMRI response to internal and external error signals. *Nature Neuroscience, 7,* 497–498.

Hooker, C. I., Germine, L. T., Knight, R. T., & D'Esposito, M. (2006). Amygdala response to facial expressions reflects emotional learning. *Journal of Neuroscience, 26,* 8915–8922.

Iversen, S. D., & Mishkin, M. (1970). Perseverative interference in monkeys following selective lesions of the inferior prefrontal convexity. *Experimental Brain Research, 11,* 376–386.

Izquierdo, A., Suda, R. K., & Murray, E. A. (2004). Bilateral orbital prefrontal cortex lesions in rhesus monkeys disrupt choices guided by both reward value and reward contingency. *Journal of Neuroscience, 24,* 7540–7548.

Johnston, J. B. (1923). Further contributions to the study of the evolution of the forebrain. *Journal of Comparative Neurology, 35,* 337–481.

Kiehl, K. A., Smith, A. M., Hare, R. D., Mendrek, A., Forster, B. B., Brink, J., *et al.* (2001). Limbic abnormalities in affective processing by criminal psychopaths as revealed by functional magnetic resonance imaging. *Biological Psychiatry, 50,* 677–684.

Knutson, B., & Cooper, J. C. (2005). Functional magnetic resonance imaging of reward prediction. *Current Opinion in Neurology, 18,* 411–417.

Kosson, D. S., Budhani, S., Nakic, M., Chen, G., Saad, Z. S., Vythilingam, M., *et al.* (2006). The role of the amygdala and rostral anterior cingulate in encoding expected outcomes during learning. *Neuroimage, 29,* 1161–1172.

Kosson, D. S., Suchy, Y., Mayer, A. R., & Libby, J. (2002). Facial affect recognition in criminal psychopaths. *Emotion, 2,* 398–411.

Kringelbach, M. L., & Rolls, E. T. (2003). Neural correlates of rapid reversal learning in a simple model of human social interaction. *Neuroimage, 20,* 1371–1383.

LaBar, K. S., Crupain, M. J., Voyvodic, J. T., & McCarthy, G. (2003). Dynamic perception of facial affect and identity in the human brain. *Cerebral Cortex, 13,* 1023–1033.

LeDoux, J. (1998). *The Emotional Brain.* New York: Weidenfeld & Nicolson.

Levenston, G. K., Patrick, C. J., Bradley, M. M., & Lang, P. J. (2000). The psychopath as observer: emotion and attention in picture processing. *Journal of Abnormal Psychology, 109,* 373–386.

Lorenz, A. R., & Newman, J. P. (2002). Deficient response modulation and emotion processing in low-anxious Caucasian psychopathic offenders: results from a lexical decision task. *Emotion, 2,* 91–104.

Lykken, D. T. (1957). A study of anxiety in the sociopathic personality. *Journal of Abnormal and Social Psychology, 55,* 6–10.

Lynam, D. R., Caspi, A., Moffitt, T. E., Loeber, R., & Stouthamer-Loeber, M. (2007). Longitudinal evidence that psychopathy scores in early adolescence predict adult psychopathy. *Journal of Abnormal Psychology, 116,* 155–165.

Marsh, A. A., Blair, K. S., Vythilingam, M., Busis, S., & Blair, R. J. (2007). Response options and expectations of reward in decision-making: the differential roles of dorsal and rostral anterior cingulate cortex. *Neuroimage, 35*(2), 979–988.

Marsh, A. A., & Blair, R. J. (2008). Deficits in facial affect recognition among antisocial populations: a meta-analysis. *Neuroscience and Biobehavioral Reviews, 32*(3), 454–465.

Marsh, A. A., Finger, E. C., Mitchell, D. G. V., Reid, M. E., Sims, C., Kosson, D. S., *et al.* (2008). Reduced amygdala response to fearful expressions in children and adolescents with callous-unemotional traits and disruptive behavior disorders. *American Journal of Psychiatry, 165*, 712–720.

Mitchell, D. G., Nakic, M., Fridberg, D., Kamel, N., Pine, D. S., & Blair, R. J. (2007). The impact of processing load on emotion. *Neuroimage, 34*, 1299–1309.

Mitchell, D. G., Richell, R. A., Leonard, A. & Blair, R. J. (2006). Emotion at the expense of cognition: psychopathic individuals outperform controls on an operant response task. *Journal of Abnormal Psychology, 115*, 559–566.

Mitchell, D. G. V., Colledge, E., Leonard, A., & Blair, R. J. R. (2002). Risky decisions and response reversal: Is there evidence of orbitofrontal cortex dysfunction in psychopathic individuals? *Neuropsychologia, 40*, 2013–2022.

Montagne, B., van Honk, J., Kessels, R. P. C., Frigerio, E., Burt, M., van Zandvoort, M. J. E., *et al.* (2005). Reduced efficiency in recognising fear in subjects scoring high on psychopathic personality characteristics. *Personality and Individual Differences, 38*, 5–11.

Montague, P. R., & Berns, G. S. (2002). Neural economics and the biological substrates of valuation. *Neuron, 36*, 265–284.

Morris, J. S., Frith, C. D., Perrett, D. I., Rowland, D., Young, A. W., Calder, A. J., *et al.* (1996). A differential response in the human amygdala to fearful and happy facial expressions. *Nature, 383*, 812–815.

Murphy, F. C., Nimmo-Smith, I., & Lawrence, A. D. (2003). Functional neuroanatomy of emotions: a meta-analysis. *Cognitive, Affective, and Behavioral Neuroscience, 3*, 207–233.

Nakic, M., Smith, B. W., Busis, S., Vythilingam, M., & Blair, R. J. (2006). The impact of affect and frequency on lexical decision: the role of the amygdala and inferior frontal cortex. *Neuroimage, 31*, 1752–1761.

Newman, J. P., & Kosson, D. S. (1986). Passive avoidance learning in psychopathic and nonpsychopathic offenders. *Journal of Abnormal Psychology, 95*, 252–256.

Newman, J. P., Patterson, C. M., & Kosson, D. S. (1987). Response perseveration in psychopaths. *Journal of Abnormal Psychology, 96*, 145–148.

O'Doherty, J., Critchley, H., Deichmann, R., & Dolan, R. J. (2003). Dissociating valence of outcome from behavioral control in human orbital and ventral prefrontal cortices. *Journal of Neuroscience, 23*, 7931–7939.

Ohira, H., Nomura, M., Ichikawa, N., Isowa, T., Iidaka, T., Sato, A., *et al.* (2006). Association of neural and physiological responses during voluntary emotion suppression. *Neuroimage, 29*, 721–733.

Padoa-Schioppa, C., & Assad, J. A. (2006). Neurons in the orbitofrontal cortex encode economic value. *Nature, 441*, 223–226.

Patrick, C. J. (ed) (2006). *Handbook of Psychopathy*. New York: Guilford Press.

Patrick, C. J., Bradley, M. M., & Lang, P. J. (1993). Emotion in the criminal psychopath: startle reflex modulation. *Journal of Abnormal Psychology, 102*, 82–92.

Pessoa, L., & Ungerleider, L. G. (2004). Neuroimaging studies of attention and the processing of emotion-laden stimuli. *Progress in Brain Research, 144*, 171–182.

Pezawas, L., Meyer-Lindenberg, A., Drabant, E. M., Verchinski, B. A., Munoz, K. E., Kolachana, B. S., *et al.* (2005). 5-HTTLPR polymorphism impacts human cingulate-amygdala interactions: a genetic susceptibility mechanism for depression. *Nature Neuroscience, 8*, 828–834.

Phelps, E. A., O'Connor, K. J., Gatenby, J. C., Gore, J. C., Grillon, C., & Davis, M. (2001). Activation of the left amygdala to a cognitive representation of fear. *Nature Neuroscience, 4*, 437–441.

Phillips, M. L., Drevets, W. C., Rauch, S. L., & Lane, R. (2003). Neurobiology of emotion perception II: implications for major psychiatric disorders. *Biological Psychiatry, 54*, 515–528.

Price, J. L. (2003). Comparative aspects of amygdala connectivity. *Annual Review of the New York Academy of Sciences, 985*, 50–58.

Rauch, S. L., Shin, L. M., & Phelps, E. A. (2006). Neurocircuitry models of posttraumatic stress disorder and extinction: human neuroimaging research—past, present, and future. *Biological Psychiatry, 60*, 376–382.

Rosenkranz, J. A., Moore, H., & Grace, A. A. (2003). The prefrontal cortex regulates lateral amygdala neuronal plasticity and responses to previously conditioned stimuli. *Journal of Neuroscience, 23*, 11054–11064.

Rushworth, M. F., Behrens, T. E., Rudebeck, P. H., & Walton, M. E. (2007). Contrasting roles for cingulate and orbitofrontal cortex in decisions and social behaviour. *Trends in Cognitive Science*, *11*, 168–176.

Schoenbaum, G., & Roesch, M. (2005). Orbitofrontal cortex, associative learning, and expectancies. *Neuron*, *47*, 633–636.

Schoenbaum, G., Setlow, B., Saddoris, M. P., & Gallagher, M. (2003). Encoding predicted outcome and acquired value in orbitofrontal cortex during cue sampling depends upon input from basolateral amygdala. *Neuron*, *39*, 855–867.

Van Honk, J., Hermans, E. J., Putman, P., Montagne, B., & Schutter, D. J. (2002). Defective somatic markers in sub-clinical psychopathy. *Neuroreport*, *13*, 1025–1027.

Whalen, P. J. (1998). Fear, vigilance, and ambiguity: initial neuroimaging studies of the human amygdala. *Current Directions in Psychological Science*, *7*, 177–188.

Whalen, P. J., McInerney, S. C., McNally, R. J., Wilhelm, S., Jenike, M. A., & Rauch, S. L. (1998). The emotional counting Stroop paradigm: a functional magnetic resonance imaging probe of the anterior cingulate affective division. *Biological Psychiatry*, *44*, 1219–1228.

Williamson, S., Harpur, T. J., & Hare, R. D. (1991). Abnormal processing of affective words by psychopaths. *Psychophysiology*, *28*, 260–273.

Winston, J. S., O'Doherty, J., & Dolan, R. J. (2003). Common and distinct neural responses during direct and incidental processing of multiple facial emotions. *Neuroimage*, *20*, 84–97.

Wootton, J. M., Frick, P. J., Shelton, K. K., & Silverthorn, P. (1997). Ineffective parenting and childhood conduct problems: the moderating role of callous-unemotional traits. *Journal of Consulting and Clinical Psychology*, *65*, 292–300.

8

Persistent violent offending among adult men:
A critical review of neuroimaging studies

Anna Plodowski, Sarah L. Gregory, and Nigel J. Blackwood

Introduction

Most criminally violent acts are committed by a small group of men who have displayed persistent aggressive behaviour from childhood (Kratzer & Hodgins, 1997). Most of these violent acts are emotionally charged and 'reactive' to a frustrating or threatening event, and are typically perpetrated by aroused, angry, and impulsive men who meet the diagnostic criteria for conduct disorder in childhood and antisocial personality disorder (ASPD) in adulthood. A minority of these violent acts are predatory, purposeful, and goal-directed: such 'instrumental' acts are typically perpetrated by men who appear fearless and low in anxiety and who meet the diagnostic criteria for psychopathy (Crick & Dodge, 1996; Cornell *et al.*, 1996; Barratt *et al.*, 1999). The distinction between the groups is clearly one of degree: thus, instrumental acts of aggression will be perpetrated by antisocial men who do not meet the criteria for psychopathy; equally, reactive acts of aggression will be perpetrated by psychopathic men (Cornell *et al.*, 1996). Nevertheless, the distinction between these types of aggression in the two clinical groups serves as a useful heuristic for neurobiological explanatory model development (see Chapter 7).

The purpose of this narrative review is to critically examine structural and functional magnetic resonance neuroimaging (sMRI and fMRI, respectively) studies in adult men distinguished from normal participants by their history of violent offending, personality traits (psychopathic traits), or clinical diagnosis (ASPD or psychopathic disorder). To put the results of such studies in context, we begin with a review of key brain areas implicated in the generation and regulation of emotional processes, abnormalities of which have been implicated in aetiological models of persistent violent offending.

Persistent violent offending and the emotional brain

The limbic structures of the amygdala, orbitofrontal cortex (OFC), and cingulate cortex are central to emotional processing (Dalgleish, 2004) and to current models of reactive and instrumental aggression (see Chapter 7). Other brain regions (the thalamus, ventral striatum, hippocampus, septum, insula, somatosensory cortices, nucleus accumbens, and brain stem) have also been implicated in the processing of emotion; however, detailed discussion of these areas is beyond the scope of this review (see Le Doux, 1996 and Rolls, 2005 for more detailed consideration).

Studies in animals have implicated the amygdala in emotional (Weiskrantz, 1956; Blanchard & Blanchard, 1972) and social (Rosvold *et al.*, 1954; Kling & Brothers, 1992) behaviours, especially those related to fear and aggression. In humans, lesion and functional neuroimaging studies suggest that the amygdala has a key role in processing social signals of emotion (particularly involving fear), in emotional conditioning, and in the consolidation of emotional memories. In processing emotional social information, functional imaging studies report amygdala activation to emotional relative to neutral faces, most reliably for fearful expressions (Morris *et al.*, 1996; Winston *et al.*, 2003). Damage to the amygdala causes deficits in recognizing 'basic' emotional expressions, again most reliably for fear (Adolphs *et al.*, 1994; Calder *et al.*, 1996), as well as impairing the ability to infer more complex 'social' emotions, such as guilt (Adolphs *et al.*, 2002). In fear-conditioning experiments, the amygdala is activated differentially in response to fear-conditioned angry faces that have been previously paired with an aversive noise, compared with angry faces that have not been paired with noise (Morris *et al.*, 1998). Damage to the amygdala results in a failure of fear conditioning to aversive stimuli (Bechara *et al.*, 1995; Angrilli *et al.*, 1996). The anterior hippocampus is also engaged by fearful situations (Kjelstrup *et al.*, 2002; Bannerman *et al.*, 2004). Both the amygdala and anterior hippocampus modulate autonomic centres, providing a basis for autonomic responses evoked by aversive stimuli. In emotional memory consolidation, damage to the amygdala impairs the usual enhanced memory for emotional aspects of stories (compared with non-emotional aspects) (Cahill *et al.*, 1995; Adolphs *et al.*, 1997). This region appears to code an interaction between the intensity and the valence of an emotional stimulus (Winston *et al.*, 2005), reflecting the overall emotional value of a stimulus for influencing adaptive behaviour (Whalen *et al.*, 2004). Amygdala hyperactivity is thought to contribute to reactive aggression by elevating basic threat circuitry sensitivity (Davidson *et al.*, 2000); amygdalar hypoactivity is thought to contribute to instrumental aggression by impacting adversely on the processing of fearful faces, aversive conditioning, and instrumental learning, deficits which in turn interfere with prosocial development (see Blair, Chapter 7).

Animal work suggests that the orbitofrontal regions (OFC and ventromedial prefrontal cortex [vmPFC]) are involved in learning the emotional and motivational value of stimuli (Rolls, 2005). Neurons in these regions can detect changes or reversals in the reward value of learned stimuli and change responses accordingly. Lesions of the orbitofrontal regions cause impairments in decision making. These are typically characterized by an inability to adapt behavioural strategies according to the consequences of decisions, leading to impulsivity (Bechara *et al.*, 1994; Winstanley *et al.*, 2004). It is thought that the OFC, incorporating inputs from the amygdala (Amaral *et al*, 1992), represents the motivational value of stimuli (or choices), which allows it to integrate and evaluate the incentive value of predicted outcomes in order to guide future behaviour (Schoenbaum *et al.*, 2003; Schoenbaum *et al.*, 2006). Whether there are distinct regions within the OFC that encode different aspects of value such as reward and punishment remains to be established. OFC hypoactivity is thought to contribute to reactive aggression through increased frustration (due to reward expectation computation failures), impulsivity, and a relative failure to down-regulate elevated responsiveness of the basic threat system (Davidson *et al.*, 2000). VmPFC hypoactivity is also thought to contribute to frustration-based reactive aggression in psychopathy via suboptimal decision making when attempting to achieve goals (see Chapter 7).

Animal, lesion, and functional neuroimaging work suggests that the anterior cingulate cortex (ACC) serves as an integration point for visceral, attentional, and emotional information that is involved in the regulation of affect and other forms of top-down control (Bush *et al.*, 2000). Patients with ACC lesions can develop impaired social judgement, blunted affect, impulsivity, disinhibition, and aggressive behaviour with minimal or no provocation (Devinsky *et al.*, 1995). The ACC has generally been conceptualized in terms of a dorsal 'cognitive' subdivision and a more rostral, ventral 'affective' subdivision. It monitors conflict between the functional state of the organism and any new information that has potential affective or motivational consequences. When such conflicts are detected, the ACC represents information about the conflict, enabling lateral prefrontal areas to 'decide' among response options. ACC activity preceding a decision encodes the integrated value of an action, in terms of either immediate gains or costs or in terms of information to aid future decision making. On the observation of an outcome, ACC activity encodes the degree to which the resulting information should influence future decisions (Rushworth & Behrens, 2008). Although ACC dysfunction is not central to current neurobiological models of reactive and instrumental aggression, it has a theoretical role in reactive aggression: activation occurs during anger arousal (including the processing of angry faces; Blair *et al.* 1999) and other negative emotions, and connections between dorsal ACC and more executive areas in the PFC suggest that it may contribute to the constraint of reactively aggressive acts.

In summary, reactively violent men are hypothesized to display deficits principally involving dysregulated processing of social threats, either through a heightened sensitivity of basic threat processing structures (medial nucleus of the amygdala, hypothalamus, dorsal periaqueductal gray; Mobbs *et al.*, 2007) or by diminished regulation of the threat response once triggered (impaired OFC function; Blair *et al*, 2005; Patrick, 2006). Instrumentally violent men display abnormalities of aversive conditioning, instrumental learning, processing of fearful expressions, and representation of reinforcement expectancy, all of which impair the socialization process. These are consistent with diminished amygdala (Adolphs *et al.*, 2005; Birbaumer *et al.*, 2005) and vmPFC (Wheeler & Fellows, 2008) activity. The key question in reviewing the extant literature at this stage of model development is the following: To what extent does the imaging literature to date support the hypothesized neurobiological distinctions between the reactive violence that typifies ASPD and the instrumental violence that typifies psychopathy?

Structural imaging studies

SMRI studies have typically employed a case-control design, scanning patients and healthy men who are usually matched on at least one characteristic (typically level of education, age, or socio-economic status).

Psychopathic disorder

The majority of the imaging studies examining structural abnormalities in psychopaths have focused on regions of interest selected *a priori*. In American populations, it is accepted practice to define psychopathy as a score of 30 or above on the *Psychopathy Checklist-Revised* (PCL-R); in European populations a score of 25 or above on the PCL-R suffices (Cooke & Michie, 1999). The first sMRI study (Raine *et al*, 2000) focused on PFC grey and white matter volumes, comparing a group of psychopathic men (mean PCL-R = 28) who met the diagnostic criteria for ASPD with substance-dependent (mean PCL-R = 20) and psychiatric control (mean PCL-R =14) groups. The psychopathic group had an 11% reduction in PFC grey matter volume compared with the psychiatric control group, and a 14% reduction compared with the substance-dependent group. By contrast, the groups did not differ on white matter PFC volumes. Those with lower grey matter volumes within the psychopathic group showed reduced skin conductance activity in response to a social stressor (participants had to spend 2 minutes preparing a speech about their faults, followed by a 2-minute period in which they gave their speech to the experimenter while being videotaped). However, this study did not delineate which subregion of the PFC is particularly reduced in volume: segmentation of the PFC into orbitofrontal, medial, and dorsolateral regions was not performed. Two significant potential confounds exist. Firstly, 33% of the psychopathic group had schizophrenia spectrum disorders, which are independently associated with frontal lobe volume decrements. In the psychiatric control group, 38% also had a co-morbid schizophrenia spectrum diagnosis, but a 'cleaner' design would have excluded such Axis 1 pathology. Secondly, the psychopathic group had significantly higher numbers of cocaine-dependent individuals compared with the substance-dependent group (66% versus 30%, respectively). Cocaine is independently associated with grey matter volume decrements in PFC structures, including the OFC and premotor cortex (Franklin *et al.*, 2002; Matochik *et al.*, 2003; Sim *et al.*, 2007).

Corpus callosum structures were investigated in a further study (Raine *et al.*, 2003), motivated both by an appreciation of the structures' role in the interhemispheric regulation of arousal and emotion and by findings of abnormal interhemispheric processing in psychopathic individuals (Hare & McPherson, 1984; Raine *et al*, 1990). Volume estimates of callosal white matter, thickness, length, and genu and splenium area were determined. The psychopathic group (mean PCL-R = 30) showed a 22% increase in estimated callosal white matter volume, a 7% increase in callosal length, and a 15% reduction in callosal thickness in comparison with a community control group. Larger callosal volumes were associated with affective and interpersonal deficits and were independent of psychosocial deficits. This result was interpreted as suggestive of a neurodevelopmental abnormality of callosal structure, due to, for example, a failure of axonal pruning and/or increased myelination of axons that survive the pruning process in adolescence. However, inferring developmental processes from purely cross-sectional data is fraught with methodological difficulties (Kraemer *et al.*, 2000). Equally, the precise relationship between such callosal abnormalities and the characteristic features of psychopathy requires further investigation using diffusion tensor imaging and connectivity analyses.

Raine's group have subsequently focused on the distinction between 'successful' psychopaths (who had evaded detection of their crimes), 'unsuccessful' psychopaths (whose crimes had been detected and who had been subsequently convicted), and control participants. PCL-R scores in both groups were greater than 23 (mean 'successful' scores = 26 and 27 respectively; mean 'unsuccessful' scores = 30 and 31, respectively). 'Unsuccessful' psychopaths, but not 'successful' psychopaths, had a 22% reduction in prefrontal grey matter volumes compared with control participants. Individual differences in psychopathy scores negatively correlated with prefrontal grey matter volumes (Yang *et al.*, 2005). This significant negative correlation between grey matter volume and psychopathy scores was observed for each of the underlying factor scores (in both Hare's 2-factor and Cooke's 3-factor models). These differences in prefrontal grey volumes remained significant after correcting for the potential confounds of age, drug and alcohol abuse/dependence, history of head injury, and socioeconomic status. There were no differences between groups in prefrontal white matter volumes. In another study by this group (Raine *et al.*, 2004), the hippocampus was chosen as an *a priori* region of interest due to its role in contextual fear conditioning and consequent social cuing (Büchel *et al.*, 1999; Strange *et al.*, 1999) together with evidence for impairments in such processes in psychopathy (Flor *et al.*, 2002). In the study of hippocampal structure, there was no significant group effect in the initial structural analysis. However, post-hoc testing (in which a laterality index was constructed by subtracting left volume from right volume and dividing by total slice volume at each slice, and estimates of anterior and posterior hippocampal volumes were computed) revealed significant laterality differences between the 'unsuccessful' and 'successful' and control groups. The 'unsuccessful' group showed an exaggerated structural hippocampal asymmetry. This laterality difference resulted from a combination of slightly decreased left and slightly increased right hippocampal volume in the unsuccessful psychopaths relative to the other two groups. The difference was again interpreted as a potential indicator of neurodevelopmental abnormalities in the 'unsuccessful' group and it was proposed that atrophy in the hippocampus may subserve impaired contextual memory of, and response to, cues leading to punishment.

Frontal and hippocampal abnormalities were further examined in Laakso's studies in which type-2 alcoholics (the group characterized by early onset, impulsive, and aggressive behaviour and social hostility; Cloninger, 1995) with co-morbid psychopathy were studied in isolation (Laakso et al., 2001) or contrasted with normal healthy men (Laakso et al., 2002). A further study (Laakso et al., 2000) in which hippocampal structure was compared between type-2 and with type-1 alcoholics (characterized by late onset, social dependency, and anxiety) will not be considered due to a lack of subject PCL-R data. Significantly reduced grey matter volumes were demonstrated in the left dorsolateral, orbitofrontal, and medial PFC in the psychopathic group (mean PCL-R score = 28) compared with a normal control group, but such differences did not survive correction for differences in education and duration of alcoholism (Laakso et al., 2002). Again, no significant differences in prefrontal white matter volumes were demonstrated. In the study of hippocampal structure (Laakso et al., 2001), posterior bilateral hippocampal volumes were shown to have a strong negative correlation with total PCL-R score. Although the former study confirms the neurotoxic effects of alcohol on prefrontal grey matter structures, it is notable that grey matter volume decrements in the study conducted by Raine et al. (2000) were even greater in the psychopathic group than in the substance-dependent control group. Equally, the control group were both less well characterized (neither their intellectual level nor PCL-R scores were examined) and matched in terms of educational background (consisting of well-educated hospital staff, their relatives, and students) than in Raine's study.

Whole brain structure has recently been examined for the first time using voxel-based morphometry (VBM) in a group of patients with neuropsychiatric disorders who satisfied the diagnostic criteria for ASPD and demonstrated high PCL-SV scores (mean = 17.8, corresponding to a PCL-R score of 26–27) compared with an age- and education-matched control group without a past history of neuropsychiatric disorder (de Oliveira-Souza et al., 2008). This study included both men and women. VBM enables a statistically principled voxel-wise between-groups comparison of grey matter volume, unconstrained by anatomical landmarks. In the whole brain comparisons, grey matter concentration was reduced in widespread areas in the psychopathic participants. In a priori defined regions of interest, grey matter concentrations were significantly ($p < 0.01$, small volume corrected for multiple comparisons) reduced in frontopolar (L > R), medial (left), and lateral (R > L) orbitofrontal areas, left anterior temporal cortex, the insula (R > L), and the superior temporal sulcus bilaterally. These decrements showed a significant negative correlation with Factor 1 scores (interpersonal-affective items) on the PCL-SV checklist. We note that the amygdala region was not defined as an a priori region of interest. Structural abnormalities in this latter region have therefore only been demonstrated in one study to date (which exists solely in abstract form, Tiihonen et al., 2000): a 20% reduction in right amygdaloid volumes was seen in a psychopathic group with 'high' scores on the interpersonal-affective factor 1 compared with violent offenders with 'moderate or low' factor 1 scores and non-violent control participants; this difference was statistically significant after adjusting for the effects of age, intelligence, and duration of alcohol abuse. There were significant negative correlations between the right amygdaloid volumes and total PCL-R ratings.

ASPD

There is a dearth of studies examining ASPD as a categorical construct with PCL-R scores of less than 25. A preliminary study compared a small sample of personality-disordered violent male offenders recruited from a high-secure hospital with healthy men (Dolan *et al.*, 2002). The majority of the personality-disordered group met the diagnostic criteria for ASPD. This group was further characterized using the Special Hospital Assessment of Personality and Socialisation (SHAPS) tool (Blackburn, 1982; subsequently known as the Antisocial Personality Questionnaire: Blackburn & Renwick, 1996), having significantly higher trait impulsivity and hostility ratings than the healthy men. PCL-R data were not collected. The use of a 0.5T mobile scanner limited the quality of images collected, providing sequence and slice thickness data that were only suitable for volume analysis for large structures (hemispheric, ventricular, frontal, and temporal volumes) without grey or white matter differentiation. Manual point-counting techniques revealed a significant 20% reduction in bilateral temporal lobe volumes in the personality-disordered group, but no significant reduction in frontal lobe volumes. A secondary subgroup analysis using planar measurements of frontal lobe subdivisions (dorsolateral, dorsomedial, and orbitofrontal) showed a significant reduction in dorsomedial prefrontal volumes in the personality-disordered group. However, this group was significantly less intelligent than the healthy comparison group, an important potential confound (see below).

Two further structural studies have compared participants with ASPD recruited from a high-secure hospital (PCL-R data not collected) with healthy men and violent and non-violent schizophrenics (Barkataki *et al.*, 2006; Narayan *et al.*, 2007). The ASPD group displayed reductions in whole brain and temporal lobe volume as well as increases in putamen volume in comparison with normal control participants (there were no IQ differences between the groups). No differences were observed in prefrontal, amygdala, or hippocampal volumes between the antisocial and normal control groups, but group sizes were small (ASPD group n = 13, community control n = 15). A similar study was conducted with the same groups, but instead focused on regional cortical thinning. Participants with ASPD showed significant thinning of the medial inferior frontal cortices bilaterally and thinning of sensory motor areas in the right hemisphere in relation to healthy comparison participants. Such a decrease in cortical thickness implies a compromise in brain structure because of changes in the characteristics and integrity of the neuropil. The cortical thickness measure may be sensitive to white matter as well as to grey matter characteristics.

The differences between ASPD and psychopathy

Only one sMRI study to date has attempted the categorical comparison between violent offenders who meet diagnostic criteria for ASPD and psychopathic disorder (mean PCL-R = 34.6), those who solely meet criteria for ASPD (mean PCL-R = 25.9), and a normal control group (mean PCL-R not recorded) (Tiihonen *et al.*, in press). The psychopathic group had more severe histories of polysubstance misuse than the other two groups. No significant differences emerged between the psychopathic and ASPD groups in whole brain analyses using VBM. This may however represent a type-2 error, because group numbers were small (ASPD n = 14, psychopathy n = 12) and a region of interest examination of key structures such as the amygdala was not performed. The offender group collectively displayed significant increases in white matter volumes in the bilateral occipital lobes, and significant volume decreases in widespread grey matter areas, including frontopolar cortex and OFC (but not the amygdala). However, we note the important potential confound of a lack of intelligence matching in the comparison between the offender participants and normal control participants (no IQ data were collected for the healthy comparison group). Substantial grey matter correlates exist with IQ, with more grey matter associated with higher IQ in widespread frontal, temporal, parietal, and occipital areas (Haier *et al.*, 2004; Colom *et al.*, 2006). Thus, the grey matter volume reductions observed in the violent offender group could in part be attributable to their lower IQ.

Functional imaging studies

FMRI studies of the psychopathic spectrum in community samples

In order to assess psychopathic traits in those without criminal records, two measures have been developed: the Psychopathic Personality Inventory (PPI; Lillienfeld & Andrews, 1996) and the Levenson Primary and Secondary Psychopathy Scales (Levenson *et al.*, 1995). Both instruments rely on self-reports and investigate both the emotional-interpersonal deficits and social deviance associated with psychopathy. Participant scores may be used either as a dimensional variable, or cut-off scores employed to generate 'high' and 'low' score groups.

In a study of facial affect processing in which healthy control participants were required to match facial affect (Gordon *et al.*, 2004), those scoring high on the emotional-interpersonal dimension of the PPI (compared to those scoring low) demonstrated reduced activity in the right inferior frontal cortex, right amygdala, and medial PFC, in trials of emotion matching compared to baseline. Unfortunately, there were insufficient trials to analyse data for specific facial emotion conditions (anger, fear, sadness, and joy). These results are consistent with the view that the emotional-interpersonal (deficient affective experience and arrogant or deceitful interpersonal behaviour) psychopathy dimension involves an impaired amygdala response to emotional stimuli. The possibility that there are distinct neural underpinnings to the individual factors of the psychopathy construct was suggested by the finding of an increased right amygdalar response for emotion matching relative to baseline in those high on the social deviance dimension.

In a study of social cooperation using the 'Prisoner's Dilemma' game (Rilling *et al.*, 2007), those participants with higher levels of psychopathic traits (according to the PPI and the Levenson Scales) defected more often and were less likely to continue cooperating after establishing mutual cooperation with a partner. They experienced more outcomes in which their cooperation was not reciprocated (the cooperate-defect outcome). After their cooperation was not reciprocated, participants scoring high in psychopathy showed less amygdala activation, suggesting that the defection of opponents was experienced as less aversive than in those with low levels of psychopathic traits. Participants higher in psychopathy (compared with low-psychopathy participants) also showed weaker activation within the OFC when choosing to cooperate (potentially reflecting a relative lack of a cooperation behaviour 'biasing' signal) and showed weaker activation within the dorsolateral prefrontal cortex (DLPFC) and rostral ACC when choosing to defect (potentially reflecting less need for the inhibition of a pre-potent 'cooperate' response in order to defect).

FMRI studies of psychopathic disorder

Aversive conditioning in psychopaths has been examined in three fMRI studies to date. In the first fMRI scanning study of its kind, neural responses during the acquisition, habituation, and extinction phases of an aversive conditioning task were examined in a psychopathic group (mean PCL-R = 28) compared with a healthy participant group (Schneider *et al.*, 2000). A differential aversive-conditioning paradigm was used with odours as unconditioned stimuli (UCS) and neutral faces as conditioned stimuli (CS). Paradoxically, the psychopathic group demonstrated superior aversive conditioning to the normal control group (contrary to the findings of other investigations of aversive conditioning; e.g., Flor *et al.*, 2002). Autonomic responses were not recorded. These factors should be taken into account when considering the counter-intuitive finding that the psychopaths showed increased amygdala activity to the presentation of the CS+ (a neutral face paired with an aversive odour) stimulus in the acquisition phase.

A preliminary study in which a small number of psychopaths were compared to social phobics and normal healthy men suggested that psychopaths showed reduced activity in the OFC, insula, and ACC in response to the CS+ in the acquisition phase (Veit *et al.*, 2002). These findings were extended in a study of aversive conditioning in a larger group of psychopaths (mean PCL-R score = 25) by the same researchers (Birbaumer *et al.*, 2005). Here, an unpleasant physical pressure on the subject's hand delivered by a short plastic tube served as the UCS and neutral faces as the CS. The psychopathic group demonstrated a lack of emotional response to the US compared with healthy men, despite a lack of differences between the groups in distinguishing the CS+ and CS−. This lack of emotional response in psychopaths included both a lack of difference in the subjective stimulus ratings between CS+ and CS− (no difference in perceived aversiveness) and a lack of a skin conductance response in the psychopathic group to the CS+ in the acquisition phase. In effect, the psychopaths failed to be aversively conditioned, and this behavioural difference must be taken into account in considering the results. The failure to be aversively conditioned was associated with reduced activity in the left amygdala, bilateral insula, ACC, and right secondary somatosensory cortex throughout the acquisition phase, suggesting that the aversive stimulus was not salient for the psychopathic group and did not elicit awareness of threat. In addition, in the second half of the acquisition phase, when anticipatory responses to the conditioned aversive stimulus are expected, psychopaths showed reduced activity in the right ventromedial OFC, suggesting a failure to anticipate punishment or to recognize a changed reinforcement value. However, as the psychopathic participants did not perform the task, we cannot know if the resulting patterns of hypoactivation caused the performance decrement, or if the performance decrement induced the abnormal pattern of activation (Price & Friston, 1999, 2003).

In an affective verbal memory task (Kiehl *et al.*, 2001), psychopaths (mean PCL-R = 33) showed reduced activation in *a priori* regions of interest including the anterior and posterior cingulate gyri, left inferior frontal gyrus, amygdala, and ventral striatum when encoding, rehearsing, and recognizing negatively valenced words in comparison to neutral words (an implicit affective-processing task), and when compared with criminal non-psychopaths (mean PCL-R = 16) and non-criminal healthy men. In a lexical decision task by psychopaths (mean PCL-R = 33) and normal control participants, Kiehl *et al.* (2004) compared responses to concrete and abstract words. The psychopathic group also showed less activation for abstract stimuli compared to concrete stimuli in the right anterior superior temporal gyrus, but this occurred in the context of behavioural differences between the groups (psychopaths were slower in naming both concrete and abstract words and less accurate in determining pseudowords).

One further study of affective processing (Muller *et al.*, 2003) contrasted the performance of psychopaths (PCL-R > 30) and control participants (PCL-R < 10) in processing a small number of positively and negatively valenced emotional pictures. No attempt was made to match the small groups other than in age. Despite similar valence and arousal ratings in the two groups, the psychopathic group showed increased activation in response to negative emotional images in widespread areas including the right amygdala, ACC, and right pre-frontal areas. This was interpreted as evidence of aberrant functional interaction between bottom-up affective processes generated by the amygdala and their top-down modulation mediated via the OFC. However, the increased activations found within these areas are inconsistent with other studies of psychopathic men (e.g., Kiehl *et al.*, 2001) and amygdala-frontal connectivity was not formally examined.

A final study (Deeley *et al.*, 2006) of six psychopathic men (mean PCL-R = 29) examined their performance of an implicit facial emotion (sad, neutral, and happy expressions) processing task in comparison with healthy men. Psychopathic men showed significantly less activation of the fusiform gyrus and cerebellum bilaterally, and the left postcentral gyrus and the cerebellum when implicitly processing fearful faces in comparison to neutral faces. The fusiform gyrus plays a critical role in processing faces (Kanwisher *et al.*, 1997; Haxby *et al.*, 2000); its activity is modulated by emotional expressions (Vuilleumier & Pourtois, 2006). Increased activity in the fusiform cortex in response to fearful (compared to neutral) faces is dependent on the integrity of the amygdala (Vuilleumier *et al.*, 2004). Thus, although there was no direct evidence of impaired amygdala activation to fearful faces in the psychopathic group compared with the normal group, the reduced fusiform gyrus activation is indirect evidence suggestive of impaired amygdalar modulation. However, confidence in such an interpretation is undermined by the small number of subjects in the study and marked age and intelligence differences between the psychopathic and healthy groups.

FMRI studies of ASPD

As in the structural literature, there is a relative dearth of studies examining participants with ASPD who do not additionally meet the criteria for psychopathic disorder. A small study of reinforcement processing in male patients with a cluster B personality disorder diagnosis (borderline and ASPDs) compared with healthy men suggested impaired OFC, DLPFC, and ACC activations in the personality-disordered groups in the rewarded versus unrewarded block comparison, and impaired medial OFC activity in the loss (punished) versus no-loss comparison (Vollm *et al.*, 2007). PCL-R data was not collected for the group. Deficits in the appropriate representation of both reward and punishment were therefore evident in the personality-disordered group.

Men with 'intermittent explosive disorder' (IED) are said to be characterized by recurrent acts of impulsive, affectively driven aggression that are disproportionate to any actual provocation. The disorder is recognised in the DSM-IV but not ICD-10 diagnostic schemes. Implicit processing of emotional faces was compared between a group of men diagnosed with IED and a group of healthy men (Coccaro *et al.*, 2007). The IED participants showed increased amygdala activation and reduced OFC activation to angry faces (but not other emotions) compared with healthy men. Such threat-related processing differences are consistent with models of reactive aggression in ASPD in which there is both elevated sensitivity of the basic threat-processing circuitry (increased amygdala activity) and diminished regulation of the threat signal once generated (reduced OFC activity).

Individuals with ASPD show impaired performance on measures of executive functioning linked to DLPFC function (e.g., the Wisconsin Card Sort Test) or ventrolateral OFC function (e.g., motor go/no-go tasks; Morgan & Lilienfeld, 2000). Function in these areas was assessed using the n-back working memory (Kumari *et al.*, 2006) and motor go/no-go response inhibition (Barkataki *et al.*, 2008) tasks in two studies of high-secure hospital violent offenders with ASPD, violent patients with schizophrenia, non-violent patients with schizophrenia, and healthy men. ASPD participants showed reduced DLPFC and dorsal ACC activity compared with healthy men in both the 1-back and 2-back conditions of the n-back task. This difference was observed in the context of similar behavioural responding in terms of accuracy and latency times. The ASPD group showed better working memory performance and greater activity in the right DLPFC than the violent schizophrenic group. ASPD participants and violent schizophrenic participants also showed reduced thalamic activation compared with healthy men in the high conflict response inhibition task (in which there were fewer no-go trials) in comparison with the low conflict response inhibition task. The violent schizophrenic group also showed significantly reduced activity in the left caudate nucleus compared with the healthy men during the low conflict response inhibition task compared with the no response inhibition (go) condition. The authors noted that the thalamus is involved in the integration of sensory information and the coordination of neural activity, and suggested that ASPD offenders may thus find it more difficult to detect and appropriately respond to stimuli that should prompt behavioural inhibition. However, the imaging results in this study are again difficult to interpret in the context of marked behavioural differences in responding between the groups: the ASPD group showed significantly poorer task performance than the healthy men, with increased numbers of errors of commission in the high conflict response inhibition task in comparison with the low conflict response inhibition task.

Methodological issues

Given the logistical difficulties in performing brain imaging studies in violent offenders, sample characteristics may not always be ideal. Nevertheless, there are some key issues that need to be addressed in future studies.

Diagnostic heterogeneity should be minimized. Considerable co-morbidity with substance misuse disorders is inevitable given the nature of the externalizing dimension, but it remains important to use reliable measures to assess both current drug use and previous substance abuse history in participants (particularly given the impact of psychoactive substances on brain structure and function). Such information can then be used either for matching purposes or to enter into multiple regression models as a covariate. IQ level is another important potential confound that must be addressed. In studies of ASPD, PCL-R data should be collected simultaneously to allow the experimenters to examine correlations with dimensional PCL-R ratings (Guay *et al.*, 2007), and to allow readers of the research to relate any demonstrated abnormalities to ASPD or to psychopathic disorder. The nature of past violence should be categorized as either reactive or instrumental to ensure that a fuller picture of the type of violence being characterized is clear. Given the different aetiologies of persistent violent offending, studies are needed that compare psychopaths, non-psychopathic ASPD offenders, non-violent offenders, and healthy participants. Finally, no study to date in adults has addressed differences within the ASPD population of trait anxiety levels, which may be particularly important given that amygdala activity varies as a function of trait anxiety (Most *et al.*, 2006).

Future directions

Genetically informed imaging designs

Investigating gene-environment interactions in antisocial behaviour in developmentally informative samples may help to clarify the nature and complexity of the aetiological risk factors involved in persistent violent offending. However, as behaviour is difficult to measure with precision, and the effects of genetic variants on behaviour can best be identified in physiological measures of brain structure and function, brain structure and function has been proposed as an important intermediate phenotype (Caspi & Moffitt, 2006). Important advances in the understanding of reactive violence have been made, particularly in understanding the role of monoamine oxidase A (MAOA) polymorphisms, their interaction with environmental factors such as maltreatment (Caspi *et al.*, 2002; Kim-Cohen *et al.*, 2006), and their impact on brain structure (e.g., Meyer-Lindenberg *et al.*, 2006) and function (Eisenberger *et al.*, 2007; Buckholtz *et al.*, 2008). Such genetically informed brain imaging investigations have yet to be performed for instrumental violence or psychopathy, given the lack of molecular genetic studies in the area to date.

Emotional processing

The affective abnormalities that contribute to the development and maintenance of persistent violent offending are likely to include emotion regulation, the role of emotion in decision making in uncertain circumstances, empathic processing, and the processing of reward and punishment information in order to inform adaptive behaviour.

Given that ASPD offenders show high levels of reactive violence, a plausible hypothesis is that this group has impairments in the ability to regulate negative emotion once it is generated. Several cognitive neuroscience paradigms have already been used to parse the processes of emotion regulation in healthy men, and these paradigms could usefully be explored in ASPD (e.g., Beauregard *et al.*, 2001; Schaeffer *et al.*, 2002; Ochsner & Gross, 2005). For instance, reinterpreting the meaning of a stimulus to change one's emotional response to it is known as *reappraisal*. Studies have found that reappraisal of negative emotion activates dorsal ACC and PFC systems that support the selection and application of reappraisal strategies, and modulate activity in appraisal systems such as the amygdala or insula in accordance with the goal of reappraisal (Ochsner *et al.*, 2002). Further, when up- or down-regulating emotion, amygdala activity was found to increase or decrease depending on the direction of the emotional regulation (Ochsner *et al.*, 2004). The strength of the amygdala coupling with the OFC and dorsomedial PFC in turn predicts the extent of attenuation of negative affect following reappraisal (Banks *et al.*, 2007). It is worth exploring the dynamic interactions between these regions in the effortful control of emotion in ASPD.

The persistence of the violent behaviour shown by ASPD and psychopathic offenders suggests a failure to learn that such behaviour has negative consequences for them personally. Regret is the emotion associated with a decision that turned out badly, elicited by a counterfactual comparison between the choice outcome (reality) and the better outcome of previously rejected alternative (what might have been), thereby potentially disposing to behavioural change (avoidance of the bad outcome). Studies in brain damaged and healthy participants suggest that the OFC is central to the representation of regret values (Camille *et al.*, 2004; Koenigs & Tranel, 2007), which in turn influence adaptive behaviour via the dorsal ACC and anterior hippocampus (Coricelli *et al.*, 2005).

Impaired empathizing is a key feature of psychopathy, and the neural substrates of empathizing have begun to be explored in healthy participants (Singer *et al.*, 2004; Singer, 2006). Empathic responses to the pain of others activate the ACC, insular cortex, and secondary somatosensory cortices, with the magnitude of activation being related to the degree of relationship to the observed person. Although it is not yet clear whether these results will generalize to the observation or imagination of others' affective states other than pain, future brain imaging research in violent offenders can usefully assess this process.

Finally, a major area that has not yet been explored in adult offenders is that of reversal learning; that is, the alteration of a behavioural response to a previously rewarded stimulus following altered reinforcement contingencies. Contingency changes in this form of instrumental learning have been found to engage the OFC in adults (Budhani *et al.*, 2007). Work to test hypotheses about the neural circuits activated by reversal learning in violent offenders (ASPD and psychopaths) is currently underway in our laboratory.

There is also a need to explore the representation and use of social norm information in guiding adaptive behaviour. A recent study in normal participants examined the behavioural and neural correlates of norm compliance using a variant of the 'ultimatum game' in which money must be shared between two participants (Spitzer *et al.*, 2007). A condition in which norm violations arising from the sharing decision could be punished was contrasted with a control condition in which punishment was impossible. The social punishment threat was very effective in inducing participants to obey the fairness norm. Participants' increase in norm compliance when punishment was possible exhibited a strong positive correlation with activations in the lateral OFC. If activation in the lateral OFC represented the punishing stimulus in the task, the strong correlation between lateral OFC activation and increases in norm compliance may have indicated that participants with a stronger subjective representation of the punishment threat showed stronger norm compliance in response to this threat. Given that psychopaths lack the ability to respond adaptively to punishment threats (e.g., Newman *et al.*, 1987), they would be expected to show less compliance with the fairness norm than healthy participants, and this diminished norm compliance should be associated with significantly lower activation in the lateral OFC.

Improved neurochemical specification of psychopathy

There is a rich animal and human literature examining the neurochemical underpinnings of reactive violence (Nelson & Trainor, 2007), with lowered serotonergic tone particularly implicated in a predisposition to reactive violence. However, instrumental violence and psychopathy remain underspecified in neurochemical terms.

One hypothesis is that the impaired amygdala function seen in psychopathy is the result of impairments in neurotransmitter function, particularly noradrenaline (Blair *et al.*, 2005), such that the formation of stimulus-punishment associations is reduced. A number of lines of evidence support this hypothesis. Administering noradrenaline antagonists in humans reduces the impact of aversive cues when making decisions (Rogers *et al.*, 2004). A heightened noradrenergic response to aversive cues has been observed in those with anxiety disorders (Charney *et al.*, 1984), showing an effect in the opposite direction to that proposed in psychopathy. Amygdala activity to emotional stimuli is also reduced by the administration of a noradrenaline antagonist (Strange & Dolan, 2004; van Stegeren *et al.*, 2005).

There are also early indications of an intriguing relationship between cortisol and psychopathy. A study measuring cortisol levels, self-reported psychopathic traits, traumatic childhood experiences, and aggression in prison inmates (Cima *et al.*, 2008) showed clear differences between psychopathic and non-psychopathic inmates in measures of cortisol function.

The psychopathic group showed the lowest diurnal cortisol levels, and the non-psychopaths the greatest daily average cortisol levels. Cortisol levels impact upon amygdala function: amygdala activity when processing emotional pictures is greater in a group with increased levels of endogenous cortisol compared with a group with lower endogenous cortisol (van Stegeren *et al.*, 2007). Such differential amygdalar activation is abolished by the administration of noradrenaline antagonists. The 'double hit' of lowered endogenous cortisol and lowered noradrenergic tone in the psychopathic group may therefore underpin the observed failure to establish aversive stimulus-punishment associations and the affective response thereto. Further studies exploring these potential interrelationships are required.

Conclusions

Detailed neurobiological models of reactive violence in ASPD and instrumental violence in psychopathy have emerged in the last decade. However, the extent to which neuroimaging studies in adult male persistent violent offenders support the proposed distinctions between these groups is limited.

In structural terms, men with psychopathy demonstrate reduced grey matter (but not white matter) volumes in the PFC; the volume decrements appear to particularly occur in frontopolar and orbitofrontal regions. Volume decrements have also been noted in the anterior temporal cortex, superior temporal sulcus, and insula in comparison with normal participants. Structural abnormalities in the corpus callosum and exaggerated hippocampal asymmetry are also observed, but no convincing structural abnormality in the amygdala in psychopathy has been demonstrated to date. Potential structural differences between the psychopathic group and the antisocial group who do not meet psychopathy criteria remain to be established. Such morphological and volumetric abnormalities may of course not necessarily relate to behaviour.

In functional terms, studies of the underlying emotional-interpersonal psychopathic trait in healthy participants suggest that impaired amygdala and OFC and/or vmPFC function is observed in the processing of facial emotions and in social cooperation tasks. In psychopathic men, reduced amygdala activation and impaired vmPFC activity is observed in aversive-conditioning tasks, but such differences are difficult to interpret given the failure of the psychopathic group to be aversively conditioned. Reduced activation is also observed in the OFC, cingulate cortex, amygdala, and ventral striatum in emotional verbal memory tasks. Potential functional differences between the psychopathic group and the antisocial group who do not meet psychopathy criteria again remain to be established.

Nevertheless, the detailed neurobiological models have been a potent spur to further studies, which will attempt to address the methodological shortcomings in the extant literature. The neural underpinnings of key processes in these disorders such as empathy, social cooperation, and the adaptive use of reward and punishment information in the social environment to guide behaviour in incompletely specified circumstances have been explored in normal populations: the implementation of such paradigms in antisocial and psychopathic men promises to move the field on from the (largely) exploratory phase reviewed within this chapter to a stage of strong inference (Platt, 1964).

Acknowledgements

Funding from the NIHR Biomedical Research Centre, South London and Maudsley NHS Foundation Trust, and Institute of Psychiatry (King's College London) is gratefully acknowledged.

References

Adolphs, R., Baron-Cohen, S., & Tranel, D. (2002). Impaired recognition of social emotions following amygdala damage. *Journal of Cognitive Neuroscience*, *14*, 1264–1274.

Adolphs, R., Cahill, L., Schul, R., & Babinsky, R. (1997). Impaired declarative memory for emotional material following bilateral amygdala damage in humans. *Learning and Memory*, *4*, 291–300.

Adolphs, R., Gosselin, F., Buchanan, T. W., Tranel, D., Schyns, P., & Damasio, A. R. (2005). A mechanism for impaired fear recognition after amygdala damage. *Nature*, *433*, 68–72.

Adolphs, R., Tranel, D., Damasio, H., & Damasio, A. (1994). Impaired recognition of emotion in facial expressions following bilateral damage to the human amygdala. *Nature*, *372*, 669–672.

Amaral, D. G., Price, J. L., Pitkanen, A., & Carmichael, S. T. (1992). In J. P. Aggleton (ed), *The Amygdala: Neurobiological Aspects of Emotion, Memory, and Mental Dysfunction* (pp. 1–66). New York: Wiley-Liss.

Angrilli, A., Mauri, A., Palomba, D., Flor, H., Birbaumer, N., Sartori, G., *et al.* (1996). Startle reflex and emotion modulation impairment after right amygdala lesion. *Brain*, *119*, 1991–2000.

Banks, S. J., Eddy, K. T., Angstadt, M., Nathan, P. J., & Luan, P. K. (2007). Amygdala-frontal connectivity during emotion regulation. *SCAN*, *2*, 303–312.

Bannerman, D. M., Rawlins, J. N., McHugh, S. B., Deacon, R. M., Yee, B. K., Bast, T., *et al.* (2004). Regional dissociations within the hippocampus—memory and anxiety. *Neuroscience and Biobehavioral Reviews*, *28*, 273–283.

Barkataki, I., Kumari, V., Das, M., Sumich, A., Taylor, P., & Sharma, T. (2008). Neural correlates of deficient response inhibition in mentally disordered violent individuals. *Behavioral Sciences and the Law*, *26*(1), 51–64.

Barkataki, I., Kumari, V., Das, M., Taylor, P., & Sharma, T. (2006). Volumetric structural brain abnormalities in men with schizophrenia or antisocial personality disorder. *Behavioral Brain Research*, *169*(2), 239–247.

Barratt, E. S., Stanford, M. S., Dowdy, L., Liebman, M. J., & Kent, T. A. (1999). Impulsive and premeditated aggression: a factor analysis of self-reported acts. *Psychiatry Research*, *86*(2), 163–173.

Beauregard, M., Levesque, J., & Bourgouin, P. (2001). Neural correlates of conscious self-regulation of emotion. *Journal of Neuroscience*, *21*, RC165:1–6.

Bechara, A., Damasio, A. R., Damasio, H., & Anderson, S. W. (1994). Insensitivity to future consequences following damage to human prefrontal cortex. *Cognition*, *50*, 7–15.

Bechara, A., Tranel, D., Damasio, H., Adolphs, R., Rockland, C., & Damasio, A. R. (1995). Double dissociation of conditioning and declarative knowledge relative to the amygdala and hippocampus in humans. *Science*, *269*, 1115–1118.

Birbaumer, N., Viet, R., Lotze, M., Erb, M., Hermann, C., Grodd, W., *et al.* (2005). Deficient fear conditioning in psychopathy: a functional magnetic resonance imaging study. *Archives of General Psychiatry*, *62*(7), 799–805.

Blackburn, R. (1982). *The Special Hospitals Assessment of Personality and Socialisation*. Liverpool, UK: Park Lane Hospital. Unpublished manuscript.

Blackburn, R., & Renwick, S. J. (1996). Rating scales for measuring the interpersonal circle in forensic psychiatric patients. *Psychological Assessment*, *8*, 76–84.

Blair, R. J. R. (2009). The amygdala and ventromedial prefrontal cortex: functional contributions and dysfunction in psychopathy. In S. Hodgins, E. Viding, & A. Plodowski (eds), *The Neurobiological Basis of Violence: Science and Rehabilitation* (pp. 123–136). Oxford: Oxford University Press.

Blair, J., Mitchell, D., & Blair, K. (2005). *The Psychopath: Emotion and the Brain*. London: Blackwell Publishing.

Blair, R. J. R., Morris, J. S., Frith, C. D., Perrett, D. I., & Dolan, R.J. (1999). Dissociable neural responses to facial expressions of sadness and anger. *Brain*, *122*, 883–893.

Blanchard, D. C., & Blanchard, R. J. (1972). Innate and conditioned reactions to threat in rats with amygdaloid lesions. *Journal of Comparative Physiology and Psychology*, *81*, 281–290.

Büchel, C., Dolan, R. J., Armony, J. L., & Friston, K. J. (1999). Amygdala-hippocampal involvement in human aversive trace conditioning revealed through event-related functional magnetic resonance imaging. *Journal of Neuroscience*, *19*(24), 10869–10876.

Buckholtz, J. W., Callicott, J. H., Kolachana, B., Hariri, A. R., Goldberg, T. E., Genderson, M., *et al.* (2008). Genetic variation in MAOA modulates ventromedial prefrontal circuitry mediating individual differences in human personality. *Molecular Psychiatry*, *13*, 313–324.

Budhani, S., Marsh, A. A., Pine, D. S., & Blair, R. J. (2007). Neural correlates of response reversal: considering acquisition. *Neuroimage*, *15*, 1754–1765.

Bush, G., Luu, P., & Posner, M. I. (2000). Cognitive and emotional influences in anterior cingulate cortex. *Trends in Cognitive Sciences*, *4*, 215–222.

Cahill, L., Babinsky, R., Markowitsch, H. J., & McGaugh, J. L. (1995). The amygdala and emotional memory. *Nature*, *377*, 295–296.

Calder, A. J., Young, A. W., Rowland, D., & Perrett, D. I. (1996). Facial emotion recognition after bilateral amygdale damage: differentially severe impairment of fear. *Cognitive Neuropsychology*, *13*, 699–745.

Camille, N., Coricelli, G., Sallet, J., Pradat-Diehl, P., Duhamel, J. R., & Sirigu, A. (2004). The involvement of the orbitofrontal cortex in the experience of regret. *Science*, *304*(5674), 1167–1170.

Caspi, A., McClay, J., Moffitt, T. E., Mill, J., Martin, J., Craig, I. W., *et al.* (2002). Role of genotype in the cycle of violence in maltreated children. *Science*, *297*(5582), 851–854.

Caspi, A., & Moffitt, T. E. (2006). Gene-environment interactions in psychiatry: joining forces with neuroscience. *Nature Reviews. Neuroscience*, *7*, 583–590.

Charney, D. S., Heninger, G. R., & Breier, A. (1984). Noradrenergic function in panic anxiety. Effects of yohimbine in healthy subjects and patients with agoraphobia and panic disorder. *Archives of General Psychiatry*, *41*(8), 751–763.

Cima, M, Smeets, T, & Jelicic M. (2008). Self-reported trauma, cortisol levels, and aggression in psychopathic and non-psychopathic prison inmates. *Biological Psychology*, *78*(1), 75–86.

Cloninger, C. R. (1995). The psychobiological regulation of social cooperation. *Nature Medicine*, *1*, 623–624.

Coccaro, E. F., McCloskey, M. S., Fitzgerald, D. A., & Phan, K. L. (2007). Amygdala and orbitofrontal reactivity to social threat in individuals with impulsive aggression. *Biological Psychiatry*, *62*(2), 168–178.

Colom, R., Jung, R. E., & Haier, R. J. (2006). Distributed brain sites for the g-factor of intelligence, *Neuroimage*, *31*, 1359–1365.

Cooke, D. J., & Michie, C. (1999) Psychopathy across cultures: North America and Scotland compared. *Journal of Abnormal Psychology*, *108*, 58–68.

Coricelli, G., Critchley, H. D., Joffily, M., O'Doherty, J. P., Sirigu, A., & Dolan, R. J. (2005). Regret and its avoidance: a neuroimaging study of choice behavior. *Nature Neuroscience*, *8*, 1255–1262.

Cornell, D. G., Warren, J., Hawk, G., Stafford, E., Oram, G., & Pine, D. (1996). Psychopathy in instrumental and reactive violent offenders. *Journal of Consulting and Clinical Psychology*, *64*(4), 783–790.

Crick, N. R., & Dodge, K. A. (1996). Social information-processing mechanisms in reactive and proactive aggression. *Child Development*, *67*(3), 993–1002.

Dalgleish, T. (2004). The emotional brain. *Nature Reviews. Neuroscience*, *5*, 583–589.

Davidson, R. J., Putnam, K. M., & Larson, C. L. (2000). Dysfunction in the neural circuitry of emotion regulation: a possible prelude to violence. *Science*, *289*, 591–594.

Deeley, Q., Daly, E., Surguladze, S., Tunstall, N., Mezey, G., Beer, D., *et al.* (2006). Facial emotion processing in criminal psychopathy. preliminary functional magnetic resonance imaging study. *British Journal of Psychiatry*, *189*, 533–539.

De Oliveira-Souza, R., Hare, R. D., Bramati, I. E., Garrido, G. J., Azevedo, I. F., Tovar-Moll, F., *et al.* (2008). Psychopathy as a disorder of the moral brain: fronto-temporo-limbic grey matter reductions demonstrated by voxel-based morphometry. *Neuroimage*, *40*(3), 1202–1213.

Devinsky, O., Morrell, M. J., & Vogt, B. A. (1995). Contributions of anterior cingulate cortex to behaviour. *Brain*, *118*, 279–306.

Dolan, M. C., Deakin, J. F. W., Roberts, N., & Anderson, I. M. (2002). Quantitative frontal and temporal structural MRI studies in personality-disordered offenders and control subjects. *Psychiatry Research: Neuroimaging*, *116*(3), 133–149.

Eisenberger, N. I., Way, B. M., Taylor, S. E., Welch, W. T., & Lieberman, M. D. (2007). Understanding genetic risk for aggression: clues from the brain's response to social exclusion. *Biological Psychiatry*, *61*, 1100–1108.

Flor, H., Birbaumer, N., Hermann, C., Ziegler, S., & Patrick, C. J. (2002). Aversive Pavlovian conditioning in psychopaths: peripheral and central correlates. *Psychophysiology*, *39*, 505–518.

Franklin, T. R., Acton, P. D., Maldjian, J. A., Gray, J. D., Croft, J. R., Dackis, C. A., *et al.* (2002). Decreased gray matter concentration in the insular, orbitofrontal, cingulate, and temporal cortices of cocaine patients. *Biological Psychiatry*, *51*(2), 134–142.

Gordon, H. L., Baird, A. A., & End, A. (2004). Functional differences among those high and low on a trait measure of psychopathy. *Biological Psychiatry*, *56*(7), 516–521.

Guay, J. P., Ruscio, P., Knight, R. A., & Hare, R.D. (2007). A taxometric analysis of the latent structure of psychopathy: evidence for dimensionality. *Journal of Abnormal Psychology*, *116*(2007), 701–716.

Haier, R. J., Jung, R. E., Yeo, R. A., Head, K., & Alkire, M. T. (2004). Structural brain variation and general intelligence. *Neuroimage*, *23*, 425–433.

Hare, R. D., & McPherson, L. M. (1984). Psychopathy and perceptual asymmetry during verbal dichotic listening. *Journal of Abnormal Psychology*, *93*, 141–149.

Haxby, J. V., Hoffman, E. A., & Gobbini, M. I. (2000). The distributed human neural system for face perception. *Trends in Cognitive Sciences*, *4*(6), 223–233.

Kanwisher, N., McDermott, J., & Chun, M. M. (1997). The fusiform face area: a module in human extrastriate cortex specialised for face perception. *Journal of Neuroscience*, *17*(11), 4302–4311.

Kiehl, K. A., Smith, A. M., Hare, R. D., Mendrek, A., Forster, B. B., Brink, J., *et al.* (2001). Limbic abnormalities in affective processing by criminal psychopaths as revealed by functional magnetic resonance imaging. *Biological Psychiatry*, *50*(9), 677–684.

Kiehl, K. A., Smith, A. M., Mendrek, A., Forster, B. B., Hare, R. D., & Liddle, P. F. (2004). Temporal lobe abnormalities in semantic processing by criminal psychopaths as revealed by functional magnetic resonance imaging. *Psychiatry Research: Neuroimaging*, *130*(1), 27–42.

Kim-Cohen, J., Caspi, A., Taylor, A., Williams, B., Newcombe, R., Craig, I. W., *et al.* (2006). MAOA, maltreatment, and gene-environment interaction predicting children's mental health: New evidence and a meta-analysis. *Molecular Psychiatry*, *11*, 903–913.

Kjelstrup, K. G., Tuvnes., F. A., Steffenach, H. A., Murison, R., Moser, E. I., & Moser, M. B. (2002). Reduced fear expression after lesions of the ventral hippocampus. *Proceedings of the National Academy of Sciences of the United States of America*, *99*(16), 10825–10830.

Kling, A. S., & Brothers, L. A. (1992). In J. P. Aggleton (ed), *The Amygdala: Neurobiological Aspects of Emotion, Memory, and Mental Dysfunction* (pp. 353–378). New York: Wiley-Liss.

Koenigs, M., & Tranel, D. (2007). Decision-making after ventromedial prefrontal damage: evidence from the ultimatum game. *Journal of Neuroscience*, *27*, 951–956.

Kraemer, H. C., Yesavage, J. A., Taylor, J. L., & Kupfer, D. (2000). How can we learn about developmental processes from cross-sectional studies, or can we? *American Journal of Psychiatry*, *157*, 163–171.

Kratzer, L., & Hodgins, S. (1997). Adult outcomes of child conduct problems: a cohort study. *Journal of Abnormal Child Psychology*, *25*(1), 65–81.

Kumari, V., Aasen, I., Taylor, P., Ffytche, D. H., Das, M., Barkataki, I., *et al.* (2006). Neural dysfunction and violence in schizophrenia: an fMRI investigation. *Schizophrenia Research*, *84*(1), 144–164.

Laakso, M. P., Gunning-Dixon, F., Vaurio, O., Repo-Tiihonen, E., Soininen, H., & Tiihonen, J. (2002). Prefrontal volumes in habitually violent subjects with antisocial personality disorder and type 2 alcoholism. *Psychiatry Research*, *114*(2), 95–102.

Laakso, M. P., Vaurio, O., Koivisto, E., Savolainen, L., Eronen, M., Aronen, H. J., *et al.* (2001). Psychopathy and the posterior hippocampus. *Behavioral Brain Research*, *118*(2), 187–193.

Laakso, M. P., Vaurio, O., Savolainen, L., Repo, E., Soininen, H., Aronen, H. J., *et al.* (2000). A volumetric MRI study of the hippocampus in type 1 and 2 alcoholism. *Behavioral Brain Research*, *109*(2), 177–186.

Le Doux, J. (1996). *The Emotional Brain*. New York: Simon and Schuster.

Levenson, M. R., Kiehl, K. A., & Fitzpatrick, C. M. (1995). Assessing psychopathic attributes in a noninstitutionalized population. *Journal of Personality and Social Psychology*, *68*(1), 151–158.

Lilienfeld, S. O., & Andrews, B. P. (1996). Development and preliminary validation of a self-report measure of psychopathic personality traits in noncriminal populations. *Journal of Personality Assessment*, *66*(3), 488–524.

Matochik, J. A., London, E. D., Eldreth, D. A., Cadet, J. L., & Bolla, K. I. (2003). Frontal cortical tissue composition in abstinent cocaine abusers: a magnetic resonance imaging study. *Neuroimage*, *19*, 1095–1102.

Meyer-Lindenberg, A., Buckholtz, J. W., Kolachana, B., Hariri, A. R., Pezawas, L., Blasi, G., *et al.* (2006). Neural mechanisms of genetic risk for impulsivity and violence in humans. *Proceedings of the National Academy of Sciences of the United States of America*, *103*(16), 6269–6274.

Mobbs, D., Petrovic, P., Marchant, J. L., Hassabis, D., Weiskopf, N., Seymour, B., *et al.* (2007). When fear is near: threat imminence elicits prefrontal-periaqueductal gray shifts in humans. *Science*, *317*, 1079–1083.

Morgan, A. B., & Lilienfield, S. O. (2000). A meta-analytic review of the relation between antisocial behavior and neuropsychological measures of executive function. *Clinical Psychology Review*, *20*, 113–136.

Morris, J. S., Frith, C. D., Perrett, D. I., Rowland, D., Young, A. W., Calder, A. J., *et al.* (1996). A differential neural response in the human amygdala to fearful and happy facial expressions. *Nature*, *383*, 812–815.

Morris, J. S., Ohman, A., & Dolan R. J. (1998). Conscious and unconscious emotional learning in the human amygdala. *Nature*, *393*, 467–470.

Most, S. B., Chun, M. M., Johnson, M. R., & Kiehl, K. A. (2006). Attentional modulation of the amygdala varies with personality. *Neuroimage*, *31*(2), 934–944.

Muller, J. L., Sommer, M., Wagner, V., Lange, K., Taschler, H., Roder, C. H., *et al.* (2003). Abnormalities in emotion processing within cortical and subcortical regions in criminal psychopaths: evidence from a functional magnetic resonance imaging study using pictures with emotional content. *Biological Psychiatry*, *54*(2), 152–162.

Narayan, V. M., Narr, K. L., Kumari, V., Woods, R. P., Thompson, P. M., Toga, A. W., *et al.* (2007). Regional cortical thinning in subjects with violent antisocial personality disorder or schizophrenia. *American Journal of Psychiatry*, *164*(9), 1418–1427.

Nelson, R. J., & Trainor, B. C. (2007). Neural mechanisms of aggression. *Nature Reviews. Neuroscience*, *8*(7), 536–546.

Newman, J. P., Patterson, C. M., & Kosson, D. S. (1987). Response perseveration in psychopaths. *Journal of Abnormal Psychology*, *96*(2), 145–148.

Ochsner, K. N., Bunge, S. A., Gross, J. J., & Gabrieli, J. D. E. (2002). Rethinking feelings: an fMRI study of the cognitive regulation of emotion. *Journal of Cognitive Neuroscience*, *14*(8), 1215–1229.

Ochsner, K. N., & Gross, J. J. (2005). The cognitive control of emotion. *Trends in Cognitive Sciences*, *9*(5), 242–249.

Ochsner, K. N., Ray, R. D., Cooper, J. C., Robertson, E. R., Chopra, S., Gabrieli, J. D. E., *et al.* (2004). For better or for worse: neural systems supporting the cognitive down- and up-regulation of negative emotion. *Neuroimage*, *23*(2), 483–499.

Patrick, C. J. (2006). Getting to the heart of psychopathy. In H. Herve, & J. Yuille (eds), *Psychopathy: Theory, Research and Social Implications*. Mahwah, NJ: Lawrence Erlbaum.

Platt, J. R. (1964). Strong inference: certain systematic methods of scientific thinking may produce much more rapid progress than others. *Science*, *146*(3642), 347–353.

Price, C. J., & Friston, K. J. (1999). Scanning patients with tasks they can perform. *Human Brain Mapping*, *8*, 102–108.

Price, C. J., & Friston, K. J. (2003). Degeneracy and redundancy in cognitive anatomy. *Trends in Cognitive Sciences*, *7*, 151–152.

Raine, A., Ishikawa, S. S., Arce, E., Lencz, T., Knuth, K. H., Bihrle, S., *et al.* (2004). Hippocampal structural asymmetry in unsuccessful psychopaths. *Biological Psychiatry*, *55*(2), 185–191.

Raine, A., Lencz, T., Bihrle, S., Lacasse, L., & Colletti, P. (2000). Reduced prefrontal gray matter volume and reduced autonomic activity in antisocial personality disorder. *Archives of General Psychiatry*, *57*(2), 119–127.

Raine, A., Lencz, T., Taylor, K., Hellige, J. B., Bihrle, S., LaCasse, L., *et al.* (2003). Corpus callosum abnormalities in psychopathic antisocial individuals. *Archives of General Psychiatry*, *60*(11), 1134–1142.

Raine, A., O'Brien, M., Smiley, N., Scerbo, A., & Chen, C. J. (1990). Reduced lateralization in verbal dichotic listening in adolescent psychopaths. *Journal of Abnormal Psychology*, *99*, 272–277.

Rilling, J. K., Glenn, A. L., Jairam, M. R., Pagnoni, G., Goldsmith, D. R., Elfenbein, H. A., *et al.* (2007). Neural correlates of social cooperation and non-cooperation as a function of psychopathy. *Biological Psychiatry*, *61*(11), 1260–1271.

Rogers, R. D., Lancaster, M., Wakeley, J., & Bhagwagar, Z. (2004) Effects of beta-adrenoceptor blockade on components of human decision-making. *Psychopharmacology*, *172*(2), 157–64.

Rolls, E. T. (2005). *Emotion Explained*. Oxford: Oxford University Press.

Rosvold, H. E., Mirsky, A. F., & Pribram, K. (1954). Influence of amygdalectomy on social behavior in monkeys. *Journal of Comparative Physiology and Psychology*, *47*, 173–178.

Rushworth, M. F., & Behrens, T. E. (2008). Choice, uncertainty and value in prefrontal and cingulate cortex. *Nature Neuroscience*, *11*(4), 389–397.

Schaefer, S. M., Jackson, D. C., Davidson, R. J., Aguirre, G. K., Kimberg, D. Y., & Thompson-Schill, S. L. (2002). Modulation of amygdalar activity by the conscious regulation of negative emotion. *Journal of Cognitive Neuroscience*, *14*, 913–921.

Schneider, F., Habel, U., Kessler, C., Posse, S., Grodd, W., & Muller-Gartner, H. W. (2000). Functional imaging of conditioned aversive emotional responses in antisocial personality disorder. *Neuropsychobiology*, *42*(4), 192–201.

Schoenbaum, G., Roesch, M. R., & Stalnaker, T. A. (2006). Orbitofrontal cortex, decision making and drug addiction. *Trends in Neurosciences*, *29*(2), 116–124.

Schoenbaum, G., Setlow, B., Saddoris, M. P., & Gallagher, M. (2003). Encoding predicted outcome and acquired value in orbitofrontal cortex during cue sampling depends upon input from basolateral amygdala. *Neuron*, *39*, 855–867.

Sim, M. E., Lyoo, I. K., Streeter, C. C., Covell, J., Sarid-Segal, O., Ciraulo, D. A., *et al.* (2007). Cerebellar gray matter volume correlates with duration of cocaine use in cocaine-dependent subjects. *Neuropsychopharmacology*, *32*(10), 2229–2237.

Singer, T. (2006). The neuronal basis and ontogeny of empathy and mind reading: review of literature and implications for future research. *Neuroscience and Biobehavioral Reviews*, *30*(6), 855–863.

Singer, T., Seymour, B., O'Doherty, J., Kaube, H., Dolan, R. J., & Frith, C. D. (2004). Empathy for pain involves the affective but not sensory components of pain. *Science*, *303*, 1157–1162.

Spitzer, M., Fischbacher, U., Herrnberger, B., Gron, G., & Fehr, E. (2007). The neural signature of social norm compliance. *Neuron*, *56*(1), 185–196.

Strange, B. A., & Dolan, R. J. (2004). Beta-adrenergic modulation of emotional memory-evoked human amygdala and hippocampal responses. *Proceedings of the National Academy of Sciences of the United States of America*, *101*(31), 11454–11458.

Strange, B. A., Fletcher, P. C., Henson, R. N., Friston, K. J., & Dolan, R. J. (1999). Segregating the functions of human hippocampus. *Proceedings of the National Academy of Sciences of the United States of America*, *96*(7), 4034–4039.

Tiihonen, J., Hodgins, S., Vaurio, O., Laakso, M., Repo, E., Soininen, H., *et al.* (2000). Amygdaloid volume loss in psychopathy. *Society for Neuroscience Abstracts*, *2017*.

Tiihonen, J., Rossi, R., Laakso, M., Hodgins, S., Testa, C., Perez, J., *et al.* (in press). Brain anatomy of persistent violent offenders: more rather than less. *Psychiatry Research: Neuroimaging*.

Van Stegeren, A. H., Goekoop, R., Everaerd, W., Scheltens, P., Barkhof, F., Kuijer, J. P. A., *et al.* (2005). Noradrenaline mediates amygdala activation in men and women during encoding of emotional material. *Neuroimage*, *24*(3), 898–909.

Van Stegeren, A. H., Wolf, O. T., Everaerd, W., Scheltens, P., Barkhof, F., & Rombouts, S. A. (2007). Endogenous cortisol level interacts with noradrenergic activation in the human amygdala. *Neurobiology of Learning and Memory*, *87*, 57–66.

Veit, R., Flor, H., Erb, M., Hermann, C., Lotze, M., Grodd, W., *et al.* (2002). Brain circuits involved in emotional learning in antisocial behaviour and social phobia in humans. *Neuroscience Letters*, *328*(3), 233–236.

Vollm, B., Richardson, P., Mckie, S., Elliott, R., Dolan, M., & Deakin, B. (2007). Neuronal correlates of reward and loss in Cluster B personality disorders: a functional magnetic resonance imaging study. *Psychiatry Research: Neuroimaging*, *156*(2), 151–167.

Vuilleumier, P., & Pourtois, G. (2007). Distributed and interactive brain mechanisms during emotion face perception: evidence from functional neuroimaging. *Neuropsychologia*, *45*(1), 174–194.

Vuilleumier, P., Richardson, M. P., Armony, J. L., Driver, J., & Dolan, R.J. (2004). Distant influences of amygdala lesion on visual cortical activation during emotional face processing. *Nature Neuroscience*, *7*(11), 1271–1278.

Weiskrantz, L. (1956). Behavioral changes associated with ablation of the amygdaloid complex in monkeys. *Journal of Comparative Physiology and Psychology*, *49*, 381–391.

Whalen, P. J., Kagan, J., Cook, R. G., Davis, F. C., Kim, H., Polis, S., *et al.* (2004). Human amygdala responsivity to masked fearful eye whites. *Science*, *306*(5704), 2061.

Wheeler, E. Z., & Fellows, L. K. (2008). The human ventromedial frontal lobe is critical for learning from negative feedback. *Brain*, *131*, 1323–1331.

Winston, J. S., Gottfried, J. A., Kilner, J. M., & Dolan, R. J. (2005). Integrated neural representations of odor intensity and affective valence in human amygdala. *Journal of Neuroscience*, *25*(39), 8903–8907.

Winston, J. S., O'Doherty, J., & Dolan, R. J. (2003). Common and distinct neural responses during direct and incidental processing of multiple facial emotions. *Neuroimage*, *20*(1), 84–97.

Winstanley, A., Theobald, D. E., Cardinal, R. N., & Robbins, T. W. (2004). Contrasting roles of baso-lateral amygdala and orbitofrontal cortex in impulsive choice. *Journal of Neuroscience*, *24*(20), 4718–4722.

Yang, Y., Raine, A., Lencz, T., Bihrle, S., LaCasse, L., & Colletti, P. (2005). Volume reduction in prefrontal gray matter in unsuccessful criminal psychopaths. *Biological Psychiatry*, *15*(57), 1103–1108.

9

Brain imaging of children with conduct disorder

Philipp Sterzer and Christina Stadler

Background

The problem of aggression and violence in modern societies has stimulated the search for factors that may predispose to aggressive behaviour. Despite the undisputable importance of socio-economic and political factors, the understanding of pathological aggression should benefit from identifying its biological basis (Davidson *et al.*, 2000). The advent and ongoing refinement of modern neuroimaging techniques such as positron emission tomography (PET) and especially structural and functional magnetic resonance imaging (sMRI and fMRI, respectively) over the past twenty years has considerably increased our knowledge about possible neural underpinnings of aggressive and violent behaviour. A number of neuroimaging studies have sought to identify structural and functional brain abnormalities in adult psychopaths and criminal offenders (for review, see McCloskey *et al.*, 2005). To further the understanding of the neurobiological factors that predispose towards aggressive and violent behaviour, it seems particularly useful to investigate individuals in whom pathological aggression manifests as early as in childhood or adolescence. The purpose of this chapter is to selectively review brain imaging studies that investigated structural and functional brain abnormalities associated with aggressive behaviour in children and adolescents.

Clinical classification of abnormal aggressive behaviour in children and adolescents

The *Diagnostic and Statistical Manual of Mental Disorders IV* (DSM-IV) classification system (American Psychiatric Association, 1994) distinguishes between the diagnoses Conduct Disorder (CD) and Oppositional Defiant Disorder (ODD), which are subsumed under disruptive behaviour disorders. They are characterized by repetitive and chronic aggressive and antisocial behaviour with a variety of implications such as school refusal, social communication problems, and legal involvement. Typical symptoms of CD range from lying, truancy, and breaking parental rules to more severe offences such as rape, assault, mugging, and breaking and entering (American Psychiatric Association, 1994). ODD is generally considered a milder disorder than CD, but is also associated with functional impairment, and in some cases progresses to CD. The prevalences of disruptive behaviour disorders are 2% for CD and 3.2% for ODD. Boys are more affected than girls (Lahey *et al.*, 1999). There is a high-risk group starting with aggressive behaviour at a particularly young age. This early onset subtype is more likely to have a non-favourable outcome and is characterized by an elevated biological risk (Moffitt *et al.*, 2008). This is acknowledged to some extent in the DSM-IV by subdividing CD into childhood- and adolescent-onset subtypes (American Psychiatric Association, 1994).

CD is not a unitary disorder. The heterogeneity of CD is reflected, firstly, by a great variety of symptoms ranging from impulsive hot-tempered quarrels to acts of cruelty to animals or stealing. A key distinction is between reactive (affective, impulsive, or defensive) and instrumental (purposeful and goal-directed) aggression, as these two types of aggression might differ in their biological basis (Kempes *et al.*, 2005). Reactive aggression is frequent in CD but is also found in many other disorders, such as depression, anxiety, bipolar disorders, and post-traumatic stress disorders (Blair, 2001, 2003, 2005). Instrumental aggression is more specific to CD but is only observed in a subgroup of CD patients. The propensity for instrumental antisocial behaviour including aggression is characteristic of psychopathic personality, which has been operationalized as 'callous-unemotional traits' in children (Frick *et al.*, 1994). Children with callous-unemotional traits show a specific neurocognitive profile, have more extreme behaviour problems, and stronger genetic risk, suggesting that this subtype of CD is mediated through different psychopathological pathways and different developmental trajectories (Moffitt *et al.*, 2008).

Neural mechanisms of emotion perception and emotion regulation

It has been suggested that the propensity for aggression and violence is associated with a deficiency in responding to emotional cues in the social environment (Davidson *et al.*, 2000; Herpertz and Sass, 2000; Blair, 2001; Raine, 2002). Several lines of evidence support this notion of a link between emotion processing and aggression. Both children and adults displaying antisocial and violent behaviour show abnormally low autonomic arousal (Blair *et al.*, 1997; Blair, 1999; Raine, 2002; Herpertz *et al.*, 2003; Loney *et al.*, 2003; Herpertz *et al.*, 2005; Herpertz *et al.*, 2007). Also, the recognition of emotional cues such as sad and fearful facial expressions is impaired in children with antisocial behaviour, especially in those with callous-unemotional traits (Blair *et al.*, 2001; Loney *et al.*, 2003). In addition, emotional shallowness and callousness have been found to be associated with several features of childhood antisocial behaviour (Frick *et al.*, 1994; Frick *et al.*, 2003).

Emotion processing in the human brain involves a complex network of brain regions including the amygdala, orbitofrontal cortex (OFC), anterior cingulate cortex (ACC), anterior insular cortex, and other interconnected regions (Dolan, 2002). Various models suggesting a failure of these brain regions that process emotional information and are involved in controlling emotional behaviour have been proposed (Damasio, 1994; Krakowski *et al.*, 1997; Morgan and Lilienfeld, 2000; Blair, 2001). These models essentially suggest that aggressive behaviour arises as a consequence of impairment in processing emotional stimuli and an inability to inhibit aggressive behaviour. Substantial evidence for these considerations has come from lesion studies. There are striking behavioural similarities between individuals with a propensity to antisocial behaviour and patients with brain lesions affecting the amygdala and prefrontal regions, especially the OFC and ACC (Damasio, 1994; Adolphs, 2003).

Brain imaging studies have confirmed the involvement of these structures in emotion processing. The amygdala is activated in response to cues that connote threat, to induced fear, and to generalized negative affect such as during watching unpleasant pictures (for review, see Phelps and LeDoux, 2005). Brain imaging has also helped to characterize the functional role of the prefrontal cortex, especially the OFC and ACC in emotion processing and regulation (Bush *et al.*, 2000; Dolan, 2002; Adolphs, 2003). The OFC seems to be tuned to assigning emotional significance to complex stimuli, such as objects and situations, and competent to trigger social emotions (Adolphs, 2003). The ACC has been implicated in executive functions (Bush *et al.*, 2000). Its dorsal part is involved in higher cognitive functions such as the modulation of attention and monitoring of response-conflicts and errors, whereas the ventrorostral ACC plays a role in the evaluation of emotional and motivational information and the regulation of emotional responses. The insular cortex, especially its anterior portion, plays a key role in emotion by providing an interface between the mapping of bodily reactions to emotional stimuli and subjective feeling states (Craig, 2002; Critchley, 2005). The anterior insula is involved in the representation not only of one's feeling states but also of the feelings of others, as demonstrated by recent fMRI studies investigating the mechanisms of empathy for pain (Singer *et al.*, 2004; Jackson *et al.*, 2005) and disgust (Wicker *et al.*, 2003) or imitation of emotional facial expression (Carr *et al.*, 2003).

Structural brain imaging in CD

Although a number of brain imaging studies have examined brain structure in adults with aggressive and antisocial behaviour (for review, see McCloskey *et al.*, 2005), less was known until recently about structural brain abnormalities in children and adolescents with disruptive behaviour disorders. The first morphometric MRI data from children with CD were reported by Bussing *et al.* (2002). These authors performed volumetric measurements of the whole brain, caudate nucleus, and the cerebellar vermis, and found a volume reduction in the latter structure in children with Attention Deficit Hyperactivity Disorder (ADHD) and in CD patients with co-morbid ADHD. No findings specific to CD and no other volumetric differences were reported. The obvious limitations of this study are that its focus was more on brain abnormalities related to ADHD and the number of CD patients was very small (n = 7). Another volumetric MRI study (Kruesi *et al.*, 2004) compared regional brain volumes in 10 children and adolescents having early onset CD with healthy controls. They found a significant reduction in total right temporal lobe volume and right temporal grey matter volume. Only a trend towards reduced prefrontal volumes in the CD group was found.

Two recent studies used voxel-based morphometry (VBM), an automated voxel-wise method for the detection of regional differences in grey or white matter (Ashburner and Friston, 2000), to assess structural brain abnormalities in children and adolescents with CD (Sterzer *et al.*, 2007; Huebner *et al.*, 2008). Sterzer *et al.* (2007) compared a group of 12 boys having CD with age- and intelligence-matched controls. Grey matter volume was significantly reduced in the bilateral anterior insular cortex and left amygdala of CD patients. Correlation analyses revealed that insular grey matter abnormalities could be attributed to aggressive behaviour. There was also a significant negative correlation between left amygdala volume and aggressive behaviour scores, but attention deficit symptoms correlated even slightly stronger with left amygdala volume. Interestingly, bilateral anterior insular grey matter volume in CD patients correlated significantly with empathy levels assessed behaviourally using an empathy questionnaire. This finding is in line with recent evidence from fMRI suggesting a crucial involvement of the anterior insula in the experience of empathy (Carr *et al.*, 2003; Wicker *et al.*, 2003; Singer *et al.*, 2004; Jackson *et al.*, 2005). This region also seems to contribute to emotional feeling states via representations of visceral arousal (Critchley *et al.*, 2004). This is particularly noteworthy in the light of the well-established abnormality in autonomic responsiveness in antisocial individuals (Blair *et al.*, 1997; Blair, 1999; Raine, 2002; Herpertz *et al.*, 2003; Loney *et al.*, 2003; Herpertz *et al.*, 2005; Herpertz *et al.*, 2007), as it suggests that a neural deficit in the anterior insula may be a linking factor between abnormal autonomic responses and the lack of empathy in CD patients.

Similar to the findings by Sterzer *et al.* (2007), volume reduction in the left amygdala, and additionally in the hippocampus and surrounding cortex of the left temporal lobe, was recently also reported by Huebner *et al.* (2008). These authors investigated grey matter abnormalities in a group of 23 boys with early onset CD compared with age- and intelligence-matched healthy controls. In addition to temporal lobe structures, reduced grey matter volume was also observed in the left OFC. In the patient group, significant inverse correlations between CD symptom severity and grey matter volumes were found in the amygdala bilaterally, the left hippocampus, parts of the right temporal cortex, prefrontal cortex, and the cerebellum (Huebner *et al.*, 2008).

Taken together, sMRI studies support the notion that aggressive and antisocial behaviour may arise as a consequence of neural deficits in brain circuits involved in emotion processing. Even though reports of structural brain abnormalities in CD are still scarce, there is now converging evidence of a neurostructural deficit in temporal lobe structures, in particular the amygdala. The neurostructural deficit in the amygdala supports the hypothesis that pathological aggression may arise from an impaired processing of emotional cues signalling the suffering of another, and also to impaired learning of cues indicating threat. A prefrontal grey matter deficit was reported in one study (Huebner *et al.*, 2008) and another study reported a trend towards reduced prefrontal volume (Kruesi *et al.*, 2004), which is in line with findings in adult psychopaths (Raine *et al.*, 2000; Yang *et al.*, 2005). Reduced grey matter in the anterior insular cortex was found to be related to aggressive behaviour and lack of empathy (Sterzer *et al.*, 2005), but was not reported (but also not explicitly tested) in other studies. Inconsistencies between studies may be due to different methodologies used (region of interest-based approaches versus voxel-wise methods such as VBM) and differences in the composition of study populations. Moreover, with the exception of the study by Huebner *et al.* (2008), sample sizes were relatively small and especially negative results must therefore be interpreted with caution.

Functional brain imaging in CD

A number of fMRI studies have examined the neural correlates of emotion processing in aggressive and antisocial adults, especially those with psychopathy (Hare *et al.*, 1991). Functional abnormalities were found in the amygdala, OFC, and ACC (Kiehl *et al.*, 2001; Veit *et al.*, 2002; Birbaumer *et al.*, 2005). More recently, the neurofunctional correlates of aggressive behaviour were also investigated in children and adolescents (Sterzer *et al.*, 2005; Stadler, Sterzer *et al.*, 2007; Marsh *et al.*, 2008). Sterzer *et al.* (2005) measured neural responses to negative affective pictures in boys with CD compared with age- and sex-matched healthy control subjects: they found a negative correlation between aggressive behaviour and responses in the left amygdala to such pictures. The inverse relationship (i.e., a positive correlation) was found with symptoms of anxiety and depression, which are often present as co-morbid conditions in CD (Loeber *et al.*, 2000). Although the latter finding is in line with the notion of an increased sensitivity to mood-congruent stimuli in negative mood states (Leppanen, 2006), the reduced responsiveness of the amygdala in aggressive individuals might reflect deficient emotion processing at the perceptual level as a neural basis for pathological aggression. Viewing of affective pictures was also accompanied by a pronounced deactivation in the ACC in CD patients compared with the controls (Sterzer *et al.*, 2005).

Of note, this abnormal activation was located in the dorsal part of the ACC, which has been implicated in cognitive rather than emotional processes (Bush *et al.*, 2000), and may thus indicate an impaired cognitive control of emotional behaviour in patients with CD, in line with the notion of a reciprocal functional relationship between the dorsal and ventrorostral ACC (Drevets and Raichle, 1998; Bush *et al.*, 2000).

In a follow-up study, the authors probed the relationship between the observed functional neural deficits in the ACC and specific temperament factors predisposing to disruptive behaviour disorders (Stadler, Sterzer *et al.*, 2007). Interestingly, the temperament dimension 'novelty seeking' (Cloninger, 1987), which comprises high impulsivity and a quick-tempered personality, was a significant predictor for ACC responses to affective pictures. Individuals with high novelty seeking are characterized by deficient behavioural control strategies and a lower level of socio-moral reasoning. The deficient activation in the dorsal ACC of patients with CD might hence be a linking factor between temperament, emotion processing, and behavioural outcome.

The recent study by Marsh *et al.* (2008) asked specifically whether neural emotion processing was deficient in children and adolescents with callous-unemotional traits. They used fMRI to assess amygdala responses to fearful and angry facial expressions in the callous-unemotional group compared with children with ADHD and healthy controls. In youths with callous-unemotional traits, amygdala activation was reduced relative to healthy comparison subjects and youths with ADHD while processing fearful expressions, but not neutral or angry expressions. Moreover, reduced functional connectivity between the amygdala and cortical regions including the ventromedial prefrontal cortex and the anterior insula was observed in callous-unemotional subjects compared with the two other groups. Symptom severity in the callous-unemotional group was negatively correlated with connectivity between the amygdala and ventromedial prefrontal cortex.

Together, the results from fMRI studies published to date show that aggressive behaviour in children and adolescents is associated with reduced amygdala responses to affective stimuli, which indicates a deficit at the level of emotional information processing. The finding of reduced amygdala responses to fearful facial expressions and reduced connectivity between the amygdala and frontal brain regions in callous-unemotional youths supports the notion that the propensity for antisocial behaviour originates from impaired processing of social distress cues. Altered responses in the dorsal ACC suggest deficient cognitive control of emotional behaviour in aggressive youths. However, this interpretation has to remain speculative for the moment, as cognitive control strategies have not been directly investigated in individuals displaying aggressive and antisocial behaviour. Up to now, there is little evidence from fMRI for the hypothesis that aggressive and antisocial behaviour may arise from an OFC dysfunction, except for the finding of reduced functional connectivity between the amygdala and medial OFC in association with callous-unemotional traits. It should be noted, however, that the fMRI studies published so far did not use tasks that are known to activate OFC, such as paradigms involving the assignment of emotional and motivational value to stimuli (Davidson *et al.*, 2000; Adolphs, 2003).

Discussion and perspectives

In recent years, an increasing number of brain imaging studies have attempted to identify the neural basis of pathological aggression and antisocial behaviour as early as in adolescence. The emerging picture from these studies suggests that juvenile antisocial behaviour can be attributed to neural deficits in limbic structures, first and foremost the amygdala, and prefrontal cortical regions including the OFC, ACC, and anterior insula. Together, these structural and functional brain imaging findings in children and adolescents are consistent with theoretical models that propose a tight link between the function of neural circuits subserving emotion processing and pathological aggression (Davidson *et al.*, 2000; Dolan, 2002; Blair, 2005). Despite the indisputable progress in the understanding of juvenile pathological aggression, this research field is still in its infancy and there are many open questions that pose challenges for future research.

Most previous imaging studies compared individuals fulfilling the diagnostic criteria for CD with healthy control subjects. Although such diagnostic classification is undoubtedly helpful for clinical purposes, it has to be kept in mind that CD is a very heterogeneous entity, encompassing a wide range of behavioural abnormalities that may have different neural substrates. This heterogeneity is reflected by the fact that CD is often associated with other co-morbid conditions (Loeber *et al.*, 2000), most notably ADHD and mood disorders. The possible relevance of these co-morbidities is illustrated by the study of Sterzer *et al.* (2005), in which blunted amygdala responses in the CD group became apparent only after statistical correction for symptoms of anxiety and depression. Along similar lines, the frequently occurring co-morbidity with ADHD has to be taken into account. Despite the high degree of co-occurrence of CD and ADHD, there is increasing evidence that they represent related but independent dimensions of abnormal behaviour in childhood and adolescents (Spencer, 2006). Another important aspect that will need more attention in future studies is that CD patients can display very different types of aggression that are likely to differ in their neuro-biological basis (Blair, 2001; Moffitt *et al.*, 2008). Both behavioural work (Blair *et al.*, 2001; Loney *et al.*, 2003) and the recent fMRI study by Marsh *et al.* (2008) indicate specific deficits in the neural circuits involved in the recognition and evaluation of emotional distress cues in children and adolescents with callous-unemotional traits-that is, the subgroup of CD characterized by instrumental rather than reactive aggression. However, little is known about the differences between the neural processes underlying more reactive forms of aggression and those related to instrumental aggression. Future research should aim at identifying the specific neural mechanisms associated with well-characterized behavioural dimensions that are theoretically and empirically founded, rather than the neural correlates of clinical diagnostic labels.

Brain imaging studies so far have focused on the neural circuits that are known to be involved in emotion processing and have provided evidence in support of current neurosci-entific theories of pathological aggression and violence (Davidson *et al.*, 2000; Herpertz and Sass, 2000; Blair, 2001; Raine, 2002). Although emotional and cognitive processes in the human brain are tightly interwoven and the distinction between them is to some degree artificial, it might still be worthwhile to further explore the more cognitive aspects of social interactions and their role in aggression and violence. For example, the ability to cognitively control emotional behaviour may be impaired especially in reactive forms of aggression (Drevets and Raichle, 1998; Sterzer *et al.*, 2005). Moreover, there is now evidence for deficits in the neural circuits subserving *emotional* empathy (Sterzer *et al.*, 2005), but the neural processes underlying *cognitive* empathy (Blair, 2005), also referred to as 'theory of mind' (Leslie, 1987), may also be impaired in aggressive individuals. FMRI has recently also provided fascinating insights into the neural basis of moral decision making, which seems to involve brain structures previously implicated in both emotional and cognitive processes (Greene *et al.*, 2001; Moll *et al.*, 2002; Borg *et al.*, 2006; Young and Saxe, 2008). Socio-moral reasoning is on a less mature level in children and adolescents with CD compared with their healthy peers (Chudzik, 2007; Stadler, Rohrmann *et al.*, 2007), but the neural mechanisms underlying impaired social reasoning in relation to aggressive and antisocial behaviour are largely unexplored and await further investigation.

An interesting avenue of neurobiological research that might yield new insights into the causes and mechanisms of aggressive and antisocial behaviour is the combination of genetic and neuroimaging research (Meyer-Lindenberg and Weinberger, 2006). Although genes have long been acknowledged as major contributors to psychiatric disorders, their mechanisms of action have long seemed elusive. The combination of genetic and neuroimaging data offers the chance to characterize the neural systems affected by risk gene variants and to elucidate the role of gene-brain interactions in psychiatric disorders. The importance of genetic factors in the development of pathological aggression is being increasingly acknowledged (Viding and Jones, 2008), and there is now first evidence in healthy subjects of alterations in the neural circuitry of emotion processing in association with a genetic variant that increases the risk of antisocial problems (Meyer-Lindenberg *et al.*, 2006). It is a challenging task for future research to further elucidate how genetic and environmental factors interact to shape the structure and function of the nervous system and thus ultimately also human social behaviour, and to identify the factors in this process that give rise to aggressive and antisocial behaviour.

Finally, it should be noted that the interpretation of neuroimaging findings in association with behavioural abnormalities is not always as straightforward as it may seem to be. Neuroimaging has undoubtedly made a substantial contribution to the understanding of psychiatric disorders and has just begun to reveal insights into the neurobiological basis of disruptive behaviour disorders in children and adolescents. Although neuroimaging can thus help to further our understanding of the pathophysiology of these disorders, results from neuroimaging should not be taken as evidence of biological deficits that represent a fateful and unchangeable condition. Especially morphological alterations are easily misinterpreted as anatomically fixed abnormalities that have a quasi-deterministic influence on behaviour. However, the nervous system is characterized by a remarkable plasticity, and sMRI has repeatedly been shown to be highly sensitive to activation-dependent changes in brain morphology (Maguire *et al.*, 2000; Draganski *et al.*, 2004). It is even more obvious that functional measures such as the fMRI signal may just represent the system's momentary functional state and can be subject to considerable change over time. It therefore remains an open question whether the structural and functional brain abnormalities found in CD indicate a neurobiological predisposition towards aggressive behaviour or whether they represent activation-dependent neuroplasticity – that is, whether they are cause or consequence of abnormal behaviour. It is an intriguing challenge for the future research to further characterize the functional role of brain imaging abnormalities in different forms of CD. It will be particularly important to differentiate between 'state' and 'trait' markers in neuroimaging, and to determine to which degree such markers can change over time, especially as a consequence of therapeutic interventions.

References

Adolphs, R. (2003). Cognitive neuroscience of human social behaviour. *Nature Reviews. Neuroscience*, *4*, 165–178.

Ashburner, J., & Friston, K. J. (2000). Voxel-based morphometry-the methods. *Neuroimage*, *11*, 805–821.

American Psychiatric Association (1994). *Diagnostic and Statistical Manual of Mental Disorders*, 4th edn (DSM-IV). Washington, DC: American Psychiatric Association.

Birbaumer, N., Veit, R., Lotze, M., Erb, M., Hermann, C., Grodd, W., *et al.* (2005). Deficient fear conditioning in psychopathy: a functional magnetic resonance imaging study. *Archives of General Psychiatry*, *62*, 799–805.

Blair, R. J. (1999). Responsiveness to distress cues in the child with psychopathic tendencies. *Personality and Individual Differences*, *27*, 135–145.

Blair, R. J. (2001). Neurocognitive models of aggression, the antisocial personality disorders, and psychopathy. *Journal of Neurology, Neurosurgery and Psychiatry, 71*, 727–731.

Blair, R. J. (2003). Neurobiological basis of psychopathy. *British Journal of Psychiatry*, *182*, 5–7.

Blair, R. J. (2005). Responding to the emotions of others: dissociating forms of empathy through the study of typical and psychiatric populations. *Consciousness and Cognition*, *14*(4), 698–718.

Blair, R. J., Colledge, E., Murray, L., & Mitchell, D. G. (2001). A selective impairment in the processing of sad and fearful expressions in children with psychopathic tendencies. *Journal of Abnormal Child Psychology*, *29*, 491–498.

Blair, R. J., Jones, L., Clark, F., & Smith, M. (1997). The psychopathic individual: a lack of responsiveness to distress cues? *Psychophysiology*, *34*, 192–198.

Borg, J. S., Hynes, C., van Horn, J., Grafton, S., & Sinnott-Armstrong, W. (2006). Consequences, action, and intention as factors in moral judgments: an fMRI investigation. *Journal of Cognitive Neuroscience*, *18*, 803–817.

Bush, G., Luu, P., & Posner, M. I. (2000). Cognitive and emotional influences in anterior cingulate cortex. *Trends in Cognitive Sciences*, *4*, 215–222.

Bussing, R., Grudnik, J., Mason, D., Wasiak, M., & Leonard, C. (2002). ADHD and conduct disorder: an MRI study in a community sample. *The World Journal of Biological Psychiatry*, *3*, 216–220.

Carr, L., Iacoboni, M., Dubeau, M. C., Mazziotta, J. C., & Lenzi, G. L. (2003). Neural mechanisms of empathy in humans: a relay from neural systems for imitation to limbic areas. *Proceedings of the National Academy of Sciences of the United States of America*, *100*, 5497–5502.

Chudzik, L. (2007). Moral judgment and conduct disorder intensity in adolescents involved in delinquency: matching controls by school grade. *Psychological Reports*, *101*, 221–236.

Cloninger, C. R. (1987). A systematic method for clinical description and classification of personality variants. A proposal. *Archives of General Psychiatry*, *44*, 573–588.

Craig, A. D. (2002). How do you feel? Interoception: the sense of the physiological condition of the body. *Nature Review. Neuroscience*, *3*, 655–666.

Critchley, H. D. (2005). Neural mechanisms of autonomic, affective, and cognitive integration. *The Journal of Comparative Neurology*, *493*, 154–166.

Critchley, H. D., Wiens, S., Rotshtein, P., Ohman, A., & Dolan, R. J. (2004). Neural systems supporting interoceptive awareness. *Nature Neuroscience*, *7*, 189–195.

Damasio, A. R. (1994). *Descartes' Error: Emotion, Rationality, and the Human Brain*. New York: Putnam (Grosset Books).

Davidson, R. J., Putnam, K. M., & Larson, C. L. (2000). Dysfunction in the neural circuitry of emotion regulation-a possible prelude to violence. *Science*, *289*, 591–594.

Dolan, R. J. (2002). Emotion, cognition, and behavior. *Science*, *298*, 1191–1194.

Draganski, B., Gaser, C., Busch, V., Schuierer, G., Bogdahn, U., & May, A. (2004). Neuroplasticity: changes in grey matter induced by training. *Nature*, *427*, 311–312.

Drevets, W. C., & Raichle, M. E. (1998). Reciprocal suppression of regional cerebral blood flow during emotional versus higher cognitive processes: implications for interactions between emotion and cognition. *Cognition and Emotion*, *12*, 353–385.

Frick, P. J., Cornell, A. H., Bodin, S. D., Dane, H. E., Barry, C. T., & Loney, B. R. (2003). Callous-unemotional traits and developmental pathways to severe conduct problems. *Developmental Psychology*, *39*, 246–260.

Frick, P. J., O'brien, B. S., Wootton, J. M., & McBurnett, K. (1994). Psychopathy and conduct problems in children. *Journal of Abnormal Psychology*, *103*, 700–707.

Greene, J. D., Sommerville, R. B., Nystrom, L. E., Darley, J. M., & Cohen, J. D. (2001). An fMRI investigation of emotional engagement in moral judgment. *Science*, *293*, 2105–2108.

Hare, R. D., Hart, S. D., & Harpur, T. J. (1991). Psychopathy and the DSM-IV criteria for antisocial personality disorder. *Journal of Abnormal Psychology*, *100*, 391–398.

Herpertz, S. C., Mueller, B., Qunaibi, M., Lichterfeld, C., Konrad, K., & Herpertz-Dahlmann, B. (2005). Response to emotional stimuli in boys with conduct disorder. *American Journal of Psychiatry*, *162*, 1100–1107.

Herpertz, S. C., Mueller, B., Wenning, B., Qunaibi, M., Lichterfeld, C., & Herpertz-Dahlmann, B. (2003). Autonomic responses in boys with externalizing disorders. *Journal of Neural Transmission*, *110*, 1181–1195.

Herpertz, S. C., & Sass, H. (2000). Emotional deficiency and psychopathy. *Behavioral Sciences and the Law*, *18*, 567–580.

Herpertz, S. C., Vloet, T., Mueller, B., Domes, G., Willmes, K., & Herpertz-Dahlmann, B. (2007). Similar autonomic responsivity in boys with conduct disorder and their fathers. *Journal of the American Academy of Child and Adolescent Psychiatry*, *46*, 535–544.

Huebner, T., Vloet, T. D., Marx, I., Konrad, K., Fink, G. R., Herpertz, S. C., et al. (2008). Morphometric brain abnormalities in boys with conduct disorder. *Journal of the American Academy of Child and Adolescent Psychiatry*, *47*(5), 540–547.

Jackson, P. L., Brunet, E., Meltzoff, A. N., & Decety, J. (2005). Empathy examined through the neural mechanisms involved in imagining how I feel versus how you feel pain. *Neuropsychologia*, *44*, 752–761.

Kempes, M., Matthys, W., de Vries, H., & van Engeland, H. (2005). Reactive and proactive aggression in children-a review of theory, findings and the relevance for child and adolescent psychiatry. *European Child and Adolescent Psychiatry*, *14*, 11–19.

Kiehl, K. A., Smith, A. M., Hare, R. D., Mendrek, A., Forster, B. B., Brink, J., et al. (2001). Limbic abnormalities in affective processing by criminal psychopaths as revealed by functional magnetic resonance imaging. *Biological Psychiatry*, *50*, 677–684.

Krakowski, M., Czobor, P., Carpenter, M. D., Libiger, J., Kunz, M., Papezova, H., et al. (1997). Community violence and inpatient assaults: neurobiological deficits. *Journal of Neuropsychiatry and Clinical Neurosciences*, *9*, 549–555.

Kruesi, M. J., Casanova, M. F., Mannheim, G., & Johnson-Bilder, A. (2004). Reduced temporal lobe volume in early onset conduct disorder. *Psychiatry Research*, *132*, 1–11.

Lahey, B. B., Goodman, S. H., Waldman, I. D., Bird, H., Canino, G., Jensen, P., et al. (1999). Relation of age of onset to the type and severity of child and adolescent conduct problems. *Journal of Abnormal Child Psychology*, *27*, 247–260.

Leppanen, J. M. (2006). Emotional information processing in mood disorders: a review of behavioral and neuroimaging findings. *Current Opinion in Psychiatry*, *19*, 34–39.

Leslie, A. K. (1987). Pretense and representation: the origins of theory of mind. *Psychological Review*, *94*, 412–426.

Loeber, R., Burke, J. D., Lahey, B. B., Winters, A., & Zera, M. (2000). Oppositional defiant and conduct disorder: a review of the past 10 years, part I. *Journal of the American Academy of Child and Adolescent Psychiatry*, *39*, 1468–1484.

Loney, B. R., Frick, P. J., Clements, C. B., Ellis, M. L., & Kerlin, K. (2003). Callous-unemotional traits, impulsivity, and emotional processing in adolescents with antisocial behavior problems. *Journal of Clinical Child and Adolescent Psychology*, *32*, 66–80.

Maguire, E. A., Gadian, D. G., Johnsrude, I. S., Good, C. D., Ashburner, J., Frackowiak, R. S., et al. (2000). Navigation-related structural change in the hippocampi of taxi drivers. *Proceedings of the National Academy of Science of the United States of America*, *97*, 4398–4403.

Marsh, A. A., Finger, E. C., Mitchell, D. G., Reid, M. E., Sims, C., Kosson, D. S., et al. (2008). Reduced amygdala response to fearful expressions in children and adolescents with callous-unemotional traits and disruptive behavior disorders. *American Journal of Psychiatry*, *165*, 712–720.

McCloskey, M. S., Phan, K. L., & Coccaro, E. F. (2005). Neuroimaging and personality disorders. *Current Psychiatry Reports*, *7*, 65–72.

Meyer-Lindenberg, A., Buckholtz, J. W., Kolachana, B. A. R. H., Pezawas, L., Blasi, G., Wabnitz, A., et al. (2006). Neural mechanisms of genetic risk for impulsivity and violence in humans. *Proceedings of the National Academy of Science of the United States of America*, *103*, 6269–6274.

Meyer-Lindenberg, A., & Weinberger, D. R. (2006). Intermediate phenotypes and genetic mechanisms of psychiatric disorders. *Nature Reviews. Neuroscience*, *7*, 818–827.

Moffitt, T. E., Arseneault, L., Jaffee, S. R., Kim-Cohen, J., Koenen, K. C., Odgers, C. L., *et al.* (2008). Research review: DSM-V conduct disorder: research needs for an evidence base. *Journal of Child Psychology and Psychiatry*, *49*, 3–33.

Moll, J., de Oliveira-Souza, R., Bramati, I. E., & Grafman, J. (2002). Functional networks in emotional moral and nonmoral social judgments. *Neuroimage*, *16*, 696–703.

Morgan, A. B., & Lilienfeld, S. O. (2000). A meta-analytic review of the relation between antisocial behavior and neuropsychological measures of executive function. *Clinical Psychology Review*, *20*, 113–136.

Phelps, E. A., & LeDoux, J. E. (2005). Contributions of the amygdala to emotion processing: from animal models to human behavior. *Neuron*, *48*, 175–187.

Raine, A. (2002). Annotation: the role of prefrontal deficits, low autonomic arousal, and early health factors in the development of antisocial and aggressive behavior in children. *Journal of Child Psychology and Psychiatry*, *43*, 417–434.

Raine, A., Lencz, T., Bihrle, S., Lacasse, L., & Colletti, P. (2000). Reduced prefrontal gray matter volume and reduced autonomic activity in antisocial personality disorder. *Archives of General Psychiatry*, *57*, 119–127, discussion 128–129.

Singer, T., Seymour, B., O'doherty, J., Kaube, H., Dolan, R. J., & Frith, C. D. (2004). Empathy for pain involves the affective but not sensory components of pain. *Science*, *303*, 1157–1162.

Spencer, T. J. (2006). ADHD and comorbidity in childhood. *Journal of Clinical Psychiatry*, *67*(Suppl 8), 27–31.

Stadler, C., Rohrmann, S., Knopf, A., & Poustka, F. (2007). [Socio-moral reasoning in boys with conduct disorder-the influence of cognitive, educational and psychosocial factors]. *Zeitschrift fur Kinder-und Jugendpsychiatrie und Psychotherapie*, *35*, 169–177, quiz 177–178.

Stadler, C., Sterzer, P., Schmeck, K., Krebs, A., Kleinschmidt, A., & Poustka, F. (2007). Reduced anterior cingulate activation in aggressive children and adolescents during affective stimulation: association with temperament traits. *Journal of Psychiatric Research*, *41*, 410–417.

Sterzer, P., Stadler, C., Krebs, A., Kleinschmidt, A., & Poustka, F. (2005). Abnormal neural responses to emotional visual stimuli in adolescents with conduct disorder. *Biological Psychiatry*, *57*, 7–15.

Sterzer, P., Stadler, C., Poustka, F., & Kleinschmidt, A. (2007). A structural neural deficit in adolescents with conduct disorder and its association with lack of empathy. *Neuroimage*, *37*, 335–342.

Veit, R., Flor, H., Erb, M., Hermann, C., Lotze, M., Grodd, W., *et al.* (2002). Brain circuits involved in emotional learning in antisocial behavior and social phobia in humans. *Neuroscience Letters*, *328*, 233–236.

Viding, E., & Jones, A. P. (2008). Cognition to genes via the brain in the study of conduct disorder. *Quarterly Journal of Experimental Psychology (Colchester)*, *61*, 171–181.

Wicker, B., Keysers, C., Plailly, J., Royet, J. P., Gallese, V., & Rizzolatti, G. (2003). Both of us disgusted in my insula: the common neural basis of seeing and feeling disgust. *Neuron*, *40*, 655–664.

Yang, Y., Raine, A., Lencz, T., Bihrle, S., Lacasse, L., & Colletti, P. (2005). Volume reduction in prefrontal gray matter in unsuccessful criminal psychopaths. *Biological Psychiatry*, *57*, 1103–1108.

Young, L., & Saxe, R. (2008). The neural basis of belief encoding and integration in moral judgment. *Neuroimage*, *40*, 1912–1920.

10

Executive functions of persistent violent offenders: A critical review of the literature

Stéphane A. De Brito and Sheilagh Hodgins

Introduction

A large body of research from diverse fields suggests that impaired neuropsychological functioning may play an important role in the aetiology of aggression and violent behaviour (Giancola, 1995; Bergvall *et al.*, 2001; Brower & Price, 2001; Séguin *et al.*, 2007). Most research has focused on the role of the prefrontal cortex (PFC) and the so-called executive functions (Morgan & Lilienfeld, 2000; Séguin & Zelazo, 2005). Executive functions are 'a collection of varying abilities that involve regulatory control over thought and behaviour in the service of goal-directed or intentional action, problem solving, and flexible shifting of actions to meet task demands' (Lesaca, 2001; p. 1). Understanding the contribution of executive functioning to violent behaviour may prove to have important implications for rehabilitation programmes.

Longitudinal, prospective studies of birth cohorts followed into adulthood that have been conducted in countries with different cultures, education, health, social, and justice systems indicate that approximately 5% of the males commit more than 70% of the violent crimes that are committed by men (Farrington & West, 1993; Kratzer & Hodgins, 1999). These repetitive violent offenders are characterized by antisocial and aggressive behaviours that onset in early childhood, escalate in severity with age, and persist across the lifespan (Farrington *et al.*, 1988; Moffitt & Caspi, 2001; Moffitt *et al.*, 2002; Fergusson *et al.*, 2005; Séguin & Zelazo, 2005). When the conduct problems and associated neuropsychological deficits that emerge in childhood are not the targets of intervention, few if any of these individuals become healthy, autonomous adults (Farrington *et al.*, 1988; Moffitt & Caspi, 2001; Moffitt *et al.*, 2002; Fergusson *et al.*, 2005). The available evidence suggests that this population of individuals, who display antisocial behaviour from early childhood through adulthood, is heterogeneous (Hodgins, 2007). Research has identified two distinct subgroups of persistent violent offenders: the majority who meet the criteria for Antisocial Personality Disorder (ASPD), as defined by the *Diagnostic and Statistical Manual of Mental Disorders* (4th edition, text revision [DSM-IV-TR]; American Psychiatric Association, 2000); and a minority who, in addition to meeting the diagnostic criteria for ASPD, meet the criteria for psychopathy as defined by the *Psychopathy Checklist-Revised* (PCL-R; Hare, 2003). Evidence indicates that ASPD and psychopathy, as defined by the PCL-R, are different disorders (Hare, 1996; Hodgins, 2007). To date, neuropsychological studies of offenders have focused largely on those with a diagnosis of psychopathy. Consequently, little is known about those with ASPD.

Chapter overview

This chapter reviews research on executive dysfunctions displayed by individuals with ASPD and psychopathy. The chapter begins by describing these two disorders and highlighting the ways in which they are similar and different. Next, executive functions (EFs) are defined and conceptual and methodological issues pertaining to this construct discussed. A brief description of the functional anatomy of the frontal lobes is then presented along with a discussion of the tests that are used to assess the functional integrity of different regions of the PFC. The following section presents the distinction between cool and hot aspects of EFs. This distinction, we propose, furthers understanding of the heterogeneity of abnormal processes that characterize persistent violent offenders. Finally, studies of EFs among individuals with ASPD and psychopathy are critically reviewed.

ASPD and psychopathy: two types of violent offenders

ASPD as defined by the DSM-IV-TR (American Psychiatric Association, 2000) is 'a pervasive pattern of disregard for and violation of the rights of others'. This diagnosis covers a range of behaviours and traits including repeated criminal acts, deceitfulness, impulsivity, repeated fights or assaults, recklessness, consistent irresponsibility, and lack of remorse. Only three symptoms are required for the diagnosis and, consequently, individuals who acquire the diagnosis present heterogeneous patterns of antisocial behaviours. The diagnosis of ASPD requires the presence of Conduct Disorder (CD) prior to age 15, and thereby, ASPD indexes a pattern of antisocial behaviour that onsets in childhood or early adolescence and remains stable across the lifespan. Evidence indicates that approximately half of the adults with ASPD display symptoms prior to age 10 and 95% before age 12 (Swanson et al., 1994). The diagnosis is firmly grounded in a large body of research from prospective, longitudinal investigations (Moffitt & Caspi, 2001; Moffitt et al., 2002; Moffitt et al., 2008).

Approximately one half of the individuals with a diagnosis of ASPD have a record of criminal offending (Robins et al., 1991; J. Samuels, personal communication, June 1, 2007). There is less consistency in the findings concerning violence. For example, the Epidemiological Catchment Area study examined 18 571 persons representative of the US population in the early 1980s and found that 85% of those with a diagnosis of ASPD engaged in violence towards others (Robins et al., 1991). In contrast, a study of a British community sample composed of 8 397 persons aged 16–74 years, found that only one half of those with ASPD reported engaging in violence towards others during the past five years, 29% reported violence towards others when intoxicated, 26% reported injuring a victim, and 23% reported five or more violent incidents (Coid et al., 2006). The difference in the results of these two studies might be due to differences in diagnostic criteria (DSM-III versus DSM-IV), diagnostic procedure (lay interviewer using the Diagnostic Interview Schedule versus self-reports on SCID II screening questionnaire), sample characteristics, and/or differences across countries and time periods (1980 and 2000).

Studies among prisoners have not consistently found ASPD to be associated with violent criminality (Hodgins & Côté, 1993; Nathan et al., 2003). For example, in a random sample of 461 prisoners from Québec with a sentence of two years or longer, those with, compared with those without ASPD, had acquired more convictions for non-violent offences, but equal numbers of convictions for violent offences (Hodgins & Côté, 1993). Importantly, this study, similar to almost all others, did not exclude inmates who would meet criteria for psychopathy from the ASPD group. More recently, it has been suggested that individuals with ASPD engage in reactive violence and not in instrumental violence (Blair et al., 2005). To test this hypothesis, we examined a representative sample of male offenders incarcerated in Scotland. We excluded those with psychopathy from among those with ASPD. Among those with ASPD, 70.6% had engaged in instrumental aggression (De Brito *et al.*, under review). These results are important as this was a random sample of incarcerated offenders and the distinction between reactive and instrumental violence was based on lifetime assessments. These results challenge the commonly held view that only psychopaths engage in instrumental aggression (Porter & Woodworth, 2006).

Among children with CD, those most at risk to develop ASPD present antisocial behaviour that is more persistent and more severe, and which includes physical aggression (Moffitt *et al.*, 1996). The earlier the onset of the physically aggressive behaviour, the more likely it is to persist into adulthood (Robins, 1966; Loeber & Stouthamer-Loeber, 1987; Maughan *et al.*, 2000; Goldstein *et al.*, 2006). In early childhood, physical aggression is common and decreases rapidly from age 2 onwards (Tremblay *et al.*, 1996). The decrease in physical aggression from toddlerhood through childhood is thought to result from a concomitant increase in EFs during this period (Zelazo & Müller, 2002; Séguin & Zelazo, 2005). It has been proposed that individuals who continue to display high levels of physical aggression from toddlerhood through childhood (approximately 4–6% of community samples) present atypical development of EFs (Séguin & Zelazo, 2005; Barker *et al.*, 2007). Taken together, the extant literature suggests that people with ASPD, compared with those without ASPD, are at increased risk to engage in violence, and equally important, that a substantial proportion of persons with ASPD do not engage in violence towards others. Although little work has been undertaken in an effort to identify the characteristics that distinguish those within this population who do engage in violence, the available evidence strongly indicates that violence in adulthood is a continuation of aggressive behaviour in childhood.

ASPD and psychopathy are distinct disorders (Hare, 1996; Patrick, 2007). Although both include a lifelong pattern of antisocial behaviour that begins in childhood, psychopathy differs markedly in that it requires, in addition, the presence of emotional impairment evidenced by a lack of empathy, callousness, shallow affect, and a failure to take responsibility for one's actions, and by an interpersonal style involving grandiosity, glibness, superficial charm, and the manipulation of others (Hart & Hare, 1996). In research and clinical practice, psychopathy is assessed with the PCL-R (Hare, 2003), a clinical rating scale consisting of 20 items. Each item is scored on a three-point rating scale based on information collected from prison files and a semi-structured interviews conducted by a trained person. Scores on the PCL-R range from 0 to 40. In North America, the cut-off for the diagnosis of psychopathy is 30 or higher, whereas in Europe it is 25 (Cooke & Michie, 1997; Hare, 2003).

Although the PCL-R was developed to assess a putatively unitary construct, early factor analytic work yielded a two-factor[1] structure indicating that the construct is underpinned

---

[1] Recently, Cooke and Michie (2001) proposed an alternative three-factor model in which items of Factor 1 are parsed into two separate, albeit correlated, factors: 'Arrogant and Deceitful Interpersonal Style' specified by glibness or superficial charm, grandiose sense of self-worth, pathological lying, and conning or manipulative; and 'Deficient Affective Experience' reflecting lack of remorse or guilt, shallow affect, callousness or lack of empathy, and failure to accept responsibility for own actions. The third factor was labelled 'Impulsive and Irresponsible Behavioural Style' and encompasses need for stimulation or proneness to boredom, irresponsibility, impulsivity, parasitic lifestyle, and lack of realistic, long-term goals. Even more recently, (Hare, 2003) proposed a four-factor model in which Factor 1 and Factor 2 are each parsed into two separate facets: Factor 1 into arrogant and deceitful interpersonal style and deficient affective experience; Factor 2 into impulsive, irresponsible, parasitic lifestyle and antisocial manifestations. The comparison between these two models is currently the focus of intense theoretical and empirical discussions (Cooke *et al.*, 2006; Hare & Neumann, 2006).

by two correlated dimensions (Hare, 2003). Factor 1 includes items indexing the emotional and interpersonal features of psychopathy (charm, grandiosity, and deceitfulness or conning; absence of remorse, empathy, and emotional depth; and blame externalization), whereas Factor 2 includes items assessing a chronic antisocial lifestyle (early behaviour problems and juvenile delinquency, impulsivity, irresponsibility, lack of long-term goals). These two factors show discriminant validity in relation to personality, behavioural, and psychophysiological measures (for a review, see Patrick, 2007). As would be expected, Factor 2 indexing a stable pattern of antisocial behaviour is strongly, selectively, and positively associated with the diagnosis of ASPD, whereas Factor 1 measuring affective traits and interpersonal style is only weakly associated with ASPD (Hare, 2003). According to Hare (2003), the prevalence of psychopathy among incarcerated convicted offenders is approximately 15–25%, whereas 50–80% of prisoners would meet the DSM diagnostic criteria for ASPD. Thus, the relationship between psychopathy and ASPD is asymmetric in that almost all individuals with a diagnosis of psychopathy would meet the criteria for a diagnosis of ASPD, whereas approximately one third of the individuals with a diagnosis of ASPD meet the criteria for psychopathy (Hart & Hare, 1996).

In sharp contrast to ASPD, a great deal of research has been conducted in various populations on the association between psychopathy and violence (for a review, see Douglas *et al.*, 2006; Porter & Woodworth, 2006). Similar to ASPD, the diagnosis of psychopathy does not require evidence of violent behaviour. In contrast to ASPD, violence is not explicitly mentioned in any of the 20 diagnostic criteria of the PCL-R. Research has shown that high scores on the PCL-R and a diagnosis of psychopathy are both related to violence. Among male offenders, those with psychopathy, compared with those without, have higher rates of convictions for violent crimes (Hare & McPherson, 1984), higher rates of aggressive behaviour both in correctional institutions and in the community, and are more likely to use weapons to injure others (Hare & McPherson, 1984; Serin, 1991). Following release from custody, offenders with psychopathy are four times more likely to reoffend than other offenders, and present at least twice the risk for violent recidivism as offenders without psychopathy (Hart *et al.*, 1988; Grann *et al.*, 1999). Taken together, the available evidence indicates a clear association between psychopathy and violence.

Defining EFs

Recently, Jurado and Rosselli (2007) noted, 'Despite the frequency with which it is mentioned in the neuropsychological literature, the concept of executive function is one that still awaits a formal definition' (p. 213). This section has by no means the pretension to present an exhaustive discussion of EFs, but will focus on aspects of EFs that will prove important for understanding the research on violent offenders. First, EFs and their functions will be defined. Second, some conceptual and methodological issues that should be borne in mind when reviewing the existing neuropsychological research on ASPD and psychopathy will be outlined.

In the past decades, many definitions of the concept of EF have been offered (for a review, see Zelazo & Müller, 2002; Jurado & Rosselli, 2007). Nevertheless, Jurado and Rosselli (2007) contend that there is some agreement in the literature and note:

'In a constantly changing environment, executive abilities allow us to shift our mind set quickly and adapt to diverse situations while at the same time inhibiting inappropriate behaviours. They enable us to create a plan, initiate its execution, and persevere on the task at hand until its completion. Executive functions mediate the ability to organize our thoughts in a goal-directed way and are therefore essential for success in school and work situations, as well as everyday living. The concept of morality and ethic behaviour also represents an executive function (Ardila & Surloff, 2004)' (p. 214).

More specifically, Rabbitt (1997) has identified some of the core features of EFs:

1. 'Executive control is necessary to deal with novel tasks that require us to formulate a goal, to plan, and to choose between alternative sequences of behaviour to reach this goal, to compare these plans in respect to their relative probabilities of success and their relative efficiency in attaining the chosen goal, to initiate the plans selected and to carry it through, amending it as necessary, until it is successful or until impending failure is recognized.' (p. 3)
2. EFs allow us, under voluntary control, to look for information in long-term memory through the formation of and execution of memory search strategies.
3. EFs play an essential role in dealing with the initiation of new sequences of behaviour and the interruption of ongoing sequences. Accordingly, they are involved in the suppression, inhibition, and replacement of automatic and habitual responses with task-appropriate responses. They also control the allocation of attention, especially in complex tasks, which have simultaneous demands.
4. EFs are essential to avoid responses that are inappropriate to the context.
5. EFs allow the strategic allocation of attention and synchronization of responses in dual-task performance.
6. EFs have a monitoring role on performance: detecting and correcting errors; altering plans deemed to be unsuccessful; identifying opportunities for new goals; formulating, selecting, initiating, and executing new plans.
7. Finally, EFs enable the attention to be sustained continuously over long periods.

Although considerable progress has been made in the field of cognitive psychology and neuropsychology, recent research on EFs still faces difficulties and a certain number of conceptual and methodological issues need to be borne in mind when assessing findings from the existing research on ASPD and psychopathy (for a review, see Royall *et al.*, 2002; Manchester *et al.*, 2004; Jurado & Rosselli, 2007). Some of these issues can be addressed by considering four dichotomies (Royall *et al.*, 2002).

Frontal lobe versus frontal system

Although EFs have traditionally been linked to the frontal lobes, and specifically the PFC, we will see in more detail in subsequent subsections that they are dependent as well on the integrity of other, posterior and subcortical, brain regions (Collette & van der Linden, 2002; Heyder *et al.*, 2004). For example, patterns of EF deficits similar to those identified in patients with cortical lesions have also been observed in patients with subcortical frontal system disorders such as Huntington's disease (Lawrence *et al.*, 1996) and Parkinson's disease (Owen *et al.*, 1993), suggesting that EFs are also supported by basal ganglia structures, such as the striatum (Chudasama & Robbins, 2006). Although lesion and brain imaging studies have contributed to furthering understanding of the localization of specific EFs within the frontal lobes (e.g., response inhibition within the orbitofrontal cortex [OFC], attentional control within the anterior cingulate cortex [ACC], working memory and rule discovery within the dorsolateral prefrontal cortex [DLPFC]), it has generally proven difficult to localize specific EFs to specific frontal regions and there are few demonstrations of double dissociations (Burgess, 1997; Royall *et al.*, 2002; Rogers, 2006). Therefore, there is presently a consensus that EFs depend on the integrity of frontal systems (i.e., frontal basal ganglia–thalamocortical networks). Frontal cortical lesions may be sufficient, but they are not necessary to cause EFs impairments, whereas frontal system damage is both sufficient and necessary for impairment of EFs (Royall *et al.*, 2002).

Frontal structure versus frontal function

EFs are often referred to as 'frontal functions'. The two terms are used interchangeably and this has often led to confusion. According to Tranel *et al.* (1994), 'this substitution is indefensible' (p. 125) because it leads to confusion between a neuroanatomical term denoting a particular region of the brain and a neuropsychological term referring to specific cognitive processes. Frontal lobe damage does not necessarily lead to executive deficits (e.g., Shallice & Burgess, 1991), and likewise, there are patients with lesions outside the frontal lobes who display EF deficits (e.g., Anderson *et al.*, 1991).

Control versus process

EFs control performance in other neuropsychological domains such as memory, language, and visuospatial processing. Therefore, it is possible that tasks that are initially considered as non-executive might in fact be sensitive to frontal system disruption. Conversely, Burgess (1997) noted that any executive task strongly implicates other non-executive processes that are not directly relevant to the target EF. Thus, poor performance on a single executive task does not automatically mean inefficient or deficient EF, but might just reflect a lesion outside the frontal system that disrupts the processes being controlled during the task (Miyake *et al.*, 2000; Royall *et al.*, 2002).

Executive function versus executive function(s)

According to Roberts *et al.* (1998), the controversy about the term 'executive function' is not so much the result of disagreements about candidate cognitive mechanisms, but more about their interrelationships. Among the many issues that remain a matter of debate is the extent to which executive function is a unitary concept reflecting one ability dependent on one underlying mechanism or separate but related abilities and brain mechanisms (Miyake *et al.*, 2000; Royall *et al.*, 2002; Jurado & Rosselli, 2007). Earlier hierarchical cognitive models (e.g., Baddeley's working memory model and Norman & Shallice's model of control of action) assumed a unitary model and did not include any distinct subfunctions or subcomponents (Miyake *et al.*, 2000). These models have been criticized on several grounds. One, they might not fully account for the complexity of the clinical data (for a review, see Zelazo & Müller, 2002; Jurado & Rosselli, 2007). There is indeed evidence that patients with frontal lobe lesions often display dissociations in their performance on measures of EFs. For example, some patients may fail on one EF measure but not on another one, whereas others might show the opposite pattern of performance (Miyake *et al.*, 2000). Two, data from factor analytic studies suggest that putative EF measures do not load on a single overarching executive factor and most studies find multiple domains such as rule discovery, working memory, attentional control, and response inhibition (Grodzinsky & Diamond, 1992). Finally, it has consistently been found that the intercorrelations between measures of EFs are low ($r = 0.40$ or less) and often not statistically significant (Miyake *et al.*, 2000).

Importantly, many widely used measures of EF are complex and might in fact index different domains of executive functioning, thus making it difficult to identify specific process(es) that are impaired. For example, the Winsconsin Card Sorting Test (WCST) is considered to be the prototypical test of executive functioning and has been one of the most widely used tests to assess EFs in antisocial populations. In this test, participants are presented with four target cards that differ in three aspects (colour, form, number) and are required to sort a series of test cards that match a target card on one of the three aspects. Through a process of trial and error, the participant must discover the sorting rule, and after 10 consecutive correct responses, the experimenter changes the sorting rule and the participant is required to learn the new rule (Milner, 1963). As noted previously, the WCST may not be sensitive to frontal lobe lesions, it taps numerous features of executive functioning, and as a result, it is difficult to determine which brain process is the origin of the errors (Delis *et al.*, 1992; Séguin & Zelazo, 2005; Jurado & Rosselli, 2007). Optimal performance on the WCST requires the ability to perform extradimensional (ED) set shifts (across perceptual dimensions, such as from colour to form, on the basis of changing reinforcement feedback), as opposed to intradimensional (ID) set shifts (shifts within a dimension such as from red to blue; Dias *et al.*, 1997), as is required in response reversal or affective shifting tasks used in many studies of violent offenders (Dolan & Park, 2002; Mitchell *et al.*, 2002). Studies of both animals and humans with frontal lobe lesions using visual discrimination-learning paradigms, such as the ID/ED set shifting (Dias *et al.*, 1996), have demonstrated that these two components of EFs are doubly dissociable: impaired ID shifting is associated with lesions in the OFC (Dias *et al.*, 1996; Fellows & Farah, 2003), whereas ED impairment is associated with damage to the DLPFC (Owen *et al.*, 1991; Dias *et al.*, 1996).

As mentioned earlier, the idea of the frontal lobes as the sole substrate of EFs has been abandoned in favour of a system view. Thus, 'executive functions do not reside in a single structure but result from the interplay of diverse cortical and subcortical neural systems' (Gazzaniga *et al.*, 1998; p. 442). Accordingly, the next section will briefly describe the functional anatomy of the frontal lobes and describe typical 'frontal' tests and executive functions.

Functional anatomy of the frontal lobes involved in executive functioning

The frontal lobes are involved in a wide range of functions such as cognitive control, language, memory, empathy, emotion regulation, decision making, behavioural inhibition, and self-monitoring (Damasio, 1994; Davidson *et al.*, 2000; Miller & Cohen, 2001; Stuss & Levine, 2002). This section briefly reviews the main cortical structures involved in EFs.

The frontal lobes represent approximately 30% of the cortical surface of the cerebrum and are located in the anterior part of the brain rostral to the central sulcus and dorsal to the lateral sulcus (Fuster, 1997). Functionally, the frontal lobes are composed of different areas and traditionally they are divided into three regions: a primary motor region, a premotor region, and a prefrontal region (the PFC) that is located anterior to the primary and association motor cortices. The PFC is further subdivided into the DLPFC, the OFC, and medial frontal or anterior cingulate cortex (the medial frontal cortex is often considered part of the ACC; see Wallis, 2007). The PFC is extensively interconnected with other cortical regions, the association cortex in the temporal, parietal, and occipital lobes, and with subcortical regions including the hippocampus, amygdala, thalamus, hypothalamus, subthalamus, septum, striatum, pons, and mesencephalon (Pandya & Barnes, 1987; Fuster, 1997). In sum, this region has a rich network of connections with widespread projections to and from almost all other parts of the brain, including most of the sensory systems,cortical and subcortical motor regions, and with limbic and midbrain structures involved in affect, memory, and reward. Consequently, it plays a central role in the control of many aspects of behaviour (Miller & Cohen, 2001).

The DLPFC

This region is composed of Brodman's areas 9, 46, and 9/46 (Petrides & Pandya, 1994). The DLPFC is extensively interconnected with the OFC and with several brain regions that allow it to play an important role in the integration of sensory and mnemonic information and the regulation of intellectual function and action. These regions are the thalamus, parts of the basal ganglia (the dorsal caudate nucleus), the hippocampus, and primary and secondary association areas, including posterior temporal, parietal, and occipital areas (Fuster, 1997). The DLPFC is involved in a wide range of EFs including, but not limited to, verbal initiatives and productivity, working memory, planning, and attentional-set shifting (Owen et al., 1993; Dias et al., 1996; Stuss & Levine, 2002; Lezak et al., 2004; Amiez & Petrides, 2007). The Controlled Word Association Test (COWAT; Benton et al., 1978) measures verbal initiative and productivity. It is one of the most sensitive tasks to assess activation deficits (Stuss & Levine, 2002). In this test, the participant is asked to generate a list of words beginning with a specific letter. Patients with lesions in the left DLPFC are impaired on this task, although lesions to other brain regions such as left parietal cortex, supplementary cortex, and left striatum also perform poorly (Stuss et al., 1998). Sentence generation and story narrative tests assess formulation deficits and are dependent on the functional integrity of the left and right DLPFC, respectively (Stuss et al., 1998).

In line with work on non-human primates, which has shown that lesions of the DLPFC give rise to impairment in working memory, results from recent neuroimaging studies in healthy adults have shown that manipulation and control of information within working memory, regardless of the nature of the stimulus information (visual non-spatial, visual spatial, auditory, etc.), is associated with increased DLPFC activity (Petrides, 2000; Amiez & Petrides, 2007). Results from one brain imaging study support the idea that the DLPFC is also important for the maintenance of information held online and that activity in this region increases when information is threatened by interference or exceeds working memory capacity (D'Esposito et al., 2000). Reversal of sequence in the digit span backwards of the Wechsler IQ tests stress manipulation and control of information held online and thus allow for an assessment of working memory (Stuss & Levine, 2002).

Planning is the ability to identify and organize the steps and elements (e.g., skills, material, other persons) needed to carry out an intention and achieve a goal (Lezak et al., 2004). It is a multifaceted activity involving conceptual activity, good impulse control, memory, and sustained attention (Lezak et al., 2004). Tests such as the Trail Making Test (TMT; Army Individual Test Battery, 1944) and the Tower of London (ToL; Shallice, 1982) are among the most widely used to assess planning abilities (Stuss & Levine, 2002; Lezak et al., 2004). The TMT is a two-part paper-and-pencil test. In part A, the participant is asked to connect pseudorandomly arranged circles as quickly as possible beginning with 1 and proceeding in a numerical sequence. In part B, the participant also connects pseudorandomly arranged circles, but alternating the order between numbers and letters (1—A—2—B—3—C ... L—13). The dependent variables are the time taken to accomplish the task and the number of errors. Patients with DLPFC lesions are slower and commit more errors on this test, compared with patients with ventral lesions or healthy adults (Stuss, Bisschop et al.,

2001; Yochim *et al.*, 2007). In the ToL, the participant is required to rearrange coloured disks on pegs from a starting position to match a target configuration (Shallice, 1982). Studies of patients with brain lesions are equivocal about the role of the DLPFC and more ventral regions in this task, whereas imaging studies have consistently shown selective DLPFC activation when performing the task (Phillips *et al.*, 2002).

Studies of both animals and humans implicate the DLPFC in the capacity to shift attention between sets as a function of contingency change (Owen *et al.*, 1993; Dias *et al.*, 1996; Rogers *et al.*, 2000). Visual discrimination-learning paradigms such as the ID/ED task (Dias *et al.*, 1996) specifically assesses different components of EFs implicit in the WCST, such as shifting attention between dimensions (ED set shifting) and shifting attention within a dimension (ID set shifting; see Rogers *et al.*, 2000 for a description of the ID/ED task). Brain imaging and lesion studies have shown that ED shifting is a function that is dissociable from ID shifting and that is dependent on the functional integrity of the DLPFC (Owen *et al.*, 1993; Rogers *et al.*, 2000).

The OFC

In this chapter, the OFC will be used to refer to Brodman's areas (BAs) 10, 11 anteriorly, 13 caudally, 14 medially, and 47/12 laterally (Carmichael & Price, 1994; Petrides & Pandya, 1994). There are three important features of the OFC. One, it is a unique region within the frontal lobe in that it receives information from all sensory modalities (Carmichael & Price, 1995). Two, it has only weak connections with motor regions, but may influence behaviour through a subcortical route, as it is strongly connected to the nucleus accumbens (Haber, 2003). Three, unlike, the DLPFC, the OFC is part of a fronto-striatal circuit that has extensive connections with the limbic system, including the amygdala, cingulate gyrus, and hippocampus (Carmichael & Price, 1995). In sum, the connections of the OFC make it a structure well suited for the integration of sensory and reward information (Kringelbach, 2005).

The OFC plays a crucial role in a wide range of EFs such as affective decision making, affective shifting (response reversal and extinction), and response inhibition (Clark *et al.*, 2004; Rolls, 2004; Kringelbach, 2005; Murray *et al.*, 2007; Wallis, 2007). Affective decision making involves the evaluation of multiple responses associated with differing probabilities of reward and punishment, followed by the selection of the optimal response (Clark *et al.*, 2004; Torralva *et al.*, 2007). Importantly, response options may be influenced by several aspects of reward and punishment such as magnitude, probability, and immediacy (i.e., the delay; Clark *et al.*, 2004). Converging evidence from studies of animals and humans with OFC lesions, and from human brain imaging studies implicates the OFC as a structure that is essential for adequate affective decision making (Clark *et al.*, 2004; Wallis, 2007).

The Iowa Gambling Task (IGT; Bechara *et al.*, 1994) is the most widely used test to assess affective decision making. In this task, participants are required to repeatedly draw a card from one of four decks (A, B, C, and D). Each card is associated with either a financial reward or punishment. Decks A and B are 'bad' in that they yield large immediate rewards, but also unpredictable, large punishments. In contrast, decks C and D are 'good' as they yield smaller immediate rewards and more predictable and limited punishments. In the long run, choosing from decks A and B is a losing strategy, because the cost–benefit ratio is larger than that of decks C and D. At the beginning of the task, participants are not aware of this and as such the task requires learning reward and punishment associations in order to perform optimally (Clark *et al.*, 2004; Fellows, 2004). As the task proceeds, healthy participants generally learn to avoid the 'bad' decks and adopt a conservative strategy of accepting smaller wins to avoid large losses.

In contrast, patients with ventromedial PFC damage persist in choosing from the high-risk decks (Bechara *et al.*, 1994). This performance profile is comparable to their real-life inability to wait for delayed reward or punishment. According to the somatic marker hypothesis, this pattern of performance is the result of a failure to produce the 'gut feeling' (somatic markers) or affective colouring that guides behaviour in healthy participants (Bechara *et al.*, 1994; Damasio, 1994). Recent evidence, however, indicates a laterality effect on the IGT, and the contribution of prefrontal regions outside the ventromedial PFC to task performance. A positron emission tomography study has shown, in addition to OFC activation, activity in the DLPFC and the ACC during this task (Ernst *et al.*, 2002). Also, performance deficits have been observed on the IGT in patients with discrete DLPFC lesions, discrete dorsomedial PFC lesions, and large PFC lesions including both dorsal and ventral aspects (Manes *et al.*, 2002). Right-sided lesions may impair performance to a greater extent than left-sided lesions (Clark *et al.*, 2003). Patients with amygdala damage are also impaired on this task, albeit due to different processes (Bechara *et al.*, 1999). Taken together, these findings support the claim that the IGT lacks specificity and taps several processes, including, but not limited to, stimulus–reinforcement learning, reversal learning, set shifting, planning, and working memory (Rogers, Owen *et al.*, 1999; Busemeyer & Stout, 2002; Clark *et al.*, 2004; Fellows & Farah, 2005a).

The OFC is crucial for adapting behaviour to change in reinforcement contingencies (Rolls, 2004). Consistent findings from studies of animals and humans indicate that the OFC is necessary for two forms of affective shifting: extinction and response reversal (Clark *et al.*, 2004; Murray *et al.*, 2007). Extinction requires the participant to stop responding to an initially rewarded stimulus when rewards cease. Adults with damage to the OFC continue to respond to a previously rewarded stimulus (Rolls *et al.*, 1994). In response reversal tasks, the participant is required to learn that one stimulus is rewarded and the other is not, but then must adapt to reversed response-reinforcement contingencies, in which the previously unrewarded stimulus is now rewarded and vice versa (Baxter & Browning, 2007). Again, adults with OFC lesions are impaired on reversal and tend to persevere in responding to the previously rewarded stimulus (Berlin *et al.*, 2004). In contrast, lesions to the DLPFC do not affect performance on either of these tasks (Rolls *et al.*, 1994; Dias *et al.*, 1996). The link between changes in day-to-day behaviour and reversal learning and extinction abilities was examined in a study of patients with brain damage. Patients with ventromedial lesions made more extinction and reversal errors and completed fewer reversals than patients with damage elsewhere in the frontal lobes or in other brain regions. These impairments were strongly associated with socially inappropriate or disinhibited behaviour (Rolls *et al.*, 1994). These findings underscore the fact that reappraisal, which involves response reversal and extinction capacities (Davidson *et al.*, 2000), is likely to play an important role in social contexts (Happaney *et al.*, 2004). It has recently been suggested that such an impairment in altering behaviour as a function of change in reinforcement contingencies may increase frustration, which in turn increases the risk for reactive aggression (Blair, 2004; see also Chapter 7).

Damage to the lateral part of the right OFC (BA 47/12; also known as ventrolateral PFC, which also encompasses parts of BAs 44 and 45) is associated with impaired response inhibition, which is 'the cognitive process required to cancel an intended movement' (Aron *et al.*, 2004; p. 170). The Go/No-go (GNG) and the Stop Task are two paradigms widely used to assess response inhibition. In the GNG, on the Go trials, the participant is required to quickly respond to one stimulus and to not respond to another stimulus. The measure of inhibitory control is the number of errors of commission (responding on No-go trials). In the Stop Task, participants are presented with a set of stimuli to which they are asked to quickly respond unless a stop signal is presented. The measure of inhibitory control is the time needed to stop the response. Both of these tests require resolution of response competitions as in affective decision-making tasks, and assess the functional integrity of the OFC. These two tests, however, differ from affective decision making in that they do not involve the resolution of response competition based on the computation of reward and punishment (Blair et al., 2005).

The ACC

The ACC, sometimes referred to as the medial frontal cortex, is located on the medial surface of the frontal lobes and includes Brodmann's areas 24, 25, 32, and 33 (Bush et al., 2000). The ACC has been shown to be involved in both emotional and cognitive processing (for a review, see Bush et al., 2000). Accordingly, it has been further subdivided into two regions: the dorsal (paralimbic) cognitive region (dACC) and the rostral-ventral (limbic) affective regions (vACC). Three aspects of ACC connections to other brain regions contribute to its prominent role in behavioural control (Paus, 2001). One, dense projections from the ACC to the motor cortex and spinal cord implicate this structure in motor control. Two, the ACC has strong reciprocal cortico-cortical connections with the DLPFC, implicating it in cognitive processing. Three, afferent links from the midline thalamus and the brainstem nuclei indicate that arousal levels are important for ACC function. This pattern of connections distinguishes the ACC from other frontocortical regions and allows it to translate intentions into actions (Paus, 2001).

Various functions such as the modulation of attention (e.g., selective attention) and EFs via influence on sensory and response selection and on conflict detection and error monitoring have been ascribed to the dACC. In contrast, the vACC is mainly involved in assessing the salience of emotional and motivational information and the regulation of emotional responses (Bush et al., 2000; Botvinick et al., 2004). Lesions in the ACC lead to perseveration and impaired selective attention as measured by the Stroop tasks (Chow & Cummings, 1999; Swick & Turken, 2002). The Stroop task assesses selective attention (Miller & Cohen, 2001; Stuss, Floden et al., 2001). There are multiple versions of the task, but the classic version consists of three conditions: (1) reading words describing colours, for example, 'red' and 'black' that are printed in black; (2) naming coloured patches using the colours identified by their written names in the first condition; and (3) naming the colour of the ink in which the name of a colour is printed when the colour is incongruent with name (i.e., 'red' printed in green). The third condition normally elicits what is called the 'Stroop' effect—a significant slowing of performance (Stuss, Floden et al., 2001). This effect arises because two processes are in conflict: a prepotent, task-irrelevant process that automatically names the word and a weaker task-relevant process that names the ink colour. Successful performance requires focusing attention on the task-relevant process and inhibiting the task-irrelevant process (Miller & Cohen, 2001). Although many neuroimaging studies have demonstrated increased activation in the dACC during performance on the Stroop task (Botvinick et al., 2004), 'the neuropsychological literature on the effects of dACC is inconsistent at best' (Fellows & Farah, 2005b; p. 788). Indeed, in line with the results of two fairly large studies of patients with brain lesions that failed to find a systematic effect of dACC damage on the size of the Stroop effect (Vendrell et al., 1995; Stuss, Floden et al., 2001), Fellows and Farah (2005b) did not observe differences on the Stroop and the Go/No-go tasks when comparing four patients with focal dACC damage with 12 age- and education-matched healthy participants. Thus, dACC functioning does not appear to be necessary for successful completion of the Stroop task.

Cool and hot executive functions: heterogeneous processes and neural substrates

It is now accepted that EFs are associated with different regions of the frontal lobes as well as distributed over a wide cerebral network, which includes subcortical regions and thalamic pathways (Heyder *et al.*, 2004; Chudasama & Robbins, 2006). Also, EFs may operate differently in different contexts (e.g., affective versus attentional set shifting). In light of this evidence, a distinction between cool and hot EFs has been proposed (Zelazo & Müller, 2002). In this heuristic framework, cool EFs refer to top-down processes that are (relatively) purely cognitive in nature and usually elicited by abstract, decontextualized problems (e.g., sorting by colour, number, or shape in the WCST). Working memory, sustained attention, attentional set shifting, and response inhibition are considered to be cool EFs. By contrast, hot EFs refer to cognitive processes that have an affective, motivational, or incentive or reward component and involve regulation (i.e., the regulation of basic limbic system functions), such as reappraising the motivational significance of a stimulus in response reversal, extinction, or affective decision-making tasks. Hot EFs include both top-down and more primitive, bottom-up processes, but the latter are more prominent in hot EFs than in cool EFs (Kelly *et al.*, 2007).

Cool and hot EFs are distinguished by the trajectories of their associated neural pathways (Zelazo & Müller, 2002; Kelly *et al.*, 2007). Indeed, cool EFs are thought to be primarily subsumed by a dorsal pathway linking the thalamus and dorsal striatum to the lateral (including inferior prefrontal) and DLPFC. Hot EFs are subserved by more ventromedial pathways connecting mesolimbic reward circuitry, including the amygdala and ventral striatum, to the OFC and medial PFC (Haber *et al.*, 2000; Haber, 2003). Admittedly, this distinction is simplistic, as most EFs include some combination of both cool and hot processes (see Manes *et al.*, 2002). Although it is impossible to design a task that is a pure measure of a hot or cool EF, it is possible to design tasks that emphasize one component over the other (Zelazo & Müller, 2002). Also, it is useful to consider a dimension of task complexity, which is orthogonal to this cool–hot dimension. Accordingly, a task such as response reversal can be considered a relatively simple measure of hot EFs, whereas the IGT is relatively complex. Similarly, the Stop Task is a relatively simple measure of cool EFs, whereas the WCST is relatively complex (Zelazo & Müller, 2002). Although response reversal and Stop tasks are both subsumed by the ventrolateral/orbitofrontal cortex (VL/OFC), the Stop task cannot be considered a measure of hot EFs, as it does not involve, similar to the response reversal task, the computation or reward/punishment.

The distinction between cool and hot EFs might prove useful in two important ways in understanding the neuropsychological deficits of persistent violent offenders. The distinction is based upon a broad conception of EFs that acknowledges the affective components (Zelazo & Müller, 2002; Ardila, 2008). Thus far, the majority of the studies on ASPD and psychopathy have focused on cool EFs. However, investigating hot EFs may be more relevant to real-world decision making (Castellanos *et al.*, 2006; Fellows, 2007). It has been suggested that this framework may potentially shed light on the role of EFs in clinical disorders that onset in childhood (Hongwanishkul *et al.*, 2005). Deficits in EFs have been observed in several disorders such as Attention-Deficit/Hyperactivity Disorder (ADHD; Barkley, 1997), autism (Russo *et al.*, 2007), and CD (Nigg & Huang-Pollock, 2003). Each of these disorders is thought to include multiple impairments in different EFs. For example, ADHD is considered to involve abnormalities in multiple neural pathways that are disso-ciable both anatomically and by neuropsychological test performance (Kelly *et al.*, 2007). It has been proposed that inattention symptoms are associated with cool EFs deficits, whereas hyperactivity or impulsivity symptoms may be more related to hot EF deficits (Castellanos *et al.*, 2006). Among individuals with a diagnosis of ADHD, some may present primarily cognitive dysfunction (cool EFs), others primarily motivational dysfunction (hot EFs), and others a combination of the two. In light of the foregoing discussion, it is thus possible that different aspects of ASPD and psychopathy might exhibit distinct associations with cool and hot EFs.

Neuropsychological evidence of executive dysfunctions in persistently violent offenders

ASPD

Little research has examined EFs among individuals with ASPD. In a meta-analysis of 39 studies that examined the association of EFs and antisocial behaviour over the past 60 years, Morgan and Lilienfeld (2000) identified only three studies of ASPD, all of which examined non-incarcerated adults (Malloy *et al.*, 1989; Gillen & Hesselbrock, 1992; Deckel *et al.*, 1996). The meta-analysis indicated weak associations between ASPD and EFs (weighted effect size $d = 0.8$). With only three studies, however, an accurate estimation of the association is not possible. We first review the three studies included in this meta-analysis.

In a sample of 182 alcoholic outpatients, a significantly higher proportion of those with ASPD (81%) compared with those without ASPD (52%) obtained scores within the impaired range on a test of general cognitive functioning. The patients with ASPD performed signifi-cantly worse on the Digit Symbol and on the immediate and delayed subtests of the revised Wechlser Memory Scale, but not on the TMT part B (Malloy *et al.*, 1989).

Gillen and Hesselbrock (1992) examined a community sample, and compared adults with ASPD (n = 34) with those without ASPD (n = 57). The participants with ASPD were unusual, with relatively high IQ scores (M = 106.5), high levels of education (M = 14.8), and no past nor current substance misuse. Few and modest differences were observed. Individuals with ASPD displayed impaired response inhibition as indicated by an increased number of perseverative responses on the Luria Motor Tasks (LMT) performed less well on the simi-larities subtest of the Wechsler Adult Intelligence Scale-Revised (WAIS-R), presented plan-ning difficulties on the part A of the TMT. No impairments were observed on the WCST, COWAT, and the Porteus Maze Test (PMT). In a subsequent study of the same participants, scores on the PMT and the LMT were inversely associated with the presence of ASPD, whereas scores on the WCST, COWAT, and TMT were not (Deckel *et al.*, 1996).

We now review three studies that have usually been considered to assess EFs among adults with psychopathy, but that have in fact examined adults with ASPD. Gorenstein (1982) compared psychiatric patients recruited from substance abuse treatment programmes, and compared those that he classified as psychopaths (n = 20) with those classified as non-psychopaths (n = 23) and with healthy students (n = 18). Patients were identified as psycho-paths if they met DSM-III diagnostic criteria for ASPD as indicated by the Research Diagnostic

Criteria (Spitzer *et al.*, 1975) and if they had a score of 27 or less on the Socialization Scale of the California Psychological Inventory (Gough, 1960). The test battery included the WCST, Stroop, Sequential Matching Memory Task (SMMT) to assess working memory, Necker cube task, and a control anagram task. Results indicated that, compared to the other patients with substance misuse problems and to students, patients with ASPD committed more perseverative errors on the WCST and more errors on the SMMT and the Necker cube. The performance of the patients with ASPD on the Stroop and the anagram task did not differ from that of the two comparison groups. Although Gorenstein concluded that the results constituted strong evidence that individuals with psychopathy have deficits in frontal lobe functions, in our view, the results of this study indicate that individuals with ASPD present deficits in EFs. In a subsequent study of 81 substance abusers assessed for psychopathy using the same criteria as Gorenstein's, Hoffman *et al.* (1987) found that those with and without ASPD did not differ on the SMMT, NC, WCST, and Mazes subtests of the Wechsler Intelligence Scale for Children. Similarly, (Sutker & Allain, 1987) compared substance abusers with and without ASPD on the WCST, PMT, and a card-based visual test indexing planning and impulse inhibition. No significant group differences were observed.

More recently, the research on ASPD and psychopathy as defined by the PCL-R has diverged into two distinct bodies of evidence. However, the studies of ASPD fail to exclude participants who would also meet the criteria for psychopathy, thereby limiting understanding of EF deficits that may be specific to ASPD. Since Morgan and Lilienfeld's meta-analysis was published, six investigations of EFs among adults with ASPD have been published. Three examined community samples and three hospitalized violent offenders.

Mazas *et al.* (2000) studied a community sample of individuals with early onset alcoholism. On the IGT, those with ASPD played less advantageously than those without ASPD, indicating a focus on immediate reward and a reduced sensitivity to punishment. Disadvantageous decision bias was also associated with the quantity of alcohol ingested and a lower IQ. Unsurprisingly, another study reported a negative correlation between ASPD symptoms and performance on the WAIS similarity subtest, but no association of symptoms with other IQ subtests nor with measures of EFs (Stevens *et al.*, 2003). Crowell *et al.* (2003) examined EFs and general cognitive abilities in a large sample (n = 336) of Vietnam War veterans divided into four groups (n = 84 each) matched on age, education, race, and general cognitive functioning: (1) ASPD-active (i.e., lifetime and current diagnosis), (2) ASPD-inactive (lifetime only), (3) psychiatric controls (matched to the ASPD-active group on all other disorders), and (4) healthy controls. Measures of EFs included the COWAT, the WCST, and the Paced Auditory Serial Addition Test that assesses sustained attention and working memory. No group differences in performance were observed on any of the tests.

In an attempt to shed light on the involvement of the DLPFC and VL/OFC in ASPD, Dolan and Park (2002) compared 29 violent patients with a DSM-IV diagnosis of ASPD recruited from a high-security forensic hospital and 20 healthy men matched for age and IQ. Importantly, the patients were screened for Axis I disorders (none had a history of substance dependence or learning disability), medication, and neurological damage, and did not present other personality disorders. Results indicated that patients with ASPD and a history of violent offending displayed planning impairments on the ToL and impairments on the ED shifting component, but not the ID shifting, of the ID/ED task. They also made more errors of commission on the GNG task indicative of difficulty in inhibiting responses. In addition, these violent patients with ASPD presented problems on the delayed-matching-to-sample task, with less accuracy on the short and medium delays, but not on the long delay, perhaps indicative of attentional problems rather than mnemonic difficulties per se. Crucially, in light of these results implicating the DLPFC and some aspects OFC functioning, the authors noted that 'the neuropsychological deficits in DSM-IV ASPD are much broader than those observed in subjects meeting the criteria for psychopathy on the PCL-R' (Dolan & Park, 2002; p. 425). This assertion seems, however, overstated. The comparison group in this study was composed of healthy men whereas most studies examining psychopathy have compared prisoners with psychopathy and prisoners without psychopathy. In addition, it is not known whether some patients in the current study met the criteria for psychopathy.

Barakataki et al. (2005) compared violent patients with ASPD (n = 14), and schizophrenia (n = 13) with non-violent patients with schizophrenia (n = 15) recruited from a high-security forensic hospital and healthy men (n = 15). The participants were screened for current substance abuse and neurological conditions, and were matched on age, ethnicity, socio-economic status, and education. The neuropsychological battery included measures of general cognitive abilities, EFs, and information processing speed. Measures of EFs included the WCST, the ToL, the Stroop, and the Executive Golf task assessing spatial strategy formation and working memory. Overall, performance of patients with ASPD did not differ significantly from that of the healthy men, except for poorer performance in processing speed. In a subsequent study on the same sample, patients with ASPD, compared to healthy men, were found to commit more errors of commission on the GNG, indicating impaired response inhibition (Barkataki et al., 2008).

Conclusions

Knowledge of EFs among adults with ASPD is limited by features of the studies reviewed. One, almost nothing is known about females. Only the studies of Malloy et al. (1989) and Mazas et al. (2000) included women, but so few that gender differences were not examined. All other studies examined men. Two, the samples studied differ markedly and included individuals recruited from the community, prisons, forensic psychiatric hospitals, outpatient psychiatric clinics, and substance abuse treatment programmes, thereby limiting an understanding of the specific associations of EFs and violent behaviour among men with ASPD. Three, no research has been published that examines individuals with ASPD while excluding those who meet diagnostic criteria for psychopathy as defined by the PCL-R (Hare, 2003), again limiting understanding of EFs and violence among men with ASPD. Four, ASPD is associated with high rates of co-morbidity with Axis I disorders and with other personality disorders (De Brito & Hodgins, in press). Most of these disorders are associated with neuropsychological impairments thereby limiting knowledge of the impairments that characterize ASPD. Distinguishing impairments associated specifically with ASPD from those specifically associated with different substance misuse disorders is particularly problematic. Almost all individuals developing ASPD begin abusing substances at a young age when the brain is still developing and continue to abuse substances through adulthood. Further, the same genes that confer vulnerability for an early onset pattern of antisocial behaviour that remains stable across the lifespan also confer vulnerability for substance misuse (Krueger et al., 2002). These genes may influence antisocial behaviour and substance misuse by reducing EFs. Thus, disentangling the associations of EFs with ASPD, substance misuse, and violent behaviour present a particular challenge that will require novel experimental designs based on the recognition of the complexity of the problem. Finally, knowledge of EFs among persons with ASPD, and the association with violence, is limited because there is little consistency in the neuropsychological tests used to assess EFs.

Notwithstanding these limitations, the studies reviewed in the preceding tentatively suggest that men with ASPD do not present general deficits of EFs (i.e., implicating both the DLPFC and OFC) as has been proposed by some authors (Dolan & Park, 2002). Rather, the most consistent finding is that men with ASPD who have a history of violent offending display a specific impairment in response inhibition as measured by the GNG task. In addition, most studies, but not all (Gorenstein, 1982; Dolan & Park, 2002), concur in demonstrating that men with ASPD, with or without histories of violent offending, do not present impairments of cool EFs subsumed by the DLPFC, as indicated their performance on the WCST.

Psychopathy

Twenty years ago, the first review of studies of frontal lobe functioning among men with antisocial behaviour concluded that EFs were not related to psychopathy based on findings from three studies (Kandel & Freed, 1989). Ten years later, five (three using PCL-R ratings) other studies have been published and included in a meta-analysis (Morgan & Lilienfeld, 2000). The meta-analysis revealed a small, but significant, overall effect ($d = 0.25$ weighted), indicating some EF deficits among offenders with psychopathy. Since the publication of this meta-analysis, there has been more research on the topic. Unfortunately, the extent to which these findings apply to psychopathy, and not ASPD, is difficult to assess, as no studies have compared these two subgroups of offenders. Also, no effort has been made to screen comparison groups for ASPD.

Hare (1984) compared three groups of offenders with low, medium, and high scores on the PCL (Hare, 1980). Performance on the Stroop and Necker cube tasks was not related to psychopathy. Analyses controlling for age, education, IQ, and substance use indicated no significant differences in performance of the three groups on the SMMT and WCST. Hart *et al.* (1990) examined two unusually large samples of offenders (n = 90, n = 167) in which participants were again divided into three groups based on PCL-R scores of low, moderate, and high. The groups did not differ on age or education. Analyses controlling for anxiety, depression, and substance use revealed no significant differences in performance of the three groups of male offenders on tests of short-term memory, intelligence, TMT, and COWAT.

The results of these two studies suggest that men with PCL-R psychopathy do not present deficits in EFs, but this conclusion is likely wrong. As noted in earlier sections, EFs are dependent on different regions of the frontal lobes and distributed over a wide cerebral network, which includes subcortical regions and thalamic pathways (Heyder *et al.*, 2004). The studies reviewed did not include tests that tap functions of different regions of the frontal lobes. These studies relied on traditional neuropsychological tests such as the WCST, COWAT, and TMT that assess cognitive (cool) aspects of EFs subsumed by the DLPFC, as opposed to more motivational (hot) aspects. These studies did not examine the associations of EFs with different facets of psychopathy. Finally, neither of these studies compared the performance of individuals with psychopathy and that of patients with brain lesions. As noted in the following, subsequent studies have overcome these weaknesses that characterized the older studies.

Lapierre *et al.* (1995) were the first to examine the performance of psychopathic offenders on a comprehensive test battery including tasks tapping VL/OFC and DLPFC functioning. The authors compared the performance of 60 male offenders, half of whom met criteria for psychopathy on the PCL-R, matched on age, education, socio-economic status, current daily cigarette consumption, and alcohol use prior incarceration. OFC measures included the GNG, the qualitative score on the PMT[2] (i.e., rule breaking indicated by the number of walls crossed and pencil lifts), and a measure of anosmia. The WCST was the only task tapping the DLPFC. Two control measures (mental rotation task and similarities) were administered to assess right and left posterorolandic functioning, respectively. In comparison with offenders without psychopathy, offenders with psychopathy made more commission errors on the GNG, performed more poorly on the qualitative, but not the quantitative, aspects of the PMT, and were more impaired on the olfactory discrimination task. Offenders with psychopathy also showed a trend towards more perseverative errors on the WCST, but performed similarly to offenders without psychopathy on a mental rotation task and a similarities task. Roussy and Toupin (2000) replicated and extended these findings by examining adolescents who had committed violent offences, comparing those with and without psychopathy. Two tasks were added: the COWAT and the Stop task to assess the DLPFC and VL/OFC, respectively. In line with Lapierre and colleagues (1995), adolescent offenders with psychopathy committed more commission errors on the GNG and the Stop task and showed a trend toward more qualitative, but not quantitative, errors on the PMT, than offenders without psychopathy. In contrast to Lapierre and colleagues findings, the adolescent offenders with and without psychopathy performed similarly on the olfactory discrimination task, the WCST, and the COWAT. The results of these two studies suggest that offenders with psychopathy show specific—cool EFs—VL/OFC impairments in response inhibition, as assessed by the GNG and the Stop tasks.

Two studies have pushed the specification of the EF deficits in psychopathy one step further by including measures tapping VL/OFC, DLPFC, and ACC functioning (Pham *et al.*, 2003; Blair *et al.*, 2006). Pham and colleagues (2003) examined 36 male offenders and compared those with and without psychopathy on the PMT, ToL, Stroop, TMT, WCST, and the D-II Cancellation test to assess sustained and selective attention. The groups were matched on age, IQ, history of substance use, and current medication. In line with the studies reviewed in the preceding (Lapierre *et al.*, 1995; Roussy & Toupin, 2000), offenders with psychopathy were not impaired on the WCST or the Stroop, but committed more qualitative errors on the PMT, more errors on the D-II test, and exhibited planning difficulties on the ToL when exposed to distractors. The authors interpreted these results as supporting their hypothesis of specific EF impairments in planning abilities and selective attention among men with psychopathy (Pham *et al.*, 2003).

Blair *et al.* (2006) examined male offenders and compared those with and without psychopathy on the Object and Spatial Alternation (OA and SA, respectively) tasks andthe reading or counting number Stroop task assessing OFC, DLPFC, and ACC functioning, respectively. In the OA task, the participant is presented with two different objects and is asked to select one of two objects on each trial, with the correct response corresponding to the object that the participant did not choose on the previous trial. In the SA task, the participant is asked to select one of two identical objects on each trial, with the correct response corresponding to the location that the participant did not choose on the previous trial. In the number Stroop task, the participant is presented with numbers on a computer screen and is asked to either count or read the numbers as quickly as possible. The number Stroop allows parametric manipulation of the level of interference and is thus more sensitive to

---

[2] As pointed out by Rogers (2006), relying on the PMT to assess OFC functioning might not be appropriate, because some studies have shown rule breaking following OFC (Levin *et al.*, 2001) and dorsolateral and dorsomedial lesion (Roberts & Wallis, 2000).

subtle impairments (Blair *et al.*, 2006). In comparison to offenders without psychopathy, offenders with psychopathy showed marked impairment on the OA task, but not on the SA task, indicative of OFC, not DLPFC, deficits. The number of reversal errors on the OA task was significantly correlated ($r = 0.40$) with scores for the affective and interpersonal factor (Factor 1 of the two-factor model) of the PCL-R. Results of the Stroop task were mixed, in that offenders with psychopathy did not significantly differ from offenders without psychopathy on the level of interference on the counting Stroop, but did show less interference on the reading task. The level of interference on the reading task was significantly correlated ($r = 0.32$) with the antisocial behaviour factor (Factor 2 of the two-factor model) of the PCL-R. According to the authors, the Stroop results reflected low levels of education rather than impairment in ACC functioning (Blair *et al.*, 2006). Group comparisons and correlational analyses provided some evidence that psychopathy, especially the emotional and interpersonal component, is related to deficits in hot EFs, as measured the OA task. Notwithstanding the lack of control for substance abuse, these results are consistent with other studies that have consistently shown that, on the standard Stroop, offenders with psychopathy display similar interference as offenders without psychopathy (Smith *et al.*, 1992; Hiatt *et al.*, 2004; Brinkley *et al.*, 2005; Dvorak-Bertsch *et al.*, 2007). Thus, these findings do not suggest dysfunction in the dACC known to be involved in conflict detection, but leave open the possibility that offenders with psychopathy present EF deficits linked to the vACC, a region that is closely connected with the amygdala and known to be associated with emotional processing (Blair *et al.*, 2006; Dvorak-Bertsch *et al.*, 2007).

Although presented as a cognitive model of psychopathy, the response-modulation hypothesis proposed by Newman and colleagues (Newman & Lorenz, 2002; Patterson & Newman, 1993) has lead to the first investigations of hot EFs among adults with psychopathy. Response modulation is 'a brief and relatively automatic shift of attention from the organization and implementation of goal-directed action to its evaluation' (Newman, 1998; p. 85). Even though the response-modulation hypothesis focuses on attention, it is based on results of animal studies showing that deficient response modulation induced by lesions in the septo-hippocampal system leads to response perseveration despite punishment or frustrative non-reward. Although Newman and colleagues did not articulate their model in an EF framework, their measure of Passive Avoidance (PA) learning (Newman & Kosson, 1986) and the one-pack Card Playing Task (CPT; Newman *et al.*, 1987) constitute measures focused on hot Efs—that is, motivational and affective processes of executive functioning thought to be subsumed by the amygdala and OFC. For example, in a study comparing stable aggressive adolescent males and non-aggressive males from the community, a strong correlation ($r = -0.58$) was observed between PA errors and EFs (LeMarquand *et al.*, 1998). This association remained after controlling for IQ and memory. Group differences in EFs accounted for the group difference in PA performance (see also Hoaken *et al.*, 2003).

The PA task presents participants with a series of eight two-digit numbers, four leading to rewards (S+) and four to punishment (S−). The participant must learn through trial and error to respond to S+ and to refrain from responding to S−. If the participant does not respond, he or she does not gain nor lose points. Dependent measures are PA errors (i.e., responses to S−) and omission errors (i.e., failure to respond to S+). PA assesses stimulus-reinforcement-based instrumental learning in which the amygdala is crucially involved (Baxter & Murray, 2002; see Chapter 7) This type of instrumental learning is disrupted by amygdala lesions (Ambrogi Lorenzini *et al.*, 1991; Takashina *et al.*, 1995; Mitchell, Fine *et al.*, 2006), but not lesions in the OFC (Mitchell, Fine *et al.*, 2006). Lesions in the OFC impair extinction as assessed by the CPT (Blair, 2004). The CPT requires participants to draw cards from a deck of 100 in which the sequence of cards associated with punishment and reward is predetermined across 10 blocks. Initially, participants keep drawing cards associated with rewards, but as the game progresses, the rate of punishments increases by 10% with every block of 10 cards from 10% to 100%. The primary dependent measure is the number of cards played.

Replicating and extending earlier findings in adolescent offenders with psychopathy (Newman et al., 1985), Newman and Kosson (1986) observed that adult male offenders with psychopathy committed more PA errors than offenders without psychopathy on a PA paradigm involving competing reward and punishment contingencies. These results have now been replicated several times (for a review, see Hiatt & Newman, 2006). Recently, using a graded reinforcement schedule, these findings were extended by Blair and colleagues (2004), who found that the performance of offenders with psychopathy on this task was modulated by the level of reward, but not by the level of punishment. This body of evidence supports models of amygdala dysfunction in men with psychopahty (Blair et al., 2005; Patrick, 2006).

Three studies using the CPT have observed extinction impairments among men with psychopathy, supporting the proposition that OFC dysfunctions characterize this disorder (Newman et al., 1987; Blair & Cipolotti, 2000; Moltó et al., 2007). In the first study, offenders with psychopathy played more cards and earned less money relative to offenders without psychopathy, only when asked to immediately play a new card but not when a five-second delay was imposed after each response (Newman et al., 1987). In a second study, Blair and Cipolotti (2000) compared the performance of two patients with OFC lesions with that of violent prisoners, half of whom met the criteria for psychopathy. The offenders with psychopathy performed worse than those without psychopathy and the patients with OFC lesions.

More recently, Moltó and colleagues (2007) replicated and extended the results of Newman's group (1987) among Spanish male prisoners divided into three groups: 9 offenders diagnosed with psychopathy (PCL-R score >30), 19 mixed (PCL-R between 20 and 30), and 11 offenders without psychopathy (PCL-R<, 20). Offenders with psychopathy played significantly more cards than the two other groups of offenders. Perseveration was related to scores on the antisocial behaviour factor (Factor 2 of the two-factor model), to scores on the impulsive and irresponsible lifestyle factor of the four-factor model, and not to the affective and interpersonal factor (Factor 1 of the two-factor model) of the disorder. These results suggest that perseveration may not be specific to psychopathy, but rather associated with externalizing disorders or with a dimension assessing externalizing problems and features (Patrick et al., in press). Contrary to Newman and colleagues' (1987) proposal that perseveration was related to the ability to reflect on negative feedback specifically, the deficit identified in this more recent study was related to a lack of reflectiveness both after punishment and after reward.

In recent years, the four-pack IGT and response reversal paradigms have increasingly been used to investigate affective decision making and the functional integrity of the OFC among offenders with psychopathy. As mentioned earlier, these paradigms are predominantly measures of hot EFs. In a sample of 157 prisoners, Schmitt et al. (1999) observed, no difference in performance on the IGT between those with low, medium, or high scores on the PCL-R, similar to Blair and Cipolotti (2000). Anxiety was related to performance on the task, as low-anxious prisoners persisted in drawing cards from the high-risk decks whereas high-anxious prisoners did not.

More recently, Mitchell et al. (2002) compared offenders with and without psychopathy on the IGT and the ID/ED tasks. Groups were matched on age and cognitive ability and excluded individuals with a diagnosis of psychosis, organic brain damage, or neurological disorders. Offenders with psychopathy, in contrast to those without, selected cards from the high-risk decks throughout the task and committed significantly more errors on the ID shift, but not on the ED shift, indicative of OFC impairment and intact DLPFC functioning (Mitchell *et al.*, 2002). Importantly, the groups were not matched on substance abuse history, an important caveat given that decision-making impairments are associated with chronic drug use (Rogers, Everitt *et al.*, 1999; Verdejo-García *et al.*, 2007) as is psychopathy (Taylor & Lang, 2006). However, the results of a recent study tend to support the idea that the group differences observed by Mitchell and colleagues may be specifically associated with psychopathy. Vassileva *et al.* (2007) studied male heroin addicts and found that those with psychopathy performed significantly more poorly than those without this disorder on the IGT. Notably, as a group, the heroin addicts with psychopathy never switched to the good decks throughout the entire task and their scores never went above zero on any of the five blocks (Vassileva *et al.*, 2007).

As noted, trait anxiety has been found to moderate the performance of individuals with psychopathy on neuropsychological tests (Hiatt & Newman, 2006). In addition, Lösel and Schmucker (2004) reported that performance on the IGT was related to attention, as measured by the D-II test, but not to psychopathy. Offenders with psychopathy and low attention capacities performed more poorly than both the attentive offenders with psychopathy and offenders without psychopathy. Interestingly, 'attentive' offenders with psychopathy performed significantly better than offenders without psychopathy. These results and those of Pham and colleagues (2003) suggest that, in addition to response inhibition difficulties, impairments in cool EFs such as attention capacities are present in some offenders with psychopathy and might impact on hot processes such as affective decision making. Also, as mentioned earlier, the results might also reflect the fact that the IGT is a complex task tapping several different processes. Methodological features of the studies such as differences in instructions, value of the reinforcers, and sample characteristics may account, at least in part, for the inconsistent results (Schmitt *et al.*, 1999; Mitchell *et al.*, 2002; Lösel & Schmucker, 2004).

Using a probabilistic response reversal paradigm, Budhani *et al.* (2006) provided further evidence that psychopathy is associated with hot EFs subsumed by the OFC. In contrast to classical response reversal paradigm (e.g., the ID set shifting component of the ID/ED task) where the contingency change is salient (i.e., one stimulus is always rewarded in the acquisition phase and then never rewarded in the reversal phase), in the probabilistic response reversal paradigm, the contingency change is probabilistic (i.e., in acquisition and reversal phases, correct and incorrect stimuli are not always rewarded or punished). Among male offenders, with and without psychopathy matched for age and IQ, no differences were found in performance in the acquisition phase, but the offenders with psychopathy displayed impairment on the reversal phase of the task for stimuli rewarded 100% and 80% of the time. The groups were not matched for history of substance misuse. A recent study reported that performance on this paradigm was impaired in chronic cocaine users (Ersche *et al.*, 2008). Thus, the impairments observed could be associated with drug abuse and have no direct link with psychopathy. A similar impairment, however, has been observed in children with callous-unemotional traits, suggesting that the deficit may be related to psychopathy (Budhani & Blair, 2005).

As mentioned earlier, an analogy has often been drawn between patients with behavioural and personality changes following OFC lesions (i.e., acquired psychopathy) and individuals with developmental psychopathy (Damasio, 1994). It has been suggested, however, that the two conditions are associated with dissociable neurocognitive deficits (Blair & Cipolotti, 2000; Blair *et al.*, 2005). Recent evidence from two studies directly comparing patients with acquired psychopathy and offenders with psychopathy have lent support to this position (Mitchell, Avny, & Blair, 2006; Mitchell, Fine *et al.*, 2006).

Mitchell, Fine, *et al.* (2006) compared the performance of male offenders with and without psychopathy, healthy men, one patient with a lesion in the left amygdala, and two patients with OFC lesions (left-sided and bilateral) on a novel task indexing stimulus-reinforcement associations and reversal learning. In the acquisition phase of the task, participants were presented on each trial with four tokens, two of one colour and two of another colour, and they were required to learn which ones yielded reward and which ones yielded punishment. In two subsequent reversal phases, each token led to the opposite consequence. In the first experiment, the patient with an amygdala lesion, performed more poorly than the patients with OFC lesions and the healthy men. In the reversal phase of the task, the two patients with OFC lesions displayed significant impairment relative to the healthy men. The offenders with psychopathy did not perform better than chance on the acquisition phase of the task, similar to the patient with an amygdala lesion.

In the second experiment, male offenders were again studied, comparing those with a diagnosis of psychopathy (≥30), those with high but subthreshold scores (21–29), and those with low scores (<21) on the PCL-R. Groups were matched for age and cognitive abilities. The offenders with psychopathy compared to those with low PCL scores were significantly impaired on the acquisition and second reversal phases. The performance of the offenders with intermediate PCL scores did not differ from that of either the offenders with psychopathy or the offenders without psychopathy in the acquisition phase. However, the offenders with intermediate PCL scores performed significantly more poorly than the offenders without psychopathy in the second reversal phase. In sum, the results of these two experiments indicate that offenders with psychopathy present stimulus-reinforcement and response reversal impairments, whereas patients with OFC lesions are impaired only on the response reversal task. Perhaps importantly, the results showed that offenders with high PCL scores not sufficient to warrant a diagnosis of psychopathy presented significant difficulty in instrumental learning.

In a subsequent study, comparing one patient with bilateral OFC lesions to five offenders with psychopathy, five offenders without psychopathy, and five healthy men, a double dissociation was observed (Mitchell, Avny, & Blair, 2006). The offenders with psychopathy exhibited stimulus-reinforcement learning (i.e., PA) deficits and intact conditional learning, whereas the patient with OFC lesions presented the opposite pattern of results. This patient was also impaired in social response reversal (i.e., modulation of one's behaviour based on social cues; see Blair & Cipolotti, 2000 for similar results), but not on the response reversal task (ID set shifting of the ID/ED task). Again, the offenders with psychopathy exhibited the reverse pattern of results. Importantly, offenders with psychopathy and patients with OFC lesions showed similar patterns of risky decision making on the IGT.

Conclusions

The findings reviewed suggest that offenders with psychopathy, as a group, do not present impairments in cool EFs subsumed by the DLPFC, as indicated by their performance on the WCST, SA, TMT, and COWAT, nor do they present impairment on EFs subsumed by the dACC, as indicated by their performance on the Stroop task. They do present, however, deficits in cool EFs subsumed by the VL/OFC such as response inhibition, as measured by the GNG and the Stop task. Investigations that have examined hot EFs are quite consistent in showing deficits on measures indexing OFC functioning such as the CPT, response reversal, and the IGT. In addition, there is evidence that offenders with psychopathy are impaired on PA learning, which can be considered a measure of hot EFs tapping the functional integrity of the amygdala.

Concluding comments

A limitation of the current literature on EFs of persistently violent offenders is the failure to distinguish those with ASPD and no or low levels of psychopathic traits and those characterized by the core affective and interpersonal features of psychopathy. Although the extant literature strongly suggests that the aetiological mechanisms promoting persistent violent behaviour in these two populations differ, neuropsychological investigations have generally failed to associate performance deficits in EFs with characteristics that distinguish these two types of offenders. Some recent studies are the exception as they have examined associations of factor scores indicative of different aspects of ASPD and psychopathy with EFs. Despite the fact that many more violent offenders present a lifelong history of antisocial behaviour but no or low levels of psychopathic traits than present psychopathy, very little research has been conducted on such offenders. Thus, based on the extant literature, it is not known if the neurocognitive impairments observed among violent offenders are associated with an early onset, lifelong pattern of antisocial behaviour, as indexed by ASPD, or psychopathic traits, or both. Future investigations that compare these two types of offenders might provide information about distinctive neurocognitive deficits.

A recent study that compared offenders with ASPD with and without psychopathy to offenders with neither disorder elegantly illustrates the promise of such an approach (Kosson *et al.*, 2006). Among the offenders with ASPD, those with psychopathy had more convictions for violent and non-violent offences and were more criminally versatile than the offenders with ASPD but without psychopathy and than the offenders with neither diagnosis. On a task requiring them to indicate if a string of letters constituted a word in English, the performance of the offenders with psychopathy was less affected by emotional words than the performance of the two other groups of offenders, consistent with a large body of evidence on offenders with psychopathy (Patrick, 2006). Finally, among the offenders who met diagnostic criteria for both psychopathy and ASPD, the less their performance was affected by emotional words, the more severe was their criminal history. By contrast, among the offenders with ASPD not co-morbid with psychopathy, the effect of emotional words on task performance was not associated with criminal activity (Kosson *et al.*, 2006).

Studies that have examined the associations between EFs and different facets of psychopathy indicate that this approach might prove important for furthering understanding of the role of EFs in promoting violent behaviour. For example, in a sample of Norwegian prisoners, Hansen *et al.* (2007) observed that high scores on the interpersonal facet of psychopathy were associated with good performance on tasks assessing sustained attention and working memory. Another study of male and female students and incarcerated offenders found that symptoms of executive dysfunction were strongly related to measures of impulsivity and antisociality, but not to psychopathy as indexed by a measure of fearless dominance, which was proposed to be protective against executive dysfunctions (Ross *et al.*, 2007).

Finally, in a sample of college students, Sellbom and Verona (2007) found that the affective and interpersonal facet of psychopathy, as measured by the Psychopathic Personality Inventory (Lilienfeld & Andrews, 1996), was associated with better performance on tests of cold EFs, whereas the social deviance facet was associated with general deficits in cold EFs and response inhibition. The results of these studies suggest that it might not be enough to distinguish between psychopaths and non-psychopaths. Impairment on cold EFs may be more strongly associated with persistent antisocial behaviour rather than psychopathy. Additional studies along these lines, but examining both cold and hot EFs, would provide valuable information about the heterogeneity of the processes involved. Poor performance on the tasks assessing hot EFs may be a distinguishing characteristic of offenders with high levels of psychopathic traits.

Neurocognitive impairments may be more associated with reactive aggression rather than with instrumental aggression. For example, in sample of violent offenders with ASPD, those who engaged in reactive aggression, compared with those who engaged in instrumental aggression, displayed poorer verbal skills (Barratt et al., 1997). This study did not examine EFs, but it is possible that underlying EF difficulties contributed to the group differences in verbal abilities (Villemarette-Pittman et al., 2003). More recently, a study of a small sample of violent offenders reported that those who engaged in reactive violence performed more poorly than those who engaged in instrumental violence on tests tapping both cold EFs (i.e., verbal and design fluency) and hot EFs (i.e., IGT; Broomhall, 2005). In this study, there was, however, no mention of exclusion criteria (e.g., history of head injury or psychotic disorder) and the groups were not matched on important potential confounds such as IQ and history of substance abuse.

The available evidence suggests that the identification of subtypes of persistent violent offenders distinguished by their performance on neuropsychological tests is an essential step in moving the field forward. Such knowledge could contribute to the development of strategies to increase participation in learning-based rehabilitation programmes and as well to increase the effectiveness of such programmes. A large body of research implicates low levels of brain serotonin among offenders who engage in impulsive and reactive violence (Brown & Linnoila, 1990; Virkkunen et al., 1995). Evidence from both animal and human studies indicates that cool and hot EFs are highly sensitive to changes in the activity of the ascending serotonin and dopamine neurotransmitter systems (Clark et al., 2004; Chudasama & Robbins, 2006). For example, reduction in central serotonergic activity impairs response reversal (Rogers, Everitt et al., 1999), whereas low doses of dopaminergic D_2 receptor agonists improve spatial working memory but impair reversal learning (Mehta et al., 2001). This line of research might prove to be useful for developing novel pharmacological interventions to improve EFs (Bechara & van der Linden, 2005).

A recent study conducted on a sample of 42 incarcerated offenders suggested that a clear delineation of EFs might help in matching available rehabilitation resources to the needs of the offenders (Mullin & Simpson, 2007). The aim of the study was to explore the extent to which an offender's executive functioning could predict outcome from the Enhanced Thinking Skills programme. Some aspects of EFs, such as attentional set shifting and planning abilities, were highly predictive of both positive and negative changes in behaviour, especially for offenders with poorer executive functioning (Mullin & Simpson, 2007).

Rehabilitation programmes that target the mechanisms underlying and contributing to repetitive violence have not been developed (see, for example, Chapter 15 by McGuire; Motiuk & Serin, 2001). Traditionally, rehabilitation programmes for violent offenders have relied on cognitive strategies and only a few have used medications. Findings from neuropsychological studies that link EF deficits to specific traits and behaviour patterns could be used to develop a two-pronged approach to rehabilitation combining pharmacological treatment with cognitive strategies. Both interventions could target deficits in EFs that are associated with violent behaviour or that limit learning not to engage in violent behaviour.

Acknowledgements

Stéphane De Brito holds a Medical Research Council Ph.D. studentship. S. Hodgins holds a Royal Society Wolfson Merit Award and funding from the NIHR Biomedical Research Centre, South London and Maudsley NHS Foundation Trust, and Institute of Psychiatry (King's College London).

References

Ambrogi Lorenzini, C., Bucherelli, C., Giachetti, A., Mugnai, L., & Tassoni, G. (1991). Effects of nucleus basolateralis amygdalae neurotoxic lesions on aversive conditioning in the rat. *Physiology and Behavior*, *49*(4), 765–770.

American Psychiatric Association (2000). *Diagnostic and Statistical Manual of Mental Disorders*, 4th edn (text revision). Washington, DC: American Psychiatric Association.

Amiez, C., & Petrides, M. (2007). Selective involvement of the mid-dorsolateral prefrontal cortex in the coding of the serial order of visual stimuli in working memory. *Proceedings of the National Academy of Sciences*, *104*(34), 13786–13791.

Anderson, S. W., Damasio, H., Jones, R. D., & Tranel, D. (1991). Wisconsin Card Sorting Test performance as a measure of frontal lobe damage. *Journal of Clinical and Experimental Neuropsychology*, *13*(6), 909–922.

Ardila, A. (2008). On the evolutionary origins of executive functions. *Brain and Cognition*, *68*(1), 92–99.

Army Individual Test Battery (1944). *Manual of Directions and Scoring*. Washington, DC: War Department, Adjutant General's Office.

Aron, A. R., Robbins, T. W., & Poldrack, R. A. (2004). Inhibition and the right inferior frontal cortex. *Trends in Cognitive Sciences*, *8*(4), 170–177.

Barkataki, I., Kumari, V., Das, M., Hill, M., Morris, R., O'Connell, P., *et al.* (2005). A neuropsychological investigation into violence and mental illness. *Schizophrenia Research*, *74*(1), 1–13.

Barkataki, I., Kumari, V., Das, M., Sumich, A., Taylor, P., & Sharma, T. (2008). Neural correlates of deficient response inhibition in mentally disordered violent individuals. *Behavioral Sciences and the Law*, *26*(1), 51–64.

Barker, E. D., Séguin, J. R., White, H. R., Bates, M. E., Lacourse, E., Carbonneau, R., *et al.* (2007). Developmental trajectories of male physical violence and theft: relations to neurocognitive performance. *Archives of General Psychiatry*, *64*(5), 592–599.

Barkley, R. A. (1997). Behavioral inhibition, sustained attention, and executive functions: constructing a unifying theory of ADHD. *Psychological Bulletin*, *121*(1), 65–94.

Barratt, E. S., Stanford, M. S., Kent, T. A., & Felthous, A. (1997). Neuropsychological and cognitive psychophysiological substrates of impulsive aggression. *Biological Psychiatry*, *41*, 1045–1061.

Baxter, M. G., & Browning, P. G. F. (2007). Two wrongs make a right: deficits in reversal learning after orbitofrontal damage are improved by amygdala ablation. *Neuron*, *54*(1), 1–3.

Baxter, M. G., & Murray, E. A. (2002). The amygdala and reward. *Nature Reviews Neuroscience*, *3*(7), 563–573.

Bechara, A., Damasio, A. R., Damasio, H., & Anderson, S. W. (1994). Insensitivity to future consequences following damage to human prefrontal cortex. *Cognition*, *50*(1-3), 7–15.

Bechara, A., Damasio, H., Damasio, A. R., & Lee, G. P. (1999). Different contributions of the human Amygdala and ventromedial prefrontal cortex to decision-making. *Journal of Neuroscience, 19*(13), 5473–5481.

Bechara, A., & van der Linden, M. (2005). Decision-making and impulse control after frontal lobe injuries. *Current Opinion in Neurology, 18*(6), 734–739.

Benton, A. L., Hamsher, K. S., & Sivan, A. B. (1978). *Multilingual Aphasia Examination*. Iowa City, IA: AJA Associates.

Bergvall, A. H., Wessely, H., Forsman, A., & Hansen, S. (2001). A deficit in attentional set-shifting of violent offenders. *Psychological Medicine, 31*(6), 1095–1105..

Berlin, H. A., Rolls, E. T., & Kischka, U. (2004). Impulsivity, time perception, emotion and reinforcement sensitivity in patients with orbitofrontal cortex lesions. *Brain, 127*(5), 1108–1126.

Blair, K. S., Newman, C., Mitchell, D. G. V., Richell, R. A., Leonard, A., Morton, J., *et al.* (2006). Differentiating among prefrontal substrates in psychopathy: neuropsychological test findings. *Neuropsychology, 20*(2), 153–165.

Blair, R. J. R. (2004). The roles of orbital frontal cortex in the modulation of antisocial behavior. *Brain and Cognition, 55*(1), 198–208.

Blair, R. J. R., & Cipolotti, L. (2000). Impaired social response reversal. A case of 'acquired sociopathy'. *Brain, 123*, 1122–1141.

Blair, R. J. R., Mitchell, D. G. V., & Blair, K. S. (2005). *The Psychopath: Emotion and the Brain.* Oxford: Blackwell.

Blair, R. J. R., Mitchell, D. G. V., Leonard, A., Budhani, S., Peschardt, K., & Newman, C. (2004). Passive avoidance learning in individuals with psychopathy: modulation by reward but not by punishment. *Personality and Individual Differences, 37*(6), 1179–1192.

Botvinick, M. M., Cohen, J. D., & Carter, C. S. (2004). Conflict monitoring and anterior cingulate cortex: an update. *Trends in Cognitive Sciences, 8*(12), 539–546.

Brinkley, C. A., Schmitt, W. A., & Newman, J. P. (2005). Semantic processing in psychopathic offenders. *Personality and Individual Differences, 38*(5), 1047–1056.

Broomhall, L. (2005). Acquired sociopathy: a neuropsychological study of executive dysfunction in violent offenders. *Psychiatry, Psychology and Law, 12*(2), 367–387.

Brower, M. C., & Price, B. H. (2001). Neuropsychiatry of frontal lobe dysfunction in violent and criminal behaviour: a critical review. *Journal of Neurology, Neurosurgery and Psychiatry, 71*(6), 720–726.

Brown, G. L., & Linnoila, M. I. (1990). CSF serotonin metabolite (5-HIAA) studies in depression, impulsivity, and violence. *Journal of Clinical Psychiatry, 51*(Suppl), 31–43.

Budhani, S., & Blair, R. J. R. (2005). Response reversal and children with psychopathic tendencies: success is a function of salience of contingency change. *Journal of Child Psychology and Psychiatry, 46*(9), 972–981.

Budhani, S., Richell, R. A., & Blair, R. J. R. (2006). Impaired reversal but intact acquisition: probabilistic response reversal deficits in adult individuals with psychopathy. *Journal of Abnormal Psychology, 115*(3), 552–558.

Burgess, P. W. (1997). Theory and methodology in executive function research. In P. Rabbitt (ed), *Methodology of Frontal and Executive Function* (pp. 81–116). Hove, UK: Psychology Press.

Busemeyer, J. R., & Stout, J. C. (2002). A contribution of cognitive decision models to clinical assessment: decomposing performance on the Bechara Gambling Task. *Psychological Assessment, 14*(3), 253–262.

Bush, G., Luu, P., & Posner, M. I. (2000). Cognitive and emotional influences in anterior cingulate cortex. *Trends in Cognitive Sciences, 4*(6), 215–222.

Carmichael, S. T., & Price, J. L. (1994). Architectonic subdivision of the orbital and medial prefrontal cortex in the macaque monkey. *Journal of Comparative Neurology, 346*(3), 366–402.

Carmichael, S. T., & Price, J. L. (1995). Limbic connections of the orbital and medial prefrontal cortex in macaque monkeys. *Journal of Comparative Neurology, 363*(4), 615–641.

Castellanos, F. X., Sonuga-Barke, E. J. S., Milham, M. P., & Tannock, R. (2006). Characterizing cognition in ADHD: beyond executive dysfunction. *Trends in Cognitive Sciences, 10*(3), 117–123.

Chow, T. W., & Cummings, J. L. (1999). Frontal-subcortical circuits. In B. L. Miller, & J. L. Cummings (eds), *The Human Frontal Lobes: Functions and Disorders* (pp. 3–26). New York: Guilford Press.

Chudasama, Y., & Robbins, T. W. (2006). Functions of frontostriatal systems in cognition: comparative neuropsychopharmacological studies in rats, monkeys and humans. *Biological Psychology*, *73*(1), 19–38.

Clark, L., Cools, R., & Robbins, T. W. (2004). The neuropsychology of ventral prefrontal cortex: decision-making and reversal learning. *Brain and Cognition*, *55*(1), 41–53.

Clark, L., Manes, F., Antoun, N., Sahakian, B. J., & Robbins, T. W. (2003). The contributions of lesion laterality and lesion volume to decision-making impairment following frontal lobe damage. *Neuropsychologia*, *41*(11), 1474–1483.

Collette, F., & van der Linden, M. (2002). Brain imaging of the central executive component of working memory. *Neuroscience and Biobehavioral Reviews*, *26*(2), 105–125.

Coid, J., Yang, M., Roberts, A., Ullrich, S., Moran, P., Bebbington, P., *et al.* (2006). Violence and psychiatric morbidity in the national household population of Britain: public health implications. *British Journal of Psychiatry*, *189*, 12–19.

Cooke, D. J., & Michie, C. (1997). An item response theory analysis of the Hare Psychopathy Checklist-Revised. *Psychological Assessment*, *9*(1), 3–14.

Cooke, D. J., & Michie, C. (2001). Refining the construct of psychopathy: towards a hierarchical model. *Psychological Assessment*, *13*(2), 171–188.

Cooke, D. J., Michie, C., & Hart, S. D. (2006). Facets of clinical psychopathy: toward clearer measurement. In *Handbook of the Psychopathy* (pp. 91–106). New York: Guilford Press.

Crowell, T. A., Kieffer, K. M., Kugeares, S., & Vanderploeg, R. D. (2003). Executive and nonexecutive neuropsychological functioning in antisocial personality disorder. *Cognitive and Behavioral Neurology*, *16*(2), 100–109.

D'Esposito, M., Postle, B. R., & Rypma, B. (2000). Prefrontal cortical contribhution to working memory: evidence from event-related fMRI. *Experimental Brain Research*, *133*(1), 3–11.

Damasio, A. R. (1994). *Descarte's Error: Emotion, Rationality and the Human Brain*. New York: Putnam.

Davidson, R. J., Putnam, K. M., & Larson, C. L. (2000). Dysfunction in the neural circuitry of emotion regulation—a possible prelude to violence. *Science*, *289*(5479), 591–594.

De Brito, S. A., & Hodgins, S. (in press). Antisocial personality. In M. McMurran, & R. Howard (eds), *Personality, Personality Disorder, and Risk of Violence*. Wiley.

De Brito, S. A., Hodgins, S., Cooke, D. J., Michie, C., & Sparkes, L. (under review). Life-long patterns of aggressive behavior among offenders: Is instrumental aggression unique to psychopathy?

Deckel, A., Hesselbrock, V., & Bauer, L. (1996). Antisocial personality disorder, childhood delinquency, and frontal brain functioning: EEG and neuropsychological findings. *Journal of Clinical Psychology*, *52*(6), 639–650.

Delis, D. C., Squire, L. R., Bihrle, A., & Massman, P. (1992). Componential analysis of problem-solving ability: performance of patients with frontal lobe damage and amnesic patients on a new sorting test. *Neuropsychologia*, *30*(8), 683–697.

Dias, R., Robbins, T. W., & Roberts, A. C. (1996). Dissociation in prefrontal cortex of affective and attentional shifts. *Nature*, *380*(6569), 69–72.

Dias, R., Robbins, T. W., & Roberts, A. C. (1997). Dissociable forms of inhibitory control within prefrontal cortex with an analog of the Wisconsin Card Sort Test: restriction to novel situations and independence from 'On-Line' Processing. *Journal of Neuroscience*, *17*(23), 9285–9297.

Dolan, M., & Park, I. (2002). The neuropsychology of antisocial personality disorder. *Psychological Medicine*, *32*(3), 417–427.

Douglas, K. S., Vincent, G. M., & Edens, J. F. (2006). Risk for criminal recidivism: the role of psychopathy. In *Handbook of the Psychopathy* (pp. 533–554). New York: Guilford Press.

Dvorak-Bertsch, J. D., Sadeh, N., Glass, S. J., Thornton, D., & Newman, J. P. (2007). Stroop tasks associated with differential activation of anterior cingulate do not differentiate psychopathic and non-psychopathic offenders. *Personality and Individual Differences*, *42*(3), 585–595.

Ernst, M., Bolla, K., Mouratidis, M., Contoreggi, C., Matochik, J. A., Kurian, V., *et al.* (2002). Decision-making in a risk-taking task: a PET study. *Neuropsychopharmacology*, *26*(5), 682–691.

Ersche, K. D., Roiser, J. P., Robbins, T. W., & Sahakian, B. J. (2008). Chronic cocaine but not chronic amphetamine use is associated with perseverative responding in humans. *Psychopharmacology*, *197*(3), 421–431.

Farrington, D. P., Gallagher, B., Morley, L., St Ledger, R. J., & West, D. J. (1988). Are there any successful men from criminogenic backgrounds? *Psychiatry, 51*(2), 116–130.

Farrington, D. P., & West, D. (1993). Criminal, penal and life histories of chronic offenders: risk and protective factors and early identification. *Criminal Behaviour and Mental Health, 3,* 492–523.

Fellows, L. K. (2004). The cognitive neuroscience of human decision making: a review and conceptual framework. *Behavioral and Cognitive Neuroscience Reviews, 3*(3), 159–172.

Fellows, L. K. (2007). Advances in understanding ventromedial prefrontal function: the accountant joins the executive. *Neurology, 68*(13), 991–995.

Fellows, L. K., & Farah, M. J. (2003). Ventromedial frontal cortex mediates affective shifting in humans: evidence from a reversal learning paradigm. *Brain, 126*(8), 1830–1837.

Fellows, L. K., & Farah, M. J. (2005a). Different underlying impairments in decision-making following ventromedial and dorsolateral frontal lobe damage in humans. *Cerebral Cortex, 15*(1), 58–63.

Fellows, L. K., & Farah, M. J. (2005b). Is anterior cingulate cortex necessary for cognitive control? *Brain, 128*(4), 788–796.

Fergusson, D. M., Horwood, L. J., & Ridder, E. M. (2005). Partner violence and mental health outcomes in a New Zealand birth cohort. *Journal of Marriage and Family, 67*(5), 1103–1119.

Fuster, J. M. (1997). *The Prefrontal Cortex: Anatomy, Physiology, and Neurophysiology of the Frontal Lobe,* 3rd edn. Philadelphia, PA: Lippincott-Raven.

Gazzaniga, M. S., Ivry, R. B., & Mangun, G. R. (1998). *Cognitive Neuroscience: The Biology of the Mind.* New York: W. W. Norton.

Giancola, P. R. (1995). Evidence for dorsolateral and orbital prefrontal cortical involvement in the expression of aggressive behavior. *Aggressive Behavior, 21*(6), 431–450.

Gillen, R., & Hesselbrock, V. (1992). Cognitive functioning, ASP, and family history of alcoholism in young men at risk for alcoholism. *Alcoholism: Clinical and Experimental Research, 16*(2), 206–214.

Goldstein, R. B., Grant, B. F., Ruan, W. J., Smith, S. M., & Saha, T. D. (2006). Antisocial personality disorder with childhood- vs adolescence-onset conduct disorder: results from the National Epidemiologic Survey on Alcohol and Related Conditions. *Journal of Nervous and Mental Disease, 194*(9), 667–675.

Gorenstein, E. E. (1982). Frontal lobe functions in psychopaths. *Journal of Abnormal Psychology, 91*(5), 368–379.

Gough, H. G. (1960). *Manual for the California Psychological Inventory,* revised edn. Palo Alto, CA: Consulting Psychologists Press.

Grann, M., Långström, N., Tengström, A., & Kullgren, G. (1999). Psychopathy (PCL-R) predicts violent recidivism among criminal offenders with personality disorders in Sweden. *Law and Human Behavior, 23*(2), 205–217.

Grodzinsky, G., & Diamond, R. (1992). Frontal lobe functioning in boys with attention deficit hyperactivity disorder. *Developmental Neuropsychology, 8,* 427–445.

Haber, S. N. (2003). The primate basal ganglia: parallel and integrative networks. *Journal of Chemical Neuroanatomy, 26*(4), 317–330.

Haber, S. N., Fudge, J. L., & McFarland, N. R. (2000). Striatonigrostriatal pathways in primates form an ascending spiral from the shell to the dorsolateral striatum. *Journal of Neuroscience, 20*(6), 2369–2382.

Hansen, A. L., Johnsen, B. H., Thornton, D., Waage, L., & Thayer, J. F. (2007). Facets of psychopathy, heart rate variability and cognitive function. *Journal of Personality Disorders, 21*(5), 568–582.

Happaney, K., Zelazo, P. D., & Stuss, D. T. (2004). Development of orbitofrontal function: current themes and future directions. *Brain and Cognition,* [Online] Available at: http://www.sciencedirect.com/science/article/B6WBY-4BVP3KK-3/1/e43d92c9088d2ae20ea11bd3666ba764.

Hare, R. D. (1980). A research scale for the assessment of psychopathy in criminal populations. *Personality and Individual Differences, 1,* 111–120.

Hare, R. D. (1984). Performance of psychopaths on cognitive tasks related to frontal lobe function. *Journal of Abnormal Psychology, 93*(2), 133–140.

Hare, R. D. (1996). Psychopathy and antisocial personality disorder: a case of diagnostic confusion. *Psychiatric Times, 13,* 39–40.

Hare, R. D. (2003). *Manual for the Revised Psychopathy Checklist*, 2nd edn. Toronto, ON: Multi-Health Systems.

Hare, R. D., & McPherson, L. M. (1984). Violent and aggressive behavior by criminal psychopaths. *International Journal of Law and Psychiatry*, *7*, 35–50.

Hare, R. D., & Neumann, C. S. (2006). The PCL-R assessment of psychopathy: development, structural properties, and new directions. In *Handbook of the Psychopathy* (pp. 58–88). New York: Guilford Press.

Hart, S. D., Forth, A. E., & Hare, R. D. (1990). Performance of criminal psychopaths on selected neuropsychological tests. *Journal of Abnormal Psychology*, *99*(4), 374–379.

Hart, S. D., & Hare, R. D. (1996). Psychopathy and antisocial personality disorder. *Current Opinion in Psychiatry*, *9*(2), 129–132.

Hart, S. D., Kropp, P. R., & Hare, R. D. (1988). Performance of male psychopaths following conditional release from prison. *Journal of Consulting and Clinical Psychology*, *56*(2), 227–232.

Heyder, K., Suchan, B., & Daum, I. (2004). Cortico-subcortical contributions to executive control. *Acta Psychologica*, *115*(2-3), 271–289.

Hiatt, K. D., & Newman, J. P. (2006). Understanding psychopathy: the cognitive side. In C. J. Patrick (ed), *The Handbook of Psychopathy* (pp. 334–352). New York: Guilford Press.

Hiatt, K. D., Schmitt, W. A., & Newman, J. P. (2004). Stroop tasks reveal abnormal selective attention among psychopathic offenders. *Neuropsychology*, *18*(1), 50–59.

Hoaken, P. N. S., Shaughnessy, V. K., & Pihl, R. O. (2003). Executive cognitive functioning and aggression: Is it an issue of impulsivity? *Aggressive Behavior*, *29*(1), 15–30.

Hodgins, S. (2007). Persistent violent offending: what do we know? *British Journal of Psychiatry*, *49*, s12–14.

Hodgins, S., & Côté, G. (1993). Major mental disorder and antisocial personality disorder: a criminal combination. *Bulletin of the American Academy of Psychiatry and the Law*, *21*(2), 155–160.

Hoffman, J. J., Hall, R. W., & Bartsch, T. W. (1987). On the relative importance of 'psychopathic' personality and alcoholism on neuropsychological measures of frontal lobe dysfunction. *Journal of Abnormal Psychology*, *96*(2), 158–160.

Hongwanishkul, D., Happaney, K. R., Lee, W. S. C., & Zelazo, P. D. (2005). Assessment of hot and cool executive function in young children: age-related changes and individual differences. *Developmental Neuropsychology*, *28*(2), 617–644.

Jurado, M., & Rosselli, M. (2007). The elusive nature of executive functions: a review of our current understanding. *Neuropsychology Review*, *17*(3), 213–233.

Kandel, E., & Freed, D. (1989). Frontal-lobe dysfunction and antisocial behavior: a review. *Journal of Clinical Psychology*, *45*(3), 404–413.

Kelly, A. M. C., Scheres, A., Sonuga-Barke, E. J., & Castellanos, F. C. (2007). Functional neuroimaging of reward and motivational pathways in ADHD. In M. A. Bellgrove, M. Fitzgerald, & M. Gill (eds), *The Handbook of Attention Deficit Hyperactivity Disorder* (pp. 209–235). Chichester: Wiley.

Kosson, D. S., Lorenz, A. R., & Newman, J. P. (2006). Effects of comorbid psychopathy on criminal offending and emotion processing in male offenders with antisocial personality disorder. *Journal of Abnormal Psychology*, *115*(4), 798–806.

Kratzer, L., & Hodgins, S. (1999). A typology of offenders: a test of Moffitt's theory among males and females from childhood to age 30. *Criminal Behaviour and Mental Health*, *9*(1), 57–73.

Kringelbach, M. L. (2005). The human orbitofrontal cortex: linking reward to hedonic experience. *Nature Review Neuroscience*, *6*(9), 691–702.

Krueger, R. F., Hicks, B. M., Patrick, C. J., Carlson, S. R., Iacono, W. G., & McGue, M. (2002). Etiologic connections among substance dependence, antisocial behavior, and personality: modeling the externalizing spectrum. *Journal of Abnormal Psychology*, *111*(3), 411–424.

Lapierre, D., Braun, C. M., & Hodgins, S. (1995). Ventral frontal deficits in psychopathy: neuropsychological test findings. *Neuropsychologia*, *33*(2), 139–151.

Lawrence, A. D., Sahakian, B. J., Hodges, J. R., Rosser, A. E., Lange, K. W., & Robbins, T. W. (1996). Executive and mnemonic functions in early Huntington's disease. *Brain*, *119*(5), 1633–1645.

LeMarquand, D. G., Pihl, R. O., Young, S. N., Tremblay, R. E., Seguin, J. R., Palmour, R. M., *et al.* (1998). Tryptophan depletion, executive functions, and disinhibition in aggressive, adolescent males. *Neuropsychopharmacology*, *19*(4), 333–341.

Lesaca, T. (2001). Executive functions in parents with ADHD. *Psychiatric Times*, *18*(11), [Online] Available at: http://www.psychiatrictimes.com/display/article/10168/53746 [retrieved 1 July 2004].

Levin, H. S., Song, J., Ewing-Cobbs, L., & Roberson, G. (2001). Porteus maze performance following traumatic brain injury in children. *Neuropsychology*, *15*(4), 557–567.

Lezak, M. D., Howieson, D. B., & Loring, D. W. (2004). *Neuropsychological Assessment*, 4th edn. New York: Oxford University Press.

Lilienfeld, S. O., & Andrews, B. P. (1996). Development and preliminary validation of a self-report measure of psychopathic personality traits in noncriminal populations. *Journal of Personality Assessment*, *66*(3), 488–524.

Loeber, R., & Stouthamer-Loeber, M. (1987). Prediction. In H. C. Quay (ed), *Handbook of Juvenile Delinquency*. New York: Wiley.

Lösel, F., & Schmucker, M. (2004). Psychopathy, risk taking, and attention: a differentiated test of the somatic marker hypothesis. *Journal of Abnormal Psychology*, *113*(4), 522–529.

Malloy, P., N, N., Rogers, S., Longabaugh, R., & Beattie, M. (1989). Risk factors for neuropsychological impairment in alcoholics: antisocial personality, age, years of drinking and gender. *Journal of Studies on Alcohol*, *50*(5), 422–426.

Manchester, D., Priestley, N., & Jackson, H. (2004). The assessment of executive functions: coming out of the office. *Brain Injury*, *18*(11), 1067–1081.

Manes, F., Sahakian, B., Clark, L., Rogers, R., Antoun, N., Aitken, M., *et al.* (2002). Decision-making processes following damage to the prefrontal cortex. *Brain*, *125*(3), 624–639.

Maughan, B., Pickles, A., Rowe, R., Costello, E. J., & Angold, A. (2000). Developmental trajectories of aggressive and non-aggressive conduct problems. *Journal of Quantitative Criminology*, *16*, 199–221.

Mazas, C. A., Finn, P. R., & Steinmetz, J. E. (2000). Decision-making biases, antisocial personality, and early-onsetalcoholism. *Alcoholism, Clinical and Experimental Research*, *24*(7), 1036–1040.

Mehta, M., Swainson, R., Ogilvie, A., Sahakian, B., & Robbins, T. (2001). Improved short-term spatial memory but impaired reversal learning following the dopamine D2 agonist bromocriptine in human volunteers. *Psychopharmacology*, *159*(1), 10–20.

Miller, E. K., & Cohen, J. D. (2001). An integrative theory of prefrontal cortex function. *Annual Review of Neuroscience*, *24*(1), 167–202.

Milner, B. (1963). Effects of different brain lesions on card sorting. *Archives of Neurology*, *9*, 90–100.

Mitchell, D. G. V., Avny, S., & Blair, R. (2006). Divergent patterns of aggressive and neurocognitive characteristics in acquired versus developmental psychopathy. *Neurocase*, *12*(3), 164–178.

Mitchell, D. G. V., Colledge, E., Leonard, A., & Blair, R. J. R. (2002). Risky decisions and response reversal: is there evidence of orbitofrontal cortex dysfunction in psychopathic individuals? *Neuropsychologia*, *40*(12), 2013–2022.

Mitchell, D. G. V., Fine, C., Richell, R. A., Newman, C., Lumsden, J., Blair, K. S., *et al.* (2006). Instrumental learning and relearning in individuals with psychopathy and in patients with lesions involving the amygdala or orbitofrontal cortex. *Neuropsychology*, *20*(3), 280–289.

Miyake, A., Friedman, N. P., Emerson, M. J., Witzki, A. H., Howerter, A., & Wager, T. D. (2000). The unity and diversity of executive functions and their contributions to complex 'Frontal Lobe' tasks: a latent variable analysis. *Cognitive Psychology*, *41*, 49–100.

Moffitt, T. E., Arseneault, L., Jaffee, S. R., Kim-Cohen, J., Koenen, K. C., Odgers, C. L., *et al.* (2008). Research review: DSM-V conduct disorder: research needs for an evidence base. *Journal of Child Psychology and Psychiatry*, *49*(1), 3–33.

Moffitt, T. E., & Caspi, A. (2001). Childhood predictors differentiate life-course persistent and adolescence-limited antisocial pathways among males and females. *Development and Psychopathology*, *13*(2), 355–375.

Moffitt, T. E., Caspi, A., Dickson, N., Silva, P., & Stanton, W. (1996). Childhood-onset versus adolescent-onset antisocial conduct problems in males: natural history from ages 3 to 18 years. *Development and Psychopathology*, *8*, 399–424.

Moffitt, T. E., Caspi, A., Harrington, H., & Milne, B. J. (2002). Males on the life-course-persistent and adolescence-limited antisocial pathways: follow-up at age 26 years. *Development and Psychopathology*, *14*(1), 179–207.

Moltó, J., Poy, R., Segarra, P., Pastor, M. C., & Montañés, S. (2007). Response perseveration in psychopaths: interpersonal/affective or social deviance traits? *Journal of Abnormal Psychology*, *116*(3), 632–637.

Morgan, A. B., & Lilienfeld, S. O. (2000). A meta-analytic review of the relation between antisocial behavior and neuropsychological measures of executive function. *Clinical Psychology Review*, *20*(1), 113–136.

Motiuk, L. L., & Serin, R. (2001). *Compendium 2000 on Effective Correctional Programming*. Ottawa, ON: Correctional Service Canada.

Mullin, S., & Simpson, J. (2007). Does executive functioning predict improvement in offenders' behaviour following enhanced thinking skills training? An exploratory study with implications for rehabilitation. *Legal and Criminological Psychology*, *12*(1), 117–131.

Murray, E. A., O'Doherty, J. P., & Schoenbaum, G. (2007). What we know and do not know about the functions of the orbitofrontal cortex after 20 years of cross-species studies. *Journal of Neuroscience*, *27*(31), 8166–8169.

Nathan, R., Rollinson, L., Harvey, K., & Hill, J. (2003). The Liverpool Violence Assessment: an investigator-based measure of serious violence. *Criminal Behaviour and Mental Health*, *13*(2), 106–120.

Newman, J. P. (1998). Psychopathic behavior: an information processing perspective. In D. J. Cooke, A. E. Forth, & R. D. Hare (eds), *Psychopathy: Theory, Research, and Implications for Society* (pp. 81–104). Dordrecht, the Netherlands: Kluwer.

Newman, J. P., & Kosson, D. S. (1986). Passive avoidance learning in psychopathic and nonpsycho-pathic offenders. *Journal of Abnormal Psychology*, *95*(3), 252–-256.

Newman, J. P., & Lorenz, A. (2002). Response modulation and emotion processing: implications for psychopathy and other dysregulatory psychopathology. In R. J. Davidson, K. Scherer, & H. H. Goldsmith (eds), *Handbook of Affective Sciences* (pp. 1043–1067). New York: Oxford University Press.

Newman, J. P., Patterson, C. M., & Kosson, D. S. (1987). Response perseveration in psychopaths. *Journal of Abnormal Psychology*, *96*(2), 145–148.

Newman, J. P., Widom, C. S., & Nathan, S. (1985). Passive avoidance in syndromes of disinhibition: psychopathy and extraversion. *Journal of Personality and Social Psychology*, *48*(5), 1316–1327.

Nigg, J. T., & Huang-Pollock, C. L. (2003). An early-onset model of the role of executive functions and intelligence in conduct disorder/delinquency. In *Causes of Conduct Disorder and Juvenile Delinquency* (pp. 227–253). New York: Guilford Press.

Owen, A. M., Roberts, A. C., Hodges, J. R., & Robbins, T. W. (1993). Contrasting mechanisms of impaired attentional set-shifting in patients with frontal lobe damage or Parkinson's disease. *Brain*, *116*(5), 1159–1175.

Owen, A. M., Roberts, A. C., Polkey, C. E., Sahakian, B. J., & Robbins, T. W. (1991). Extra-dimensional versus intra-dimensional set shifting performance following frontal lobe excisions, temporal lobe excisions or amygdalo-hippocampectomy in man. *Neuropsychologia*, *29*(10), 993–1006.

Pandya, D. N., & Barnes, C. L. (1987). Architecture and connections of the frontal lobe. In E. Perecman (ed), *The Frontal Lobes Revisited* (pp. 41–72). New York: IBRN.

Patrick, C. J. (2006). Getting to the heart of psychopathy. In *The Psychopath: Theory, Research, and Practice* (pp. 207–252). Mahwah, NJ: Lawrence Erlbaum Associates Publishers.

Patrick, C. J. (2007). Antisocial personality disorder and psychopathy. In W. O'Donohue, K. A. Fowler, & S. O. Lilienfeld (eds), *Handbook of Personality Disorder*. New York: Sage.

Patrick, C. J., Curtin, J. J., & Krueger, R. F. (in press). The externalizing spectrum: structure and mechanisms. In D. Barch (ed), *Cognitive and Affective Neuroscience of Psychopathology*. New York: Oxford University Press.

Patterson, C. M., & Newman, J. P. (1993). Reflectivity and learning from aversive events: toward a psychological mechanism for the syndromes of disinhibition. *Psychological Review*, *100*(4), 716–736.

Paus, T. (2001). Primate anterior cingulate cortex: where motor control, drive and cognition interface. *Nature Reviews. Neuroscience*, *2*(6), 417–424.

Petrides, M. (2000). Dissociable roles of mid-dorsolateral prefrontal and anterior inferotemporal cortex in visual working memory. *Journal of Neuroscience*, *20*(19), 7496–7503.

Petrides, M., & Pandya, D. N. (1994). Comparative architectonic analysis of the human and the macaque frontal cortex. In F. Boller, & J. Grafman (eds), *Handbook of Neuropsychology* (pp. 17–58). Amsterdam, the Netherlands: Elsevier.

Pham, T. H., Vanderstukken, O., Philippot, P., & van der Linden, M. (2003). Selective attention and executive functions deficits among criminal psychopaths. *Aggressive Behavior*, *29*(5), 393–405.

Phillips, L. A., MacPherson, S. E. S., & Della Salla, S. (2002). Age, cognition, and emotion: the role of anatomical segregation in the frontal lobes. In J. Grafman (ed), *Handbook of Neuropsychology*, Vol. 7, 2nd edn (pp. 73–98). Amsterdam, the Netherlands: Elsevier Science.

Porter, S., & Woodworth, M. (2006). Psychopathy and aggression. In *Handbook of the Psychopathy* (pp. 481–494). New York: Guilford Press.

Rabbitt, P. (ed) (1997). Introduction: methodologies and models in the study of executive function. In *Methodology of Frontal and Executive Function* (pp. 1–38). Hove, UK: Psychology Press.

Roberts, A. C., Robbins, T. W., & Weiskrantz, L. (1998). Discussions and conclusions. In A. C. Roberts, T. W. Robbins, & L. Weiskrantz (eds), *The Prefrontal Cortex: Executive and Cognitive Functions* (pp. 221–242). Oxford: Oxford University Press.

Roberts, A. C., & Wallis, J. D. (2000). Inhibitory control and affective processing in the prefrontal cortex: neuropsychological studies in the common marmoset. *Cerebral Cortex*, *10*(3), 252–262.

Robins, L. N. (1966). *Deviant Children Grown Up: A Sociological and Psychiatric Study of Sociopathic Personality*. Baltimore, MD: Williams & Wilkins.

Robins, L. N., Tipp, J., & Przybeck, T. (1991). Antisocial personality. In L. N. Robins, & D. A. Regier (eds), *Psychiatric Disorders in America: The Epidemiological Catchement Area Study* (pp. 258–290). New York: The Free Press.

Rogers, R. D. (2006). The functional architectures of the frontal lobes psychopathy: implications for research with psychopathic offenders. In C. J. Patrick (ed), *Handbook of Psychopathy* (pp. 313–333). New York: Guilford Press.

Rogers, R. D., Andrews, T. C., Grasby, P. M., Brooks, D. J., & Robbins, T. W. (2000). Contrasting cortical and subcortical activations produced by attentional-set shifting and reversal learning in humans. *Journal of Cognitive Neuroscience*, *12*(1), 142–162.

Rogers, R. D., Everitt, B. J., Baldacchino, A., Blackshaw, A. J., Swainson, R., Wynne, K., *et al.* (1999). Dissociable deficits in the decision-making cognition of chronic amphetamine abusers, opiateabusers, patients with focal damage to prefrontal cortex, and tryptophan-depleted normal volunteers: evidence for monoaminergic mechanisms. *Neuropsychopharmacology*, *20*(4), 322–339.

Rogers, R. D., Owen, A. M., Middleton, H. C., Williams, E. J., Pickard, J. D., Sahakian, B. J., *et al.* (1999). Choosing between small, likely rewards and large, unlikely rewards activates inferior and orbital prefrontal cortex. *Journal of Neuroscience*, *19*(20), 9029–9038.

Rolls, E. T. (2004). The functions of the orbitofrontal cortex. *Brain and Cognition*, *55*, 11–29.

Rolls, E. T., Hornak, J., Wade, D., & McGrath, J. (1994). Emotion-related learning in patients with social and emotional changes associated with frontal lobe damage. *Journal of Neurology, Neurosurgery and Psychiatry*, *57*(12), 1518–1524.

Ross, S. R., Benning, S. D., & Adams, Z. (2007). Symptoms of executive dysfunction are endemic to secondary psychopathy: an examination in criminal offenders and noninstitutionalized young adults. *Journal of Personality Disorders*, *21*(4), 384–399.

Roussy, S., & Toupin, J. (2000). Behavioral inhibition deficits in juvenile psychopaths. *Aggressive Behavior*, *26*(6), 413–424.

Royall, D. R., Lauterbach, E. C., Cummings, J. L., Reeve, A., Rummans, T. A., Kaufer, D. I., *et al.* (2002). Executive control function: a review of its promise and challenges for clinical research. A report from the committee on research of the American Neuropsychiatric Association. *Journal of Neuropsychiatry and Clinical Neurosciences*, *14*(4), 377–405.

Russo, N., Flanagan, T., Iarocci, G., Berringer, D., Zelazo, P. D., & Burack, J. A. (2007). Deconstructing executive deficits among persons with autism: implications for cognitive neuroscience. *Brain and Cognition*, *65*(1), 77–86.

Schmitt, W. A., Brinkley, C. A., & Newman, J. P. (1999). Testing Damasio's somatic marker hypothesis with psychopathic individuals: risk takers or risk averse? *Journal of Abnormal Psychology*, *108*(3), 538–543.

Séguin, J., Sylvers, P., & Lilienfeld, S. (2007). The neuropsychology of violence. In D. J. Flannery, A. T. Vazsonyi, & I. D. Waldman (eds), *The Cambridge Handbook of Violent Behavior and Aggression* (pp. 187–214). New York: Cambridge University Press.

Séguin, J., & Zelazo, P. (2005). Executive function in early physical aggression. In R. E. Tremblay, W. H. Willard, & J. Archer (eds), *Developmental Origins of Aggression* (pp. 307–329). New York: Guilford Press.

Sellbom, M., & Verona, E. (2007). Neuropsychological correlates of psychopathic traits in a non-incarcerated sample. *Journal of Research in Personality*, *41*(2), 276–294.

Serin, R. C. (1991). Psychopathy and violence in criminals. *Journal of Interpersonal Violence*, *6*(4), 423–431.

Shallice, T. (1982). Specific impairments of planning. *Philosophical Transactions of the Royal Society of London: Series B, Biological Sciences*, *298*(1089), 199–209.

Shallice, T., & Burgess, P. W. (1991). Higher-order cognitive impairments and frontal lobe lesions. In H. S. Levin, H. M. Eisenberg, & A. L. Benton (eds), *Frontal Lobe Function and Dysfunction* (pp. 125–138). Oxford: Oxford University Press.

Smith, S. S., Arnett, P. A., & Newman, J. P. (1992). Neuropsychological differentiation of psychopathic and nonpsychopathic criminal offenders. *Personality and Individual Differences*, *13*(11), 1233–1243.

Spitzer, R. L., Endicott, J., & Robins, E. (1975). Preliminary report of the reliability of Research Diagnostic Criteria applied to psychiatric case records. In A. Sudilovsky, S. Gershan, & B. Beer (eds), *Predictability in Psychopharmacology: Preclinical and Clinical Correlations*. New York: Raven Press.

Stevens, M. C., Kaplan, R. F., & Hesselbrock, V. M. (2003). Executive-cognitive functioning in the development of antisocial personality disorder. *Addictive Behaviors*, *28*(2), 285–300.

Stuss, D. T., Alexander, M. P., Hamer, L., Palumbo, C., Dempster, R., Binns, M., *et al.* (1998). The effects of focal anterior and posterior brain lesions on verbal fluency. *Journal of the International Neuropsychological Society*, *4*(3), 265–278.

Stuss, D. T., Bisschop, S. M., Alexander, M. P., Levine, B., Katz, D., & Izukawa, D. (2001). The Trail Making Test: a study in focal lesion patients. *Psychological Assessment*, *13*(2), 230–239.

Stuss, D. T., Floden, D., Alexander, M. P., Levine, B., & Katz, D. (2001). Stroop performance in focal lesion patients: dissociation of processes and frontal lobe lesion location. *Neuropsychologia*, *39*(8), 771–786.

Stuss, D. T., & Levine, B. (2002). Adult clinical neuropsychology: lessons from studies of the frontal lobes. *Annual Review of Psychology*, *53*(1), 401–433.

Sutker, P. B., & Allain Jr., A. N. (1987). Cognitive abstraction, shifting, and control: clinical sample comparisons of psychopaths and nonpsychopaths. *Journal of Abnormal Psychology*, *96*(1), 73–75.

Swanson, M. C., Bland, R. C., & Newman, S. C. (1994). Epidemiology of psychiatric disorders in Edmonton. antisocial personality disorders. *Acta Psychiatrica Scandinavica*, *376*, 63–70.

Swick, D., & Turken, A. U. (2002). Dissociation between conflict detection and error monitoring in the human anterior cingulate cortex. *Proceedings of the National Academy of Sciences*, *99*(25), 16354–16359.

Takashina, K., Saito, H., & Nishiyama, N. (1995). Preferential impairment of avoidance performances in amygdala-lesioned mice. *Japanese Journal of Pharmacology*, *67*(2), 107–115.

Taylor, J., & Lang, A. (2006). Psychopathy and substance use disorders. In C. J. Patrick (ed), *Handbook of Psychopathy* (pp. 495–511). New York: Guilford Press.

Torralva, T. Kipps, C. M., Hodges, J. R., Clark, L., Bekinschtein, T., Roca, M., *et al.* (2007). The relationship between affective decision-making and theory of mind in the frontal variant of fronto-temporal dementia. *Neuropsychologia*, *45*(2), 342–349.

Tranel, D., Anderson, S. W., & Benton, A. (1994). Development of the concepts of 'executive function' and its relationship to the frontal lobes. In F. Boller, & J. Grafman (eds), *Handbook of Neuropsychology* (Vol. 9). Amsterdam, the Netherlands: Elsevier.

Tremblay, R. E., Boulerice, B., Harden, P. W., McDuff, P., Perusse, D., Pihl, R. O., *et al.* (1996). Do children in Canada become more aggressive as they approach adolescence? In R. E. Tremblay, B. Boulerice, P. W. Harden, P. McDuff, D. Perusse, D. Phil, *et al.* (eds), *Growing Up in Canada* (pp. 127–137). Ottawa, ON: Statistics Canada.

Vassileva, J., Petkova, P., Georgiev, S., Martin, E. M., Tersiyski, R., Raycheva, M., *et al.* (2007). Impaired decision-making in psychopathic heroin addicts. *Drug and Alcohol Dependence, 86*(2-3), 287–289.

Vendrell, P., Junqué, C., Pujol, J., Jurado, M. A., Molet, J., & Grafman, J. (1995). The role of prefrontal regions in the Stroop task. *Neuropsychologia, 33*(3), 341–352.

Verdejo-García, A. J., Perales, J. C., & Pérez-García, M. (2007). Cognitive impulsivity in cocaine and heroin polysubstance abusers. *Addictive Behaviors, 32*(5), 950–966.

Villemarette-Pittman, N. R., Stanford, M. S., & Greve, K. W. (2003). Language and executive function in self-reported impulsive aggression. *Personality and Individual Differences, 34*(8), 1533–1544.

Virkkunen, M., Goldman, D., Nielsen, D. A., & Linnoila, M. (1995). Low brain serotonin turnover rate (low CSF 5-HIAA) and impulsive violence. *Journal of Psychiatry and Neuroscience, 20*(4), 271–275.

Wallis, J. D. (2007). Orbitofrontal cortex and its contribution to decision-making. *Annual Review of Neuroscience, 30*(1), 31–56.

Yochim, B., Baldo, J., Nelson, A., & Delis, D. C. (2007). D-KEFS Trail Making Test performance in patients with lateral prefrontal cortex lesions. *Journal of the International Neuropsychological Society, 13*(4), 704–709.

Zelazo, P. D., & Müller, U. (2002). Executive function in typical and atypical development In U. Goswami (ed), *Handbook of Childhood Cognitive Development* (pp. 445–469). Malden, MA: Blackwell.

11

The neuroendocrinology of antisocial behaviour

Stephanie H. M. van Goozen and Graeme Fairchild

Introduction

Antisocial behaviour is an issue of significant social and clinical concern. When committed by young people, it is an issue of *increasing* concern. Although environmental factors have traditionally attracted most attention in explaining the origin and persistence of antisocial behaviour, it is important not to overlook the vulnerability of the individual in the development of antisocial behaviour. Relatively few studies have been conducted on the neuroendocrine factors involved in the development of antisocial behaviour in children. In this chapter, we explain how stress and androgenic hormones could be important factors in the behavioural problems of antisocial individuals. We will show that cortisol has been found to be significantly inversely related to severity of antisocial behaviour and can predict antisocial behaviour over time. We will also show that the role of androgens in aggression is less clear, and that there is currently only limited data suggesting that testosterone, or indeed other androgenic hormones, is particularly involved in violent behaviour or the prediction of antisocial behaviour over time.

Causal factors of early onset antisocial behaviour

Children who show antisocial behaviour from an early age have an increased risk of showing violently aggressive and other forms of criminal behaviour in adolescence and adulthood. The percentages found in the various studies range between 35 and 75%. Thus early onset antisocial behaviour is an important predictor of chronic and increasingly more serious forms of violent behaviour (Loeber & Hay, 1997; Fombonne *et al.*, 2001). Conduct problems in childhood also predict a host of other negative outcomes in adulthood, such as substance abuse and dependence (Kazdin, 1995), early pregnancy in antisocial girls (Bardone *et al.*, 1998), persistent health problems (Bardone *et al.*, 1998), and depression. Both dispositional, child-specific (i.e., genetic, temperamental) factors and social factors contribute to the development and maintenance of antisocial behaviour, although most research interest has focused on social factors. For example, life circumstances (e.g., bad neighbourhoods), stress in the family due to adverse life events, and parental relationship problems and psychopathology all play a role (Conger *et al.*, 1994; Moffitt, 2005). These factors are likely to result in the affective neglect of the child (Erel & Burman, 1995). However, not all children exposed to social adversity develop antisocial behaviour, and some children become antisocial despite a favourable social background. There is a growing literature showing that certain children have an increased risk of developing psychiatric disorders, and this predisposition is presumably partly biologically determined. Specifically, research suggests that a number of different biological factors may be involved in antisocial behaviour, and that these factors could play a role in the development, severity, and maintenance of such behaviour over time. An understanding of these factors should generate hypotheses concerning the underlying neurobiological mechanisms and aetiology of antisocial behaviour.

Neuroendocrine features of antisocial behaviour

In line with findings from aggressive adults with Antisocial Personality Disorder (Woodman *et al.*, 1978; Virkunnen, 1985), which is preceded by Conduct Disorder (CD) in childhood (Robins, 1978; American Psychiatric Association, 1994), there is convincing evidence for changes in the functioning of several interrelated neuroendocrine systems in individuals with antisocial behaviour. We will first focus on the androgens, testosterone and dehydroepiandros-terone (DHEA), before discussing in detail the role of the hypothalamic-pituitary-adrenal (HPA) axis and cortisol in particular.

Testosterone and aggression

The rationale for considering androgens to be involved in aggressive behaviour is that males have both higher concentrations of androgens and higher levels of physical aggression than females. Criminological studies reveal a similar clear-cut sex difference: men are more prone to using physical violence and are more often the victims of physical aggression themselves. Biological explanations have linked these findings to the social dominance of the male and consequently to testosterone, the most important male sex hormone. Although an association between androgens and aggression has been clearly established in animals (e.g., Higley *et al.*, 1996), the evidence in humans is less clear-cut (Archer, 1991; Archer *et al.*, 2005).

Gender differences in aggression

If one investigates behaviours that show marked differences between men and women, it is clear that gonadal hormones may play an important role. Boys and girls are exposed prena-tally to different levels of sex hormones, a situation which is reprised from puberty onwards when vast disparities in the level of hormones are again evident.

The process of sexual differentiation refers not only to the formation of the internal and external genitals, but also to the differentiation of the brain into male or female. Prenatal exposure to sex steroids of gonadal origin organizes the neural circuits of the developing brain (Goy & McEwen, 1980; Collaer & Hines, 1995; Hines, 2004). What evidence is there to support the claim that male and female brains are different?

In humans, a number of hypothalamic nuclei have been reported to be sexually dimorphic with respect to size and/or shape (see Hines, 2004 for a recent overview). These sex differ-ences in the hypothalamus may underlie important sex differences in behaviour. Moreover, recent studies on the distribution of oestrogen receptor (OR) alpha and beta immunoreac-tivity in cerebral regions probably significant for cerebral sexual differentiation, such as hypothalamic nuclei, indicate potential sex differences in both OR alpha and beta expression patterns suggestive of 'activational' rather than 'organizational' effects (Kruijver *et al.*, 2002, 2003). Beyond that, findings suggest that XY and XX cerebral cells have different patterns of gene expression influencing differentiation and function independently of the masculinizing effects of gonadal secretions. For example, a direct male-specific effect on the brain of the Y-linked male-determining *SRY* gene has been demonstrated that precedes the influence of gonadal hormones (Dewing *et al.*, 2003). However, although progress has been made in our understanding of the extent of sex differences in the brain, the mechanisms by which sexually dimorphic structures are formed remain poorly understood. Moreover, our understanding of the origin of sex differences in behaviour is complicated by the fact that such differences are not only manifestations of the organizing and activating effects of sex hormones, but also the result of interactions between these hormonal influences on behaviour, on the one hand, and social influences on the individual during various phases of development, on the other (van Goozen, 2005).

One can assume that socialization processes start early; so, if one wants to study gender differences in behaviour as a result of sex differences in prenatal hormonal exposure (i.e., brain organization), these behaviours have to be studied at an early age. Boys and girls differ in play styles and toy preference: Boys are more energetic and active, and show more aggressive and destructive behaviour, involving so-called rough-and-tumble play, a form of play-aggression that has also been observed to be sex-dependent in monkeys (Hines & Green, 1991). Some of these gender differences have been reported as early as 12 months of age (Hines, 2004). Recently, Hines et al. (2002), in a large population-based study, found a relationship between testosterone levels, as measured in the blood samples of pregnant women, and gender role behaviour in 3.5-year-old girls: as maternal testosterone levels increased, so did masculine-typical gender role behaviour. No relationships between hormones and gender role behaviour were found in boys. The largest gender differences in behaviour, however, are manifested in the years that follow, and this is a strong argument for the influence of socialization, modelling, and norms and values.

Reviews of studies of girls exposed prenatally to excessive androgens conclude that certain aspects of gender-related behaviour are influenced by prenatal hormones, particularly gender role behaviour, but there does not appear to be a clear influence on aggression (e.g., Berenbaum & Resnick, 1997; Hines, 2004). It remains possible, however, that the fact that boys and girls are born with sexually dimorphic brains and are raised post-natally in different environments ultimately contributes to gender-specific patterns of normal and abnormal behaviour. There are clear gender differences in the prevalence rates for psychopathology, with females being more prone to develop internalizing disorders, such as depression, anxiety, and eating disorders, and males showing a greater tendency to develop externalizing disorders, such as CD (Cyranowski et al., 2000). Although these patterns of gender-differentiated psychopathology are already observed in childhood, they become even more pronounced in adolescence. At the moment we do not know why this should be the case, although the fact that male and female brains are differently organized due to the distinctive patterns of prenatal sex hormone exposure and are differently activated from the start of puberty onwards could be important factors that should be taken into consideration. Future research on the interplay between genes, biology, life experience, and development (e.g., pubertal transition) is needed to understand patterns of change and continuity in childhood and adolescent psychopathology.

Activating effects of testosterone on normal aggression
Correlations in men between androgens and self-reports of aggressive behaviour or scores on aggression inventories are generally low (Meyer-Bahlburg, et al. 1974). For example, in one study, a correlation of 0.28 was found between total testosterone and scores on a physical aggre-ssion subscale; the correlation with free testosterone was even lower at 0.14 (Gladue, 1991). A study relevant to the issue of whether pubertal increases in testosterone levels produce an increase in physical aggression is that by Halpern et al. (1994). They found no

evidence of either an increase in aggression or an association between testosterone and aggression in a three-year longitudinal study of 100 teenage boys (aged 12–13 at study entry) going through puberty. Generally, studies of normal children and adolescents have yielded mixed results (for negative results, see Granger *et al.*, 2003; Maras *et al.*, 2003; for positive results, see van Bokhoven *et al.*, 2006). Furthermore, recent evidence indicates that testosterone levels are related to social dominance, rather than aggression per se (Mazur & Booth, 1998; Rowe *et al.*, 2004; van Bokhoven *et al.*, 2006). Thus, high testosterone levels may be associated with peer-group leadership, both within groups of normal children and antisocial groups, such as gangs (Rowe *et al.*, 2004).

Most of the studies on activating effects have been correlational in design, thereby limiting the possibility of establishing a causal role for testosterone in eliciting aggression. A more compelling line of research is the one that examines the effects of testosterone administration or depletion on aggression. Finkelstein *et al.* (1997) investigated the effects of testosterone administration on aggression in hormone-deficient (puberty-delayed) adolescents. The data demonstrated significant testosterone effects, specifically on physical aggression and aggressive impulses in boys (and similar effects were found after oestrogen administration in teenage girls). O'Connor *et al.* (2002) studied the effects of exogenous testosterone on aggression and mood in 30 eugonadal and 8 hypogonadal men. No significant increases on a range of aggression measures and no testosterone-related mood effects were observed in the eugonadal men. However, significant positive mood effects were found in the hypogonadal group. A subsequent study also found no increase in aggressive behaviour in eugonadal men following testosterone administration, although there was a small, but significant, increase in ratings of anger and hostility two weeks after treatment (O'Connor *et al.*, 2004). Another group of human participants that is interesting from the standpoint of the study of activating effects of testosterone on aggression are transsexuals. In the process of the sex reassignment procedure, these patients are treated with high doses of so-called opposite sex hormones. In two studies, it was found that when female-to-male transsexuals received high doses of androgens their anger and aggression proneness increased, whereas the reverse occurred in male-to-female transsexuals receiving anti-androgens and oestrogens (van Goozen *et al.*, 1994; van Goozen *et al.*, 1995). It is nevertheless clear that the evidence of a link between androgens and aggression is much weaker in humans than in animals (Archer, 1991). The results seem to be clearer when the relation is studied in younger (i.e., prepubertal) age groups (Schaal *et al.*, 1996). This could be because social restrictions on aggression are still limited at a younger age, and behaviour has yet to be shaped. It is also possible that a stronger relationship is found in more serious aggression. Next, we will examine whether testosterone levels are higher in clinical or criminological individuals with high levels of antisocial behaviour.

Testosterone and severe antisocial behaviour or aggression
Present or past aggressive behaviour has sometimes been found to correlate with testosterone concentrations. Dabbs and colleagues (1987) measured salivary testosterone in 89 male prison inmates and found that testosterone was related to type of crime: men convicted for violent crimes (murder, rape, robbery) had higher testosterone levels than men convicted for non-violent crimes (e.g., theft or burglary). In late adolescents and adults, elevated testosterone levels in the cerebrospinal fluid (CSF), plasma, and saliva have been linked to antisocial behaviour and violent crime (e.g., Ehrenkranz *et al.*, 1974; Dabbs *et al.*, 1987; Dabbs & Morris, 1990; Dabbs *et al.*, 1991; Virkkunen *et al.*, 1994; Banks & Dabbs, 1996).

With respect to children with CD, not many studies have focused on testosterone. Constantino *et al.* (1993) measured testosterone in the plasma of 18 highly aggressive boys and 11 controls (aged between 4 and 10 years) and found neither a group difference in testosterone nor a relationship between testosterone and the children's Child Behaviour Checklist (CBCL; Achenbach, 1991) aggression scores. Although the authors concluded that these findings raise questions about inferences from adult studies that testosterone may play a causal role in the development of aggression, an explanation for the negative results could lie in the composition of the groups, because 10 of the 18 aggressive boys had a co-morbid diagnosis of psychotic disorder. Psychosis has been considered an exclusion criterion in some studies (Kruesi *et al.*, 1990), because aggression as a temporary symptom of psychosis is clearly different from aggression as observed in children with a psychiatric diagnosis of CD, let alone in normally developing children. Van Goozen and colleagues (1998) also found no difference in plasma testosterone between boys with CD (n = 15) and normal controls (n = 25; all participants were between 8 and 12 years of age), and there were no significant relationships between testosterone and CBCL ratings of aggression and delinquency. Similarly, a recent study found no differences in morning salivary testosterone levels between control boys and those with either conduct problems, high levels of callous-unemotional (CU) traits, or a combination of these features (Loney *et al.*, 2006). And finally, Scerbo and Kolko (1994) measured saliva testosterone in 40 7–14-year-old clinic-referred disruptive children and found significant positive relationships between testosterone and staff- and teacher-rated aggression, after taking age and physical characteristics into account, but no differences in mean levels for children with or without CD, Oppositional Defiant Disorder (ODD), or Attention Deficit Hyperactivity Disorder (ADHD).

It has recently been reported that CSF testosterone levels and monoamine oxidase A (*MAOA*) genotype interact to predict antisocial behaviour (Sjöberg *et al.*, 2008). Thus, testosterone levels were only elevated in patients with antisocial personality disorder relative to controls, in the subgroup of participants expressing the low-activity form of the *MAOA* gene. If it can be replicated, this finding may explain why studies investigating relationships between testosterone and aggressive or antisocial behaviour have yielded such mixed results, because the low-activity polymorphism of the *MAOA* gene is only found in 35% of the population. As well as assessing the *MAOA* genotype to confirm this observation, it is recommended that future studies of testosterone-behaviour relationships in clinical or forensic groups obtain measures of social dominance given the findings discussed in the preceding.

DHEA

In prepubertal children, an important part of the androgenic activity is of adrenal rather than gonadal origin. From around the age of 6, children exhibit a gradual increase in androgens of adrenal origin, a period called the adrenarche (Parker, 1999), and it is not until puberty that gonadal androgens, such as testosterone, become important. Therefore, it is quite likely that the testosterone-aggression relationship does not emerge until after puberty, and research in prepubertal children should therefore also focus on adrenal androgens, such as DHEA, its sulphate (DHEA-S), and androstenedione. Of these, DHEA and DHEA-S are particularly interesting because they are also endogenously synthesized by the brain and act as neurosteroids (Robel & Baulieu, 1994), they increase neuronal excitability, enhance neuronal plasticity, and have neuroprotective properties (Wolf & Kirschbaum, 1999); finally, DHEA-S has $GABA_A$ antagonistic (i.e., neuroexcitatory) actions and could contribute to increased aggression (Majewska *et al.*, 1990; Majewska, 1992). One would therefore expect to find elevated DHEA and DHEA-S levels in individuals who are aggressive.

Few studies have focused on the role of adrenal androgens in antisocial behaviour. Interestingly, a pattern of DHEA hyposecretion has been found in youngsters with major depression (Goodyer *et al.*, 1996) whereas higher levels of DHEA-S have been found in those with CD (Dmitrieva *et al.*, 2001). The previously mentioned study by Constantino *et al.* (1993) found no relationship between DHEA-S and aggression; but, as noted in the preceding subsection, there are some grounds for treating this null finding with caution. Van Goozen *et al.* (1998a) found that DHEA-S levels were significantly higher in boys with CD than normal controls and were also strongly related to aggression and delinquency scores; differences between the two groups in androstenedione and testosterone were marginally significant and not significant, respectively. However, no data on developmental status were collected and no psychiatric control group was included. One could speculate that if higher adrenal androgen levels reflect adrenal response to stress, and if chronic stress stimulates adrenal development and secretion, it is possible that elevated DHEA-S levels would also be found in other psychiatric groups as a result of stress associated with having a psychiatric disorder. The aim of a subsequent study (van Goozen *et al.*, 2000) was to investigate DHEA-S levels in a new group of prepubertal children with CD, typically developing children, and psychiatric controls, including a group of children with ADHD. DHEA-S levels were examined in relation to developmental status, psychiatric diagnosis, and intensity of aggression and delinquency during the preceding 6 months as rated by parents or care workers. The results confirmed the findings of the earlier study in that the CD group again had significantly higher levels of DHEA-S than the normal control group, but it was also found that their levels were higher than those of the psychiatric controls.

The observed positive relation observed between CD or antisocial behaviour, on the one hand, and plasma levels of DHEA-S, on the other, is of interest. As mentioned in the preceding, higher endogeneous levels of this neuroexcitatory steroid may contribute to more aggression because of its $GABA_A$ antagonistic actions (Majewska, 1992). It is also possible that higher DHEA-S levels contribute to a larger pool of endogeneous testosterone. However, when measuring different androgenic hormones (i.e., testosterone, DHEA-S, and androstenedione) in children with CD, we found that the relation between aggressive behavioural problems and DHEA-S was stronger than that for testosterone, suggesting a more important role for central nervous system excitatory mechanisms in aggressive behaviour of children (van Goozen *et al.*, 1998a).

A recent study by Pajer *et al.* (2006) found no difference between adolescent girls with CD and matched controls in terms of plasma DHEA, DHEA-S, androstenedione, oestradiol or testosterone. The only group difference found was a significantly lower cortisol: DHEA ratio in girls with CD, relative to controls. This supports the concept of 'functional hypocortisolaemia' in CD (see later), whereby moderate reductions in cortisol are exacerbated by increases in DHEA, which has weak antiglucocorticoid properties. Finally, a comparison of girls with aggressive CD versus those with non-aggressive CD showed that free testosterone levels were elevated in the former group.

The role of androgens in emotion processing

Although the evidence for a role of testosterone in serious antisocial behaviour is at present unclear (e.g., Archer *et al.*, 2005), a different issue is that most supportive data involving antisocial adults are not very recent and come from one group in particular (i.e., Dabbs' group).

Although not directly relevant to our current goal-explaining the role of hormones in the aetiology of serious antisocial behaviour-a recent line of research explores the role of testosterone administration in emotion processing.

Exogenous testosterone administration has been shown to attenuate fear-potentiated startle (Hermans *et al.*, 2006) and reduce unconscious attentional biases to fearful facial stimuli in an emotional Stroop task (van Honk *et al.*, 2005). However, testosterone administration did not alter conscious awareness of the contingencies of the startle experiment, as measured by subjective fear states, or self-reported anxiety during the emotional Stroop task. These results, together with data showing that testosterone administration impairs performance on the Iowa Gambling Task (van Honk *et al.*, 2004), have been interpreted as evidence that testosterone reduces unconscious or implicit processing of punishment cues, causing a shift towards preferential processing of reward signals in the environment. This view that testosterone enhances activity of approach-related motivational systems may have implications for the development of aggressive and antisocial behaviour, explaining why antisocial individuals with high testosterone levels may show punishment insensitivity. One caveat is that all of these studies involved sublingual administration of relatively high doses of testosterone to young women, so it is unclear (a) whether similar effects would be obtained in males and (b) whether changes in endogenous testosterone within the physiological range would induce similar psychological effects.

To examine whether the same relationships hold between *physiological* testosterone concentrations and emotion-processing biases, Wirth and Schultheiss (2007) examined the relationship between endogenous testosterone levels and performance on a dot-probe task involving anger or neutral faces. They reported a negative correlation between testosterone levels and attentional bias towards subthreshold (i.e., presented too rapidly for conscious awareness) anger faces, again suggesting that testosterone reduces aversion to unconscious threat signals. Although these observations are interesting and potentially relevant, further research is needed to understand whether testosterone-mediated biases in unconscious emotion processing are relevant to social behaviour in the real world and, crucially, whether there is any relationship between these biases and aggressive behaviour or reward sensitivity in ecologically valid tasks; that is, does this apparent shift in sensitivity to punishment cues partly mediate the effects of elevated testosterone on aggressive behaviour? A prediction arising from the data presented earlier showing an interaction between *MAOA* genotype and testosterone levels in the prediction of antisocial personality disorder is that these processing biases should be particularly apparent in those with the low-activity form of the *MAOA* gene.

The HPA axis system

From everyday life, we know that stress is a primary factor in promoting aggression in humans. The principal endocrine system that mediates the effects of stress on behaviour is the HPA axis. Cortisol secretion represents the final step in a neuroendocrine cascade beginning in the paraventricular nucleus (PVN) of the hypothalamus. In response to activation by limbic, cortical, and other afferent inputs, corticotropin-releasing hormone (CRH) is released into the portal venous system by the PVN. CRH stimulates the release of adrenocorticotropic hormone (ACTH) from the anterior pituitary, which in turn leads to activation of the adrenal glands, resulting in the synthesis and release of cortisol. Once secreted into general circulation, cortisol acts on a variety of target cells to mobilize the physiological response to stress. Cortisol also crosses the blood-brain barrier to act at sites in the central nervous system, where it activates negative-feedback mechanisms that inhibit the release of CRH and ACTH, thereby reducing HPA axis activity (e.g., Chrousos & Gold, 1992).

In addition to its role in mediating the stress response, the HPA axis exhibits a marked circadian rhythm, which is synchronized with the activity cycle. Cortisol levels reach their peak approximately 30 minutes after waking and decline throughout the day, reaching their lowest point in the evening, at the end of the activity phase. Thus, cortisol levels fluctuate by as much as eightfold during the day (Netherton *et al.*, 2004). It is therefore crucial to control for time of day, relative to the individual's waking time, both in studies of basal (resting) cortisol levels and in studies assessing the effects of stress on cortisol secretion. Furthermore, there is some evidence that the HPA axis is more responsive to stress in the afternoon or evening. Finally, it has recently been noted that cortisol levels increase by approximately 60% in the 30 minutes after waking (Pruessner *et al.*, 1997; Clow *et al.*, 2004). This has been termed the *cortisol awakening response* (CAR) and appears to be influenced by genetic factors (Wüst *et al.*, 2000). As a result, in evaluating studies that relate HPA axis activity to certain forms of behaviour (e.g., aggression or CD), the temporal complexity of the cortisol signal needs to be acknowledged.

There are clear indications that stress plays an important role in explaining individual differences in antisocial behaviour. One starting point of research on the relationship between stress and antisocial behaviour is that aggressive individuals are less sensitive to the stressful or punishing consequences of their actions. This can be deduced from the fact that these individuals more often engage in risky, stressful, or dangerous situations than other people. If this is true, there are two possible explanations for a relationship between lower stress sensitivity and antisocial behaviour. One theory claims that antisocial individuals have low levels of fear (Raine, 1996). A relative lack of fear would lead to antisocial or delinquent behaviour because one is less sensitive to the negative consequences of one's own or other people's behaviour in general and the experience of receiving punishment in particular. If this is the case, the implications for the treatment of these problem behaviours are clear. It would mean that antisocial individuals have problems in conditioning; therefore, pointing out the negative consequences of their behaviour or punishing unacceptable behaviour are both likely to have little or no effect.

A different theory involving stress focuses on sensation seeking (Zuckerman, 1979). Here, it is argued that a certain level of stress is needed in order to feel pleasant and that too little or too much stress is experienced as aversive. Antisocial individuals are considered to have an elevated threshold for stress: they are easily bored and are not put-off by situations that the average person finds too exciting, stressful, or dangerous.

What evidence is there that a dysfunctional HPA axis system plays a role in antisocial behaviour? A large number of studies have investigated relationships between the end product of HPA axis activation, the stress hormone cortisol, and antisocial and aggressive behaviour. Studies of antisocial adults clearly show an inverse relationship between cortisol levels and the magnitude of behavioural deviation (e.g., Woodman *et al.*, 1978; Virkkunen, 1985; Bergman & Brismar, 1994). Only four studies measured ACTH or CRH in aggressive or antisocial individuals. Virkkunen and Linnoila (1993) and Virkkunen *et al.* (1994) found lower levels of ACTH in the CSF of alcoholic, impulsive offenders with antisocial personality disorder compared to healthy controls, but no differences in CSF CRH levels. Susman *et al.* (1999) reported that CRH levels were lower in pregnant teenage mothers with CD compared to teenage mothers without symptoms of CD. In contrast, Dmitrieva *et al.* (2001) found *higher* plasma ACTH levels in adolescents with CD.

Studies of antisocial children or adolescents have yielded mixed results. Some studies have found associations between reduced basal cortisol concentrations and aggressive behaviour or CD (e.g., Vanyukov *et al.*, 1993; van Goozen, Matthys, Cohen-Kettenis, Gispen-de Wied *et al.*, 1998; McBurnett *et al.*, 2000; Pajer *et al.*, 2001; Shoal *et al.*, 2003); other studies found no such relationship (e.g., Kruesi *et al.*, 1989; Schulz *et al.*, 1997; van Goozen *et al.*, 2000; Azar *et al.*, 2004) or even a positive relationship (van Bokhoven *et al.*, 2005; Sondeijker *et al*, 2007). McBurnett *et al.* (1991) found that anxious children with CD had higher cortisol levels than children with CD alone, although there was no group difference between the CD and control participants.

Using up-to-date saliva-collection methodology, a recent study showed that the CAR was blunted in 12–14-year-old boys with an ODD or CD diagnosis relative to matched controls (Popma, Doreleijers *et al*, 2007). The ODD or CD group also showed a slower decline in cortisol levels across the day, suggestive of a flatter circadian rhythm. Future studies that seek to compare aggressive and non-aggressive groups in terms of basal cortisol secretion should adopt similar designs, controlling for waking time and collecting multiple samples across the day, expressed in relation to waking time. Studies may also consider obtaining samples over several consecutive days to examine intra-individual stability (Wüst *et al.*, 2000; Goodyer *et al.*, 2001). In this manner, a more consistent picture of group differences in basal cortisol secretion would be achieved.

In the majority of the studies referred to in the preceding, the findings have been correlational in nature, with the result that it has not been possible to draw causal inferences between low cortisol concentrations and antisocial behaviour. There have been very few studies with a design capable of showing that low cortisol levels *precede* the onset of antisocial or aggressive behaviour and can therefore be used to predict which individuals will exhibit a pervasive pattern of antisocial behaviour throughout adolescence and into adulthood. The study that comes closest to demonstrating a longitudinal, albeit non-causal, link between low cortisol levels and aggressive behaviour is that by Shoal *et al.* (2003). This five-year longitudinal study investigated the relationship between cortisol at age 10–12 years and aggressive behaviour, as measured using the Youth Self-Report scale (Achenbach, 1991), at age 15-17 years. The results showed that low cortisol was moderately predictive of aggressive behaviour five years later, and further, that this relationship appeared to be mediated by the effects of cortisol on a personality variable the authors termed 'low self-control' (Shoal *et al.*, 2003). A further study with a longitudinal component was performed by McBurnett *et al.* (2000): they demonstrated that clinic-referred boys with consistently low cortisol levels in samples obtained two years apart showed the highest levels of aggressive CD symptoms over time. A limitation of this study was that it failed to control for the time of day of saliva collection, which is problematic due to the marked diurnal rhythm of cortisol.

Another point of interest is that basal glucocorticoid concentrations have been reported to be moderately heritable in humans (Meikle *et al.*, 1988; Inglis *et al.*, 1999); so it seems unlikely that basal cortisol levels could fall after the onset of antisocial behaviour. Finally, it should be noted that parental antisocial personality symptom counts have been shown to be inversely related to cortisol concentrations in their children (Vanyukov *et al.*, 1993). This suggests that HPA axis dysfunction may be involved in the intergenerational transmission of antisocial behaviour and provides further, indirect evidence that cortisol plays a role in the aetiology of antisocial behaviour.

Findings of reduced basal levels of cortisol in antisocial individuals could support the stimulation-seeking theory: antisocial children seek out stressful situations (e.g., fights) in order to increase their aversive, low basal cortisol levels. On the other hand, the more often these children get involved in stressful situations, the more likely they are to habituate to these stimuli and to subsequently show a blunted cortisol response to stress. The effect of frequent exposure (i.e., habituation) but also a lack of anticipatory fear, as suggested by the fearlessness theory, would be better studied under stressful conditions.

Accordingly, a number of studies have shown that the cortisol response to psychosocial stress is attenuated in children and prepubertal adolescents with conduct problems (van Goozen et al., 1998b; van Goozen et al., 2000; Popma et al., 2006). We noted earlier that aggressive individuals might differ from normal individuals in both respects: a low tonic stress level could lead to the fact that the individual does not avoid stressful events, or may even actively seek them out. On the other hand, low stress responsivity could indicate that one is fearless and less sensitive to the aversive consequences of negative events. We have found in our challenge studies that the stress-induced increase in salivary cortisol observed in normal controls is attenuated in children with CD (van Goozen et al., 1998b; van Goozen et al., 2000). Although increased cortisol reactivity to stress has been found in relation to aggressive behaviour, this has only been reported in healthy subjects and community samples (Gerra et al., 1997; Scarpa et al., 2000). These results suggest that a pattern of low cortisol reactivity during stress may be a specific characteristic of early onset antisocial individuals. Indeed, Snoek et al. (2004) found that child psychiatric patients suffering from ADHD showed a normal, stress-induced cortisol response whereas children with CD did not.

It is also important to note that another recent study showed that antisocial children with a blunted cortisol response to psychosocial stress showed the least improvement following a therapeutic intervention (van de Wiel et al., 2004). Children with CD who had similar levels of externalizing behaviours to cortisol non-responders before treatment, but who exhibited a normal cortisol stress response to psychosocial challenge, responded more favourably to treatment. These findings show that, despite manifesting similar levels of aggressive or oppositional behaviour as their antisocial peers, the children with attenuated HPA axis reactivity had a poorer prognosis. An impairment of HPA axis functioning may prevent the types of cognitive or emotional processing that play a critical role in therapeutic processes, and the prognosis for individuals with serious antisocial behaviour therefore appears more favourable when their cortisol reactivity to stress is preserved (van Goozen et al., 2007).

It is known that children who show antisocial behaviour from an early age, and children with CD in particular, have often been exposed to adverse rearing circumstances involving neglect, abuse, and domestic violence; but it is also true that their own problem behaviour elicits negative or harsh responses from peers, siblings, and parents that might be experienced as stressful (Kazdin, 1995). It could be that frequent exposure to stressful situations has resulted in a habituation among these children to (some types of) stress, and as a result, they show low stress reactivity (van Goozen et al., 2007). In this context, it is important to study the individual interpretation of the stressful event in order to elicit whether the subjective (emotional) experience of antisocial children is in line with their biological reactivity. In our studies, children with CD who fail to show a cortisol response during stress subjectively report and display intense emotions (i.e., they report increased levels of anger and react more aggressively towards their opponent), a pattern suggestive of a mismatch between subjective and physiological arousal (Snoek et al., 2004; van Goozen et al., 2000). Given the argument that blunted cortisol reactivity could partly explain stress habituation, future studies may also usefully explore links between chronic exposure to different forms of stress and cortisol hyporeactivity. It would be of particular interest to examine whether similar relationships hold in controls and those with CD (with or without high levels of CU traits).

Cortisol and psychopathic personality traits

Relatively little research has examined the role of variation in psychopathic (or more specifically, CU) traits in moderating the effect of antisocial behaviour on cortisol secretion. Preliminary work suggests that adolescents with high levels of CU traits may have reduced basal cortisol levels compared to controls (Loney *et al.*, 2006). Surprisingly, participants who were high on CU traits but low on conduct problems had lower cortisol levels than participants low on CU traits but high on conduct problems. Furthermore, these findings were specific to males. Although these findings are intriguing, only one cortisol sample was collected, at 9 a.m., so the group differences are difficult to interpret. It is not clear whether they relate to group differences in CARs or time of awakening, or reflect stable differences in cortisol secretion in high-CU trait participants, which would be observed across the diurnal cycle.

In a subsequent study by the same group in young adults, this association between high-CU traits and reduced basal cortisol levels was not replicated, although cortisol responses to social stress were reported to be attenuated in high-CU relative to low-CU male subjects (O'Leary *et al.*, 2007). Because only one post-stress sample was obtained, the study leaves open the possibility that presence of high-CU traits affects the latency of the stress response, but the response is otherwise normal. In addition, it is unknown whether the high-CU subjects found the social stressor stressful at all, because no subjective measures of stress were collected. Therefore, it remains unclear whether the cortisol data reflect a cortisol *stress* response. Finally, as the stressor used in that study was ineffective in eliciting cortisol secretion in female participants, it was not possible to test whether a similar effect of CU traits was seen in females.

A recent study that characterized the diurnal cortisol profile of prisoners and controls reported higher cortisol levels at 8 a.m. in non-psychopathic prisoners relative to psychopathic prisoners, although neither group differed significantly from controls (Cima *et al.*, 2008). Unfortunately, the authors' failure to obtain samples relative to waking time or to screen systematically for psychiatric disorders means that this finding is somewhat difficult to interpret. The difference could be due to group differences in waking time, magnitude of CAR, or co-morbid psychiatric illness, which may influence the CAR. No group differences were seen in terms of diurnal slope values or estimates of total cortisol secretion across the day, although the daily average value for cortisol across four assessment points was higher in non-psychopathic prisoners than controls (Cima *et al.*, 2008), largely due to the 8 a.m. difference. The authors interpreted their data as stronger evidence for HPA axis hyperarousal in non-psychopathic criminals, than for hypoarousal in psychopathic criminals.

In summary, although a handful of studies suggest it may be important to consider variation in psychopathic traits in studies of hormone-behaviour relationships, this possibility needs to be tested further using improved measures of endocrine activity. Similarly, those interested in investigating relationships between aggressive or antisocial behaviour and hormone secretion may wish to add measures of psychopathic personality traits to their assessment batteries, because these personality traits may exert a moderating influence.

Animal models of stress-induced and pathological aggression

Animal models have been shown to be extremely useful in our understanding of human psychopathological conditions. However, how stress mechanisms and the mechanisms involved in aggression interact on a neurobiological level has only recently become clear. Kruk *et al.* (2004) demonstrated a fast positive-feedback loop between the adrenocortical stress response and one of the brain areas involved in defensive aggression (i.e., the hypothalamus). Specifically, stimulation of the aggressive area in the hypothalamus rapidly activated the HPA axis, even in the absence of an opponent. Hypothalamic aggression was also quickly facilitated by an injection of corticosterone (the main stress hormone in rodents). These findings have clear implications for aggression regulation and treatment. For example, regulation of the adrenocortical stress response with certain anxiolytics, which reduce different stress-induced behaviours, may be effective in counteracting acute stress-precipitated violence (Kruk *et al.*, 2004). Thus, in normal animals and humans, so-called 'reactive' aggression is potentiated by high levels of arousal, an effect that is partly mediated by elevations in corticosteroid concentrations.

We described evidence that 'pathological' aggression appears to be related to HPA axis hyporeactivity. How, then, can these apparently opposing findings be reconciled? Haller and colleagues have developed a 'hypoarousal-driven aggression' model in animals, which is intended to mimic human pathological aggression. They showed that rats with low concentrations of circulating corticosterone and no ability to initiate HPA axis responses exhibit abnormal levels of aggressiveness and attempt to inflict the maximum amount of damage to their opponent in a resident/intruder fighting situation (Haller *et al.*, 2001; Halász *et al.*, 2002; Haller *et al.*, 2004). This is in contrast to control animals who, when confronted with a smaller opponent, give 'attack signals' as a warning before engaging in aggression, and then normally attack less vulnerable parts of the opponent's body (Blanchard & Blanchard, 1977). Acute injections of corticosterone (mimicking the increase normally seen during aggressive encounters in rats) prior to exposure to the fighting situation were shown to prevent this abnormal pattern of aggressive behaviour (Haller *et al.*, 2001). The authors concluded that an acute increase in cortisol is important in making the correct interpretation of the type of social conflict one is dealing with. If one fails to initiate an acute cortisol response, it may be more difficult to evaluate the true nature of the conflict. Halász *et al.* (2002) concluded that abnormal aggressiveness due to glucocorticoid hypofunction is related to increased sensitivity to stressors and fear-eliciting stimuli, possibly in the sense that signals coming from the opponents are misinterpreted, resulting in a behavioural response that is characteristic of more critical, defensive situations.

These findings have clear implications for human pathological aggression. It is possible that glucocorticoid hyporeactivity in antisocial individuals enhances their stress reactions, resulting in an overreaction that could lead to abnormal aggression. The animal findings also fit with findings on social-information-processing deficits in antisocial children (e.g., Milich & Dodge, 1984). Thus, antisocial children may interpret negative emotional situations incorrectly leading to more extreme, impulsive, and aggressive behaviour.

Although caution should be exercised in extrapolating from animal models to human behaviour, it is possible to speculate that reduced basal cortisol levels and/or a failure in the ability of antisocial individuals to activate their HPA axis in response to stress may underlie their persistent aggressive behaviour: they are more sensitive to provocation, but at the same time do not comprehend (i.e., cognitively) or experience (physiologically) the negative consequences of their behaviour. The animal studies also suggest that if a normal pattern of cortisol reactivity to stress were reinstated, this might reduce the level of aggression shown by antisocial individuals. At the same time, we acknowledge that it may be difficult to achieve this normalization given that it is well established that HPA axis function is shaped by events occurring in early life (Liu *et al.*, 1997; Plotsky *et al.*, 2005).

Because the evidence of reduced basal cortisol in antisocial or aggressive groups is very mixed, whereas cortisol hyporeactivity has been reported in several studies, it may be necessary to develop animal models that show better construct validity with human aggressive behaviour (i.e., the effects on corticosteroid secretion should be selective to the physiological response to aggressive conflict and other forms of stress, rather than affecting the entire circadian profile). This may be achieved by selectively breeding animals that show an attenuated corticosterone response in conflict situations, or identifying polymorphisms of the glucocorticoid receptor that confer reduced physiological sensitivity to stress or cause hypersensitivity of negative feedback mechanisms.

To summarize, several studies support the notion that HPA axis activity is important in explaining the differences between antisocial, conduct-disordered, and normal individuals. A major limitation of most of the existing studies that have been carried out is, however, that they have only measured the end product of the HPA axis. Although the measurement of salivary cortisol provides us with information on HPA axis reactivity, cortisol is secreted by the adrenals and therefore reflects a relatively late response. It would be instructive to investigate the functioning of higher levels of the HPA axis, for example, at the level of the pituitary (ACTH) and/or the hypothalamus (CRH). This could be achieved via CRH challenge tests to examine the sensitivity of pituitary CRH receptors, for example. An important, unresolved question relates to the origin of the cortisol hyporeactivity shown by individuals with CD: is this a result of HPA axis dysfunction (e.g., hypersensitive negative-feedback mechanisms that rapidly curtail the stress response or decreased sensitivity of pituitary CRH receptors), or rather due to deficient corticolimbic activation of the HPA axis? In the studies discussed earlier, subjective responses to stress were normal or even increased in participants with CD, relative to controls, but this does not preclude the possibility that limbic mechanisms involved in initiating the HPA axis response were impaired. This issue could be examined by directly comparing the efficacy of physiological and psychological stressors to elicit cortisol responses in the same individuals.

Relevant to this, a distinction has been made in the animal literature between 'systemic' stressors, which involve a physiological threat (e.g., hypoxia), and 'processive' stressors, which require emotional or psychological interpretation and appear to be relayed via limbic forebrain circuits (Herman & Cullinan, 1997). It seems plausible that CD is associated with reduced sensitivity to processive, rather than systemic, stressors, possibly as a result of corticolimbic network dysfunction or volume loss (Sterzer et al., 2005; Sterzer et al., 2007). Supporting this view, preliminary evidence suggests that ODD or CD is associated with normal cortisol and cardiovascular reactivity during physical exercise (Jansen et al., 1999). This distinction between 'processive' and 'systemic' stressors in CD clearly requires further investigation.

Relationships between neuroendocrine variables

As well as the absolute level of a specific circulating hormone, the balance between different hormones may also be important in the aetiology of aggression or CD. Popma, Vermeiren et al. (2007) recently demonstrated an interaction between cortisol and testosterone in relation to aggressive behaviour in adolescents, such that testosterone and overt aggressive behaviour were only positively correlated in participants with low basal cortisol levels. There was no relationship between testosterone and aggression in those with high basal cortisol levels. Dabbs et al. (1991) also reported a stronger relationship between testosterone levels and violence in male adolescents with low cortisol levels, compared to those with high cortisol levels. These findings have been interpreted as evidence that high cortisol levels may be protective against aggression, and buffer the effects of other risk factors, possibly by increasing anxiety levels or 'behavioural inhibition' (Kagan et al., 1988).

Implications of neuroendocrine findings

An understanding of the hormonal factors involved in antisocial behaviour should generate hypotheses concerning both the underlying neurobiological mechanisms and the aetiology of antisocial behaviour (van Goozen et al., 2007). Furthermore, biological studies of antisocial behaviour could lead to new approaches in the treatment of psychiatric conditions associated with aggression. Such approaches might involve pharmacological interventions to manipulate indirectly or perhaps even directly the biological substrates of aggression, or lead to hypotheses that influence the content of psychotherapy.

For example, one prediction arising from Haller's animal model of pathological aggression is that reinstatement of normal HPA axis functioning should ameliorate some forms of antisocial behaviour and enhance the response to therapeutic interventions. By restoring stress response systems to a relatively normal state of activity, it may be possible to repair the apparent disjunction between strong emotional reactions (often inappropriate or seemingly out of proportion to the precipitating conditions) and weak or non-existent physiological responses to situations that normally elicit anger, embarrassment, or fear. This connection between the cognitive and emotional components of an experience and the accompanying physiological reaction may be crucial for some aspects of emotional regulation and development. It may also be important from a clinical perspective given data indicating that individuals with intact cortisol reactivity respond more favourably to psychological treatment (van de Wiel et al., 2004). The importance of experiencing 'somatic feedback' in decision-making and risk-taking behaviour has been outlined by other authors (Damasio et al., 1990).

The neurobiological perspective could be applied to personality assessment and indicate that the underlying deficits of an antisocial individual are such that, for example, interventions involving 'empathy induction' (if it has been established that the individual is unresponsive to self-experienced or observed fear or sadness) or 'learning from punishment' (making use of time-out or response cost) are unlikely to work. This perspective could also be applied to risk assessment. For example, once the sensitivity of psychosocial stress tests has reached a sufficiently high level for detecting probable non-response to psychological treatment, these could be used in the future to guide allocation of treatment resources. If it can be verified that individuals who fail to show a cortisol response during psychosocial stress are resistant to current forms of treatment, it makes sense to develop new treatment approaches for these individuals, possibly involving a pharmacological component, and preferentially direct currently available psychological treatments to those who show a normal pattern of cortisol reactivity. The implication of such a neurobiological approach is that one should cease investing public finances in so-called 'blanket approaches' and replace these with targeted interventions that take the individual's personality and neurobiological profile into account. An investigation of neurobiological mechanisms involved in serious antisocial behaviour will identify not only different subgroups of antisocials in whom different causal processes initiate and maintain problem behaviour, but also interventions that specifically target the deficits presented by each subgroup.

Conclusion

Aggressive and antisocial behaviour, especially when it is already evident in childhood, is often persistent and difficult to treat. Although behavioural interventions have been shown to be effective in milder forms of these disorders, their efficacy in more seriously disturbed individuals is limited. This is partly due to the fact that we lack knowledge of the underlying cognitive and emotional problems of these individuals and the neurobiological causes of these difficulties. Knowing that antisocial behaviour in children is persistent and difficult to treat, it is interesting and relevant to note that HPA axis disturbances are found in children because these systems are also implicated in serious antisocial behaviour in adults (van Goozen *et al.*, 2007).

At present, we do not know what causes this pattern of impairments, although it is clear that genetic factors are involved in modulating HPA axis reactivity (Wüst *et al.*, 2000; DeRijk *et al.*, 2006; Kumsta *et al.*, 2007). An important line of research in animals suggests that early stressful experiences (prenatal and perinatal) affect the development of the brain in the first years of life. Knowing that many antisocial children have problematic backgrounds, it seems possible that they have been exposed to severe stress and that these experiences have had a permanent effect on the development of their stress systems, including the HPA axis. There is a clear need for long-term follow-up research from a very early age onwards, in order to shed more light on this issue.

A study of the neurobiological factors involved in aggression may help to explain why some antisocial individuals profit from psychological interventions whereas others do not. There are promising data from a small number of studies showing that neurobiological factors, including those discussed in this review, differ between those antisocial children who persist and those who desist from engaging in antisocial behaviour (van de Wiel *et al.*, 2004).

Studies examining whether cortisol hyporeactivity precedes the onset of aggressive behaviour or CD are needed to show that neuroendocrine factors play a causal role in the development of these conditions. For example, it is possible that changes in cortisol reactivity are simply a consequence of chronically engaging in antisocial behaviour. We also need to understand more about the physiological origin of cortisol hyporeactivity to stress in antisocial populations; for example, is it due to a fundamental dysfunction of the HPA axis or alternatively to abnormalities in corticolimbic innervation of the HPA axis?

And finally, if it is the case that antisocial behaviour is characterized by neurobiological impairments, pharmacological interventions should be taken into consideration as a treatment option. One should realize that impairments of HPA axis functioning, such as the ones discussed here, may disrupt the types of cognitive or emotional processing that normally play a critical role in therapeutic interventions. Thus, individuals with antisocial behaviour and either low basal cortisol levels or attenuated cortisol reactivity may be more effectively treated using pharmacologically based therapies that reinstate normal HPA axis functioning, perhaps as a precursor or an adjunct to psychological forms of treatment. These are clearly important lines of future research.

References

Achenbach, T. (1991). *Manual for the Youth Self Report and 1991 Profile*. Burlington, VT: Department of Psychiatry, University of Vermont.

Archer, J. (1991). The influence of testosterone on human aggression. *British Journal of Psychology*, *82*, 1–28.

Archer, J., Graham-Kevan, N., & Davies, M. (2005). Testosterone and aggression: a reanalysis of Book, Starzyk, and Quinsey's (2001) study. *Aggression and Violent Behavior*, *10*, 241–261.

Azar, R., Zoccolillo, M., Paquette, D., Quiros, E., Baltzer, F., & Tremblay, R. E. (2004). Cortisol levels and conduct disorder in adolescent mothers. *Journal of the American Academy of Child and Adolescent Psychiatry*, *43*, 461–468.

Bardone, A. M., Moffitt, T. E., Caspi, A., Dickson, N., Stanton, W. R., & Silva, P. A. (1998). Adult physical health outcomes of adolescent girls with conduct disorder, depression and anxiety. *Journal of the American Academy of Child and Adolescent Psychiatry, 37*, 594–601.

Berenbaum, S. A., & Resnick, S. M. (1997). Early androgen effects on aggression in children and adults with congenital adrenal hyperplasia. *Psychoneuroendocrinology, 22*, 505–515.

Bergman, B., & Brismar, B. (1994). Hormone levels and personality traits in abusive and suicidal male alcoholics. *Alcoholism, Clinical and Experimental Research, 18*, 311–316.

Blanchard, R. J., & Blanchard, D. C. (1977). Aggressive behavior in the rat. *Behavioral Biology, 21*, 197–224.

Chrousos, G. P., & Gold, P. W. (1992). The concepts of stress and stress system disorders. Overview of physical and behavioral homeostasis. *Journal of the American Medical Association, 267*, 1244–1252.

Cima, M., Smeets, T., & Jelicic, M. (2008). Self-reported trauma, cortisol levels, and aggression in psychopathic and non-psychopathic prison inmates. *Biological Psychology, 78*, 75–86.

Clow, A., Thorn, L., Evans, P., & Huckleridge, F. (2004). The awakening cortisol response: methodological issues and significance. *Stress, 7*, 29–37.

Collaer, M. L. & Hines, M. (1995). Human behavioural sex differences: a role for gondal hormones during early development? *Psychological Bulletin, 118*, 55–107.

Conger, R. D., Ge, X., Elder, G. H., Lorenz, F. O., & Simons, R. L. (1994). Economic stress, coercive family process, and developmental problems of adolescents. *Child Development, 65*, 541–561.

Constantino, J. N., Grosz, D., Saenger, P., Chandler, D. W., Nandi, R., & Earls, F. J. (1993). Testosterone and aggression in children. *Journal of the American Academy of Child and Adolescent Psychiatry, 32*, 1217–1222.

Cyranowski, J. M., Frank, E., Young, E., & Shear, K. (2000). Adolescent onset of the gender difference in lifetime rates of major depression. *Archives of General Psychiatry, 57*, 21–27.

Banks, T., & Dabbs, J. M. (1996). Salivary testosterone and cortisol in a delinquent and violent urban subculture. *Journal of Social Psychology, 136*, 49–56.

Dabbs, J. M., Frady, R. L., Carr, T. S., & Besch, N. F. (1987). Saliva testosterone and criminal violence in young adult prison inmates. *Psychosomatic Medicine, 49*, 174–182.

Dabbs Jr., J. M., Jurkovic, G. J., & Frady, R. L. (1991). Salivary testosterone and cortisol among late adolescent male offenders. *Journal of Abnormal Child Psychology, 19*, 469–478.

Dabbs, J. M., & Morris, R. (1990). Testosterone, social class, and antisocial behavior in a sample of 4462 men. *Psychological Science, 1*, 209–211.

Damasio, A. R., Tranel, D., & Damasio, H. (1990). Individuals with sociopathic behavior caused by frontal damage fail to respond autonomically to social stimuli. *Behavior Brain Research, 14*, 81–94.

DeRijk, R. H., Wüst, S., Meijer, O. C., Zennaro, M. C., Federenko, I. S., Hellhammer, D. H., *et al.* (2006). A common polymorphism in the mineralocorticoid receptor modulates stress responsiveness. *The Journal of Clinical Endocrinology and Metabolism, 91*, 5083–5089.

Dewing, P., Shi, T., Horvath, S., & Vilain, E. (2003). Sexually dimorphic gene expression in mouse brain precedes gonadal differentiation. *Molecular Brain Research, 118*, 82–90.

Dmitrieva, T. N., Oades, R. D., Hauffa, B. P., & Eggers, C. (2001). Dehydro-epiandrosterone sulphate and corticotropin levels are high in young male patients with conduct disorder: comparisons for growth factors, thyroid and gonadal hormones. *Neuropsychobiology, 43*, 134–140.

Ehrenkrantz, J., Bliss, E., Sheard, M. (1974). Plasma testosterone: correlations with aggressive behavior and social dominance in man. *Psychosomatic Medicine, 36*, 469–475.

Erel, O., & Burman, B. (1995). Interrelatedness of marital relations and parent-child relations: a meta-analytic review. *Psychological Bulletin, 118*, 108–132.

Finkelstein, J. W., Susman, E. J., Chinchilli, V. M., Kunselman, S. J., D'Arcangelo, M. R., Schwab, J., *et al.* (1997). Estrogen or testosterone increases self-reported aggressive behaviors in hypogonadal adolescents. *Journal of Clinical Endocrinology and Metabolism, 82*, 2433–2438.

Fombonne, E., Wostear, G., Cooper, V., Harrington, R., & Rutter, M. (2001). The Maudsley long-term follow-up of child and adolescent depression. I. Psychiatric outcomes in adulthood. *British Journal of Psychiatry, 179*, 210–217.

Gerra, G., Zaimovic, A., Avanzini, P., Chittolini, B., Giucastro, G., Palladino, M., *et al.* (1997). Neurotransmitter-neuroendocrine responses to experimentally induced aggression in humans: influence of personality variable. *Psychiatry Research, 66*, 33–43.

Gladue, B.A. (1991). Aggressive behavioral characteristics, hormones, and sexual orientation in men and women. *Aggressive Behavior, 17*, 313–326.

Goodyer, I. M., Herbert, J., Altham, P. M. E., Pearson, J., Secher, S., & Shiers, S. (1996). Adrenal secretion during major depression in 8 to 16 year olds, I: Altered diurnal rhythms in salivary cortisol and dehydroepiandrosterone (DHEA) at presentation. *Psychological Medicine, 26*, 245–256.

Goodyer, I. M., Park, R. J., Netherton, C. M., & Herbert, J. (2001). Possible role of cortisol and DHEA in human development and psychopathology. *British Journal of Psychiatry, 177*, 243–249.

Goy, R. W., & McEwen, B. S. (1980). *Sexual Differentiation of the Brain*. Cambridge, MA: MIT Press.

Granger, D. A., Shirtcliff, E. A., Zahn-Waxler, C., Usher, B., Klimes-Dougan, B., & Hastings, P. (2003). Salivary testosterone diurnal variation and psychopathology in adolescent males and females: individual differences and developmental effects. *Development and Psychopathology, 15*, 431–449.

Halász, J., Liposits, Z., Kruk, M. R., & Haller, J. (2002). Neural background of glucocorticoid dysfunction-induced abnormal aggression in rats: involvement of fear- and stress-related structures. *European Journal of Neuroscience, 15*, 561–569.

Haller, J., Halász, J., Mikics, E., & Kruk, M. R. (2004). Chronic glucocorticoid deficiency-induced abnormal aggression, autonomic hypoarousal, and social deficit in rats. *Journal of Neuroendocrinology, 16*, 550–557.

Haller, J., van de Schraaf, J., & Kruk, M. R. (2001). Deviant forms of aggression in glucocorticoid hyporeactive rats: a model for 'pathological' aggression? *Journal of Neuroendocrinology, 13*, 102–107.

Halpern, C. T., Udry, R., Campbell, B., & Suchindran, C. (1994). Relationships between aggression and pubertal increases in testosterone: a panel analysis of adolescent males. *Social Biology, 40*, 8–24.

Herman, J. P., & Cullinan, W. E. (1997). Neurocircuitry of stress: central control of the hypothalamo-pituitary-adrenal axis. *Trends in Neuroscience, 20*, 78–84.

Hermans, E. J., Putnam, P., Baas, J. M., Koppeschaar, H. P., & van Honk, J. (2006). A single administration of testosterone reduces fear-potentiated startle in humans. *Biological Psychiatry, 59*, 872–874.

Higley, J. D., Mehlman, P. T., Poland, R. E., Taub, D. M., Vickers, J., Suomi, S. J., *et al.* (1996). CSF testosterone and 5-HIAA correlate with different types of aggressive behaviours. *Biological Psychiatry, 40*, 1067–1082.

Hines, M. (2004). *Brain Gender*. New York: Oxford University Press.

Hines, M., Golombok, S., Rust, J., Johnston, K. J., Golding, J., and the Avon Longitudinal Study of Parents and Children study team (2002). Testosterone during pregnancy and gender role behavior of preschool children: a longitudinal, population study. *Child Development, 73*, 1678–1687.

Hines, M., & Green, R. (1991). Human hormonal and neural correlates of sex-typed behaviors. *Review of Psychiatry, 10*, 536–555.

Inglis, G. C., Ingram, M. C., Holloway, C. D., Swan, L., Birnie, D., Hillis, W. S., *et al.* (1999) Familial pattern of corticosteroids and their metabolism in adult human subjects—the Scottish Adult Twin Study. *Journal of Clinical Endocrinology and Metabolism, 84*, 4132–4137.

Jansen, L. M. C., Gispen-de-Wied, C. C., Jasen, M. A., van der Gaag, R. J., Matthys, W., & van Engeland, H. (1999). Pituitary-adrenal reactivity in a child psychiatric population: salivary cortisol response to stressors. *European Neuropsychopharmacology, 9*, 67–75.

Kagan, J., Reznick, J. S., & Snidman, N. (1988). Biological bases of childhood shyness. *Science, 240*, 167–171.

Kazdin, A. (1995). *Conduct Disorders in Childhood and Adolescence*, 2nd edn. Thousand Oaks, CA: Sage.

Kruesi, M. J., Rapoport, J. L., Hamburger, S., Hibbs, E., Potter, W. Z., Lenane, M., *et al.* (1990). Cerebrospinal fluid monoamine metabolites, aggression, and impulsivity in disruptive behavior disorders of children and adolescents. *Archives of General Psychiatry, 47*, 419–426.

Kruesi, M. J., Schmidt, M. E., Donelly, M., Hibbs, E. D., & Hamburger, S. D. (1989). Urinary free cortisol output and disruptive behavior in children. *Journal of the American Academy of Child and Adolescent Psychiatry, 28*, 441–443.

Kruijver, F. P., Balesar, R., Espila, A. M., Unmehopa, U. A., & Swaab, D. F. (2002). Estrogen receptor-alpha distribution in the human hypothalamus in relation to sex and endocrine status. *The Journal of Comparative Neurology, 454*, 115–139.

Kruijver, F. P., Balesar, R., Espila, A. M., Unmehopa, U. A., & Swaab, D. F. (2003). Estrogen-receptor-ß distribution in the human hypothalamus: similarities and differences with ERα distribution. *The Journal of Comparative Neurology, 466*, 251–277.

Kruk, M. R., Halasz, J., Meelis, W., & Haller, J. (2004). Fast positive feedback between the adrenocortical stress response and a brain mechanism involved in aggressive behavior. *Behavioral Neuroscience, 118*, 1062–1070.

Kumsta, R., Entringer, S., Koper, J. W., van Rossum, E. F., Hellhammer, D. H., & Wüst, S. (2007). Sex-specific associations between common glucocorticoid receptor gene variants and hypothalamus-pituitary-adrenal axis responses to psychosocial stress. *Biological Psychiatry, 62*, 863–869.

Loeber, R., & Hay, D. F. (1997). Key issues in the development of aggression and violence from childhood to early adulthood. *Annual Review of Psychology, 48*, 371–410.

Loney, B. R., Butler, M., Lima, E., Counts, C., & Eckel, L. (2006). The relation between salivary cortisol, callous-unemotional traits, and conduct problems in an adolescent non-referred sample. *Journal of Child Psychology and Psychiatry, 47*, 30–36.

Liu, D., Diorio, J., Tannebaum, B., Caldji, C., Francis, D., Freedman, A., *et al.* (1997). Maternal care, hippocampal glucocorticoid receptors, and hypothalamic-pituitary-adrenal responses to stress. *Science, 277*, 1659–1662.

Majewska, M. D. (1992). Neurosteroids: endogeneous bimodal modulators of the GABAa receptor. Mechanisms of action and physiological significance. *Progress in Neurobiology, 38*, 379–395.

Majewska, M. D., Demirgoren, S., Spivak, C. E., & London, E. D. (1990). The neurosteroid dehydroepiandrosterone sulfate is an allosteric antagonist of the GABA$_A$ receptor. *Brain Research, 526*, 143–146.

Maras, A., Laucht, M., Gerdes, D., Wilhelm, C., Lewicka, S., Haack, D., *et al.* (2003). Association of testosterone and dihydrotestosterone with externalizing behavior in adolescent boys and girls. *Psychoneuroendocrinology, 28*, 932–940.

Mazur, A., & Booth, A. (1998). Testosterone and dominance in men. *Behavioral and Brain Sciences, 21*, 353–397.

McBurnett, K., Lahey, B. B., Frick, P. J., Risch, C., Loeber, R., Hart, E. L., *et al.* (1991). Anxiety, inhibition, and conduct disorder in children: II. Relation to salivary cortisol. *Journal of the American Academy of Child and Adolescent Psychiatry, 30*, 192–196.

McBurnett, K., Lahey, B. B., Rathouz, P. J., & Loeber, R. (2000). Low salivary cortisol and persistent aggression in boys referred for disruptive behavior. *Archives of General Psychiatry, 57*, 38–43.

Meikle, A. W., Stringham, J. D., Woodward, M. G., & Bishop, D. T. (1988) Heritability of variation of plasma cortisol levels. *Metabolism, 37*, 514–517.

Meyer-Bahlburg, H. F. L., Boon, D. A., Sharma, M., & Edwards, J. A. (1974). Aggressiveness and testosterone measures in man. *Psychosomatic Medicine, 36*, 269–274.

Milich, R., & Dodge, K. (1984). Social information processing in child psychiatric populations. *Journal of Abnormal Child Psychology, 12*, 471–490.

Netherton, C., Goodyer, I. M., Tamplin, A., & Herbert, J. (2004). Salivary cortisol and dehydroepiandrosterone in relation to puberty and gender. *Psychoneuroendocrinology, 29*, 125–140.

O'Connor, D. B., Archer, J., Hair, W. M. & Wu, F. C. W. (2002). Exogenous testosterone, aggression, and mood in eugonadal and hypogonadal men. *Physiology and Behavior, 75*, 557–566.

O'Connor, D. B., Archer, J., & Wu, F.C.W. (2004). Effects of testosterone on mood, aggression, and sexual behavior in young men: a double-blind, placebo-controlled, cross-over study. *Journal of Clinical Endocrinology and Metabolism, 89*, 2837–2845.

O'Leary, M., Loney, B. R., & Eckel, L. A. (2007). Gender differences in the association between psychopathic personality traits and cortisol response to induced stress. *Psychoneuroendocrinology*, *32*, 183–191.

Pajer, K., Gardner, W., Rubin, R. T., Perel, J., & Neal, S. (2001). Decreased cortisol levels in adolescent girls with conduct disorder. *Archives of General Psychiatry*, *58*, 297–302.

Pajer, K., Tabbah, R., Gardner, W., Rubin, R. T., Czambel, R. K., & Wang, Y. (2006). Adrenal androgen and gonadal hormone levels in adolescent girls with conduct disorder. *Psychoneuroendocrinology*, *31*, 1245–1256.

Parker Jr., C. R. (1999). Dehydroepiandrosterone and dehydroepiandrosterone sulfate production in the human adrenal during development and aging. *Steroids*, *64*, 640–647.

Plotsky, P. M., Thrivrikraman, K. V., Nemeroff, C. B., Caldji, C., Sharma, S., & Meaney, M. J. (2005). Long-term consequences of neonatal rearing on central corticotropin-releasing factor systems in adult male rat offspring. *Neuropsychopharmacology*, *30*, 2192–2204.

Popma, A. R., Doreleijers, T. A. H., Jansen, L. M. C., van Goozen, S. H., van Engeland, H., & Vermeiren, R. (2007). The diurnal cortisol cycle in delinquent male adolescents and normal controls. *Neuropsychopharmacology*, *32*, 1622–1628.

Popma, A. R., Jansen, L. M. C., Vermeiren, R., Steiner, H., Raine, A., van Goozen, S. H. M., *et al.* (2006). Hypothalamus-pituitary-adrenal axis and autonomic activity during stress in delinquent male adolescents and controls. *Psychoneuroendocrinology*, *31*, 948–957.

Popma, A. R., Vermeiren, R., Geluk, C. A. M. L, Rinne, T., van den Brink, W., Knol, D. L., *et al.* (2007). Cortisol moderates the relationship between testosterone and aggression in delinquent male adolescents. *Biological Psychiatry*, *61*, 405–411.

Pruessner, J. C., Wolf, O. T., Hellhammer, D. H., Buske-Kirschbaum, A., von Auer, K., Jobst, S., *et al.* (1997). Free cortisol levels after awakening: a reliable biological marker for the assessment of adrenocortical activity. *Life Sciences*, *61*, 2539–2549.

Raine, A. (1996). Autonomic nervous system activity and violence. In D. M. Stoff, & R. B. Cairns (eds), *Aggression and Violence: Genetic, Neurobiological and Biological Perspectives* (pp. 145–168). Mahwah, NJ: Lawrence Erlbaum Associates.

Robel, P., & Baulieu, E. E. (1994). Neurosteroids: biosynthesis and function. *Trends in Endocrinology and Metabolism*, *5*, 1–8.

Robins, L. N. (1978). Sturdy childhood predictors of adult antisocial behavior: replications from longitudinal studies. *Psychological Medicine*, *8*, 611–622.

Rowe, R., Maughan, B., Worthman, C. M., Costello, E. J., & Angold, A. (2004). Testosterone, antisocial behavior, and social dominance in boys: pubertal development and biosocial interaction. *Biological Psychiatry*, *55*, 546–552.

Scarpa, A., Fikretoglu, D., & Luscher, K. (2000). Community violence exposure in a young adult sample: II. Psychophysiology and aggressive behavior. *Journal of Community Psychology*, *28*, 417–425.

Scerbo, A. S., & Kolko, D. J. (1994). Salivary testosterone and cortisol in disruptive children: relationship to aggressive, hyperactive, and internalizing behaviors. *Journal of the American Academy of Child and Adolescent Psychiatry*, *33*, 1174–1184.

Schaal, B., Tremblay, R., Soussignan, R., & Susman, E. (1996). Male testosterone linked to high social dominance but low physical aggression in early adolescence. *Journal of the Academy of Child and Adolescent Psychiatry*, *34*, 1322–1330.

Schulz, K. P., Halperin, J. M., Newcorn, J. H., Sharma, V., & Gabriel, S. (1997). Plasma cortisol and aggression in boys with ADHD. *Journal of the American Academy of Child and Adolescent Psychiatry*, *36*, 605–609.

Shoal, G. D., Giancola, P. R., & Kirillova, G. P. (2003). Salivary cortisol, personality, and aggressive behavior in adolescent boys: a 5-year longitudinal study. *Journal of the American Academy of Child and Adolescent Psychiatry*, *42*, 1101–1107.

Sjöberg, R. L., Ducci, F., Barr, C. S., Newman, T. K., Dell'Osso, L., Virkunnen, M., *et al.* (2008). A non-additive interaction of a functional MAO-A VNTR and testosterone predicts antisocial behavior. *Neuropsychopharmacology*, *33*, 425–430.

Snoek, H., van Goozen, S. H. M., Matthys, W., Buitelaar, J. K., & van Engeland, H. (2004). Stress responsivity in children with externalizing behavior disorders. *Development and Psychopathology*, *16*, 389–406.

Sondeijker, F. E., Ferdinand, R. F., Oldehinkel, A. J., Veenstra, R., Tiemeier, H., Ormel, J., *et al.* (2007). Disruptive behaviors and HPA-axis activity in young adolescent boys and girls from the general population. *Journal of Psychiatric Research*, *41*, 570–578.

Sterzer, P., Stadler, C., Krebs, A., Kleinschmidt, A., & Poustka, F. (2005). Abnormal neural responses to emotional visual stimuli in adolescents with conduct disorder. *Biological Psychiatry*, *57*, 7–15.

Sterzer, P., Stadler, C., Poustka, F., & Kleinschmidt, A. (2007). A structural neural deficit in adolescents with conduct disorder and its association with lack of empathy. *Neuroimage*, *37*, 335–342.

Susman, E. J., Schmeelk, K. H., Worrall, B. K., Granger, D. A., Ponirakis, A., & Chrousos, G. P. (1999). Corticotropin-releasing hormone and cortisol: longitudinal associations with depression and antisocial behavior in pregnant adolescents. *Journal of the American Academy of Child and Adolescent Psychiatry*, *38*, 460–467.

Van Bokhoven, I., van Goozen, S. H. M., van Engeland, H., Schaal, B., Arseneault, L., Séguin, J.R., *et al.* (2005). Salivary cortisol and aggression in a population-based longitudinal study of adolescent males. *Journal of Neural Transmission*, *112*, 1083–1096.

Van Bokhoven, I., van Goozen, S. H. M., van Engeland, H., Schaal, B., Arseneault, L., Séguin, J. R., *et al.* (2006). Salivary testosterone and aggression, delinquency, and social dominance in a population-based longitudinal study of adolescent males. *Hormones and Behavior*, *50*, 118–125.

Van de Wiel, N. M. H., van Goozen, S. H. M., Matthys, W., Snoek, H., & van Engeland, H. (2004). Cortisol and treatment effect in children with disruptive behavior disorders: a preliminary study. *Journal of the American Academy of Child and Adolescent Psychiatry*, *43*, 1011–1018.

Van Goozen, S. H. M. (2005). Hormones and the developmental origins of aggression. In R. E. Tremblay, W. W. Hartup, & J. Archers (eds), *Developmental Origins of Aggression* (pp. 281–306). New York: Guilford Press.

Van Goozen, S. H. M., Cohen-Kettenis, P. T., Gooren, L. J. G., Frijda, N. H., & van de Poll, N. E. (1995). Gender differences in behaviour: activating effects of cross-sex hormones. *Psychoneuroendocrinology*, *20*, 343–363.

Van Goozen, S. H. M., Fairchild, G., Snoek, H., & Harold, G. T. (2007). The evidence for a neurobiological model of childhood antisocial behavior. *Psychological Bulletin*, *133*, 149–182.

Van Goozen, S. H. M., Frijda, N. H., & van de Poll, N. E. (1994). Anger and aggression in women: influence of sports choice and testosterone administration. *Aggressive Behavior*, *20*, 213–222.

Van Goozen, S. H. M., Matthys, W., Cohen-Kettenis, P. T., Buitelaar, J. K., & van Engeland, H. (2000). Hypothalamic-pituitary-adrenal axis and autonomic nervous system activity in disruptive children and matched controls. *Journal of the American Academy of Child and Adolescent Psychiatry*, *39*, 1438–1445.

Van Goozen, S. H. M., Matthys, W., Cohen-Kettenis, P. T., Thijssen, J. H. H., & van Engeland, H. (1998a). Adrenal androgens and aggression in conduct disorder prepubertal boys and normal controls. *Biological Psychiatry*, *43*, 156–158.

Van Goozen, S. H. M., Matthys, W., Cohen-Kettenis, P. T., Gispen-de Wied, C., Wiegant, V. M., & van Engeland, H. (1998b). Salivary cortisol and cardiovascular activity during stress in oppositional-defiant disorder boys and normal controls. *Biological Psychiatry*, *43*, 531–539.

Van Honk, J., Peper, J. S., & Schutter, D. J. L.G. (2005). Testosterone reduces unconscious fear but not consciously experienced anxiety: implications for the disorders of fear and anxiety. *Biological Psychiatry*, *58*, 218–225.

Van Honk, J., Schutter, D. J., Hermans, E. J., Putnam, P., Tuiten, A., & Koppeschaar, H. (2004). Testosterone shifts the balance between sensitivity for punishment and reward in healthy young women. *Psychoneuroendocrinology*, *29*, 937–943.

Vanyukov, M. M., Moss, H. B., Plail, J. A., Blackson, T., Mezzich, A. C., & Tarter, R. E. (1993). Antisocial symptoms in preadolescent boys and in their parents: associations with cortisol. *Psychiatry Research*, *46*, 9–17.

Virkkunen, M. (1985). Urinary free cortisol secretion in habitually violent offenders. *Acta Psychiatrica Scandinavica*, *72*, 40–44.

Virkkunen, M., & Linnoila, M. (1993). Brain serotonin, type II alcoholism and impulsive violence. *Journal of Studies on Alcohol*, *11*(Suppl), 163–169.

Virkkunen, M., Rawlings, R., Tokola, R., Poland, R. E., Guidotti, A., Nemeroff, C., *et al.* (1994). CSF biochemistries, glucose metabolism, and diurnal activity rhythms in alcoholic, violent offenders, fire setters and healthy volunteers. *Archives of General Psychiatry*, *51*, 28–33.

Wirth, M. M., & Schultheiss, O. C. (2007). Basal testosterone moderates responses to anger faces in humans. *Physiology and Behavior*, *90*, 496–505.

Wolf, O. T., & Kirschbaum, C. (1999). Actions of dehydroepiandrosterone and its sulfate in the central nervous system: effects on cognition and emotion in animals and humans. *Brain Research Review*, *30*, 264–288.

Woodman, D. D., Hinton, J. W., & O'Neill, M. T. (1978). Cortisol secretion and stress in maximum security hospital patients. *Journal of Psychosomatic Research*, *22*, 133–136.

Wüst, S., Federenko, I., Hellhammer, D. H., & Kirschbaum, C. (2000). Genetic factors, perceived chronic stress, and the free cortisol response to awakening. *Psychoneuroendocrinology*, *25*, 707–720.

Zuckerman, M. (1979). *Sensation Seeking: Beyond the Optimum Level of Arousal*. Hillsdale, NJ: Lawrence Erlbaum Associates.

12

From markers to mechanisms: Using psychophysiological measures to elucidate basic processes underlying aggressive externalizing behaviour

Christopher J. Patrick and Edward M. Bernat

Introduction

The brain is the essential common pathway through which heredity and experience operate to shape core psychological processes that determine behaviour. Understanding the behaviour of persistently violent individuals thus requires consideration of phenomena at varying levels of analysis: genes and environments; nervous system anatomy and physiology; neural representations and networks; perceptual, cognitive, and affective functions; and overt action and its regulation. Psychophysiological approaches to the study of aggression fill a crucial niche in this analytic hierarchy by providing information about brain and bodily responses associated with ongoing psychological and behavioural processes in time. The aim of this chapter is to provide a framework for thinking about findings from existing published studies of this kind, and to highlight in particular the unique contribution that advanced electrocortical (EEG/ERP) measurement techniques can make to our understanding of neuropsychological processing dynamics underlying impulsive aggressive behaviour.

The chapter begins with an overview of alternative methodological approaches to investigating the neurobiological bases of aggressive behavior, highlighting the key role that psychophysiological studies can play in this area of research. Next, it provides a brief overview of major lines of evidence emerging from psychophysiological investigations of aggressive and violent behaviour that have been published to date. The third section presents a broad conceptual framework for interpreting available evidence from studies of this kind. The fourth section describes new research by our laboratory group investigating basic cognitive-affective processing differences in aggressive externalizing individuals using electrocortical (brain potential response) measures. This work, conducted from the standpoint of an integrative hierarchical model of impulse control ('externalizing') problems, capitalizes on the fine-grained measurement afforded by electroencephalography (EEG) in the domains of both frequency and time to elucidate the dynamics of brain processing deviations associated with impulsive aggressive behaviour in high-externalizing individuals. The chapter ends with a discussion of how these findings can be interpreted in relation to the conceptual model described in section 3 and of the implications this model has for clinical interventions with impulsive-aggressive individuals.

Approaches to investigating the neurobiological bases of aggressive behaviour: the role of psychophysiological measurement

A variety of different methodological approaches exist for studying the role that neurobiological factors play in violent and aggressive behaviour. These approaches contribute to knowledge in differing, but complementary ways. They can be grouped according to the particular sorts of questions they address regarding violent or aggressive behaviour.

One approach consists of *aetiological studies*. Studies of this kind address the question: 'What constitutional and environmental factors contribute *causally* to the occurrence of violence or aggression?' For example, behavioural genetic studies address this question by comparing the degree of similarity in tendencies towards aggression between identical and fraternal twins, or between identical twins who are reared in the same versus differing family environments. Studies of this type can be used to estimate the proportion of variance in a behavioural phenotype that is attributable to additive genetic influence compared with shared (family) or non-shared environmental influence. Twin research designs can also be used to test for moderating effects of varying environments on the proportional contribution of genetic factors to a behavioural phenotype (cf. Purcell, 2002).

Molecular genetic studies provide another means for investigating aetiologic contributions to behavioural phenotypes such as aggression—contributions made by specific genes or gene sequences, or by interactions between specific genes and environmental factors (e.g., Caspi *et al.*, 2002). In addition to behavioural and molecular genetic investigations, a third approach to investigating aetiologic contributions of neurobiological variables to aggressive behaviour is longitudinal developmental research. Studies of this kind provide a basis for inferring aetiologic influences because temporal relations between putative causal factors and outcome variables can be specified with precision in quantitative models of longitudinal data (cf. Card & Little, 2007).

Behavioral genetic, molecular genetic, and longitudinal studies are crucial to understanding the role of hereditary and environmental factors (and their interactions) in the genesis of aggressive tendencies. However, in addition, it is important to understand what neurobiological systems are affected by these basic aetiologic factors and how individual differences in the structure and functioning of neurobiological systems dispose to and give rise to aggressive actions. To do so, it is necessary to measure characteristics of neurobiological systems within individuals. Psychophysiological (including neuroimaging) and neurochemical assessment methods provide this capability.

In this regard, a second type of approach to the investigation of neurobiological factors in aggressive behaviour consists of *marker* studies. The basic question addressed by studies of this type is: 'What biological differences are characteristic of aggressive individuals compared with non-aggressive individuals?' Methods for addressing this question include (1) peripheral and electrocortical psychophysiology (to index visceral and/or autonomic, somatic and/or muscular, and brain activity differences); (2) structural and functional neuroimaging (to detect differences in brain anatomy and brain activity); and (3) neurochemical assays (to assess differences in brain neurotransmitter levels and activity). Some biological variables on which individuals who exhibit (or are at risk for) aggressive behaviour differ reliably from non-aggressive individuals include resting heart rate levels, amplitude of brain event-related potential (ERP) responses, volume and activity in specific brain regions, and levels of the brain neurotransmitter serotonin. Marker studies are valuable because they point to biological systems and functions that may be targets of genetic and/or environmental influence and because they can provide biologically based indicators of vulnerability that can be used to identify candidates for prevention programmes.

A third type of approach to investigating neurobiological factors in aggression consists of *process* studies. The question addressed by studies of this type is: 'How do aggressive individuals differ in their psychological processing of stimuli and events?' The emphasis is on understanding the functional role that neurobiological reactivity differences play in dispositions towards aggression and in instigating aggressive acts. Cognitive and affective psychophysiology studies contribute to understanding at this level by measuring brain activation within a performance task designed to index some specific psychological process or processes. The focus of such studies is on understanding differences in online cognitive or emotional processing that appear relevant to some clinical phenomenon of interest, such as aggression. Measurement techniques used to study brain activity associated with online processing include functional neuroimaging (positron emission tomography [PET], functional magnetic resonance imaging [fMRI]), and EEG/ERP recording.

These brain measurement techniques each have relative advantages and disadvantages. fMRI provides fine-grained spatial resolution, which permits activity to be precisely localized within specific regions of the brain, but its temporal resolution is limited. EEG provides fine-grained resolution in both temporal and spectral (frequency) domains, but its spatial resolution is limited in comparison to fMRI. However, the spatial resolution of EEG can be improved through multi-electrode, dense-array recording, which provides for more precise estimation of signal sources at and below the brain's surface ('source modelling'). The resolution of EEG can be improved even further by referencing EEG data to structural or functional neuroimaging data collected from the same participant, either concurrently or in separate test sessions. In conjunction with continuous measurement of activity along dimensions of time and frequency, this technique provides for even finer-grained localization of underlying sources of brain activity ('source imaging') because EEG source models can be constrained to accommodate known neuroanatomic structures or regions of brain activation established by MRI recording.

The next section provides a brief overview of findings from studies that have used psychophysiological measurement techniques to investigate neurobiological factors contributing to the behaviour of persistently aggressive individuals. It will be seen that most published studies of this sort, including the majority of the studies that have employed neuroimaging methods, fall into the category of marker studies.

Overview of findings from autonomic, electrocortical, and brain imaging studies of aggressive individuals

Autonomic response measures: cardiovascular and electrodermal activity

Children and adolescents exhibiting antisocial behaviour (i.e., conduct problems encompassing non-aggressive as well as aggressive behaviour) show consistent evidence of lower resting autonomic activity levels-most notably heart rate (HR), but also to some extent skin conductance (SC)—compared with control youth (Lorber, 2004; Ortiz & Raine, 2004). The finding of low resting HR is especially robust among children exhibiting aggression (Scarpa & Raine, 1997). Findings for autonomic *reactivity* to stressful stimuli have been more mixed, but as a whole the available findings point to *enhanced* HR and SC response to stressors in children exhibiting aggressive conduct problems specifically (Lorber, 2004)—particularly in those exhibiting *reactive* aggression; proactively aggressive children if anything tend to show attenuated reactivity to stressors compared with control children (Hubbard *et al.*, 2002). In addition, studies of parasympathetic versus sympathetic mediation of cardiovascular activity have yielded some evidence of weaker vagal-parasympathetic regulation of HR activity in children and adolescents exhibiting aggressive conduct problems (Mezzacappa *et al*., 1997; Beauchaine *et al*., 2001). Taken together, these findings are consistent with the idea that aggression in children entails difficulties regulating anger and other emotional reactions—with consequent enhancement of defensive reactivity under conditions of threat.

One focus of research with adults has been on differences in autonomic (particularly cardiac) activity in individuals high on aggression-related traits such as hostility, anger expression, and Type A personality. Significant effects when obtained have generally been in the direction of heightened autonomic reactivity to stressful events in high trait-aggressive individuals, particularly during interpersonal stress (e.g., Suls & Wan, 1993; Smith & Gallo, 1999; Peters *et al*., 2003). Studies comparing autonomic reactivity in adults with and without a history of violent behaviour have yielded less consistent results. For example, physiological studies of men who have assaulted their romantic partners have not revealed consistent differences in relation to non-assaultive men (Gottman *et al*., 1995; Meehan *et al*., 2001; Babcock *et al*., 2004). Fewer studies have examined physiological response differences in individuals with a history of physical abuse towards children. One study by Frodi and Lamb (1980) reported enhanced autonomic reactivity to infant emotional displays (both smiling and crying) in women with a history of abuse compared to non-abusive women.

Most published studies involving autonomic response qualify as marker studies because they have focused on detecting simple reactivity differences between aggressive and non-aggressive individuals. In some cases, speculative inferences have been made about underlying psychological processes based on the use of particular measures (e.g., cardiac variability as an index of vagal regulation) or particular stimulus manipulations (e.g., aversive versus non-aversive cues, interpersonal versus physical stressors). However, studies of this kind have for the most part not set out to measure specific processing differences online. One exception is recent work by Verona and colleagues examining the mediating role of negative emotional activation in enhancing punitive behaviour among aggression-prone individuals (e.g., Verona *et al*., 2002; Verona & Curtin, 2006).

In summary, aggressive children and adolescents consistently exhibit lower baseline levels of autonomic arousal but higher autonomic reactivity to stressful events. Similarly, research with adult samples has generally indicated enhanced autonomic reactivity to stressors (interpersonal stressors in particular) in hostile-aggressive individuals. In contrast, markedly different results are evident in psychophysiological studies of psychopathy. Most recent work of this kind has focused on incarcerated offenders assessed using Hare's *Psychopathy Checklist-Revised* (PCL-R). Adult psychopathic offenders, relative to non-psychopaths, show *reduced* electrodermal response to aversive cues and during anticipation of stressful events (Hare, 1978; Arnett, 1997; Lorber, 2004), and normal HR reactivity (Lorber, 2004). They also tend to show normal baseline levels of HR and electrodermal arousal (Hare, 1978; Arnett, 1997; but see Hansen *et al*., 2007).

These contrasting results are noteworthy because psychopathy—in particular, the antisocial deviance ('Factor 2'; Hare, 2003) features, which consist of tendencies towards impulsivity, recklessness, and aggression—is reliably associated with increased violence and violent recidivism in offender samples (Hemphill *et al*., 1998; Walters, 2003; Porter & Woodworth, 2006). However, a PCL-R diagnosis of psychopathy also requires the presence of affective-interpersonal features, including absence of remorse or empathy, shallow affect, glibness and grandiosity, and manipulativeness (Hare, 2003). Although at odds with results for impulsive-aggressive individuals, the finding of reduced autonomic (especially electrodermal) reactivity to stressors fits with the idea that psychopathy (in particular, its affective-interpersonal features) is associated with reduced fear capacity (Patrick, 1994; Lykken, 1995; Patrick, 2007; Frick & White, 2008). The affective-interpersonal features of psychopathy are also more related to instrumental or proactive aggression (Porter & Woodworth, 2006) than to the impulsive or reactive type of aggression that has been emphasized historically in physiological studies. Thus, individuals possessing the core-affective features of psychopathy need to be considered separately from other types of violent offenders in attempting to understand neurobiological substrates of aggressive behaviour.

Electrocortical response measures: EEG and ERP

Early EEG studies of violent criminal offenders revealed evidence of enhanced cortical slow-wave activity in brain areas including frontal and temporal regions, particularly in the delta (<4 Hz) frequency range (cf. Volavka, 1990). Subsequent studies successfully replicated this finding, with longitudinal research demonstrating that increased slow-wave EEG activity in adolescence predicted later emergence of antisocial behaviour (i.e., criminal convictions) in adulthood (Raine *et al.*, 1990). Theoretical interpretations of this enhanced slow-wave EEG have focused on cortical immaturity resulting in impaired inhibitory control (Volavka, 1990), and cortical underarousal that predisposes towards compensatory stimulation seeking (Raine *et al.*, 1990).

In addition, associations with aggression have been reported for various components of the ERP. The most consistent finding has been reduced amplitude of P300 response to intermittent target stimuli in oddball tasks. Diminished P300 has been reported especially among individuals exhibiting aggression of the impulsive type (e.g., Barratt *et al.*, 1997b; Branchey *et al.*, 1988; Gerstle *et al.*, 1998). Reduced P300 amplitude has also been reported in individuals diagnosed with antisocial personality (Bauer *et al.*, 1994), a disorder that often includes impulsive aggressive behaviour. In addition, however, reduced P300 has been found for a variety of other impulse control problems, most notably alcohol dependence (cf. Polich *et al.*, 1994)—but also drug dependence, nicotine dependence, child conduct disorder, and attention deficit hyperactivity disorder (cf. Iacono *et al.*, 2002). The implication is that reduced P300 amplitude may reflect something these disorders have in common, rather than what is unique to any one of them. As discussed in the third section of this chapter, reduced P300 amplitude appears to be an indicator of the broad 'externalizing' factor (Krueger, 1999) that these disorders share. We hypothesize that this broad factor, which has been conceptualized as a dispositional vulnerability to impulse control problems of various kinds (Krueger *et al.*, 2002), represents a key to understanding aggressive behaviour—in particular, impulsive or reactive aggression.

In contrast with findings from studies of impulsive aggressive individuals, Stanford *et al.* (2003) reported no difference in P300 amplitude to auditory target stimuli in psychiatric outpatients characterized as 'premeditated aggressors' compared with controls. Similarly, Barratt *et al.* (1997b) found no evidence of a relationship between premeditated aggression and P300. Results from these studies indicate that the association between reduced P300 and aggression may be specific to individuals who manifest aggression of an impulsive nature. Studies examining the association between psychopathy and P300 amplitude have yielded mixed results, with some showing a negative association, others a positive association, and still others no association (see reviews by Raine, 1989, 1993, along with more recent work by

Kiehl *et al.*, 1999).[1] As noted earlier, these inconsistent findings could reflect the fact that a diagnosis of psychopathy includes affective-interpersonal features in addition to antisocial deviance symptoms. The affective-interpersonal features, which tend to be associated more with proactive rather than impulsive aggression, may moderate the association between psychopathy and brain potential response in some samples.

As with studies using autonomic measures, most published EEG and ERP studies of aggressive individuals consist of marker studies aimed at detecting differences in brain activity at rest or in simple task procedures. Given the fine-grained information available from EEG and/or ERP measurement in time and frequency domains (cf. second last section of this chapter), together with advances in EEG source localization methods, there is potentially much to be learned in the future from process-oriented studies of aggression-prone individuals using electrocortical measures.

Neuroimaging measures: CT, SPECT, PET, and MRI

Three older neuroimaging studies involving violent psychiatric patients and homicide offenders that employed computerized tomography (CT), a technique in which fluctuations in X-ray beams passed through the brain are used to index brain structure, reported evidence of abnormalities in temporal (Tonkonogy, 1991; Wong *et al.*, 1994) and frontal brain regions (Blake *et al.*, 1995). More recent studies using single photon emission computerized tomography (SPECT)-a procedure in which photons emitted by a radioactive isotope injected into the brain are measured to index regional activity—have also yielded consistent evidence of abnormalities in the prefrontal cortex and the temporal lobes. Three studies that used SPECT to assess brain activity at rest in psychiatric patients exhibiting severe antagonism, physical attack, or property destruction (Amen *et al.*, 1996; Hirono *et al.*, 2000) or impulsive violent offenders (Soderstrom *et al.*, 2000) found evidence of reduced blood flow in both the prefrontal cortex and the temporal lobes (left temporal lobe, specifically, in 2 of the 3 studies). In contrast with reductions evident in these brain regions, Amen *et al.* (1996) reported *increased* activity in basal ganglia and subcortical (limbic) regions in an aggressive patient sample. One other SPECT study (Kuruoglu *et al.*, 1996) reported reduced blood flow in frontal brain regions in alcoholic individuals with co-morbid antisocial personality compared with non-alcoholic controls. SPECT has also been used to examine differences in neurotransmitter function in impulsively violent offenders, with findings indicating abnormal dopaminergic neurotransmission in the striatum and diminished serotonin transporter density in the midbrain (Tiihonen *et al.*, 1995; Tiihonen *et al.*, 1997).

Studies employing PET comprise the largest number of published neuroimaging studies of aggression to date. PET, similar to SPECT, relies on measurement of particles (positrons) from an injected radioisotope to index neural activity or neurotransmitter function in specific brain regions. Most PET studies have reported evidence of prefrontal brain dysfunction

---

[1] Relations with psychopathy have been reported for other components of the ERP besides P300. For example, studies by Kiehl and colleagues have yielded evidence of an abnormal late negativity, maximal over frontocentral scalp regions, among high PCL-R scoring offenders within a variety of stimulus-processing and decision-making tasks (for an overview Relations with psychopathy have been reported for other components of the ERP besides P300. For example, studies by Kiehl and colleagues have yielded evidence of an abnormal late negativity, maximal over frontocentral scalp regions, among high PCL-R scoring offenders within a variety of stimulus-processing and decision-making tasks (for an overview of this work, see Kiehl et al., 2006).

in violent individuals compared with controls (for a detailed review, see Patrick & Verona, 2007). Some of these have measured brain activity at rest (e.g., Volkow & Tancredi, 1987), others during simple (e.g., continuous performance) tasks designed to activate the prefrontal cortex (e.g., Raine *et al.*, 1994; Raine *et al.*, 1997). Raine *et al.* (1998) subgrouped 41 convicted murderers into predatory (proactive) and affective (impulsive) subgroups based on the nature of their crimes, and found that prefrontal dysfunction was specific to the affective subgroup. Other studies that have used PET to assess brain reactivity to drugs in impulsive-aggressive patients (e.g., Siever *et al.*, 1999; New *et al.*, 2002) have reported blunted reactivity to serotonin agonists (as evidenced by lower levels of glucose metabolism) in regions of prefrontal cortex, particularly orbitofrontal and ventromedial regions. Additional brain regions implicated in these and other PET imaging studies include the temporal cortex, anterior cingulate cortex, and to a lesser degree, the hippocampus and amygdala.

With regard to the amygdala and hippocampus, Raine *et al.* (1997) found evidence of abnormal asymmetry (i.e., decreased left side versus increased right side function) in both of these structures in murderers compared with controls. In a PET study of serotonin binding potential, Parsey *et al.* (2002) reported a negative association between reported lifetime aggression and binding in brain regions including the amygdala (but not hippocampus). George *et al.* (2004) examined domestic abusers with co-morbid alcoholism and reported decreased correlations between glucose activity in the amygdala and glucose activity in various cortical structures in comparison with non-violent controls. These authors interpreted these decreased associations as reflecting a lack of cortical input to the amygdala associated with increased sensitivity to environmental stressors in impulsively violent individuals.

Studies using structural magnetic resonance imaging (sMRI) to investigate neuroanatomic differences associated with impulsive aggressive behaviour have yielded less consistent results than PET studies. Two studies—one involving temporal lobe epilepsy patients with aggressive-assaultive behaviour (Woermann *et al.*, 2000) and the other female patients diagnosed with borderline personality disorder (van Elst *et al.*, 2003)—reported reduced grey matter volume in the prefrontal cortex, with the latter study also reporting volume reductions in the anterior cingulate cortex, hippocampus, and amygdala. Dolan *et al.* (2002) found a significant reduction in temporal lobe volume in impulsive-aggressive patients compared with controls but no reduction in frontal lobe volume, and two other studies that examined subcortical structures (Laakso *et al.*, 2000; van Elst *et al.*, 2000) found no difference between violent and non-violent patient groups in hippocampal or amygdala volume.

Few studies of violent individuals have been conducted using fMRI. Raine *et al.* (2001) examined brain activation during a working memory task in small groups of community participants with histories of serious violent behaviour and/or early abuse (n = 4–5) relative to a healthy control group (n = 9). Compared with controls, violent individuals who had been abused as children showed reduced right hemisphere activation (particularly in right temporal regions), whereas abused individuals without violence showed lower left, but higher right activation of the superior temporal gyrus. Both these groups also showed generally reduced cortical activation during task processing, particularly in the left hemisphere. The authors interpreted these findings as indicating a unique role of right hemisphere dysfunction, when combined with exposure to early abuse, in violent behaviour. However, these findings must be considered tentative due to the small sample sizes.

Other published neuroimaging studies have examined brain differences in individuals diagnosed as psychopathic using Hare's (2003) PCL-R (for a review, see Raine & Yang, 2006). The findings of these studies are difficult to compare with those already reviewed because they did not focus specifically on aggressive behaviour, and because individuals diagnosed as psychopathic differ from individuals who primarily exhibit impulsive (reactive) aggression. In particular, psychopathy is theorized to involve a deficiency in negative affectivity (in particular, anxiety or fear; Patrick, 1994; Lykken, 1995) and it has been theorized that psychopaths differ from other aggressive-antisocial individuals in subcortical brain structures that mediate basic emotional processing (e.g., the amygdala; Intrator *et al.*, 1997; Blair, 2006; Frick & White, 2008). The few neuroimaging studies that have separated violent offender participants into emotionally overreactive versus predatory-psychopathic subgroups (e.g., Raine *et al.*, 1998) have reported differing patterns of results for these groups. For these reasons, it is important to consider psychophysiological (including neuroimaging) findings for impulsively violent individuals separately from findings for individuals diagnosed as psychopathic or exhibiting mainly predatory (proactive) aggression.

From the foregoing summary, it is apparent that most published neuroimaging studies of aggressive individuals qualify as marker studies. These studies point to deviations in the structure and functioning of frontal, temporal, and anterior cingulate brain regions in impulsive-aggressive individuals, but the nature of the cognitive and affective processing deficits arising from these brain abnormalities remains unclear. Accordingly, there is a great need for PET and neuroimaging studies that target specific processes underlying aggressive behaviour. As an illustration of this, Pietrini *et al.* (2000) reported evidence of decreased blood flow in the prefrontal cortex (particularly, in the ventromedial region) in healthy control participants during imagery of a scenario in which they expressed unrestrained aggressive behaviour in comparison with imagery of a neutral scene. In contrast, Drexler *et al.* (2000) reported *increased* activity in the inferior frontal cortex during imagery of a personal anger scene versus a neutral scene in a different control sample. The fact that participants in the Pietrini *et al.* study imagined themselves actively aggressing may account for the difference in findings across these two studies: activation of the ventromedial prefrontal cortex may occur primarily during anger states in which aggressive urges are suppressed rather than enacted (cf. Davidson *et al.*, 2000).

An integrative conceptual framework for interpreting results from psychophysiological studies of aggression and violence

To provide a basis for thinking integratively about existing research on the psychophysiology of aggression, two conceptual models are considered: (i) a hierarchical model of externalizing syndromes that conceives of various types of impulse control problems, including aggressive-antisocial behaviour, as manifestations of a common dispositional vulnerability, and (ii) a neurobiological model that views persistent aggression as arising from dysfunction in a set of interconnected brain systems (including the prefrontal cortex, anterior cingulate cortex, and amygdala) that function to regulate affective states, including anger.

Hierarchical model of the externalizing spectrum

An integrative, hierarchical model of the externalizing spectrum—encompassing child and adult antisocial deviance, alcohol and drug dependence, and impulsive personality traits— has recently been developed to account for the systematic covariance (co-morbidity) known to exist among these phenomena. The foundation for this model was a behaviour genetic study by Krueger *et al.* (2002). These authors performed confirmatory factor analyses on diagnostic and psychometric data from a large mixed-gender sample of monozygotic and dizygotic twins (n = 1048) recruited from the community. Variables in the analysis included symptom scores for four DSM disorders (child conduct disorder, adult antisocial behaviour, alcohol dependence, and drug dependence) along with a self-report measure of disinhibitory personality traits consisting of reversed scores on the Constraint factor of Tellegen's (1982) Multidimensional Personality Questionnaire. The best-fitting model of the data was a common pathways model in which a shared general factor (externalizing) contributed aetiologically to all primary variables in the model. Over 80% of the variance in this common factor was found to be attributable to additive genetic influence. Non-shared environmental influence accounted for most of the residual variance in each primary variable not accounted for by the broad externalizing factor—although for conduct disorder a significant contribution was also found for shared environment. Based on these findings, Krueger *et al.* (2002) advanced a hierarchical model in which a largely heritable general vulnerability contributes to the development of various traits and disorders in the externalizing spectrum, but the distinctive expression of this underlying vulnerability (i.e., as disinhibitory personality traits, antisocial behaviour of different sorts, or as alcohol or drug problems) is determined by other specific aetiologic influences.

Krueger *et al.* (2007) extended this work by undertaking a more comprehensive analysis of personality trait and behavioural constructs within the domain of externalizing. Self-report items were developed to index constructs embodied in the diagnostic criteria for conduct disorder, adult antisocial behaviour, alcohol dependence, drug dependence (cf. Krueger *et al.*, 2002), along with other constructs (e.g., impulsivity and aggression of varying types, non-conformity, stimulation seeking) identified as relevant to externalizing through a review of existing literatures. Quantitative methods including item response modelling and confirmatory factor analysis were applied across multiple rounds of data collection to refine the item set as well as clarify the nature of constructs linked to the broad externalizing factor. The final result was a set of 23 constructs, each assessed by a distinctive scale. Confirmatory factor analyses of these 23 construct scales yielded evidence of one superordinate factor ('Externalizing') on which all scales loaded, and two subordinate factors that accounted for residual variance in particular scales. The two subordinate factors were independent from one another statistically, and independent also from the superordinate externalizing factor. Table 12.1 lists the 23 scales of the Externalizing inventory along with loadings of each scale on the general Externalizing factor and on each of the two subfactors. It can be seen that all of the scales loaded 0.45 or higher on the general factor, with irresponsibility and problematic impulsivity scales demonstrating the highest loadings. The table also shows that variance in some of the scales not accounted for by the general Externalizing factor was associated with one or the other subfactor. One subordinate factor was defined by residual variance in subscales measuring aggression (all three types), callousness, excitement seeking, rebelliousness, and (low) honesty; the other subfactor was defined by residual variance in subscales indexing alcohol or drug use and substance-related problems. It is important to note that the variance defining each of these subfactors consisted of residual variance from particular scales unrelated (orthogonal) to the broad externalizing factor.

The findings of this research provide further support for the idea that a broad dispositional factor contributes to the emergence of a wide range of externalizing problems as well as to disinhibitory personality traits that have been linked to such problems. In addition, the findings of this work have important implications for conceptualization and understanding of aggressive behaviour. A sizable portion of the variance in all three types of aggression represented in the Externalizing inventory was accounted for by the general factor on which all scales loaded. In addition, residual variance in each aggression scale went towards defining a separate, statistically independent factor on which low empathy (callousness) and excitement seeking also loaded prominently. Notably, among the three aggression scales, it was the physical aggression scale (which emphasizes reactive or angry aggressive tendencies more so than proactive or instrumental tendencies) that loaded most strongly on the general Externalizing factor (i.e., 0.74 versus 0.62–0.65), whereas it was the relational aggression scale (which emphasizes proactive or instrumental aggressive tendencies in particular) that loaded most strongly on the callous-aggression subfactor (i.e., 0.68 versus 0.41–0.55).

The findings of this research are consistent with the idea that differing types of aggressive behaviour are interrelated (e.g., Bushman & Anderson, 2001), yet meaningfully distinct from one another (e.g., Dodge, 1991). The findings of Krueger *et al.* (2007) suggest that a general propensity towards impulse control problems contributes to aggression in varying forms-in particular, to physically aggressive acts prompted by provocation or stress. From this standpoint, the broad externalizing factor represents an important target of investigation in the study of impulsive-reactive aggression in particular. In addition, a separate propensity involving deficient empathy and stimulation-seeking tendencies appears to contribute independently to aggressive behaviour—particularly aggression that involves instrumental coercion and abuse of others. Other constructs that loaded to some degree on this callous-aggression subfactor included dishonesty, fraudulence, rebelliousness, and a tendency to externalize blame (Table 12.1). These various features are reminiscent of the core affective-interpersonal component of psychopathy in Hare's PCL-R, which tends to be associated more so with proactive or instrumental aggression than with reactive or impulsive aggression. This callous-aggression subfactor may be important for reconciling divergences in findings for aggressive individuals diagnosed as psychopathic compared with those low in core psychopathic features. For example, Frick and White (2008) have proposed that callous-unemotional tendencies (which are associated with diminished anxiety and fearfuless, and proactive forms of aggression) comprise a distinct aetiologic pathway, distinct from general disinhibitory tendencies, to conduct problems and antisocial deviance later in life.

In sum, the hierarchical model of externalizing traits and behaviours provides a framework for isolating distinctive factors contributing to varying subtypes of aggression that can be targeted separately in neurobiological studies.

Neurobiological model of impulsive aggression

The other model we consider is the neurobiological model of aggressive behaviour formulated by Davidson and colleagues (2000). In this model, impulsive aggression is viewed as arising from dysfunction in set of interrelated brain structures that function to regulate emotional processing and reactivity—including the prefrontal cortex (in particular, its orbitofrontal and ventromedial subdivisions), the anterior cingulate cortex, and subcortical-limbic structures (in particular, the amygdala, hippocampus, and hypothalamus). The subcortical elements of this circuit play a primary role in activating emotional states, whereas the anterior cingulate cortex and prefrontal cortex operate to detect circumstances under which affective control is needed and to implement control processes, respectively. From the standpoint of this model, repetitive episodes of impulsive aggression (as tend to be characteristic of high-externalizing individuals) reflect a breakdown in the normal capacity to recognize and respond to signals of possible provocation as they arise and/or to modulate defensive reactivity in the face of immediate provocation or threat.

Table 12.1 Loadings of 23 scales of the Externalizing inventory on general factor and residual subfactors.

Externalizing scale	General factor	First subfactor	Second subfactor
Irresponsibility	**0.93**	0.00	−0.01
Dependability	**−0.66**	−0.15	0.00
Problematic impulsivity	**0.91**	0.00	−0.04
Impatient urgency	**0.73**	0.22	0.00
Planful control	**−0.66**	−0.07	0.00
Theft	**0.87**	0.00	0.13
Alienation	**0.49**	0.01	0.00
Blame externalization	**0.51**	0.24	0.00
Relational aggression	**0.62**	**0.68**	0.00
Destructive aggression	**0.65**	**0.55**	0.00
Physical aggression	**0.74**	0.41	0.00
Empathy	**−0.48**	**−0.55**	0.00
Excitement seeking	**0.56**	0.46	0.00
Rebelliousness	**0.79**	0.31	0.00
Boredom proneness	**0.59**	−0.31	0.00
Honesty	**−0.54**	**−0.31**	0.00
Fraud	**0.87**	0.26	0.00
Marijuana use	**0.73**	0.00	**0.61**
Marijuana problems	**0.75**	0.00	**0.48**
Other drug use	**0.79**	0.00	**0.49**
Other drug problems	**0.87**	0.00	**0.30**
Alcohol use	**0.45**	0.00	**0.36**
Alcohol problems	**0.69**	0.00	0.24

Note: Loading coefficients reflect standardized parameter estimates from a hierarchical model with two subfactors fit using semi-parametric maximum likelihood estimation (for details, see Krueger *et al.*, 2007). Loadings higher than greater than +/–0.30 are bolded. Loadings listed as zero to two decimal values were fixed at this value and not estimated.

Interpretation of results from existing psychophysiological studies

A number of consistent findings have emerged from psychophysiological studies of aggression and aggressive individuals. One is the finding of low baseline HR, including work by Raine *et al.* demonstrating that low resting HR prospectively predicts the emergence of antisocial deviance in at-risk individuals. Reduced baseline HR has been interpreted as reflecting low dispositional arousal, which is assumed to promote stimulation seeking and disinhibited behaviour (Raine, 1993, 2002; Ortiz & Raine, 2004). However, this interpretation remains speculative, as no research has yet been conducted to directly assess the functional role of low cardiac arousal in the disinhibited behaviour of antisocial-aggressive individuals.

Two consistent findings from the electrocortical literature are those of enhanced EEG slow wave activity and reduced P300 brain potential response in antisocial-aggressive individuals.

Enhanced EEG slow wave, similar to low resting HR, has been theorized to reflect low dispositional arousal that motivates stimulation seeking (Eysenck, 1967; Zuckerman, 1979). Differing interpretations have been attached to the finding of reduced P300 response amplitude in individuals with externalizing problems (e.g., Iacono, 1998; Begleiter & Porjesz, 1999). One interpretation that fits with the evidence for low resting HR and enhanced EEG slow wave, as well as with evidence for diminished non-specific electrodermal actvity (cf. Raine, 1993), is that anticipatory and preparatory activities are reduced in such individuals, resulting in a more stimulus-driven processing style (Taylor *et al.*, 1999). Relevant to this, Malone *et al.* (2002) reported that high-externalizing individuals showed reduced vigilance, as indexed by alpha-band EEG activity, prior to the occurrence of stimuli in a visual oddball task in which reduced P300 was observed.

Although findings pertaining to P300 amplitude reduction in antisocial-aggressive individuals have been emphasized in this review, it should be noted that, historically, reduced P300 has been investigated more extensively as an indicator of risk for alcohol problems (cf. Polich *et al.*, 1994). Reports of reduced P300 amplitude in relation to other externalizing syndromes (e.g., conduct disorder, antisocial personality, drug dependence) have appeared more recently. These more recent findings raised the possibility that P300 amplitude reduction might reflect a disposition towards externalizing problems generally rather than to specific problem(s) within this spectrum. Patrick *et al.* (2006) tested this hypothesis in a large sample of adolescent male twins and found that the general factor representing the overlap among various externalizing syndromes (conduct disorder, adult antisocial behaviour, and alcohol, nicotine, and other drug dependence) fully accounted for bivariate associations between individual syndromes and reduced P300 amplitude. In a follow-up study that capitalized on the twin composition of this sample, Hicks *et al.* (2007) undertook biometric analyses to examine the aetiologic basis of the relationship between externalizing and P300 amplitude and established that the relationship was mediated primarily by genes.

This work is important because it demonstrates that a known physiological indicator of impulsive aggressive behaviour, reduced P300 response amplitude, is in fact an endophenotype marker of the externalizing vulnerability factor that contributes to various problems of impulse control, including impulsive or reactive aggression. In turn, this raises the question of whether low resting HR and increased EEG slow-wave activity are specific to antisocial-aggressive individuals, or if these physiological indicators might be associated with externalizing vulnerability more generally. To address this question, it will be valuable in future research to systematically investigate relations between these physiological indicators and other problems that fall within the externalizing spectrum (e.g., alcohol, drug, and nicotine dependence). In addition, the finding that P300 represents a marker of general externalizing vulnerability rather than an indicator of specific problems within this spectrum highlights the importance of the broad externalizing factor as a target for investigation in the study of aggressive behaviour. This broad factor plays an important role in aggression of various forms (physical, relational, destructive; Krueger *et al.*, 2007) and, as illustrated in the next section, the hierarchical model of externalizing provides a strategy for isolating this broad aetiologic factor and investigating its correlates and mechanisms separately from other aetiologic variables.

In contrast with findings of reduced autonomic and electrocortical arousal at rest and in simple stimulus processing tasks, other research has demonstrated *enhanced* phasic reactivity to stressful or aversive stimuli in hostile, aggressive, and abusive individuals—including enhanced cardiac and skin conductance reactivity to stressors, poor regulation of autonomic activity during anticipation of aversive events, and reduced cardiac vagal tone.

Furthermore, some evidence exists to indicate that this pattern of heightened reactivity to aversive cues or events, such as reduced P300 brain response, may be generally characteristic of individuals with impulse control problems, rather than specific to impulsive aggressive individuals (Taylor *et al.*, 1999). Although the finding of enhanced reactivity to phasic stressors might seem inconsistent with data indicating low resting activation levels, the aforementioned hypothesis that externalizing (including proneness to impulsive-aggressive) entails a reactive, stimulus-driven processing style provides a framework for interpreting this overall configuration of results. From this perspective, high-externalizing individuals are more reactive to immediate stressors or challenges because they anticipate and prepare for them less effectively. This configuration of results is also consistent with Davidson *et al.*'s (2000) neurobiological conceptualization of impulsive aggression: aggression-prone individuals are impaired in conflict-detection and/or emotion-regulation systems that mediate normal anticipation of events and proactive coping efforts; as a function of this, they exhibit reduced levels of activation until stressors or challenges are actually encountered. Indeed, it can be argued that impairments in the regulatory circuitry identified by Davidson *et al.* underlie the impulsive aggressive tendencies of individuals high on the broad externalizing factor.

A further point is that these findings for impulsive-aggression (and externalizing more generally) are clearly at odds with findings for the syndrome of psychopathy. Adult psychopathic offenders do not show reliable differences in resting autonomic activity levels or P300 brain potential response (Raine, 1993), whereas they do show consistent reductions in phasic reactivity to aversive cues, including diminished SC response (cf. Hare, 1978; Arnett, 1997) and startle reflex potentiation (cf. Patrick, 1994, 2007). The explanation for this divergence in findings almost certainly lies in the distinction between the affective-interpersonal versus the antisocial deviance features of psychopathy: it is the latter features that reflect heightened externalizing tendencies, including aggression and impulsiveness (Patrick *et al.*, 2005; Patrick, 2007). However, most EEG and/or ERP and brain imaging studies have not examined effects for these two components of psychopathy separately (for exceptions, see: Laakso *et al.*, 2001; de Oliveira-Souza *et al.*, 2008). This is a crucial issue that needs to be addressed systematically in future research. Related to this, it will be important in future research to systematically examine alternative forms of aggression associated with differing underlying motives (e.g., proactive-instrumental versus reactive-impulsive) in relation to these two psychopathy factors in order to clarify relations with neurobiological measures. In particular, it is the impulsive-reactive subtype that appears to be most related to externalizing and to impairments in brain systems that govern emotion regulation. It will also be valuable in future studies to include multiple measures of physiological response (peripheral-autonomic along with electrocortical; EEG together with structural or functional neuroimaging) so that findings for different measures can be directly compared within the same task procedures.

With regard to neuroimaging studies, research of this kind-together with research on serotonin system function in aggressive individuals and studies of patients with lesions to distinct regions of the prefrontal cortex—served as the basis empirical basis for Davidson *et al.*'s (2000) neurobiological model of aggression. As described earlier, these authors postulated that impulsive aggressive behaviour arises from dysfunction in frontocortical and limbic brain regions that mediate affective reactivity and regulation. Specifically, these authors proposed that (1) the orbitomedial prefrontal cortex, which connects directly with limbic structures as well as other regions of the frontal cortex, plays a crucial role in regulating (i.e., maintaining, inhibiting, or enhancing) emotional states activated by subcortical structures such as the amygdala; and (2) the anterior cingulate cortex functions to signal the need for regulatory control on the part of the prefrontal cortex by detecting conflict among competing goals and response dispositions. Consistent with this formulation, neuroimaging studies have consistently yielded evidence of reduced activity in prefrontal brain regions (including the orbitomedial cortex) in aggressive individuals, together with some evidence of reduced activity in the anterior cingulate cortex. The finding that high-externalizing individuals show reduced brain error-related negativity (ERN) following incorrect responses in a speeded performance task (see the next section) lends further support to the idea that impaired anterior cingulate function plays a role in impulsive aggression.

It bears mention again that most published psychophysiological studies of aggressive individuals to date (including neuroimaging studies) qualify as marker studies, in that they have focused either on differences in brain structure or differences in physiological activity at rest or in simple stimulus tasks. A pressing need exists for process-oriented studies aimed at elucidating differences in online cognitive and affective processing with functional relevance to aggression—including cortical psychophysiology studies that capitalize on the fine-grained temporal and frequency information afforded by EEG and/or ERP, and functional neuroimaging studies that capitalize on the fine-grained spatial information provided by MRI. The next section describes some examples of research of this kind by our lab group.

From markers to mechanisms: using cortical event-related potentials to identify processes underlying the aggressive behaviour of high-externalizing individuals

This section describes new investigative work by our laboratory group that build on findings from prior published research identifying electrocortical (ERP) indicators of aggressive-externalizing tendencies. This work capitalizes on the fine-grained information provided by EEG measurement in both time and frequency domains to elucidate differences in online processing of semantic and emotional information associated with externalizing tendencies. This work, which points to externalizing-related impairments in anterior brain systems governing post-perceptual elaborative processing of stimulus events (including affective events), has implications for our understanding of impulsive-reactive aggression in particular.

Post-processing of discrete stimulus events: P300 brain potential response

As noted earlier, recent published work has demonstrated that reduced P300 amplitude is a reliable brain response marker of the general externalizing factor that underlies impulse control problems of various kinds (Patrick *et al.*, 2006) and that the association between P300 and externalizing is mediated largely by genetic influences (Hicks *et al.*, 2007). The implication is that reduced P300 directly reflects some alteration in brain function associated with the broad, predominantly heritable vulnerability to disorders within the externalizing spectrum. What might the finding of reduced P300 response tell us about the brain mechanisms underlying this broad vulnerability? Although the P300 has been characterized for some time as a distributed brain response reflecting activity in multiple brain regions, more recent research on the neutral generators underlying P300 response supports the idea that prefrontal brain regions play a particularly important role (see, for example, Dien *et al.*, 2003; Nieuwenhuis *et al.*, 2005). In addition, new research by our laboratory group has yielded evidence of an enhanced relationship between externalizing scores and P300 amplitude at frontocentral compared with parietal scalp sites, particularly for novel task stimuli that are known to preferentially activate anterior brain regions.

The task procedure we have used to further investigate reduced P300 in relation to externalizing is a three-stimulus variant of the rotated heads oddball task (Bernat *et al.*, 2003). In addition to non-target oval (70% of trials) and target 'head' stimuli (15% of trials), the task includes infrequent novel stimuli (15% of trials) requiring no response. The novel stimuli consist of pleasant, neutral, and unpleasant picture stimuli selected from the International Affective Picture System (IAPS; Center for the Study of Emotion and Attention, 1999). All task stimuli occur for 100 ms, and because the primary task is to detect and respond to the target heads, the novel picture stimuli are processed incidentally. Target stimuli in a task of this kind are known to elicit a P300 response that is maximal at parietal scalp sites. In contrast, novel stimuli evoke a P300 response, termed the 'novelty P3' (Courchesne *et al.*, 1975) or P3a response (Squires *et al.*, 1975) to distinguish it from the target P300 (P3) response, that is maximal at frontocentral scalp sites. With regard to generators, evidence exists for a role of the lateral prefrontal cortex in the processing of novel stimuli (see Newenhuis *et al.*, 2005) and ERP source localization work has additionally identified the anterior cingulate cortex (ACC) as contributing to the novelty P3 response (Dien *et al.*, 2003). Functional neuroimaging research also implicates these two regions in novel stimulus processing, consistent with the idea that frontal brain regions are involved in the allocation of attentional resources to novel stimuli, as well as the processing of affective cues (Yamaski *et al.*, 2002; Fichtenholtz *et al.*, 2004). The use of emotional and neutral pictures as incidental, novel stimuli in this 3-stimulus oddball task thus provided us with an opportunity to assess automatic affective processing in a context in which diminished cognitive-elaborative processing (as indexed by P300 response) has reliably been observed.

The strategy we have used to select subjects for recent studies of externalizing using this task procedure is to administer a 100-item screening version of the Externalizing Inventory (Krueger *et al.*, 2007) to students in large undergraduate classes. Scores on this screening version correlate very highly ($r = 0.98$) with scores on the full, 415-item Externalizing inventory. Individuals in the lowest and highest quartiles of the overall score distribution are oversampled to provide Low-Externalizing (EXT) and High-Externalizing groups of adequate size, and in addition, individuals among the middle 50% of scorers are included to provide for supplementary correlational analyses in which the full distribution of EXT scores is represented. Using this strategy, a total of 149 participants were selected and tested in the 3-stimulus oddball task: 34 (21 female) in the Low-EXT group, 61 (34 female) in the High-EXT group, and 54 (34 female) intermediate scorers. Brain activity was recorded from 64 scalp sites, including frontal and central as well as parietal sites.

This work has yielded a number of important findings. First, we replicated the finding of reduced P3 amplitude to target (head) stimuli in this task, both in the extreme groups analysis and in the correlational analysis involving the full participant sample ($N = 149$). High-Externalizing participants showed significantly smaller P3 amplitude than Low-Externalizing participants at varying scalp sites, and significant negative correlations were evident between Externalizing scores and P3 amplitude in the sample as a whole at varying sites. This finding is important because it confirms that high scores on the Externalizing Inventory, similar to high scores on the externalizing factor computed from DSM diagnostic symptoms, are associated with reduced P3 brain response. Fig. 12.1 depicts average target P3 waveforms for low- and high-externalizing groups at representative anterior (midline frontocentral; FCz) and posterior (midline parietal; Pz) scalp sites, along with the topography of the P3/ Externalizing association across all sites. Notably, consistent with the hypothesis that reduced P3 in externalizing individuals reflects a deviation in frontal brain processing, the negative association between externalizing scores and target P3 response was stronger at the

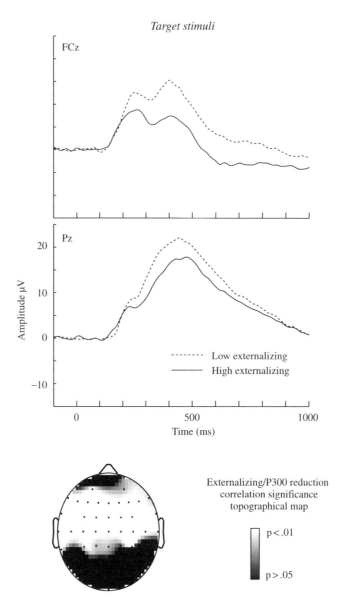

Fig. 12.1 Average ERP waveforms at frontocentral (FCz; upper plot) and parietal (Pz; lower plot) scalp sites for target stimuli in a visual oddball task, depicting reductions in P3 response amplitude for subgroups of high- (n = 61) versus low-externalizing participants (n = 34) as defined by scores on a 100-item screening version of the Externalizing Inventory (Krueger *et al.*, 2007). High- and low-externalizing groups were formed by oversampling from the top and bottom 25% of scorers in an undergraduate screening pool. The target stimuli were schematic 'head' stimuli calling for a button-press response. The statistical map at the bottom depicts the scalp topography distribution of the negative relationship between externalizing factor scores and P3 amplitude in the test sample as a whole (N = 149). From the topographic maps, it can be seen that the negative association between externalizing and P3 is most robust at anterior scalp sites.

FCz recording site than at the Pz site, $rs = -0.27$ and -0.12, respectively, and generally most robust at anterior scalp sites (see Fig. 12.1, bottom statistical-topographic map). A second key finding was that a parallel negative association was evident for novel (picture) stimuli as well, both in the extreme (High versus Low Externalizing) groups analysis and in the correlational analysis employing all subjects. As with target stimuli, the negative association for novel stimuli was stronger at FCz ($r = -0.27$) than at PCz ($r = -0.14$).

A further notable finding had to do with comparative brain responses to novel picture stimuli that were affective (pleasant or unpleasant) compared with neutral. Analyses of brain potential responses to affective pictures in relation to neutral pictures have consistently revealed a positive slow-wave component extending far beyond the P3 in time (e.g., Cuthbert et al., Schupp, Bradley, Birbaumer, & Lang, 2000; Schupp, et al., 2004). In order to examine effects for this affective EEG slow-wave component separately from the P3 response, a time-frequency signal decomposition was undertaken. Time-frequency decomposition (cf. Bernat et al., 2005) is a statistical technique that isolates ERP components through concurrent evaluation of activity in both time and frequency domains; the technique provides an effective way to separate brain signals that overlap in time but have distinctive frequency characteristics. For participants as a whole, the results of this decomposition revealed that a slow-wave (subdelta frequency) component, distinguishable from the higher-frequency (delta) component associated with the P3 response to pictures in general, accounted for most of the positive amplitude difference between affective and neutral pictures. Comparisons of Low- and High-Externalizing participant groups in terms of these two distinctive frequency components revealed that the effect of Externalizing was restricted to the higher-frequency (delta) P3 component; the slow-wave (subdelta) affect-differentiation component showed no significant difference in relation to Externalizing.

To summarize, High-Externalizing participants in this study showed no reduction in brain response differentiation between pictures that were affective compared with pictures that were neutral, despite showing an overall reduction in amplitude of P3 response to novel picture stimuli. This result indicates that even though high-externalizing individuals showed a generally attenuated cortical response to the novel picture stimuli (particularly at anterior scalp sites), these individuals nonetheless showed normal processing of the affective content of the pleasant and unpleasant pictures-suggesting an intact subcortical-affect processing system. As discussed in the final section, our interpretation of this dissociation in effects for differing ERP components is that high-externalizing individuals show normal reactivity to immediate perceptual and emotional features of explicit stimulus events, but impaired elaborative-associative processing of stimulus input in conjunction with basic perceptual and affective processing. This impairment results in weaker integration of current stimulus information with preexisting brain representations and lesser reliance on past experiences and future goals in the guidance of current behaviour.

Monitoring performance and outcomes of decision making: brain error-related negativities

In other work employing undergraduate participants pre-selected according to scores on the Externalizing inventory, we have examined negative-polarity scalp potentials associated with errors in responding and with loss-related feedback. In a recent published study (Hall et al., 2007), we reported a robust association between externalizing scores and reduced amplitude of the response-locked error-related negativity (r-ERN), a negative deflection of the ERP that occurs following errors in a performance task. The r-ERN is maximal at frontocentral scalp sites and has been characterized as a neurophysiological index of endogenous action monitoring-that is, of the brain's automatic capacity to monitor behavioural performance online and to initiate corrective action as needed (Gehring *et al.*, 1995; Carter *et al.*, 1998). Evidence from EEG source localization work indicates that the primary neural generator of the r-ERN is the anterior cingulate cortex (Dehaene *et al.*, 1994), a brain structure that has been implicated in self-monitoring and behavioural regulation (Bush *et al.*, 2000).

Using the 100-item Externalizing Inventory as a basis for subject selection and oversampling high and low scorers from a large undergraduate screening pool, Hall *et al.* (2007) evaluated the association between r-ERN amplitude and externalizing in 92 participants comprising 22 Low-Externalizing individuals, 38 High-Externalizing individuals, and 32 intermediate scorers. Consistent with prediction, r-ERN amplitude was significantly reduced in the High-Externalizing group (Fig. 12.2, upper line plot). Time-frequency analysis was used to isolate distinctive components of the response-locked ERP following commission of errors. This analysis yielded a dominant first component reflecting oscillatory activity within the theta frequency band (4–7 Hz). The peak of this theta activity component coincided in time with the peak of the r-ERN and showed a similar midline-central scalp distribution (Fig. 12.2, middle color plot). Further, a source localization analysis placed the source of this theta component squarely within the region of the anterior cingulate cortex. Paralleling results for r-ERN peak, the theta response to errors was maximal at electrode Cz, with theta activity significantly attenuated in the High-Externalizing group (Fig. 12.2, bottom statistical-topographic map).

The findings of this study demonstrate a relationship between reduced r-ERN response and externalizing tendencies that implies a weakness in the brain's capacity to automatically detect performance errors during online processing. A weakness in this capacity could contribute to problems that high-externalizing individuals show in learning from and adjust responding as a function of errors, and perhaps also to failures in regulating impulsive-aggressive actions. Notably, scores on the Externalizing Inventory in this study sample were correlated quite highly ($r = 0.69$) with scores on a measure of negative-affective aggression, the Aggression scale of Tellegen's (1982) MPQ. Given evidence for the anterior cingulate cortex as the primary generator of the r-ERN, the observed reduction in r-ERN response could reflect a deficit in anterior cingulate cortex functioning specifically. Alternatively, it could reflect impaired processing in other regions of the brain that participate with the anterior cingulate cortex in endogenous action monitoring.

To evaluate these competing alternatives, we undertook a follow-up study in which we examined brain responses to externally presented loss feedback in a decision-making task (Bernat *et al.*, 2008). The procedure we used was a simulated gambling task developed by Gehring and Willoughby (2002) in which participants choose between two numeric options and receive explicit visual feedback subsequently on whether their choice resulted in a monetary gain or a loss. The dependent measure of interest in this study was the feedback error-related negativity (f-ERN), an enhanced brain negativity that occurs following the presentation of monetary-loss or negative-performance feedback. Similar to the r-ERN, the f-ERN has been localized to the anterior cingulate cortex (Miltner *et al.*, 1997; Holroyd *et al.*, 2004), and a prominent theoretic model (the reinforcement learning theory; Holroyd & Coles, 2002) proposes that a common neural process—involving input from the mesencephalic dopamine system to the anterior cingulate cortex signalling that an outcome is 'worse than expected'-gives rise to both the r-ERN and the f-ERN. Nonetheless, it is important to note that the r-ERN occurs following error responses in the absence of explicit feedback, whereas the f-ERN occurs following presentation of explicit loss feedback. Although the anterior cingulate cortex may generate similar brain negativities following the

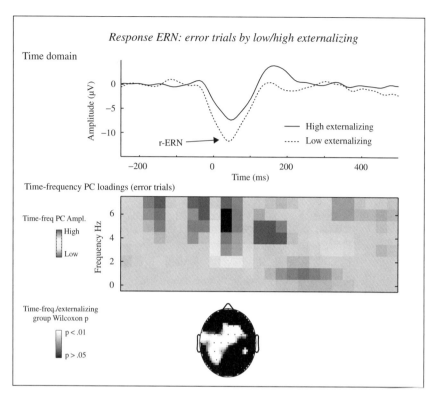

Fig. 12.2 Time–domain and time–frequency (TF) representations of response error-related negativity (r-ERN) differences for subgroups of high- (n = 38) versus low-externalizing participants (n = 22) as defined by scores on a 100-item screening version of the Externalizing Inventory (Krueger *et al.*, 2007). High and low externalizing groups were formed by oversampling from the top and bottom 25% of scorers in an undergraduate screening pool. **Top** (line plot): Average response-locked ERP waveforms at the midline central (Cz) scalp site for trials of a flanker task in which participants made incorrect responses, depicting reduced amplitude of the r-ERN for participants high on externalizing. The r-ERN is visible as a prominent negative deflection that peaks around 50 ms post-response. **Middle** (colour-surface plot; see Colour Plate Section, for colour version of this plot): TF representation of a principal component, derived from a TF decomposition of EEG activity following response errors, that accounted for much of variance (~64%) in r-ERN response amplitude; as indicated, signal power of this r-ERN component was concentrated in the theta (4–7 Hz) frequency band. **Bottom** (statistical map): Scalp topography distribution of externalizing group differences (high-externalizing group minus low-externalizing group) in scores on the r-ERN/theta component derived from the TF decomposition. The peak of this response-locked increase in theta energy coincided in time with the r-ERN waveform response and had a similar frontocentral scalp maximum.

occurrence of each type of event, it seems likely that other brain regions are differentially recruited in the endogenous detection of errors compared with the processing of exogenous feedback.

The participant sample for this study of brain reactivity to loss feedback (f-ERN) consisted of 149 undergraduate participants selected from a larger screening sample, with oversampling of individuals identified as low and high in externalizing tendencies (n = 40 and n = 57, respectively) as indexed by the 100-item Externalizing inventory. This sample incorporated the 92 individuals who participated in the Hall *et al.* (2007) study of r-ERN response.

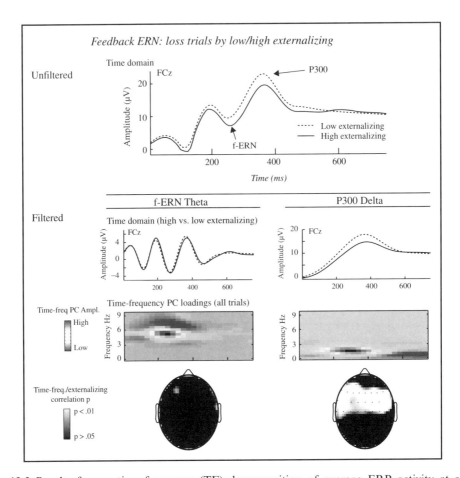

Fig. 12.3 Results from a time–frequency (TF) decomposition of average ERP activity at scalp site Cz following loss feedback stimuli, depicted separately for subgroups of high- (n = 59) versus low-externalizing participants (n = 42) as defined by scores on a 100-item screening version of the Externalizing Inventory (Krueger *et al.*, 2007). High- and low-externalizing groups were formed by oversampling from the top and bottom 25% of scorers in an undergraduate screening pool. Waveform plot (top): Average unfiltered ERP activity following loss feedback stimuli for these high- and low-externalizing subgroups. Waveform plots (second level): Average time–domain ERP activity following loss feedback stimuli for these extreme subgroups, frequency-filtered (3rd order Butterworth) to capture activity in the theta (3–9 Hz bandpass) range corresponding to f-ERN response (left plot) and activity in the delta (3 Hz low pass) range corresponding to the P3 response (right plot). Colour-surface plots (third level; see Colour Plate Section, for colour version of this plot): Principal component scores reflecting the f-ERN/theta and P3/delta activity contained in the ERP signal, derived from a TF decomposition of average EEG activity following loss trials. Statistical maps (bottom level): Scalp topography distributions, for the overall study sample (N = 154) that included these extreme subgroups, of correlations between externalizing scores and (1) scores on the f-ERN/theta component derived from the TF decomposition (left map) and (2) scores on the P3/delta component (right map). From the topographic maps, it can be seen that the association between externalizing and ERP response following loss feedback evident in the top waveform plot is attributable to reduced EEG activity within the delta (P3) frequency range at anterior scalp sites.

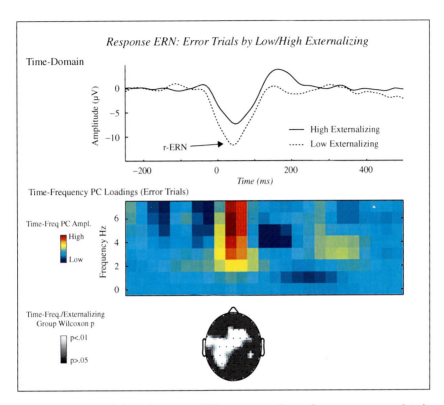

Fig. 12.2 Time–domain and time–frequency (TF) representations of response error-related negativity (r-ERN) differences for subgroups of high- (n = 38) versus low-externalizing participants (n = 22) as defined by scores on a 100-item screening version of the Externalizing Inventory (Krueger *et al.*, 2007). High and low externalizing groups were formed by oversampling from the top and bottom 25% of scorers in an undergraduate screening pool. **Top** (line plot): Average response-locked ERP waveforms at the midline central (Cz) scalp site for trials of a flanker task in which participants made incorrect responses, depicting reduced amplitude of the r-ERN for participants high on externalizing. The r-ERN is visible as a prominent negative deflection that peaks around 50 ms post-response. **Middle** (colour-surface plot): TF representation of a principal component, derived from a TF decomposition of EEG activity following response errors, that accounted for much of variance (~64%) in r-ERN response amplitude; as indicated, signal power of this r-ERN component was concentrated in the theta (4–7 Hz) frequency band. **Bottom** (statistical map): Scalp topography distribution of externalizing group differences (high-externalizing group minus low-externalizing group) in scores on the r-ERN/theta component derived from the TF decomposition. The peak of this response-locked increase in theta energy coincided in time with the r-ERN waveform response and had a similar frontocentral scalp maximum.

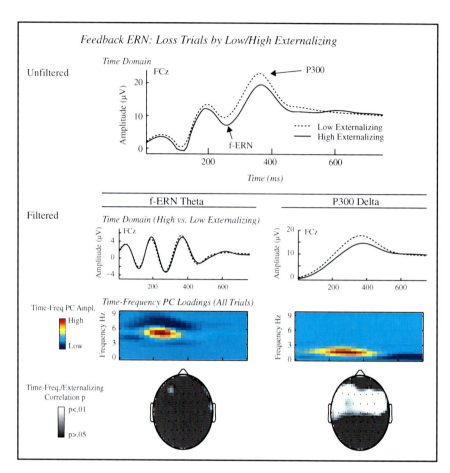

Fig. 12.3 Results from a time–frequency (TF) decomposition of average ERP activity at scalp site Cz following loss feedback stimuli, depicted separately for subgroups of high- (n = 59) versus low-externalizing participants (n = 42) as defined by scores on a 100-item screening version of the Externalizing Inventory (Krueger *et al.*, 2007). High- and low-externalizing groups were formed by oversampling from the top and bottom 25% of scorers in an undergraduate screening pool. Waveform plot (top): Average unfiltered ERP activity following loss feedback stimuli for these high- and low-externalizing subgroups. Waveform plots (second level): Average time–domain ERP activity following loss feedback stimuli for these extreme subgroups, frequency-filtered (3rd order Butterworth) to capture activity in the theta (3–9 Hz bandpass) range corresponding to f-ERN response (left plot) and activity in the delta (3 Hz low pass) range corresponding to the P3 response (right plot). Colour-surface plots (third level): Principal component scores reflecting the f-ERN/theta and P3/delta activity contained in the ERP signal, derived from a TF decomposition of average EEG activity following loss trials. Statistical maps (bottom level): Scalp topography distributions, for the overall study sample (N = 154) that included these extreme subgroups, of correlations between externalizing scores and (1) scores on the f-ERN/theta component derived from the TF decomposition (left map) and (2) scores on the P3/delta component (right map). From the topographic maps, it can be seen that the association between externalizing and ERP response following loss feedback evident in the top waveform plot is attributable to reduced EEG activity within the delta (P3) frequency range at anterior scalp sites.

The upper line plot of Fig. 12.3 depicts average ERP responses following presentation of loss feedback in Low- versus High-Externalizing participants. It can be seen that the ERP waveform in this case includes an earlier negativity reflecting the f-ERN, and a somewhat later (but overlapping) positivity reflecting the P300 response to the feedback stimulus. Time-frequency decomposition, as described earlier, was used to separate these two overlapping ERP components. The decomposition yielded evidence of two highly distinct spectral components, one a higher-frequency theta component (mirroring the r-ERN) that corresponded to the f-ERN, and the other a lower-frequency delta component corresponding to the P300 response. Although High-Externalizing participants showed reduced amplitude of P300-delta response compared with Low-Externalizing participants, the groups did not differ in oscillatory activity within the theta range corresponding to the f-ERN response (Fig. 12.3, middle line plots, and lower colour-surface and statistical-topographic plots).

The findings of this study thus showed a clear divergence from those of the Hall *et al.* (2007) study. In response to explicit negative (loss) feedback in the forced decision-making task of this study, high externalizing was associated with a general reduction in delta activity reflecting P300. This finding is consistent with extensive prior evidence, described earlier, for reduced P300 reactivity to meaningful stimuli in performance tasks of various kinds. However, whereas high-externalizing participants showed markedly reduced r-ERN following performance errors in the Hall *et al.* investigation, high externalizing was associated with no discernable reduction in theta activity reflecting f-ERN-despite the fact that the test sample for the f-ERN was markedly larger (N = 149) and incorporated all participants from the Hall *et al.* study. The implication is that tendencies towards externalizing do not reflect a deficit in anterior cingulate cortex function per se, but rather processing impairments in other brain regions crucial for endogenous action monitoring but not for registration of external performance feedback. Nonetheless, despite showing normal f-ERN reactivity to the motivational (loss) component of feedback in the choice task, high-externalizing individuals evidenced a significant reduction in P300 response to the exact same feedback cue-indicating diminished associative-elaborative processing of loss feedback. This dissociation parallels the finding, described earlier, of reduced delta P3 response in the three-stimulus oddball task to novel picture stimuli as a whole despite intact subdelta slow-wave differentiation between affective versus neutral picture stimuli.

Theoretical interpretations and implications for clinical intervention

The findings just described illustrate how psychophysiological research aimed at identifying basic brain response indicators can be extended to elucidate our understanding of neuropsychological processing deviations underlying aggressive-externalizing tendencies. P300 amplitude reduction has long been recognized as an indicator of risk for alcohol problems, and recent research has established reduced P300 as a genetically based, endophenotypic marker of externalizing tendencies more generally. Our follow-up research investigating P300 responses to novel picture stimuli as well as target stimuli indicates that P300 is pervasively reduced in high-externalizing individuals in relation to visual stimuli of varying types. However, we found a salient dissociation in brain reactivity to brief novel picture stimuli: Whereas high-externalizing individuals showed diminished delta/P300 response to picture stimuli in general, they showed a normal enhancement of low frequency (subdelta) activity response to affective versus neutral pictures—indicating intact low-level recognition of and responsiveness to the motivational significance of the affective picture stimuli (cf. Lang *et al.*, 1997).

Reduced ERN has been identified more recently as an indicator of externalizing, although a prior research base (e.g., Dikman & Allen, 2000; Ridderinkhoff *et al.*, 2002; Pailing & Segalowitz, 2004) pointed to the likelihood of this association being found. Our follow-up research investigating brain responses to feedback stimuli yielded two results of major interest. First, in contrast with the findings of reduced r-ERN response following errors in a speeded performance task (Hall *et al.*, 2007), high-externalizing individuals did not showed reduced f-ERN response in relation to explicit feedback signalling loss. This result is important because it indicates that reduced r-ERN is not attributable to a deficit in anterior cingulate cortex function per se, but rather impaired processing in other brain regions that contribute to endogenous action monitoring in contexts where explicit performance feedback is not available. A second notable result was that high-externalizing individuals showed attenuated delta/P300 reactivity to loss feedback stimuli despite showing intact theta/f-ERN reactivity. This dissociation parallels what we found for brain responses to novel picture stimuli: High externalizing individuals demonstrated intact brain response to the basic motivational content of feedback stimuli, but impaired delta/P300 reactivity to these same feedback stimuli.

What do these striking dissociations between basic affective reactivity and P300 brain response mean? In thinking about the implications of these findings for our understanding of processes underlying the aggressive behaviour of persistently violent individuals, it is useful to revisit some of the major points arising from prior published work reviewed in earlier sections. One key point is that the type of aggressive behaviour most closely associated with general tendencies toward externalizing is impulsive or reactive aggression—that is, aggression that reflects a weakly regulated response to immediate threat or provocation. Callous-aggressive behaviour entailing strategic exploitation or victimization of others represents a phenotypically distinguishable phemonenon (Krueger *et al.*, 2007) with potentially distinctive aetiologic underpinnings. As described in the second section of this chapter, individuals diagnosed as psychopathic differ in patterns of peripheral and brain response from individuals who are primarily impulsive-aggressive, and it has been suggested that the callous-aggressive behaviour of psychopathic individuals arises from a core deficiency in emotional processing (Patrick *et al.*, 1997; Blair, 2006; Frick & White, 2008).

Individuals who are impulsively aggressive show lower levels of autonomic arousal at rest, but enhanced autonomic reactivity to immediate stressors. In terms of EEG and/or ERP response, impulsive-aggressive individuals show evidence of enhanced electrocortical slow-wave activity (indicative of diminished cortical arousal) at rest, and (as noted for externalizing syndromes in general) diminished P300 response to non-stressful stimuli. With regard to brain morphology and activation, impulsively violent individuals show evidence of reduced grey matter volume in frontal and temporal lobe regions especially, along with reduced activity in these regions at rest, during performance of simple processing tasks, and in response to a pharmacologic challenge (e.g., administration of a serotonin agonist). Evidence of reduced anterior cingulate cortex activation has also been reported in some studies, but as highlighted in our work on externalizing, differences in this activation in some processing tasks may be secondary to impairments in other brain regions that interact with the anterior cingulate cortex. In addition, some studies have revealed evidence of abnormal function in limbic (amygdala, hippocampus) regions, including evidence of reduced functional connectivity between cortical and limbic regions. An important caveat with this literature, however, is that aggressive behaviour in many studies is defined generically (e.g., on the basis of violent convictions, or aggressive ward reports), without clear assessment of the type(s) of violence engaged in.

Nonetheless, the findings of these existing studies provide a useful background against which to interpret findings from the ERP studies reported in the preceding section. An integrative interpretation that accommodates results from both the novelty-P300 and the f-ERN studies is that performance of these tasks entails processing along two parallel streams: a lower stream along which immediate stimulus features are processed, prompting actions as required by the task, and a higher stream along which deeper elaborative processing occurs (i.e., beyond what is required by the immediate demands of the task). Processing of the motivational significance of task stimuli (reflected in the subdelta slow-wave component of response to pictures in the novelty P300 task, and the theta f-ERN component of response to loss feedback in the f-ERN task) occurs via the lower stream, whereas cognitive-associative processing of task stimuli (reflected in the delta P300 response) occurs via the higher stream. We hypothesize that this higher stream (1) involves comparing and integrating transient cognitive or affective representations stored in long-term memory (cf. Ericsson & Kinsch, 1995); (2) is instantiated by an anterior brain circuit that includes the prefrontal cortex and anterior cingulate cortex; and (3) is fundamental to anticipation, reflection, and self-regulation of affect and behaviour.

The findings of this work have intriguing implications for clinical treatment of aggressive behaviour. Impulsive (reactive) violence, involving unconstrained expression of negative affect in the form of physical attack, represents part of the general propensity towards externalizing problems (cf. Krueger et al., 2007). As such, processing impairments that underlie the general propensity towards externalizing problems represent an important target for intervention with impulsive aggressive individuals. The findings of the novelty P300 and f-ERN studies indicate that concrete, motivationally relevant feedback is likely to be processed by high-externalizing individuals at a basic (lower-stream) level and effective in the immediate term. However, for effects of feedback to persist outside the treatment context, deeper processing of feedback information is required-processing that will contribute to the formation of neural representations capable of influencing future behaviour. From this perspective, a key goal of treatment with aggressive-externalizing individuals would be to improve extended working memory function (cf. Ericsson & Kinsch, 1995) in the service of anticipation, planning, and self-control. There is some evidence that pharmacologic agents that show effectiveness in reducing impulsive-aggressive behaviour do so by altering brain processing deficits associated with general externalizing tendencies (e.g., Barratt et al., 1997a; New et al., 2004). In the future, pharmacologic agents of this sort may prove effective as adjuncts to psychological treatment of aggressive-externalizing individuals—just as antidepressant drugs have come to be regarded as key allies in the psychological treatment of depression.

Acknowledgements

The authors were supported by grants MH52384, MH65137, and MH072850 from the National Institute of Mental Health, Grant R01 AA12164 from the National Institute on Alcohol Abuse and Alcoholism, and funds from the Hathaway endowment at the University of Minnesota.

References

Amen, D. G., Stubblefield, M., Carmichael, B., & Thisted, R. (1996). Brain SPECT findings and aggressiveness. *Annals of Clinical Psychiatry*, *8*, 129–137.

Arnett, P.A. (1997). Autonomic responsivity in psychopaths: a critical review and theoretical proposal. *Clinical Psychology Review*, *17*, 903–936.

Babcock, J. C., Green, C. E., Webb, S. A., & Graham, K.H. (2004). A second failure to replicate the Gottman et al. (1995) typology of men who abuse intimate partners and possible reasons why. *Journal of Family Psychology*, *18*, 396–400.

Barratt, E. S., Stanford, M. S., Felthous, A. R., & Kent, T. A. (1997a). The effects of phenytoin on impulsive and premeditated aggression: a controlled study. *Journal of Clinical Psychopharmacology*, *17*, 341–349.

Barratt, E. S., Stanford, M. S., Kent, T. A., & Felthous, A. R. (1997b). Neuropsychological and cognitive psychophysiological substrates of impulsive aggression. *Biological Psychiatry*, *41*, 1045–1061.

Bauer, L. O., O'Connor, S., & Hesselbrock, V. M. (1994). Frontal P300 decrements in antisocial personality disorder. *Alcoholism: Clinical and Experimental Research*, *18*, 1300–1305.

Beauchaine, T. P., Katkin, E. S., Strassberg, Z., & Snarr, J. (2001). Disinhibitory psychopathology in male adolescents: discriminating conduct disorder from attention-deficit/hyperactivity disorder through concurrent assessment of multiple autonomic states. *Journal of Abnormal Psychology*, *110*, 610–624.

Begleiter, H., & Porjesz, B. (1999). What is inherited in the predisposition toward alcoholism? A proposed model. *Alcholism: Clinical and Experimental Research*, *23*, 1125–1135.

Bernat, E. M., Williams, W. J., et al. (2005). Decomposing ERP time-frequency energy using PCA. *Clin Neurophysiol*, *116*(6), 1314–1334.

Blair, R. J. R. (2006). Subcortical brain systems in psychopathy: the amygdala and associated structures. In C. J. Patrick (ed), *Handbook of Psychopathy* (pp. 296–312). New York: Guilford Press.

Blake, P. Y., Pincus, J. H., & Buckner, C. (1995). Neurological abnormalities in murderers. *Neurology*, *45*, 1641–1647.

Branchey, M. H., Buydens-Branchey, L., & Lieber, C. S. (1988). P3 in alcoholics with disordered regulation of aggression. *Psychiatry Research*, *25*, 49–58.

Bush, G., Luu, P., et al. (2000). Cognitive and emotional influences in anterior cingulate cortex. *Trends in Cognitive Sciences*, *4*(6), 215–222.

Bushman, B. J. & Anderson, C. A. (2001). Is it time to pull the plug on the hostile versus instrumental aggression dichotomy? *Psychological Review*, *108*, 273–279.

Card, N. A., & Little, T. D. (2007). Longitudinal modeling of developmental processes. *International Journal of Behavioral Development*, *31*, 297–302.

Carter, C. S., Braver, T. S., *et al.* (1998). Anterior cingulate cortex, error detection, and the online monitoring of performance. *Science*, *280*(5364), 747–749.

Caspi, A., McClay, J., Moffitt, T. E., Mill, J., Martin, J., Craig, I. W. *et al.* (2002). Role of genotype in the cycle of violence in maltreated children. *Science*, *297*, 851–854.

Courchesne, E., Hillyard, S. A., *et al.* (1975). Stimulus novelty, task relevance and the visual evoked potential in man. *Electroencephalogr Clin Neurophysiol*, *39*(2), 131–143.

Davidson, R. J., Putnam, K. M., & Larson, C. L. (2000). Dysfunction in the neural circuitry of emotion regulation—a possible prelude to violence. *Science*, *289*, 591–594.

De Oliveira-Souza, R., Hare, R. D., Bramati, I. E., Garrido, G. J., Ignácio, F. A., Tovar-Moll, F., *et al.* (2008). Psychopathy as a disorder of the moral brain, Fronto-temporo-limbic grey matter reductions demonstrated by voxel-based morphometry. *Neuroimage*, *40*(3), 1202–1213.

Dehaene, S., Posner, M., *et al.* (1994). Localization of a neural system for error detection and compensation. *Psychological Science*, *5*(5), 303–305.

Dien, J., Spencer, K., *et al.* (2003). Localization of the event-related potential novelty response as defined by principal components analysis. *Cognitive Brain Research*, *17*(3), 637–650.

Dikman, Z. V., & Allen, J. J. B. (2000). Error monitoring during reward and avoidance learning in high- and low-socialized individuals. *Psychophysiology*, *37*, 43–54.

Dodge, K. (1991). The structure and function of reactive and proactive aggression. In D. J. Pepler, & K. H. Rubin (eds), *The Development and Treatment of Childhood Aggression* (pp. 201–248). New York: Lawrence Erlbaum Associates.

Dolan, M. C., Deakin, J. F. W., Roberts, N., & Anderson, I. M. (2002). Quantitative frontal and temporal structural MRI studies in personality-disordered offenders and control subjects. *Psychiatry Research Neuroimaging, 116*, 133–149.

Drexler, K., Schweitzer, J. B., Quinn, C. K., Gross, R., Ely, T. D., Muhammad, F., *et al.* (2000). Neural activity related to anger in cocaine-dependent men: a possible link to violence and relapse. *American Journal of Addictions, 9*, 331–339.

Ericsson, K., & Kinsch, W. (1995). Long-term working memory. *Psychological Review, 102*(2), 211–245.

Eysenck, H. J. (1967). *The Biological Basis of Personality*. Springfield, IL: Charles C. Thomas.

Fichtenholtz, H. M., Dean, H. L., *et al.* (2004). Emotion-attention network interactions during a visual oddball task. *Brain Res Cogn Brain Res, 20*(1), 67–80.

Frick, P. J., & White, S. F. (2008). The importance of callous-unemotional traits for developmental models of aggressive and antisocial behavior. *Journal of Child Psychology and Psychiatry, 49*, 359–375.

Frodi, A. M., & Lamb, M. E. (1980). Child abusers' responses to infant smiles and cries. *Child Development, 51*, 238–241.

George, D. T., Rawlings, R. R., Williams, W. A., Phillips, M. J., Fong, G., Kerich, M. *et al.* (2004). A select group of perpetrators of domestic violence: evidence of decreased metabolism in the right hypothalamus and reduced relationships between cortical/subcortical brain structures in position emission tomography. *Psychiatry Research: Neuroimaging, 130*, 11–25.

Gerstle, J. E., Mathias, C. W., & Stanford, M. S. (1998). Auditory P300 and self-reported impulsive aggression. *Progress in NeuroPsychopharmacology and Biological Psychiatry, 22*, 575–583.

Gehring, W. J., Coles, M. G., *et al.* (1995). A brain potential manifestation of error-related processing. *Electroencephalogr Clin Neurophysiol Suppl, 44*, 261–272.

Gehring, W. J., & Willoughby, A. R. (2002). The medial frontal cortex and the rapid processing of monetary gains and losses. *Science, 295*(5563), 2279–2282.

Gottman, J. M., Jacobson, N. S., Rushe, R. H., Shortt, J. W., Babcock, J., La Taillade, J. J., *et al.* (1995). The relationship between heart rate reactivity, emotionally aggressive behavior, and general violence in batterers. *Journal of Family Psychology, 9*, 227–248.

Hall, J. R., Bernat, E. M., *et al.* (2007). Externalizing psychopathology and the error-related negativity. *Psychol Sci, 18*(4), 326–333.

Hansen, A. L., Johnsen, B. H., Thornton, D., Waage, L., & Thayer, J. F. (2007). Facets of psychopathy, heart rate variability and cognitive function. *Journal of Personality Disorders, 21*, 568–582.

Hare, R. D. (1978). Electrodermal and cardiovascular correlates of psychopathy. In R. D. Hare, & D. Schalling (eds), *Psychopathic Behavior: Approaches to Research* (pp. 107–143). Chichester, UK: Wiley.

Hare, R. D. (2003). *Manual for the Hare Psychopathy Checklist-Revised*, 2nd edn. Toronto, ON: Multi-Health Systems.

Hemphill, J. F., Hare, R. D., & Wong, S. (1998). Psychopathy and recidivism: a review. *Legal and Criminological Psychology, 3*, 139–170.

Hicks, B. M., Bernat, E., Malone, S. M., Iacono, W. G., Patrick, C. J., Krueger, R. F., *et al.* (2007). Genes mediate the association between P3 amplitude and externalizing disorders. *Psychophysiology, 44*, 98–105.

Hirono, N., Mega, M. S., Dinov, I. D., Mishkin, F., & Cummings, J. L. (2000). Left fronto-temporal hypoperfusion in associated with aggression in patients with dementia. *Archives of Neurology, 57*, 861–866.

Holroyd, C. B., & Coles, M. G. (2002). The neural basis of human error processing, reinforcement learning, dopamine, and the error-related negativity. *Psychol Rev, 109*(4), 679–709.

Hubbard, J. A., Smithmyer, C. M., Ramsden, S. R., Parker, E. H., Flanagan, K. D., Dearing, K. F., *et al.* (2002). Observational, physiological, and self-report measures of children's anger: relations to reactive versus proactive aggression. *Child Development, 73*, 1101–1118.

Iacono, W. G. (1998). Identifying psychophysiological risk for psychopathology: examples from substance abuse and schizophrenia research. *Psychophysiology, 35*, 621–637.

Iacono, W. G., Carlson, S. R., Malone, S. M., & McGue, M. (2002). P3 event-related potential amplitude and risk for disinhibitory disorders in adolescent boys. *Archives of General Psychiatry, 59*, 750–757.

Intrator, J., Hare, R., Stritzke, P., & Brichtswein, K. (1997). A brain imaging (single photon emission computerized tomography) study of semantic and affective processing in psychopaths. *Biological Psychiatry*, *42*, 96–103.

Kiehl, K. A., Hare, R. D., Liddle, P. F., & McDonald, J. J. (1999). Reduced P300 responses in criminal psychopaths during a visual oddball task. *Biological Psychiatry*, *45*, 1498–1507.

Kiehl, K. A., Bates, A. T., Laurens, K. R., Hare, R. D., & Liddle, P. F. (2006). Brain potentials implicate temporal lobe abnormalities in criminal psychopaths. *Journal of Abnormal Psychology*, *115*, 443–453.

Krueger, R. F. (1999). The structure of common mental disorders. *Archives of General Psychiatry*, *56*, 921–926.

Krueger, R. F., Hicks, B., Patrick, C. J., Carlson, S., Iacono, W. G., & McGue, M. (2002). Etiologic connections among substance dependence, antisocial behavior, and personality: modeling the externalizing spectrum. *Journal of Abnormal Psychology*, *111*, 411–424.

Krueger, R. F., Markon, K. E., Patrick, C. J., Benning, S. D., & Kramer, M. (2007). Linking antisocial behavior, substance use, and personality: an integrative quantitative model of the adult externalizing spectrum. *Journal of Abnormal Psychology*, *116*, 645–666.

Kuruoglu, A. C., Arikan, Z., Vural, G., & Karatas, M. (1996). Single photon emission computerised tomography in chronic alcoholism: antisocial personality disorder may be associated with decreased frontal perfusion. *British Journal of Psychiatry*, *169*, 348–354.

Laakso, M. P., Vaurio, O., Koivisto, E., Savolainen, L., Eronen, M., & Aronen, H. J. (2001). Psychopathy and the posterior hippocampus. *Behavioural Brain Research*, *118*, 187–193.

Laakso, M. P., Vaurio, O., Savolainen, L., Repo, E., Soininen, H., Aronen, H. J., et al. (2000). A volumetric MRI study of the hippocampus in type 1 and 2 alcoholism. *Behavioural and Brain Research*, *109*, 177–186.

Lang, P. J., Bradley, M. M., & Cuthbert, B. N. (1997). Motivated attention: affect, activation, and action. In P. J. Lang, R. F. Simons, & M. T. Balaban (eds), *Attention and Orienting: Sensory and Motivational Processes* (pp. 97–135). Mahwah, NJ: Lawrence Erlbaum Associates, Inc.

Lorber, M. F. (2004). Psychophysiology of aggression, psychopathy, and conduct problems: a meta-analysis. *Psychological Bulletin*, *130*, 531–552.

Lykken, D. T. (1995). *The Antisocial Personalities*. Hillsdale, NJ: Erlbaum.

Malone, S. M., Bernat, E., Patrick, C. J., & Iacono, W. G. (2002). P300 and prestimulus EEG power: relationship to externalizing psychopathology in adolescent males. *Psychophysiology*, *39*, S54.

Meehan, J. C., Holtzworth-Munroe, A., & Herron, K. (2001). Maritally violent men's heart rate reactivity to martial interactions: a failure to replicate the Gottman et al. (1995) typology. *Journal of Family Psychology*, *15*, 394–408.

Mezzacappa, E., Tremblay, R. E., Kindlon, D., Saul, J. P., Arseneault, L., Seguin, J., et al. (1997). Anxiety, antisocial behavior and heart rate regulation in adolescent males. *Journal of Child Psychology and Psychiatry*, *38*, 457–469.

Miltner, W., Braun, C., et al. (1997). Event-related brain potentials following incorrect feedback in a time-estimation task, evidence for a HGeneric neural system for error detection. *Journal of Cognitive Neuroscience*, *9*(6), 788–798.

New, A. S., Buchsbaum, M. S., Hazlett, E. A., Goodman, M., Koenigsberg, H. W., Lo, J., et al. (2004). Fluoxetine increases relative metabolic rate in prefrontal cortex in impulsive aggression. *Psychopharmacology*, *176*, 451–458.

New, A. S., Hazlett, E. A., Buchsbaum, M. S., Goodman, M., Reynolds, D., Mitropoulou, V., et al. (2002). Blunted prefrontal cortical superscript 1-sup-8 fluorodeoxyglucose positron emission tomography response to meta-chlorophenylpiperazine in impulsive aggression. *Archives of General Psychiatry*, *59*, 621–629.

Nieuwenhuis, S., Aston-Jones, G., et al. (2005). Decision making, the P3, and the locus coeruleus-norepinephrine system. *Psychol Bull*, *131*(4), 510–32.

Ortiz, J., & Raine, A. (2004). Heart rate level and antisocial behavior in children and adolescents: a meta-analysis. *Journal of the American Academy of Child and Adolescent Psychiatry*, *43*, 154–162.

Pailing, P. E., & Segalowitz, S. J. (2004). The error-related negativity as a state and trait measure: motivation, personality, and ERPs in response to errors. *Psychophysiology*, *41*, 84–95.

Parsey, R. V., Oquendo, M. A., Simpson, N. R., Ogden, R. T., van Heertum, R., Arango, V., *et al.* (2002). Effects of sex, age, and aggressive traits in man on brain serotonin 5-HT-sub(1A) receptor binding potential measured by PET using [C-11]WAY-100635. *Brain Research, 954,* 173–182.

Patrick, C. J. (1994). Emotion and psychopathy: startling new insights. *Psychophysiology, 31,* 319–330.

Patrick, C. J. (2007). Getting to the heart of psychopathy. In H. Hervé, & J. C. Yuille (eds), *The Psychopath: Theory, Research, and Social Implications* (pp. 207–252). Hillsdale, NJ: Lawrence Erlbaum Associates.

Patrick, C. J., Bernat, E., Malone, S. M., Iacono, W. G., Krueger, R. F., & McGue, M. K. (2006). P300 amplitude as an indicator of externalizing in adolescent males. *Psychophysiology, 43,* 84–92.

Patrick, C. J., Hicks, B. M., Krueger, R. F., & Lang, A. R. (2005). Relations between psychopathy facets and externalizing in a criminal offender sample. *Journal of Personality Disorders, 19,* 339–356.

Patrick, C. J., & Verona, E. (2007). The psychophysiology of aggression: autonomic, electrocortical, and neuro-imaging findings. In D. Flannery, A. Vazsonyi, & I. Waldman (eds), *Cambridge Handbook of Violent Behavior* (pp. 111–150). New York: Cambridge University Press.

Patrick, C. J., Zempolich, K. A., & Levenston, G. K. (1997). Emotionality and violent behavior in psychopaths: a biosocial analysis. In A. Raine, P. A. Brennan, D. P. Farrington, & S. A. Mednick (eds), *Biosocial Bases of Violence* (pp. 145–161). New York: Plenum.

Peters, M. L., Godaert, G. L. R., Ballieux, R. E., & Heijnen, C. J. (2003). Moderation of physiological stress responses by personality traits and daily hassles: less flexibility of immune system responses. *Biological Psychology, 65,* 21–48.

Pietrini, P., Guazzelli, M., Basso, G., Jaffe, K, & Grafman, J. (2000). Neural correlates of imaginal aggressive behavior assessed by positron emission tomography in healthy subjects. *American Journal of Psychiatry, 157,* 1772–1781.

Polich, J., Pollock, V. E., & Bloom, F. E. (1994). Meta-analysis of P300 amplitude from males at risk for alcoholism. *Psychological Bulletin, 115,* 55–73.

Porter, S., & Woodworth, M. (2006). Psychopathy and aggression. In C. J. Patrick (ed), *Handbook of Psychopathy* (pp. 481–494). New York: Guilford Press.

Purcell, S. (2002). Variance component models for gene-environment interaction in twin analysis. *Twin Research, 5,* 554–571.

Raine, A. (1989). Evoked potentials and psychopathy. *International Journal of Psychophysiology, 8,* 1–16.

Raine, A. (1993). *The Psychopathology of Crime.* San Diego, CA: Academic Press.

Raine, A., Buchsbaum, M., & LaCasse, L. (1997). Brain abnormalities in murderers indicated by positron emission tomography. *Biological Psychiatry, 42,* 495–508.

Raine, A., Buchsbaum, M. S., Stanley, J., Lottenberg, S., Abel, L., & Stoddard, J. (1994). Selective reductions in pre-frontal glucose metabolism in murderers. *Biological Psychiatry, 36,* 365–373.

Raine, A., Meloy, J. R., Bihrle, S., Stoddard, J., LaCasse, L., & Buchsbaum, M. S. (1998). Reduced prefrontal and increased subcortical brain functioning assessed using positron emission tomography in predatory and affective murderers. *Behavioral Sciences and the Law, 16,* 319–332.

Raine, A., Park, S., Lencz, T., Bihrle, S., LaCasse, L., Widom, C. S., *et al.* (2001). Reduced right hemisphere activation in severely abused violent offenders during a working memory task: an fMRI study. *Aggressive Behavior, 27,* 111–129.

Raine, A., Venables, P. H., & Williams, M. (1990). Relationships between N1, P300, and CNV recorded at age 15 and criminal behavior at age 24. *Psychophysiology, 27,* 567–575.

Raine, A., & Yang, Y. (2006). The neuroanatomical bases of psychopathy: a review of brain imaging findings. In C. J. Patrick (ed), *Handbook of Psychopathy* (pp. 278–295). New York: Guilford Press.

Ridderinkhoff, K. R., de Vlugt, Y., Bramlage, A., Spaan, M., Elton, M., Snel, J., *et al.* (2002). Alcohol consumption impairs detection of performance errors in mediofrontal cortex. *Science, 298,* 2209–2211.

Scarpa, A., & Raine, A. (1997). Psychophysiology of anger and violent behavior. *The Psychiatric Clinics of North America, 20,* 375–394.

Siever, L. J., Buchsbaum, M. S., New, A. S., Spiegel-Cohen, J., Wei, T., Hazlett, E. A., *et al.* (1999). D,l-Fenfluramine response in impulsive personality disorder assessed with [18F] flurodeoxyglucose positron emission tomography. *Neuropsychopharmacology*, *20*, 413–423.

Smith, T. W., & Gallo, L. C. (1999). Hostility and cardiovascular reactivity during marital interaction. *Psychosomatic Medicine*, *61*, 436–445.

Soderstrom, H., Tullberg, M., Wikkelsoe, C., Ekholm, S., & Forsman, A. (2000). Reduced regional cerebral blood flow in non-psychotic violent offenders. *Psychiatry Research: Neuroimaging*, *98*, 29–41.

Squires, N. K., Squires, K. C., *et al.* (1975). Two varieties of long-latency positive waves evoked by unpredictable auditory stimuli in man. *Electroencephalogr Clin Neurophysiol*, *38*(4), 387–401.

Stanford, M. S., Houston, R. J., Villemarette-Pittman, N. R., & Greve, K. W. (2003). Premeditated aggression: clinical assessment and cognitive psychophysiology. *Personality and Individual Differences*, *34*, 773–781.

Suls, J. & Wan, C. K. (1993). The relationship between trait hostility and cardiovascular reactivity: a quantitative review and analysis. *Psychophysiology*, *30*, 615–626.

Taylor, J., Carlson, S. R., Iacono, W. G., Lykken, D. T., & McGue, M. (1999). Individual differences in electrodermal responsivity to predictable aversive stimuli and substance dependence. *Psychophysiology*, *36*, 193–198.

Tellegen, A. (1982). *Brief manual for the Multidimensional Personality Questionnaire*. Unpublished manuscript, University of Minnesota.

Tiihonen, J., Kuikka, J., Bergstrom, K., Hakola, P., Karhu, J., Ryynanen, O. P., *et al.* (1995). Altered striatal dopamine re-uptake site densities in habitually violent and non-violent alcoholics. *Nature Medicine*, *1*, 654–657.

Tiihonen, J., Kuikka, J. T., Bergstrom, K. A., Karhu, J., Viinamaki, H., Lehtonen, J., *et al.* (1997). Single-photon emission tomography imaging of monoamine transporters in impulsive violent behaviour. *European Journal of Nuclear Medicine and Molecular Imaging*, *24*, 1253–1260.

Tonkonogy, J. M. (1991). Violence and temporal lobe lesion: head CT and MRI data. *Journal of Neuropsychiatry and Clinical Neurosciences*, *3*, 189–196.

Van Elst, L. T., Hesslinger, B., Thiel, T., Geiger, E., Haegele, K., Lemieux, L., *et al.* (2003). Frontolimbic brain abnormalities in patients with borderline personality disorder: a volumetric magnetic resonance imaging study. *Biological Psychiatry*, *54*, 163–171.

Van Elst, L. T. Woermann, F. G., Lemieux, L., Thompson, P. J., & Trimble, M. R. (2000). Affective aggression in patients with temporal lobe epilepsy: a quantitative MRI study of the amygdala. *Brain*, *123*, 234–243.

Verona, E., & Curtin, J.J. (2006). Gender differences in the negative affective priming of aggression. *Emotion*, *6*, 115–124.

Verona, E., Patrick, C. J., & Lang, A. R. (2002). A direct assessment of the role of state and trait negative emotion in aggressive behavior. *Journal of Abnormal Psychology*, *111*, 249–258.

Volavka, J. (1990). Aggression, electroencephalography, and evoked potentials: a critical review. *Neuropsychiatry, Neuropsychology, and Behavioral Neurology*, 3, 249–259.

Volkow, N. D., & Tancredi, L. (1987). Neural substrates of violent behaviour: a preliminary study with positron emission tomography. *British Journal of Psychiatry*, *151*, 668–673.

Walters, G. (2003). Predicting institutional adjustment and recidivism with the Psychopathy Checklist factor scores: a meta-analysis. *Law and Human Behavior*, *27*, 541–558.

Woermann, F. G., van Elst, L. T., Koepp, M. J., Free, S. L., Thompson, P. J., Trimble, M. R., *et al.* (2000). Reduction of frontal neocortical grey matter associated with affective aggression in patients with temporal lobe epilepsy: an objective voxel by voxel analysis of automatically segmented MRI. *Journal of Neurology, Neurosurgery, & Psychiatry*, *68*, 162–169.

Wong, M. T. H., Lumsden, J., Fenton, G. W., & Fenwick, P. B. C. (1994). Electroencephalography, computed tomography and violence ratings of male patients in a maximum-security mental hospital. *Acta Psychiatrica Scandinavica*, *90*, 97–101.

Yamasaki, H., LaBar, K. S., & McCarthy, G. (2002). Dissociable prefrontal brain systems for attention and emotion. *Proceedings of the National Academy of Sciences*, 11447–11451.

Zuckerman, M. (1979). *Sensation Seeking: Beyond the Optimal Level of Arousal*. Hillsdale, NJ: Erlbaum.

13

Quantitative genetic studies of antisocial behaviour

Essi Viding, Henrik Larsson, and Alice P. Jones

Background

Each year over 1.6 million people are killed through violence, and violence prevention is one of the most important global concerns (Krug *et al.*, 2002). Governmental bodies everywhere in the Western world, including the United Kingdom, prioritize for prevention of antisocial behaviour (Bailey, 2002; Department for Employment and Skills, 2003). The political, social, or economic risk factors for antisocial behaviour (AB) are well studied; but more recently, the awareness has grown that biological risk factors, which may explain individual differences in predisposition to violence, also need to be explored. Furthermore, many environmental risk factors that are traditionally thought to be social may actually reflect genetic vulnerability (Moffitt, 2005). Finally, the vulnerability factors and their 'modus operandi' may differ for different subtypes of antisocial behaviour. Thus, the question is not really, 'Is it in their genes?' or 'What environmental factors are to blame?' It is, How do genetic and environmental factors interact to produce specific types of antisocial behaviour.

This chapter will provide a broad and selective review of twin and adoption research into the nature and nurture of AB. Twin and adoption research has been important in not only demonstrating the relative importance of genetic and environmental factors to AB , but also in increasing our understanding of the aetiological differences between subtypes of individuals with AB and how gene–environment interplay works.

Twin and adoption methods

The twin method is a natural experiment that relies on the different levels of genetic relatedness between monozygotic (MZ) and dizygotic (DZ) twins to estimate the contribution of genetic and environmental factors to individual differences, or extreme scores in a phenotype of interest. Phenotypes include any behaviour or characteristic that is measured separately for each twin, such as twins' scores on an AB checklist. The basic premise of the twin method is this: if identical twins, who share 100% of their genetic material, appear more similar on an AB measure than fraternal twins, who share on average 50% of their genetic material (similar to any siblings), then we infer that there are genetic influences on AB. Identical twins' genetic similarity is twice that of fraternal twins. If nothing apart from genes influences behaviour, then we would expect the identical twins to be twice as similar with respect to the AB measure when compared with fraternal twins. Shared environmental influences (environmental influences that make twins similar to each other) are inferred if fraternal twins appear more similar than is expected from sharing 50% of their genes. Finally, if identical twins are not 100% similar on the measure of AB (as would be expected if only genes influenced a trait), non-shared environmental influences (environmental influences that make twins different from each other) are inferred. The non-shared environmental estimate also includes measurement error.

In adoption studies, the occurrence of behaviour or trait may be compared between adoptive relatives and biological relatives. For example, one can compare adoptees whose biological parents and/or siblings are with or without AB, or study adoptees reared by adoptive parents and/or siblings with or without AB. Genetic influences are indicated by the association between the adoptee and biological relative on measures of AB; environmental influences are indicated by the association between the adoptee and adoptive relative on measures of AB. Because adoptions have become less common since the 1970s, most quantitative genetic studies designed in recent years use the twin method.

For both twin and adoption data, statistical model-fitting techniques and regression analyses methods incorporating genetic relatedness parameters are used to investigate the aetiology of the phenotype of choice. These techniques will not be covered here and an interested reader is referred to Plomin *et al.* (2008). It is important to remember that heritability and environmental variance estimates derived from both twin and adoption data pertain to a particular population at a particular time; should the environmental circumstances change dramatically, so would the proportion of variance accounted for by genetic and environmental factors. It is equally important to note that no heritability or environmental statistic concerns a single individual but instead reflects the contribution of genetic and environmental influences to individual differences or group differences on a behaviour or trait. Finally, simple heritability and environmental variance estimates also reflect gene-environment interplay. Ingenious study designs, such as 'children of twins', enable researchers to conduct more fine-grain study on the gene-environment interplay (see the section on gene-environment correlation).

Several concerns have been raised regarding both twin and adoption methods. Just to mention a few, twin studies have been criticized on account of the equal environments assumption (EEA) and representativeness of twins, whereas adoption studies have been criticized on account of representativeness of adoptive families and resultant restricted environmental variance. It is beyond the scope of this chapter to deal with these issues in detail and an interested reader is referred to Rutter (2005; pp. 41–44). However, a brief consideration of the concerns is warranted here. The EEA for AB assumes that the environmental variance with MZ and DZ twins will be the same with respect to the environments that influence that behaviour. In other words, the expectation is that MZ and DZ twins share environment to the same extent. Analyses that have specifically tested the EEA by introducing environmental similarity measures (sharing friends, sharing classes, dressing alike, and perceived zygosity) to a twin model have found scarce evidence for violation of EEA when assessing behavioural problems (Cronk *et al.*, 2002). This is hardly surprising as factors such as dressing alike are unlikely to represent an environment that will influence AB.

An often heard objection to the EEA refers to the fact that MZ twins are more likely to share a chorion, which critics of the twin method assume makes their prenatal environment more similar than that of DZ twins. In fact, the opposite is true, with monochorionic MZ twins more likely to differ in birth weight (result of the 'transfusion syndrome' and the following differences in availability of placental blood). To the extent that data are available, chorionicity and its consequences do not seem to threaten the logic of the twin method (Rutter, 2005; p. 42). Rutter (2005; p. 43) highlights that there are genetic effects on exposure to those environments that perpetuate (via an environmental main effect) the development of behavioural problems. Some of the difference in similarity between MZ and DZ pairs may thus be due to MZ twins (who share all their genes) being exposed to more of the similar environmental risk events. More research is required to study this phenomenon; but, although it would inflate the heritability estimate somewhat, the magnitude of this EEA violation is unlikely to be sufficient to cast doubt on the whole twin strategy. Critics of the twin method have also highlighted that there may be important twin-singleton differences that would jeopardize the conclusions from the twin studies. Although twins are delayed in language development and twin pregnancies are associated with increased rate of obstetric complications, neither concern is particularly relevant for twin data on AB. Twins with obstetric complications are routinely excluded from twin analyses and language delay found in twins is very mild, representing variation in the normal range. It has been rightly pointed out that adoptive families are often carefully selected and represent only a small range of possible home environments (Moffitt, 2005). Given the limitations of both twin and adoption methods, it is important to collate data across studies and methodologies.

Quantitative genetic studies of AB

Quantitative genetic studies can be used to estimate the heritability of AB. These studies have also gone beyond reporting simple heritability estimates and investigated aetiology of different subtypes of AB and co-morbidity. Recent meta-analyses of twin and adoption studies of AB suggest moderate heritability and non-shared environmental influence, as well as modest shared environmental influence on AB in general (Rhee & Waldman, 2002; Waldman & Rhee, 2006).

The magnitude of heritability estimate has been shown to vary as a function of operationalization (what criteria are used to define AB), assessment method, age, zygosity determination method, gender, and whether twin or adoption design was used (see Fig. 13.1). The magnitude of heritability estimate can also vary as a function of subtype (see Fig. 13.2). The magnitude differences in heritability and environmental estimates could reflect several things. For example, different operationalization methods may produce different heritability and environmental estimates as they involve distinct age groups (e.g., child and conduct disorder versus adult and criminality), as well as use of varying assessment tools (e.g., symptom count versus arrest record). The differences in the magnitude of estimated heritability and environmental estimates can thus reflect a real finding associated with the developmental period or type of AB measured, but could also reflect different levels of measurement error associated with each operationalization. Different assessment methods are also likely to have different levels of measurement error associated with them. Studies where zygosity is determined by blood generally report much lower sample sizes than studies where zygosity is determined by a questionnaire. The low sample size in turn limits the power of the statistical analyses and introduces sample size-dependent measurement error.

Gender does not appear to influence the aetiology of individual differences in AB. Thus, although there are mean differences in the average number of ABs displayed by boys and girls (with boys displaying a larger number than girls), the source of this mean difference is likely to result from factors that shift the distribution for the boys towards the risk cut-off. A recent study suggests that genetic and environmental influences on delinquency have less effect on the population variation in delinquency among girls and that girls require greater causal liability for expression of delinquency than boys (van Hulle et al., 2007). Different heritability and environmental estimates in twin versus adoption studies could relate to different sample size (twin studies are usually much larger), different assessment instruments (in twin studies, both twins receive the same age-appropriate instruments; in parent adoption studies, the child and the parent receive different age-appropriate instruments), and restricted variance in environmental risk factors in the adoptive families. However, what is

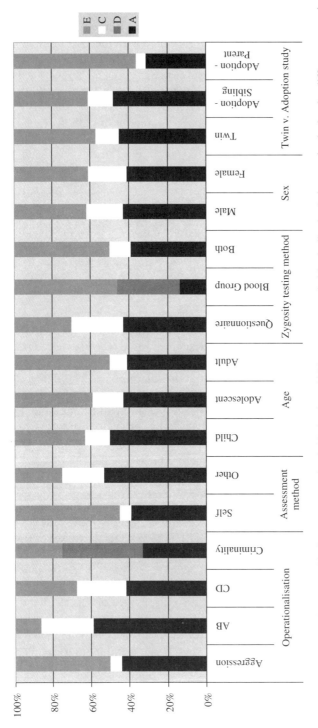

Fig. 13.1 Genetic and environmental influences on antisocial behaviour (AB) appear remarkably similar in their magnitude despite different operationalization methods, assessment methods, age of assessment, zygosity assessment methods, gender of the participants, or whether twin versus adoption design was used. This figure represents a selection of the statistics reported in the meta-analysis by Rhee and Waldman (2002). A, additive genetic influences; D, dominant genetic influences; C, shared environmental influences; E, non-shared environmental influences.

striking is the considerable similarity in heritability estimates (mostly in the range of 40-50%) irrespective of the operationalization, assessment method, age, zygosity determination method, gender, or study design used (Fig. 13.1).

Subtyping by callous-unemotional (CU)traits appears to index a large difference in the heritability of AB (Viding *et al.*, 2005; Viding *et al.*, 2008; see Fig. 13.2.). These findings from our research group are still relatively new and will require replication. We first studied teacher ratings of CU traits and AB in approximately 7500 7-year-old twins from the Twins Early Development Study (TEDS; Viding *et al.*, 2005). We separated children with elevated levels of AB (in the top 10% for the TEDS sample) into AB/CU+ and AB/CU–groups based on their CU score (in the top 10% or not). AB in children with AB/CU+ was under strong genetic influence (heritability of 0.81) and no influence of shared environment. In contrast, such behaviour in children without elevated levels of CU traits showed moderate genetic influence (heritability of 0.30) and substantial environmental influence (shared environmental influence = 0.34, non-shared environmental influence = 0.36; see Fig. 13.2).

We have recently replicated the finding of different heritability magnitude for the AB/CU+ and AB/CU– groups using the nine-year teacher data (Viding *et al.*, 2008). This difference in heritability magnitude holds even after hyperactivity scores of the children are controlled for, suggesting that the result is not driven by any differences in hyperactivity between the two groups. In summary, our research with pre-adolescent twins suggests that although the

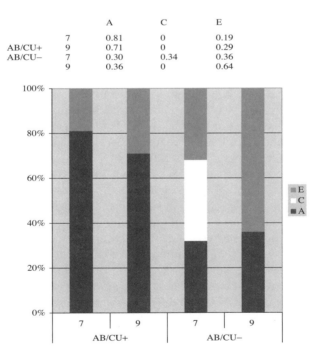

		A	C	E
AB/CU+	7	0.81	0	0.19
	9	0.71	0	0.29
AB/CU–	7	0.30	0.34	0.36
	9	0.36	0	0.64

Fig. 13.2 The heritability of antisocial behaviour (AB) appears to be strong in those children with elevated levels of both antisocial behaviour and callous-unemotional (CU) traits (AB/CU+). In contrast, children with antisocial behaviour, but lower levels of CU traits (AB/CU–) show a strong environmental influence on their antisocial behaviour (Viding *et al.*, 2005; Viding *et al.*, 2008). This finding holds even when the contribution of co-occurring hyperactivity is controlled for in the analyses (Viding *et al.*, 2008). A, additive genetic influences; C, shared environmental influences; E, non-shared environmental influences.

CU subtype is genetically vulnerable to AB, the non-CU subtype manifests a more strongly environmental aetiology to their AB (Viding *et al.*, 2005; Viding *et al.*, 2008). Other research has also suggested that heritability of AB may vary by subtype. For example, early onset AB appears more heritable than adolescent AB (e.g., Taylor, Iacono, & McGue, 2000; Taylor, McGue, & Iacono, 2000; Arseneault *et al.*, 2003); conduct disturbance coupled with hyperactivity shows strong genetic influence, but conduct disturbance without hyperactivity is associated with shared environmental influences (Silberg, Meyer, *et al.*, 1996); and finally, aggressive AB appears more heritable than non-aggressive AB (Eley *et al.*, 1999, 2003).

Recent quantitative genetic work also suggest that co-occurrence of AB and CU (Krueger *et al.*, 2002; Taylor *et al.*, 2003; Larsson *et al.*, 2007; Viding *et al.*, 2007), Conduct Disorder and Oppositional Defiant Disorder (Dick *et al.*, 2005), Attention Deficit/Hyperactivity Disorder (ADHD) or hyperactivity and Conduct Disorder (Silberg, Rutter, *et al.*, 1996; Thapar *et al.*, 2001; Nadder *et al.*, 2002), as well as AB and substance abuse behaviours (Krueger *et al.*, 2002) are due to common genetic factors. This research has implications for molecular genetic research. We should expect that pleiotropy (the same genes influencing many traits) and any genes showing an association with AB are also likely to influence a host of other problem behaviours

Are environmental risk factors truly environmental?

Although it is well established what environment factors are associated with AB, it is still unclear whether these factors are causal (Moffitt, 2005). This is partly explained by the fact that many studies cannot control for the potential impact of genetic influences on the correlation between a putative environmental risk factor and an antisocial outcome. This has led several researchers to conclude that the study of AB is 'stuck in the risk factor stage' (Hinshaw, 2002; Moffitt, 2005). One way to further examine the causal role of environmental risk factors in the development of such behaviour is to use genetically sensitive twin and adoption designs to control for the confounding effects of parents' or children's genes on putative environmental measures (Moffitt, 2005).

A powerful way of studying whether a risk factor has an environmentally mediated effect on children's AB is to use the MZ-twin differences method. Because MZ twins share all their segregating genes and their environment, links between MZ-twin differences in an environmental risk factor and subsequent AB can thus be attributed to non-shared environmental processes. Careful and deliberate hypothesis testing using this design usually involves three steps: (1) documenting a non-shared environmental component in individual differences in the child outcome (e.g., AB), (2) identifying specific, theoretically informative, environmental risk factors that vary between siblings and are correlated with the child outcome, (e.g., negative parenting), and (3) correlating MZ-twin differences in the environmental risk factor with MZ-differences in the child outcome.

Several studies have reported that MZ-twin differences in negative parenting are correlated with MZ-twin differences in AB (Asbury *et al.*, 2003; Caspi *et al.*, 2004; Burt *et al.*, 2006). As a prime example, Caspi and colleagues (2004) used a longitudinal twin differences design to compare identical twins discordant for teacher-rated AB (i.e., identical twins who differ on AB outcome). They demonstrated that mothers' negative emotional attitudes towards their children were associated with children's AB. This association was not purely due to child effects (i.e., an effect of children's behaviour on parental treatment). In addition, the discordant identical twins design ruled out that the association between maternal-expressed emotion and children's AB was genetically mediated, as this emotion predicted differences between genetically identical individuals. Thus, these findings suggest maternal-expressed emotion is an environmentally mediated risk factor, and possibly an environmental cause for AB.

There are other ways to demonstrate an environmental main effect on AB. If an MZ mother's parenting predicts a child's AB better than an MZ aunt's parenting, then parenting has an environmental effect. On the other hand, if the MZ aunt's and the MZ mother's parenting predict the children's AB to the same extent, then parents' genes are responsible for the association between parenting and such behaviour. If the adoptive parent's bad parenting increases the adoptee's AB over and above the genetic influence from the biological parents' AB, this again demonstrates a main effect of environment on such behaviour. For a comprehensive discussion of study of environment in the context of quantitative genetic designs, the reader is referred to Moffitt (2005).

In summary, quantitative genetic studies have been useful in strongly demonstrating that environmental factors play an important role in individual differences of AB. Non-shared, or child–specific, environmental factors appear to be particularly important in bringing about such behaviour. In addition to the study of environmental main effects on this behaviour, quantitative genetic studies have also been instrumental in mapping out the effects of gene–environment interplay on AB.

Gene-environment interplay

There are now several ongoing twin and adoption studies that have included well-defined measures of putative environmental risk factors. These enable sophisticated extended twin models to test developmental hypothesis about different patterns of gene–environment interplay in AB (Moffitt, 2005). Two broad types of gene–environment interplay operate to bring about such behaviour: gene–environment correlation (rGE) and gene–environment interaction (GxE).

Risk environments may be a reflection of the parent's or child's genotype (Moffitt, 2005), a phenomenon known as rGE. In short, rGE refers to genetic effects on individual differences in liability to exposure to environmental risk (Rutter, 2005). Different types of rGE are passive, evocative, and active rGE. *Passive* rGE is a result of parents providing their children with both genes and with environments that are correlated with genetically influenced characteristics of parents. *Evocative* rGE appears when a child's inherited characteristics evoke a response from their environment. *Active* rGE refers to active genetically driven child choices of the particular environments. These phenomena are reviewed extensively in Moffitt (2005) and the reader is referred to this paper. However, a synopsis of the types of study designs that have demonstrated rGE effects on AB is presented here. To our knowledge, research is still required on active rGE, but several studies have shown passive and evocative rGE effects.

Adoption studies are a means of removing most passive rGE as adopted children are provided with environments by unrelated parents. As adoption studies show heritable effects on AB, this suggests that twin heritability estimates cannot just be a function of passive rGE (e.g., Cadoret *et al.*, 1995). However, if we were to ask whether passive rGE exists, we would be asking whether the effect of the genes the parents share with their child and also influence negative parenting confound the association between negative parenting and children's AB. Studies that have examined the parenting of adult MZ and DZ twins (Niederhiser *et al.*, 2004) or the parenting of adult MZ twins reared apart (Plomin *et al.*, 1989) have demonstrated that parenting strategies show a modest genetic influence.

The Children of Twin (CoT) design (e.g., D'Onofrio *et al.*, 2003) has been put forward as an alternative to the adoption design to distinguish the direct effect of negative parenting from parent-child associations due to genetic effects. In other words, the CoT can be used to study whether the genetic effects go on to mediate the association between parenting and children's AB; that is, to assess the potential impact of passive rGE on AB. The CoT design compares the offspring of MZ and DZ twins who differ in their genetic and environmental risk. Appropriate statistical analyses, therefore, provide the opportunity for detecting and quantifying environmental risk factors that are specific to the measured factor (e.g., negative parenting), genetic confound, and environmental confounds that twins share.

Using this approach, Harden *et al.* (2007) showed that the effect of parents' genes on marital conflict mediated the association between marital conflict and children's AB. D'Onofrio *et al.* (2007) used the same design and found an environmentally mediated role of parental AB on behavioural problems in male offspring. In contrast, common genetic risk confounds the entire intergenerational transmission in female offspring. The potential of this design is great, but there are also some noteworthy limitations. For example, this study design requires large sample sizes for more detailed analyses of family relationships and CoT models that include only one parent present potential problems (e.g., divorce: Eaves *et al.*, Silberg & Maes, 2005). Adoption designs could also be used to demonstrate passive rGE. Passive rGE exists if biological parents' parenting predicts that their adopted-away child will also parent poorly. This study design would show that negative parenting is genetically transmitted, in the absence of social transmission. Currently, no such studies exist due to difficulty in obtaining intergenerational parenting data in adoption studies.

If we were to ask whether evocative rGE exists, we would be asking whether a genetic child effect confounds the association between bad parenting and children's AB. The first step to assess evocative rGE is to compare MZ and DZ twins' ratings of the parental treatment they receive. Such studies have demonstrated that genetic child effects on parenting exist (Pike *et al.*, 1996; Neiderhiser *et al.*, 2004), although the finding may partly be due to the MZ twins more similar perception of parenting. These studies did not, however, explore what it is that children do to provoke negative parenting. Twin studies that also include children's AB as a measured variable are needed to more directly assess evocative rGE. Such multivariate twin designs assess to what extent Twin A's AB predicts the negative parenting Twin B's receives and vice versa. If the correlation between Twin A's AB and Twin B's experience of negative parenting is higher among MZ pairs than DZ pairs, then this would support evocative rGE processes. Existing research indicates that children's genes account for most of the relationship between negative parenting within the normal range and AB (Neiderhiser *et al.*, 1999; Larsson *et al.*, 2008) , but not between more extreme forms of parenting (i.e., maltreatment) and AB (Jaffee *et al.*, 2004).

Adoptee designs provide a different opportunity to explore the potential importance of evocative rGE for AB (Ge *et al.*, 1996; O'Connor *et al.*, 1998). One example of such study found that children at higher genetic risk of AB (i.e., those with antisocial biological parents) are more likely to receive punitive parenting from their adoptive parents than those children without genetic risk of such behaviour (O'Connor *et al.* 1998). However, the results also showed an association between negative parenting and AB, after the impact of evocative rGE was controlled for, which highlights the role of environmentally mediated parent effects.

GxE refers to genetically influenced individual differences in the sensitivity to specific environmental factors (Rutter, 2005). Within the twin design, GxE can be demonstrated when response to environmental risk occurs as a function of genetic vulnerability (Kendler *et al.*, 1995). MZ twins whose co-twin is affected with a disorder are at the highest risk to develop any disorder that has a genetic component, which responds to environmental risk. DZ twins whose co-twin is affected are at the second-highest risk to develop the disorder. DZ twins with an unaffected co-twin are less vulnerable, but show a higher genetic risk than MZ twins with an unaffected co-twin. Comparing twins with different levels of genetic vulnerability, Jaffee *et al.* (2005) studied child conduct problems in physically maltreated and non-maltreated individuals. In line with the GxE hypothesis, they found that maltreated MZ twins with an affected (i.e., antisocial) co-twin were at the highest risk to develop conduct problems after physical maltreatment, whereas MZ twins with unaffected co-twins showed the lowest risk to develop conduct problems. DZ twins with affected and un-affected co-twins fell in between the two types of MZ pairs, as predicted. Adoption studies generally demonstrate that the combination of a genetic predisposition (Antisocial Personality Disorder and/or alcohol abuse or dependence in biological parents) and a high-risk environment (adverse adoptive home environment with stress and discord) leads to greater pathology than what would be expected from either factor acting alone or both in an additive combination (Cadoret *et al.*, Yates, Troughton, Woodworth, & Stewart, 1995).

In short, twin and adoption designs have demonstrated that genetic effects on individual differences in liability to exposure to environmental risk (rGE) and genetically influenced individual differences in the sensitivity to specific environmental factors (GxE) are important in explaining variance in AB. GxE research on such behaviour is now moving beyond quantitative genetic designs onto studying the effects of specific genes (e.g., *MAOA*) in response to environmental risk (e.g., Caspi *et al.*, 2002; Kim-Cohen *et al.*, 2006). This research suggests that the main effects of individual genes and environmental factors can be small, but that GxE effects are bigger. The challenge for the social scientists is to perfect environmental measurement, which is always going to be more ambiguous than determining someone's genotype or twin zygosity status. More studies of environmental effects in the abnormal range are required and environmental influences beyond the family need to be studied in more detail both within the twin and adoption framework and in study designs including measured genotypes. These are the future challenges of quantitative genetic research.

Translational implications of quantitative genetic research

Publication of results from twin and adoption data can often make sensational headlines, largely due to misunderstanding of what the heritability statistic represents. A recent Academy of Medical Sciences working group report highlights that science should be integrated into policymaking by, for example, embedding researchers into policy teams and providing senior civil servants with scientific training (Academy of Medical Sciences, 2007). It is important to engage with policymakers to ensure that the nature of the heritability statistic is understood. A heritability estimate of 70% does not mean that a single individual is at a 70% risk to develop a disorder or that a disorder outcome is nearly inevitable. It merely means that 70% of the individual or group differences in the population (at that particular time) are influenced by genetic differences among individuals. It is also important to highlight that no genes directly code for AB. Instead, genes code for proteins that influence characteristics such as neurocognitive vulnerabilities that may in turn increase risk of AB.

In this section, we focus our discussion to prevention and treatment of AB in child populations. Antisocial Personality Disorder does not suddenly manifest itself as a complete problem in adulthood; rather, it has its origins and early indicators in childhood and adolescence. Research has demonstrated robust trajectories of AB, and strong links between delinquency, Conduct Disorder and later Antisocial Personality Disorder have been reported (Moffitt, 2003). Given the high burden and cost of AB, novel prevention and treatment approaches for at-risk children are imperative. Early intervention strategies have potentially substantial cost benefits for the taxpayer. High-quality early intervention has been shown to be cost-effective in the United States (Schweinhart & Weikart, 1998), and has been highly recommended by Romeo et al. (2006) in a study explicitly investigating the economic cost of severe AB in children.

Research into environmental risk factors within quantitative genetic designs has highlighted a number of important issues. First of all, the implicit assumption within social sciences research that risk environments have a main effect on behaviour appears to be true for some important social risk factors, such as parenting and maltreatment. It has also been shown that for children with vulnerable genotype, this genotype will react with risk environments, the phenomenon known as GxE. Furthermore, at least one of the parents will share the risk genes for AB, and thus, the parental genotype can also contribute to a less-than-optimal rearing environment, a phenomenon known as passive rGE. It is also possible that a child with a certain genotype is more likely to evoke negative parenting, a phenomenon known as evocative rGE. Parenting programmes, such as those outlined in the NICE guidelines, are targeted to changing parental response to difficult behaviours that children with conduct problems exhibit (http://www.nice.org.uk/guidance/index.jsp?action=byID&o=11584). Mapping out the environmental risk profile and the potential challenges to ameliorating such profile is extremely important for successful intervention. This notion has also been implemented with results in programmes such as Multi-Systemic Therapy (Schaeffer & Borduin, 2005). It is also noteworthy that simple interventions, such as nurse-visit programmes, can be extremely successful in breaking the association between maltreatment and AB (Olds et al., 1997; Eckenrode et al., 2001). This suggests that genetic risk can be effectively moderated by environmental intervention and enables us to think about treatment as a positive form of GxE. However, at-risk families should be monitored and helped regardless of the child's or parent's genotype. Does the genetic information therefore add anything? We would argue that even if environmental interventions are already provided, the scope to make them better lies within better understanding of the mechanisms of gene-environment interplay.

Quantitative genetic research can also help in isolating disorders or patterns that may require distinct forms of intervention. For example, current quantitative genetic research supports the notion of subtyping antisocial children on CU traits (Viding et al., 2005; Viding et al., 2008). Aetiologically heterogeneous samples may explain why intervention programmes can sometimes have mixed results in their success (Frick, 2001; Hawes & Dadds, 2005). Some children seem to respond to well-timed, early prevention and treatment whereas others do not. We would suggest that the root of this may lie in aetiological differences and concomitant differences in cognitive profile of distinct subtypes of children with AB. It is particularly challenging to map out the cognitive profiles and make predictions about treatment approaches that capitalize on what is known about cognitive strengths and weaknesses. For example, children with CU traits are strong on self-interest and get motivated by rewards, but do not characteristically process others' distress or react to punishment (Blair *et al.*, 2006). These are cognitive strengths and limitations that have to be worked with to produce change in behaviour. There may also eventually be scope for pharmacogenetic interventions (i.e., medical interventions tailored to suit genotype-driven response to drugs) that support cognitive-behavioural and family approaches, provided that the research suggests that such interventions enhance the success of these therapeutic programmes.

Summary

Both genetic vulnerability and environmental factors account for variance in AB. Of the environmental risk factors, those that act in a child-specific manner, such as negative parenting, appear to be most important for the development of AB. Genetic effects on individual differences in liability to exposure to environmental risk (gene-environment correlation) and genetically influenced individual differences in the sensitivity to specific environmental factors (gene-environment interaction) both operate to increase liability to AB. Future research must concentrate on better understanding the mechanisms of gene-environment interplay and on translating such understanding to improved intervention programmes. Quantitative genetic research can also improve the understanding of different subtypes of AB and the resultant scope and limitations for tailored interventions.

Acknowledgements

The writing of this chapter was supported by grants from the Medical Research Council (G0401170) and the Department of Health FMH Programme (MRD 12-37) to E.V. H.L. was supported by a postdoctoral stipend from the Swedish Brain Foundation.

References

Academy of Medical Sciences (2007). Identifying the environmental causes of disease: How should we decide what to believe and when to take action? [Online], Available at: http://www.acmedsci.ac.uk/p47prid50.html.

Arseneault, L., Moffitt, T. E., Caspi, A., Taylor, A., Rijsdijk, F. V., Jaffee, S. R., *et al.* (2003). Strong genetic effects on cross-situational antisocial behaviour among 5-year-old children according to mothers, teachers, examiner-observers, and twins' self-reports. *Journal of Child Psychology and Psychiatry*, *44*, 832–848.

Asbury, K., Dunn, J. F., Pike, A., & Plomin, R. (2003). Nonshared environmental influences on individual differences in early behavioral development: a monozygotic twin differences study. *Child Development*, *74*, 933–943.

Bailey, S. (2002). Treatment of delinquents. In M. Rutter, & E. Taylor (eds), *Child and Adolescent Psychiatry: Modern Approaches* (pp. 1019–1037). Oxford: Blackwell Scientific.

Blair, R. J. R., Peschardt, K. S., Budhani, S., Mitchell, D. G. V., & Pine, D. S. (2006). The development of psychopathy. *Journal of Child Psychology and Psychiatry*, *47*, 262–275.

Burt, S. A., McGue, M., Iacono, W. G., & Krueger, R. F. (2006). Differential parent-child relationships and adolescent externalizing symptoms: cross-lagged analyses within a monozygotic twin differences design. *Developmental Psychology*, *42*, 1289–1298.

Cadoret, R. J., Yates, W. R., Troughton, E., Woodworth, G., & Stewart, M. A. (1995). Genetic-environmental interaction in the genesis of aggressivity and conduct disorders. *Archives of General Psychiatry*, *52*, 916–924.

Caspi, A., McClay, J., Moffitt, T. E., Mill, J., Martin, J., Craig, I. W., *et al.* (2002). Role of genotype in the cycle of violence in maltreated children. *Science, 297,* 851–854.

Caspi, A., Moffitt, T. E., Morgan, J., Rutter, M., Taylor, A., Arsenault, L., *et al.* (2004). Maternal expressed emotion predicts children's antisocial behaviour problems: using MZ-twin differences to identify environmental effects on behavioural development. *Developmental Psychology, 40,* 149–161.

Cronk, N. J., Slutske, W. S., Madden, P. A., Bucholz, K. K., Reich, W., & Heath, A. C. (2002). Emotional and behavioral problems among female twins: an evaluation of the equal environments assumption. *Journal of the American Academy of Child and Adolescent Psychiatry, 41,* 829–837.

Department for Education and Skills (2003). *Every Child Matters Green Paper.* London: Her Majesty's Stationery Office.

Dick, D. M., Viken, R. J., Kaprio, J., Pulkkinen, L., & Rose, R. J. (2005). Understanding the covariation among childhood externalizing symptoms: genetic and environmental influences on conduct disorder, attention deficit hyperactivity disorder, and oppositional defiant disorder symptoms. *Journal of Abnormal Child Psychology, 33,* 219–229.

D'Onofrio, B. M., Slutske, W. S., Turkheimer, E., Emery, R. E., Harden, K. P., Heath, A. C., *et al.* (2007). Intergenerational transmission of childhood conduct problems: a Children of Twins Study. *Archives of General Psychiatry, 64,* 820–829.

D'Onofrio, B. M., Turkheimer, E., Eaves, L. J., Corey, L. A., Berg, K., Solaas, M. H., *et al.* (2003). The role of the Children of Twins design in elucidating causal relations between parent characteristics and child outcomes. *Journal of Child Psychology and Psychiatry, 44,* 1130–1144.

Eaves, L. J., Silberg, J. L., & Maes, H. H. (2005). Revisiting the children of twins: can they be used to resolve the environmental effects of dyadic parental treatment on child behavior? *Twin Research and Human Genetics, 8,* 283–290.

Eckenrode, J., Zielinski, D., Smith, E., Marcynyszyn, L. A., Henderson Jr., C. R., Kitzman, H., *et al.* (2001). Child maltreatment and the early onset of problem behaviors: can a program of nurse home visitation break the link? *Development and Psychopathology, 13,* 873–890.

Eley, T. C., Lichtenstein, P., & Moffitt, T. E. (2003). A longitudinal behavioral genetic analysis of the etiology of aggressive and non-aggressive antisocial behavior. *Development and Psychopathology, 15,* 383–402.

Eley, T. C., Lichtenstein, P., & Stevenson, J. (1999). Sex differences in the etiology of aggressive and nonaggressive antisocial behavior: results from two twin studies. *Child Development, 70,* 155–168.

Frick, P. J. (2001). Effective interventions for children and adolescents with conduct disorder. *Canadian Journal of Psychiatry, 46,* 597–608.

Ge, X., Conger, R. D., Cadoret, R. J., Neiderhiser, J. M., Yates, W., Troughton, E., *et al.* (1996). The developmental interface between nature and nurture: a mutual influence model of child antisocial behavior and parent behaviors. *Developmental Psychology, 32,* 574–589.

Harden, K. P., Turkheimer, E., Emery, R. E., D'Onofrio, B. M., Slutske, W. S., Heath, A. C., *et al.* (2007). Marital conflict and conduct problems in Children of Twins. *Child Development, 78,* 1–18.

Hawes, D. J., & Dadds, M. R. (2005). The treatment of conduct problems in children with callous-unemotional traits. *Journal of Consulting and Clinical Psychology, 73,* 737–741.

Hinshaw, S. P. (2002). Process, mechanism, and explanation related to externalizing behavior in developmental psychopathology. *Journal of Abnormal Child Psychology, 30,* 431–446.

Jaffee, S. R, Caspi, A., Moffitt, T. E., Dodge, K. A., Rutter, M., Taylor, A., *et al.* (2005). Nature × nurture: genetic vulnerabilities interact with physical maltreatment to promote conduct problems. *Development and Psychopathology, 17,* 67–84.

Jaffee, S. R., Caspi, A., Moffitt, T. E., Polo-Tomas, M., Price, T. S., & Taylor, A. (2004). The limits of child effects: evidence for genetically mediated child effects on corporal punishment but not on physical maltreatment. *Developmental Psychology, 40,* 1047–1058.

Kendler, K. S., Kessler, R. C., Walters, E. E., MacLean, C., Neale, M. C., Heath, A. C., *et al.* (1995). Stressful life events, genetic liability, and onset of an episode of major depression in women. *American Journal of Psychiatry, 152,* 833–842.

Krueger, R. F., Hicks, B. M., Patrick, C. J., Carlson, S. R., Iacono, W. G., & McGue, M. (2002). Etiologic connections among substance dependence, antisocial behavior, and personality: modeling the externalizing spectrum. *Journal of Abnormal Psychology, 111,* 411–424.

Krug, E. G., Dahlberg, L., Mercy, J., Zwi, A., & Lozano, R. (2002). *World Report on Violence and Health*. Geneva: WHO Library.

Larsson, H., Tuvblad, C., Rijsdijk, F., Andershed, H., Grann, M., & Lichtenstein, P. (2007). A common genetic factor explains the association between psychopathic personality and antisocial behaviour. *Psychological Medicine*, *37*, 15–26.

Larsson, H., Viding, E., Rijsdijk, F. V., & Plomin, R. (2008). Relationships between parental negativity and childhood antisocial behavior over time: a bidirectional effect model in a longitudinal genetically informative design. *Journal of Abnormal Child Psychology*, *36*(5), 633–645.

Moffitt, T. E. (2003). Life-course-persistent and adolescence-limited antisocial behavior. In B. B. Lahey, T. E. Moffitt, & A. Caspi (eds), *Causes of Conduct Disorder and Juvenile Delinquency*. New York: Guilford Press.

Moffitt, T. E. (2005). The new look of behavioral genetics in developmental psychopathology: gene-environment interplay in antisocial behaviors. *Psychological Bulletin*, *131*, 533–554.

Nadder, T. S, Rutter, M., Silberg, J. L., Maes, H. H., & Eaves, L. J. (2002). Genetic effects on the variation and covariation of attention deficit-hyperactivity disorder (ADHD) and oppositional-defiant disorder/conduct disorder (ODD/CD) symptomatologies across informant and occasion of measurement. *Psychological Medicine*, *32*, 39–53.

Neiderhiser, J. M., Reiss, D., Hetherington, E. M., & Plomin, R. (1999). Relationships between parenting and adolescent adjustment over time: genetic and environmental contributions. *Developmental Psychology*, *35*, 680–692.

Neiderhiser, J. M., Reiss, D., Pedersen, N., Lichtenstein, P., Spotts, E. L., Hansson, K., *et al.* (2004). Genetic and environmental influences on mothering of adolescents: a comparison of two samples. *Developmental Psychology*, *40*, 335–351.

O'Connor, T. G., Deater-Deckard, K., Fulker, D., Rutter, M., & Plomin, R. (1998). Genotype–environment correlations in late childhood and early adolescence: antisocial behavioral problems and coercive parenting. *Developmental Psychology*, *34*, 970–981.

Olds, D. L., Eckenrode, J., Henderson Jr., C. R., Kitzman, H., Powers, J., Cole, R., *et al.* (1997). Long-term effects of home visitation on maternal life course and child abuse and neglect. Fifteen-year follow-up of a randomized trial. *The Journal of the American Medical Association*, *278*, 637–643.

Pike, A., McGuire, S., Hetherington, E. M., Reiss, D., & Plomin, R. (1996). Family environment and adolescent depression and antisocial behavior: a multivariate genetic analysis. *Developmental Psychology*, *32*, 590–603.

Plomin, R., DeFries, J., McClearn, G., & McGuffin, P. (2008). *Behavioral Genetics*, 5th edn. New York: Worth Publishers.

Plomin, R., McClearn, G. E., Pedersen, N. L., Nesselroade, J. R., & Bergeman, C. S. (1989). Genetic influence on adults' ratings of their current family environment. *Journal of Marriage and the Family*, *51*, 791–803.

Rhee, S. H., & Waldman, I. D. (2002). Genetic and environmental influences on antisocial behavior: a meta-analysis of twin and adoption studies. *Psychological Bulletin*, *128*, 490–529.

Romeo, R., Knapp, M., & Scott, S. (2006). Economic cost of severe antisocial behaviour in children and who pays for it. *British Journal of Psychiatry*, *188*, 547–553.

Rutter, M. (2005). *Genes and Behavior: Nature–Nurture Interplay Explained*. Oxford: Blackwell Publishing.

Schaeffer, C. M., & Borduin, C. M. (2005). Long-term follow-up to a randomized clinical trial of multisystemic therapy with serious and violent juvenile offenders. *Journal of Consulting and Clinical Psychology*, *73*, 445–453.

Schweinhart, L. J., & Weikart, D. P. (1998). High/Scope Perry Preschool Program effects at age twenty-seven. In J. Crane (ed), *Social Programs That Work* (pp. 148–162). New York: Russell Sage Foundation.

Silberg, J., Meyer, J., Pickles, A., Simonoff, E., Eaves, L., Hewitt, J., *et al.* (1996). Heterogeneity among juvenile antisocial behaviours: findings from the Virginia Twin Study of Adolescent Behavioural Development. *Ciba Foundation Symposium*, *194*, 76–86.

Silberg, J., Rutter, M., Meyer, J., Maes, H., Hewitt, J., Simonoff, E., *et al.* (1996). Genetic and environmental influences on the covariation between hyperactivity and conduct disturbance in juvenile twins. *Journal of Child Psychology and Psychiatry*, *37*, 803–816.

Taylor, J., Loney, B. R., Bobadilla, I., Iacono, W. G., & McGue, M. (2003). Genetic and environmental influences on psychopathy traits dimensions in a community sample of male twins. *Journal of Abnormal Child Psychology*, *31*, 633–645.

Taylor, J., Iacono, W. G., & McGue, M. (2000). Evidence for a genetic etiology of early-onset delinquency. *Journal of Abnormal Psychology*, *109*, 634–643.

Taylor, J., McGue, M., & Iacono, W. G. (2000). Sex differences, assortative mating, and cultural transmission effects on adolescent delinquency: a twin family study. *Journal of Child Psychology and Psychiatry*, *41*, 433–440.

Thapar, A., Harrington, R., & McGuffin, P. (2001). Examining the comorbidity of ADHD-related behaviours and conduct problems using a twin study design. *British Journal of Psychiatry*, *179*, 224–229.

Van Hulle, C. A., Rodgers, J. L., D'Ononfriou, B. M., Waldman, I. D., & Lahey, B. B. (2007). Sex differences in the causes of self-reported adolescent delinquency. *Journal of Abnormal Psychology*, *116*, 236–248.

Viding, E., Blair, R. J. R., Moffitt, T. E., & Plomin, R. (2005). Evidence for substantial genetic risk for psychopathy in 7-year-olds. *Journal of Child Psychology and Psychiatry*, *46*, 592–597.

Viding, E., Frick, P. J., & Plomin, R. (2007). Aetiology of the relationship between callous-unemotional traits and conduct problems in childhood. *British Journal of Psychiatry*, *190*, s33–s38.

Viding, E., Jones, A. P., Frick, P., Moffitt, T. E., & Plomin, R. (2008). Genetic and phenotypic investigation to early risk factors for conduct problems in children with and without psychopathic tendencies. *Developmental Science*, *11*, 17–22.

Waldman, I. D., & Rhee, S. H. (2006) Genetic and environmental influences on psychopathy and antisocial behavior. In C. J. Patrick (ed), *Handbook of Psychopathy* (pp. 205–28). New York: Guilford.

14

Gene–brain associations: The example of *MAOA*

Joshua W. Buckholtz and Andreas Meyer-Lindenberg

Since the beginning of recorded history, humans have noted (and lamented) the existence of individuals whose actions consistently contravene widely shared sentiments about appropriate behavior (social norms) and who thus pose a threat to social order and community peace (Cleckley, 1988). Furthermore, it was understood even in ancient times that the propensity toward antisocial behaviour 'breeds true' in families, and moreover, that the inheritance of antisocial traits was especially pronounced in men[1]. In the 1980's, this long-held notion of heritable contributions to personality was confirmed by studies of twins reared apart, which provided powerful evidence for a strong genetic component to individual variation in a variety of human traits (Bouchard *et al.*, 1990), including those linked to antisocial behaviour (Grove *et al.*, 1990; Viding *et al.*, 2005; Koenig *et al.*, 2007; Viding *et al.*, 2007). Similar to most other psychiatric phenotypes However, antisocial behaviour is genetically complex, meaning that multiple genetic variants are likely to contribute to the associated traits in interaction with one another (epistasis) and with the environment. Clues as to which specific gene or set of genes might account for this inherited variation were not forthcoming until Brunner's landmark finding of a single, rare, genetic mutation associated with antisocial behaviour in a large Dutch kindred (Brunner, Nelen, Breakefield*et al.*, 1993). This study implicated the first (and, to date, most compelling) candidate susceptibility gene for human antisocial behaviour, *MAOA*.

MAOA encodes the mitochondrial catabolic enzyme monoamine oxidase A (MAO-A), which catalyzes the oxidative deamination of biogenic amines, making it a critical regulator of neurotransmitter signalling at monoaminergic synapses throughout the brain (Shih, Chen, & Ridd, 1999). *MAOA* and *MAOB* (encoding the isoform MAO-B) map to adjacent sites on chromosome Xp11.23; each are comprised of 15 exons and demonstrate matching exon-intron organization, suggesting their derivation from the same ancestral gene by a duplication event (Grimsby *et al.*, 1991). The monoamine oxidases are localized to the outer mitochondrial membrane in the presynaptic terminal of monoamine projection neurons (MAO-A; Westlund *et al.*, 1993; Arai *et al.*, 2002) and in astroctyes (MAO-A and MAO-B; Levitt *et al.*, 1982; Westlund *et al.*, 1988) where they are positioned to regulate both the amount of intracellular substrate available for release and the extrasynaptic inactivation of monoamine neurotransmitters.

In addition to considerable divergence in regional expression and activity (Westlund *et al.*, 1985, Fowler *et al.*, 1987; Willoughby *et al.*, 1988; Saura, Bleuel *et al.*, 1996; Saura, Nadal *et al.*, 1996; Jahng *et al.*, 1997), other key differences between the two isoforms are critical and instructive. First, MAO-A is thought to preferentially catabolize serotonin (5-HT) and norepinephrine (NE); although dopamine (DA) is a good substrate for both

---

[1] For example, in the Old Testament book of Deuteronomy (25:17–19), the Jewish people are commanded to slay the 'sons of Amalek' in each generation, as'wickedness' was thought to be inherited in this pedigree.

isoforms of MAO, the relative importance of MAO-A in regulating 5-HT and NE versus DA is underscored by the finding that *MAOA* knockout mice show drastically increased brain 5-HT and NE compared to wild-type, but only negligibly increased DA (Cases *et al.*, 1995; Shih, 2004). No such changes are evident in *MAOB* knockouts (Grimsby *et al.*, 1997). Furthermore, *MAOA* and *MAOB* knockout mice demonstrate distinct behavioural and neuromorphological phenotypes (discussed later). Finally, the developmental trajectories of MAO-A and MAO-B expression are quite different: MAO-A expression precedes MAO-B, and whereas MAO-A is present at adult levels at birth, and is the critical enzyme in mono-amine catabolism ante partum, MAO-B appears only post-natally and subsequently exhibits a striking increase (Tsang *et al.*, 1986; Strolin Benedetti *et al.*, 1992; Nicotra *et al.*, 2004).

Both human and animal studies point to a functional role for MAO-A in impulsive-aggressive behaviour. In a landmark study, Brunner examined a large Dutch kindred that was notorious for the high levels of reactive aggression demonstrated by some of its males. The characteristic behavioural phenotype, which stretched back for many generations, included mild mental retardation; predisposition to aggressive outbursts, especially in response to frustration, anger, and fear; and violent impulsive behaviour, such as rape, assault and attempted murder, arson, and exhibitionism (Brunner, Nelen, van Zandvoort *et al.*, 1993). Affected individuals demonstrated alterations in monoamine metabolism (Brunner, Nelen, Breakefield *et al.*, 1993; Abeling *et al.*, 1998), and females in this family were asymptomatic, which suggested that the heritable factor was X-linked (Brunner, Nelen, van Zandvoort *et al.*, 1993). Sequencing and linkage analysis revealed the culprit to be a point mutation (C936T) in the eighth exon of the *MAOA* gene, present in all affected individuals, which results in a premature stop codon–representing, in hemizygous males, a functional *MAOA* knockout (Brunner, Nelen, Breakefield *et al.*, 1993).

Subsequent genetic deletion studies have recapitulated the aggressive phenotype demon-strated in this human kindred and, by showing alterations in brain structure and function that relate to developmentally specific changes in 5-HT and NE metabolism, suggest mecha-nisms for the influence of *MAOA* on behaviour. Male *MAOA* knockout mice are hyperag-gressive and show dramatically elevated 5-HT (ninefold increase in pups, twofold increase in adults) and NE (twofold increase in pups and adults) and much smaller increases in DA (pups only; Cases *et al.*, 1995). The marked aggressive behaviour in these animals likely results from excess 5-HT, as it is blocked by the 5-HT2A antagonist ketanserin, as well as tetrabenazine, which depletes presynaptic monoamine stores (Shih *et al.*, 1999). *MAOA* knockouts also show selectively altered emotional (fear) learning in the context of normal motor learning (Kim *et al.*, 1997). An adverse influence of excess 5-HT during development is further suggested by the finding that *MAOA*-deficient mice show cytoarchitectonic changes in sensory cortex. These alterations are developmentally specific; pharmacological (clorgyline) attenuation of MAO-A replicates the phenotype only when administered during a critical developmental window. Furthermore, pharmacological depletion of 5-HT, but not of catecholamines, rescues the phenotype in *MAOA*-deficient animals (Cases *et al.*, 1996). Notably forebrain specific expression of *MAOA* rescues the behavioural, metabolic, and structural effects of *MAOA* deletion (Chen *et al.*, 2007).

These findings are consonant with a growing body of literature implicating elevated 5-HT during ontogeny in the development adult affective illness(Gingrich *et al.*, 2003; Ansorge *et al.*, 2004; Gross & Hen, 2004; Ansorge *et al.*, 2007,) and reinforce the established link between impulsive violence and alterations in 5-HT metabolism (Linnoila *et al.*, 1983; Brown & Linnoila, 1990; Virkkunen & Linnoila, 1990; Linnoila *et al.*, 1994; Virkkunen *et al.*, 1995; Krakowski, 2003). Thus, *MAOA* may represent a possible genetic pathway that accounts for the long-standing and frequently replicated observation that low serotonergic turnover (indicated by low cerebrospinal fluid [CSF] concentrations of the 5HT metabolite 5-hydroxyindoleacetic acid [5-HIAA]) strongly predicts high rates of aggression, particularly impulsive violence (Linnoila *et al.*, 1983; Virkkunen & Linnoila, 1990, 1993; Virkkunen *et al.*, 1995; Soderstrom *et al.*, 2001).

Although the human functional knockout described by Brunner and colleagues is rare, several relatively common polymorphisms have been identified in the *MAOA* gene, including a dinucleotide repeat in intron 2, single nucleotide polymorphisms (SNPs) in exons 8 (rs6323) and 14 (rs1801291), and a number of intronic SNPs (Balciuniene *et al.*, 2002; Pinsonneault *et al.*, 2006). However, the greatest degree of interest has been generated by Sabol and colleagues' discovery of a common, likely functional, variable number tandem repeat (VNTR) polymorphism in the upstream region of the gene. The *MAOA* u-VNTR is a 30 bp repeat that has been shown to impact transcription in an *in vitro* heterologous expression system; the presence of 3.5 or 4 repeats is associated with relatively higher *MAOA* expression (and are thus referred to as *MAOA*-H alleles), whereas the presence of 3 repeats (and also, possibly, 5 repeats, but see reference 43 for a contradictory report) results in relatively lower expression (*MAOA*-L alleles; Sabol *et al.*, 1998; Deckert *et al.*, 1999). However, the relevance of these *in vitro* changes to *in vivo* MAO-A expression and activity have yet to be confirmed; a recent study (Fowler *et al.*, 2006) found no correspondence between *MAOA*-uVNTR and MAO-A activity, assessed with radiolabelled clorgyline during positron emission tomography (PET).

The discovery of common functional variants in the *MAOA* gene, especially the *MAOA* u-VNTR, was greeted with great enthusiasm by behavioural geneticists, who immediately began the search for associations of this variant with behaviour and temperament. Given Brunner's linkage of altered *MAOA* function to antisocial behaviour, special emphasis was placed on finding associations to manifest behaviour and to traits that are empirically and conceptually related to aggression and impulsivity. A number of behavioural instruments and temperament measures have been used; however, mixed effects in terms of statistical significance, subscale heterogeneity, and allelic directionality for these associations render interpretation difficult. For example, six studies have examined the relationship between variation at the *MAOA* u-VNTR and NEO-PI traits, with the following results: positive association to the A2 ('Straightforwardness') subscale only in healthy individuals (Rosenberg *et al.*, 2006); Neuroticism (*MAOA*-H > *MAOA*-L) and Conscientiousness (*MAOA*-L>*MAOA*-H) in individuals with histrionic personality disorder, with no significant effect in healthy individuals or those with borderline personality disorder or antisocial personality disorder (Jacob *et al.*, 2005); Openness (*MAOA*-L , *MAOA*-H) in healthy males (Samochowiec *et al.*, 2004); peer-assessed Neuroticism (*MAOA*-H>*MAOA*-L) in healthy males; and two reports that were completely negative for association (Garpenstrand *et al.*, 2002; Tochigi *et al.*, 2006).

Associations to Tridimensional Personality Questionnaire and Temperament and Character Inventory (TPQ/TCI)-assessed personality traits are similarly mixed (Garpenstrand *et al.*, 2002; Samochowiec *et al.*, 2004; Jacob *et al.*, 2005; Contini *et al.*, 2006; Kim *et al.*, 2006), as are those using self-report assessments of aggression and impulsivity in adults (Manuck *et al.*, 2000; Koller *et al.*, 2003) and children (Beitchman *et al.*, 2004), although two studies support association of the *MAOA*-L allele to antisocial behaviour in alcoholics (Samochowiec *et al.*, 1999; Contini *et al.*, 2006). In addition, Guo and colleagues (2008) found a significant association of the rare *MAOA* VNTR '2 repeat' allele with delinquency in adolescents and young adults. Notably, a recent study found an interaction between *MAOA* genotype and CSF testosterone on antisocial behaviour, suggesting that genotype may interact with biological trait variables in determining risk for violence (Sjoberg *et al.*, 2007).

Other investigators have taken a different tack in examining the impact of the *MAOA* u-VNTR on brain and behaviour by utilizing clinical biomarkers for impulsivity and aggression, such as low CSF 5-HIAA (Linnoila *et al.*, 1983; Brown & Linnoila, 1990; Virkkunen & Linnoila, 1993; Mehlman *et al.*, 1994; Virkkunen *et al.*, 1995; Higley *et al.*, 1996; Higley & Linnoila, 1997; Stanley *et al.*, 2000; Soderstrom *et al.*, 2001; Daderman & Lidberg, 2002) and prolactin response to fenfluramine (Coccaro, 1989; Coccaro *et al.*, 1989; Fishbein *et al.*, 1989; Coccaro *et al.*, 1994; Coccaro *et al.*, 1997; Manuck *et al.*, 1998; Stanley *et al.*, 2000), in lieu of or in addition to diagnostic or self-report measures. Such biologically intermediate phenotypes hold promise in marking the neurobiological impact of *MAOA* genetic variation and confirming its potential relevance for individual differences in neurotransmitter function and metabolism in humans; however, given the conflicting findings to date (Manuck *et al.*, 1998; Jonsson *et al.*, 2000; Williams *et al.*, 2003; Zalsman *et al.*, 2005; Ducci *et al.*, 2006), we must conclude that this promise remains unfulfilled with respect to these particular phenotypes.

Although clinical, trait, and biomarker associations are mixed, the examination of gene-environment interactions in the context of risk of impulsive violence has revealed a fairly consistent effect of the *MAOA*-L allele in predisposing antisocial behaviour in males who experience early life adversity. In their path-breaking study of the *MAOA* genotype, childhood abuse, and adult violence, Caspi and colleagues (2002) found that, although genotype alone was not associated with antisocial behaviour, *MAOA* genotype mediated the impact of early life maltreatment on the development of antisocial behaviour later in life, with *MAOA*-L males significantly more susceptible to the effects of abuse and *MAOA*-H males relatively protected. This effect held for each of four distinct measures of impulsively violent behaviour: Conduct Disorder diagnosis (ages 10–18), adult violent convictions, self-reported disposition towards violence, and scores on an informant-reported Antisocial Personality Disorder symptom scale (Caspi *et al.*, 2002). Subsequent studies, including one meta-analysis (Kim-Cohen *et al.*, 2006), have independently replicated and extended this finding in new cohorts and with additional measures of impulsive violence (Foley *et al.*, 2004; Huang *et al.*, 2004; Nilsson *et al.*, 2006; Widom & Brzustowicz, 2006; Frazzetto *et al.*, 2007; Ducci *et al.*, 2008), although the predicted effect did not reach nominal significance in three groups (Haberstick *et al.*, 2005; Huizinga *et al.*, 2006; Prichard *et al.*, 2008). Intriguingly, one study of gene-environment interactions in non-human primates has also implicated the *MAOA*-L allele in amplifying the effect of early life experience on aggressive behaviour (Newman *et al.*, 2005); this same group has reported a significant impact of *MAOA* promoter variation on interspecies differences in aggression and social hierarchy in macaques, suggesting evolutionary mechanisms (Wendland, Hampe *et al.*, 2006; Wendland, Lesch *et al.*, 2006).

The advent of non-invasive functional and structural imaging techniques has allowed the development of a second, complimentary approach to characterizing a role for *MAOA* genetic variation in susceptibility to antisocial behaviour: the neural intermediate phenotype strategy. The intermediate phenotype (Gottesman & Gould, 2003) approach is motivated by the knowledge that the effect sizes for risk alleles implicated in neuropsychiatric illness are likely to be small, owing to the often subtle biological changes produced by, for example, alterations in transcriptional efficiency resulting from gene promoter polymorphisms. By studying quantitative biological traits that are closer to the level of a variant's putative direct physiological effect, the ability to detect such an effect is enhanced, as genetic penetrance will be greater at the level of the intermediate phenotype than at the level of manifest behaviour and/or diagnosis, and the genetic architecture is likely to be simpler (Meyer-Lindenberg & Weinberger, 2006). Functional and structural neuroimaging have been particularly useful in characterizing the impact of disease-associated alleles on risk for psychosis, affective illness, and personality disorders, by elucidating their influence on complex neural circuitry underlying cognition (Egan *et al.*, 2001; Fan *et al.*, 2003; Egan *et al.*, 2004; Gothelf *et al.*, 2005; Ho *et al.*, 2005; Meyer-Lindenberg, Kohn *et al.*, 2005; Passamonti *et al.*, 2005; McIntosh *et al.*, 2006; Ohnishi *et al.*, 2006; Addington *et al.*, 2007; Buckholtz *et al.*, 2007; Meyer-Lindenberg *et al.*, 2007), memory (Egan *et al.*, 2003; Hariri *et al.*, 2003; Pezawas *et al.*, 2004; Callicott *et al.*, 2005; Szeszko *et al.*, 2005; Bueller *et al.*, 2006; Hashimoto *et al.*, 2006; Ho *et al.*, 2006), and emotion regulation (Hariri*et al.*, 2002; Zubieta *et al.*, 2003; Brown *et al.*, 2005; Meyer-Lindenberg, Hariri *et al.*, 2005; Pezawas *et al.*, 2005; Smolka *et al.*, 2005; Bishop *et al.*, 2006; Neumann *et al.*, 2006; Drabant *et al.*, 2006; Eisenberger *et al.*, 2007; Smolka *et al.*, 2007).

Studies of candidate gene effects on brain structure and function are aided by parallel comparisons of these neuroimaging parameters in illness versus health. Overlap between a neural phenotype demonstrated by affected subjects, compared to healthy controls, and one shown by healthy individuals who possess a putative risk allele strengthens the argument that the allele is plausibly related to disease susceptibility and contributes to risk by adversely impacting brain activation, connectivity, and/or morphology. Therefore, although healthy subjects are often used in gene-imaging analyses to reduce genetic complexity and avoid potential disease-related confounds (e.g., current medication effects, history of drug abuse), such studies benefit from an understanding of how the condition itself manifests in the neuroimaging modalities under investigation. In the case of impulsive aggression, a relatively consistent picture has emerged implicating dysregulated corticolimbic circuitry for emotional inhibitory control that is strongly mediated by serotonergic function (Lee & Coccaro, 2001; Bufkin & Luttrell, 2005; Frankle *et al.*, 2005). Neuroimaging studies in highly impulsively aggressive patients, including adults diagnosed with intermittent explosive disorder (Best *et al.*, 2002; Coccaro *et al.*, 2007), adolescents with Conduct Disorder (Sterzer *et al.*, 2005; Stadler *et al.*, 2007), and convicted murderers (Raine *et al.*, 1994; Raine *et al.*, 1997; Raine *et al.*, 1998), implicate hyperreactive amygdala in the context of reduced recruitment of the orbital and medial prefrontal cortex, especially anterior cingulate cortex, during emotional engagement. These converge well with preclinical studies that have identified, both anatomically(Amaral & Price, 1984; Carmichael & Price, 1995; Carmichael & Price, 1996; Cavada *et al.*, 2000; Ongur & Price, 2000; Ghashghaei & Barbas, 2002; Stefanacci & Amaral, 2002) and functionally (Rosenkranz & Grace, 2001; Quirk *et al.*, 2003; Rosenkranz *et al.*, 2003; Schoenbaum *et al.*, 2003; Sotres-Bayon *et al.*, 2004; Likhtik *et al.*, 2005; Quirk & Beer, 2006; Sotres-Bayon *et al.*, 2006,), amygdalo-orbito-/medial-frontal circuits for emotion regulation and social cognition, as well as with over a century of lesion studies that have demonstrated violent impulsive behaviour[2] resulting from damage to these circuits (Butter & Snyder, 1972; Anderson *et al.*, 1999; Blair & Cipolotti, 2000; Clark & Manes, 2004; Machado & Bachevalier, 2006; Goursaud & Bachevalier, 2007).

To examine a potential role for the *MAOA* u-VNTR in contributing to risk for impulsive violence, investigators have examined the impact of this genetic variant on the structure, function, and connectivity of the circuits identified in patient studies by using functional imaging during

---

[2] so-called 'pseudo-psychopath' or 'acquired psychopathy', in contrast to 'developmental' psychopathy which, unlike these lesion-induced disorders, is characterized by primarily instrumental or goal-directed aggression; Blair, 2001.

experimental tasks that index inhibitory control, affective arousal, and emotional memory. Based on the genetic deletion and gene-environment interaction studies described in the preceding, special focus has been given to the *MAOA* u-VNTR: specifically, if the low-expression (*MAOA*-L) allele accounts for some of the variance in risk of impulsive-aggressive behaviour, it should bias cognitive and emotional information processing, even in neuropsychiatrically healthy subjects with no history of impulsive-aggression, towards a pattern reminiscent of that seen in ill subjects. This would be consistent with a model of risk wherein multiple genes, each of small effect size, impact susceptibility in a non-deterministic fashion by exerting a relatively deleterious influence over neural circuits that subserve cognitive domains impaired in the disorder.

In the first such study, Fan and colleagues (2003) found decreased anterior cingulate activation (and slightly increased reaction times, but no difference in error rates) during a combined attentional-orienting/conflict-resolution task in *MAOA*-L versus *MAOA*-H subjects. Passamonti *et al.* (2006) also studied executive cognition in *MAOA*-L subjects and found decreased ventrolateral prefrontal recruitment during a go/no-go task in *MAOA*-L compared with *MAOA*-H individuals, highlighting another brain region implicated in response inhibition. The magnitude of ventrolateral activation predicted increased scores on the Barrat Impulsivity Scale (BIS-11). Using genetic deletion mapping and voxel-based morphometry (VBM), a magnetic resonance imaging (MRI)-based method for analyzing between-group neurostructural differences (Ashburner & Friston, 2000), Good and colleagues (*Good et al.*, 2003) found morphometric changes in the orbitofrontal cortex and amygdala of women with Turner syndrome (45,X) and those with partial deletions of the X-chromosome that encompassed the *MAOA* gene. These women were also relatively impaired at facial expression recognition, a function modulated by the amygdala (Adolphs *et al.*, 1994).

Building on these findings, and with the aim of extending the investigation of *MAOA* genetic variation into the domain of emotional regulation and social cognition, our group used VBM and functional imaging during tasks that involve affective arousal, emotional memory, and cognitive inhibitory control. In a large sample of healthy individuals (n = 97), we found profound morphological differences throughout the limbic system (including cingulate gyrus, amygdala, hippocampus, in addition to changes in telencephalic and neocortical structures) in *MAOA*-L subjects, with these individuals demonstrating, on average, an 8% decrease in grey matter volume relative to *MAOA*-H subjects. In addition, we found an unhypothesized, but pronounced, gene-sex interaction, with *MAOA*-L men showing, on average, an 11% increase in lateral orbitofrontal volume compared to *MAOA*-H men; no such genotype-dependent differences were evident in women. Using fMRI, we found highly significant genotype-related differences in brain function. During the perceptual matching of fearful and angry faces (implicit emotion processing), *MAOA*-L subjects showed exaggerated limbic and paralimbic (amygdala and insula) activation, with diminished recruitment of prefrontal regulatory regions (i.e., the orbitofrontal and anterior cingulate cortices). We then tested the *MAOA* u-VNTR for an impact on the neural substrates of emotional memory and found a specific effect on aversive memory retrieval, such that *MAOA*-L subjects have significantly greater activation in the amygdala and hippocampus during the recall of negatively valenced, but not neutral, visual scenes. In the case of the hippocampus, we found a significant genotype-sex interaction, with *MAOA*-L men showing greater activation than *MAOA*-H men, but no significant differences between genotypes in women. We examined cognitive inhibitory control with a go/no-go variant of the Erikson flanker task (Blasi *et al.*, 2006) and, consistent with prior reports, found reduced dorsal cingulate activation (a region of maximal structural change) in *MAOA*-L men versus *MAOA*-H men, with no genotype-related differences in women. Of note, Lee and Ham (2008) have recently replicated our finding of altered limbic response to affective stimuli in *MAOA*-L individuals, using sad and angry facial expressions.

Although these highly significant regional structural and functional changes were remarkable, a critical test of the relevance of these findings is whether or not they predict relevant aspects of behaviour. Therefore, we were also interested in characterizing the consequence of *MAOA* genetic variation at the level of neural circuits, with the aim of demonstrating that an influence of *MAOA* u-VNTR on such circuits influences individual differences in temperamental traits that are conceptually and empirically related to impulsive aggression. Such traits are stable stimulus-response patterns that characterize individual behaviour, mediate risk for physical and psychiatric illness (Maunder & Hunter, 2001; Smith *et al.*, 2004; DeLongis & Holtzman, 2005), and predict measures of antisocial behaviour (including criminal arrests; Widiger & Lynam, 1998; Gullone & Moore, 2000; Lynam & Widiger, 2001; Miller *et al.*, 2001; Samuels *et al.*, 2004). We hypothesized that, similar to findings in genetic risk for major depressive illness, genotype would be more penetrant at the level of the neural circuit intermediate phenotype than at the level of self-report (Hariri *et al.*, 2005; Pezawas *et al.*, 2005; Meyer-Lindenberg & Weinberger, 2006). Furthermore, we predicted that the influence of genotype on personality would be mediated through the impact of genotype on activation and connectivity of brain circuitry for emotion and social cognition.

To this end, we first examined functional connectivity, a measure of linear regional fMRI signal covariation, during the facial emotion processing task, with a focus on structures that co-activate with, and hence might regulate, the amygdala. We identified the ventromedial prefrontal cortex (Brodmann area 10; vmPFC) as a region where functional connectivity was modified by genotype in a sex-specific fashion: *MAOA*-L men showed stronger amygdala-vmPFC functional coupling than *MAOA*-H men, whereas no effect of genotype was evident in women (Buckholtz *et al.*, 2008). The observation of connectivity between these regions was surprising, given the relative absence of direct anatomical connections between the vmPFC and amygdala (Amaral & Price, 1984; Carmichael & Price, 1995; Carmichael & Price, 1996; Ongur & Price, 2000; Ghashghaei & Barbas, 2002; Stefanacci & Amaral, 2002; Ghashghaei *et al.*, 2007). Thus, we hypothesized that another region that is directly connected to both the vmPFC and amygdala might mediate the observed functional coupling. Using individual amygdala-vmPFC connectivity parameters as regression covariates, we identified the perigenual anterior cingulate – a structure that is robustly interconnected with both the amygdala (Carmichael & Price, 1995) and the vmPFC (Ongur & Price, 2000) – as the region where activity tracked the degree of amygdala-vmPFC linkage.

Given our finding that vmPFC-amygdala coupling appeared to serve a regulatory function (vmPFC-amygdala functional connectivity correlated with the magnitude of amygdala dysregulation in *MAOA*-L men, explaining >30% of the interindividual variance in amygdala activation), we posited a model whereby the vmPFC is brought online in *MAOA*-L males as a second-level emotion regulation node to provide compensatory support to the perigenual cingulate, the structure and function of which is compromised in these individuals. This hypothesis was supported by path analysis to parse the effective (directional) connections within this amygdala-cingulate-vmPFC circuit: we found that the vmPFC regulates amygdala activation indirectly via an input to the perigenual cingulate, which sends an inhibitory projection to amygdala (Buckholtz *et al.*, 2008). These findings recapitulate preclinical and human studies that have elaborated a critical role for the perigenual cingulate in providing inhibitory cortical feedback to amygdala (Quirk *et al.*, 2003; Rosenkranz *et al.*, 2003). This circuit has been implicated as a neural substrate for fear extinction (Phelps *et al.*, 2004;

Sotres-Bayon et al., 2006) and affect regulation (Ochsner et al., 2002; Ochsner et al., 2004), is involved in individual differences in temperament (Zald et al., 2002; Keightley et al., 2003; Pezawas et al., 2005; Most et al., 2006), and may be dysfunctional in mood disorders (Mayberg et al., 1999; Anand et al., 2005). Importantly, this region is highly sensitive to modulation by 5-HT, as it has the greatest density of 5-HT receptors in human cortex (Varnas et al., 2004). This finding converges with other studies of genetic variation in 5-HT signalling (e.g., utilizing 5HTTLPR, a functional promoter VNTR in the 5-HT transporter gene *SLC6A4*, and a regulatory variant in *TPH2*, encoding the 5-HT anabolic enzyme tryptophan hydroxylase), which have shown aberrant amygdala activation (Brown et al., 2005; Canli et al., 2005; Hariri et al., 2005) and alterations in amygdala-cingulate (Pezawas et al., 2005) and amygdala-vmPFC (Heinz et al., 2005) connectivity in individuals possessing the allele associated with higher synaptic 5-HT, suggesting a unique developmental vulnerability of this circuit to changes in 5-HT during ontogeny.

To test the prediction that the neural circuit properties affected by *MAOA* genetic variation might predict individual trait differences, we extracted amygdala-VMPFC functional connectivity values and correlated these with individual subject scores on the NEO-PI (Costa & McCrae, 1992) and TPQ (Cloninger, 1987; Cloninger et al., 1993), two highly reliable measures of cardinal personality traits. The NEO-PI indexes five such traits, each with several subscales – Openness, Conscientiousness, Extraversion, Agreeableness, and Neuroticism – whereas the TPQ gauges three traits that are mediated, in Cloninger's model, by different neurotransmitters-Harm Avoidance (5-HT), Novelty Seeking (DA), and Reward Dependence (NE).In *MAOA*-L males, the magnitude of vmPFC-amygdala connectivity predicted increased Harm Avoidance and decreased Reward Dependence scores on the TPQ, and increased Angry Hostility (an Agreeableness subscale) scores on the NEO-PI. A striking feature of this finding is the correspondence between the putative neurobiological basis of the traits impacted by *MAOA* u-VNTR-associated functional connectivity and the neurotransmitters that are developmentally regulated by *MAOA* (Harm Avoidance-5-HT and Reward Dependence-NE). Notably, a control analysis using a genetic variant that impacts cortical DA, and which has been previously associated with amygdala-orbitofrontal functional connectivity linked to TPQ Novelty Seeking (COMT val158met; Drabant et al., 2006), did not cause alterations in this circuit (Buckholtz et al., 2008). Viewed categorically, the personality pattern associated with *MAOA*-linked differences in neural circuitry (high Harm Avoidance, low Reward Dependence, and high Angry Hostility) marks individuals with enhanced reactivity to threat cues; increased tendency to experience anger, frustration, and bitterness; and reduced sensitivity to cues that elicit and maintain prosocial behaviour – consistent with the neural signature of a risk factor of reactive aggression.

A previous study has shown that variation within one of these 'normal' personality dimensions (Angry Hostility) is associated with criminal arrest history; the likelihood of arrest increase dimensionally with increasing Angry Hostility scores (Samuels et al., 2004). As Angry Hostility is also represented in the Five Factor Model (FFM) characterizations of Antisocial Personality Disorder and psychopathy proposed by Widiger and Lynam (Widiger & Lynam, 1998; Lynam & Widiger, 2001), and predicts risk-taking judgments and behaviour in adolescents (Gullone & Moore, 2000), our findings accord with some prior research delineating the underlying personality structure of antisocial behaviour and raise the possibility that the pattern of emotional information processing we observe in healthy *MAOA*-L allele carriers may predispose them to personality traits that are similar to those seen in individuals who have committed or are at risk of committing antisocial acts.

We then used path analysis to test the hypothesis that vmPFC-amygdala functional connectivity mediates the relationship between genotype and personality. Two path models were created: a direct model and a mediated model. In the direct model, *MAOA* genotype had a direct path to temperament scores and a direct path vmPFC-amygdala functional connectivity (which itself had a direct path to temperament scores). In the mediated model, the input from *MAOA* genotype to personality was mediated exclusively by vmPFC-amygdala functional connectivity. Comparison of chi-square values for each of the models (a test for non-rejection of the null hypothesis that the correlation structure predicted by the model fit the observations) and Bollen's relative fit index showed that the mediated model fit the data better, and using a bootstrapping analysis to create confidence intervals for individual path coefficients, we found that the coefficients for the direct paths from genotype to personality scores were not significantly different than zero. By showing that the effects of *MAOA* genetic variation are more penetrant at the level of a neurobiological endophenotype (fMRI-assessed corticolimbic circuit function) than at the level of manifest behaviour, but that the changes indexed by the phenotype are relatable in a conceptually consistent way to such behaviour, this finding provides a validation of the intermediate phenotype approach in assessing the impact of neuropsychiatric risk genes (Buckholtz *et al.*, 2008).

A consistent feature in our neuroimaging studies of *MAOA* genetic variation is the greater impact of the *MAOA*-L allele on brain structure, function, and connectivity in men compared with women, a finding that resonates with the much greater incidence of antisocial behaviour and impulsive violence in this population (Moffitt *et al.*, 2001; Moffitt, 2006). Given that *MAOA* is located on the X chromosome, a simple gene-dosage effect might at first appear compelling. However, several factors weigh against this interpretation. Similar gender-dependent (males only) effects on amygdala-vmPFC connectivity have been shown in studies of a variant within the gene for the 5-HT transporter (Heinz *et al.*, 2005; Pezawas *et al.*, 2005), which is located on an autosomal gene. Moreover, our *in vivo* fMRI evidence suggests X inactivation of the *MAOA* gene, as female *MAOA*-L heterozygotes have a task-related neural response that is intermediate to that of female homozygotes (who are similar to hemizygous males). It is possible that the differential effects of the *MAOA*-L allele in women may involve a direct regulation of *MAOA* function by oestrogen, a known modulator of brain *MAOA* activity (Chakravorty & Halbreich, 1997; Holschneider *et al.*, 1998). Furthermore, oestrogen receptors are densely expressed in the amygdala, cingulated, and orbitofrontal cortex (MacLusky *et al.*, 1986), where they are able to regulate *MAOA* transcription (Gundlah *et al.*, 2002). Alternatively, or in addition, testosterone, long suspected to play a role in human aggression (Book *et al.*, 2001), may act in males through several glucocorticoid or androgen response elements in the *MAOA* promoter to influence transcription (Ou *et al.*, 2006). Such an influence might account for the recent finding of an interaction between CSF testosterone and *MAOA* genotype on male antisocial behaviour (Sjoberg *et al.*, 2007). Clearly, further study is needed to determine a precise mechanism underlying the consistent observation that females are relatively protected against (or men are particularly vulnerable to) the deleterious effects of the *MAOA*-L allele.

On the whole, our findings suggest that the *MAOA*-L allele specifically contributes to an impulsive or reactive dimension of aggression that is more common in antisocial behaviuor and intermittent-explosive disorder, rather than the instrumental or goal-directed style of aggression often linked to psychopathy (Blair, 2001, Ramirez & Andreu, 2006). Instrumental aggression has been linked to diminished neural responsiveness to affective cues and reduced orbitofrontal volume (Blair, 2004, 2005), the opposite pattern to that evinced by *MAOA*-L men.

Although the distinction between reactive and instrumental aggression may not be clear-cut in all, or even most, violent offenders, our data argue for a genetic dissociation between the two. Therefore, we offer a model of genetic risk for violence whereby distinct risk factors for reactive and instrumental aggression may exert their effects by impacting (at least partially) discrete neural systems, unique influences on which may be separable via multimodal neuroimaging.

We speculate that linkage between the *MAOA*-L-mediated alterations in corticolimbic structure, function, connectivity, and individual differences in temperament may relate to the proposed role of this circuitry in social cognition and affect regulation. The amygdala is involved in detecting social signals (e.g., affective facial expressions) and, by virtue of its connectivity with the prefrontal cortex, mediates the impact of these signals on attention and motivated behaviour (Zald, 2003; Phelps, 2006). The vmPFC is active during decision making under conditions of uncertainty and plays a role in context-dependent emotional decision making; damage to this region affects both of these abilities (Bechara, 2001; Davidson, 2002; Krawczyk, 2002; Volz *et al.*, 2006). The vmPFC, by virtue of its diverse heteromodal inputs, is able to provide context to ambiguity, facilitating resolution of the motivational significance of a stimulus under conditions of uncertainty (Mesulam, 1998; Price, 2005). The requirement for such resolution may be increased in *MAOA*-L subjects, as the amygdala, which signals ambiguous environmental threat (Davis & Whalen, 2001; Whalen *et al.*, 2001), is relatively unconstrained by its primary regulatory circuitry and hyperreactivity in *MAOA*-L individuals. Corticolimbic circuit dysfunction, resulting in persistent amygdala activation to social stimuli in *MAOA*-L men, may bias these individuals to misattribute hostile intent in the presence of ambiguous social cues, a predisposition seen in adolescent boys with high rates of reactive aggression (Crick & Dodge, 1996; Hudley & Friday, 1996; Schwartz *et al.*, 1998; Hubbard *et al.*, 2001).

Further evidence for aberrant social cognition resulting from *MAOA* genetic variation is gleaned from the recent demonstration by Eisenberger and colleagues (2007) of an exaggerated neural response to perceived social rejection in *MAOA*-L individuals; there, as here, brain activation mediated the relationship between genotype and temperament (trait aggression). In that study, trait social hypersensitivity mediated this relationship as well, suggesting that genotype-dependent sociocognitive alterations are involved in genetic predisposition to aggression. These phenomena, combined with poor behavioural controls resulting from deleterious changes in the structure and function of circuits subserving cognitive inhibitory control (Fan *et al.*, 2003; Passamonti *et al.*, 2005; Meyer-Lindenberg *et al.*, 2006), may prejudice *MAOA*-L subjects towards a more emotionally reactive personality type. We therefore propose that the *MAOA* genotype may modify an individual's socioaffective scaffold, the basic neural equipment for social and emotional experience. We suggest that, by altering 5-HT and NE levels during a critical window for the development of corticolimbic circuitry, the *MAOA*-L allele-induced developmental changes labilizes critical circuitry for affect and action regulation, which renders these individuals more vulnerable to the influence of adverse early life environment. In a supportive environment, increased threat sensitivity, diminished capacity for emotion regulation, and enhanced fear memory in *MAOA*-L men might only manifest subclinically as a temperamental variation; however, these same characteristics in an abusive childhood environment – one that may be typified by the presence of physical threat, a constant sense of fear, diminished external demand – for emotion regulation, and poor behavioural modelling-may translate to manifest aggression and impulsive violence in the adult. Moreover, early life experience – particularly maternal care – has been shown to dramatically impact neural pathways for stress sensitivity and emotional reactivity by modifying limbic glucocorticoid signalling (Weaver *et al.*, 2004). As glucocorticoids regulate *MAOA* expression through the promoter response elements mentioned earlier, this might represent a neural pathway for the observed interaction between *MAOA* genotype and childhood maltreatment. Thus, genetics might contribute to 'loading the gun', but in the absence of environmental challenges will rarely if ever by itself 'pull the trigger' (Buckholtz & Meyer-Lindenberg, 2008).

In closing, it is important to re-emphasize that our data and others reaffirm the fact that in the complex causal structure of impulsive violence, the *MAOA* u-VNTR contributes only a small amount of risk. Although it is not a 'violence gene' *per se,* the *MAOA*-L allele biases brain development towards alterations in function and structure that are associated with individual differences in personality that may predispose, in combination with other factors, the development of antisocial behaviour. However, considered on its own, the *MAOA*-L allele is completely compatible with psychiatric health. The main utility of this approach is therefore less in the claim to have isolated a genetic risk factor that is, by itself, predictive of behaviour, than in using this genetic variant as a tool for discovery of neural systems linked to impulsive violence, furthering our biological understanding of this complex and relevant phenomenon. Further different word advances in understanding of the neural mechanisms by which *MAOA* exerts its influence on behaviour awaits large-scale, multimodal imaging studies of the interplay between gene and the environment. In addition, given the small risk effect size of one genetic variant in isolation, multimarker (haplotype) and gene-gene interaction analysis of statistical and functional epistasis will be key to unraveling the manner by which individual genetic background, modified by experience, translates into individual behaviour.

References

Abeling, N. G., van Gennip, A. H., van Cruchten, A. G., Overmars, H., & Brunner, H. G. (1998). Monoamine oxidase A deficiency: biogenic amine metabolites in random urine samples. *Journal of Neural Transmission. Supplementum, 52*, 9–15.

Addington, A. M., Gornick, M. C., Shaw, P., Seal, J., Gogtay, N., Greenstein, D., *et al.* (2007). Neuregulin 1 (8p12) and childhood-onset schizophrenia: susceptibility haplotypes for diagnosis and brain developmental trajectories. *Molecular Psychiatry, 12*, 195–205.

Adolphs, R., Tranel, D., Damasio, H., & Damasio, A. (1994). Impaired recognition of emotion in facial expressions following bilateral damage to the human amygdala. *Nature, 372*, 669–672.

Amaral, D. G., & Price, J. L. (1984). Amygdalo-cortical projections in the monkey (Macaca fascicularis). *The Journal of Comparative Neurology, 230*, 465–496.

Anand, A., Li, Y., Wang, Y., Wu, J., Gao, S., Bukhari, L., *et al.* (2005). Activity and connectivity of brain mood regulating circuit in depression: a functional magnetic resonance study. *Biological Psychiatry, 57*, 1079–1088.

Anderson, S. W., Bechara, A., Damasio, H., Tranel, D., & Damasio, A. R. (1999). Impairment of social and moral behavior related to early damage in human prefrontal cortex. *Nature Neuroscience, 2*, 1032–1037.

Ansorge, M. S., Hen, R., & Gingrich, J. A. (2007). Neurodevelopmental origins of depressive disorders. *Current Opinion in Pharmacology, 7*, 8–17.

Ansorge, M. S., Zhou, M., Lira, A., Hen, R., & Gingrich, J. A. (2004). Early-life blockade of the 5-HT transporter alters emotional behavior in adult mice. *Science, 306*, 879–881.

Arai, R., Karasawa, N., Kurokawa, K., Kanai, H., Horiike, K., & Ito, A. (2002). Differential subcellular location of mitochondria in rat serotonergic neurons depends on the presence and the absence of monoamine oxidase type B. *Neuroscience, 114*, 825–835.

Ashburner, J., & Friston, K. J. (2000). Voxel-based morphometry—the methods. *Neuroimage, 11*, 805–821.

Balciuniene, J., Emilsson, L., Oreland, L., Pettersson, U., & Jazin, E. (2002). Investigation of the functional effect of monoamine oxidase polymorphisms in human brain. *Human Genetics*, *110*, 1–7.

Bechara, A. (2001). Neurobiology of decision-making: risk and reward. *Seminars in Clinical Neuropsychiatry*, *6*, 205–216.

Beitchman, J. H., Mik, H. M., Ehtesham, S., Douglas, L., & Kennedy, J. L. (2004). MAOA and persistent, pervasive childhood aggression. *Molecular Psychiatry*, *9*, 546–547.

Best, M., Williams, J. M., & Coccaro, E. F. (2002) Evidence for a dysfunctional prefrontal circuit in patients with an impulsive aggressive disorder. *Proceedings of the National Academy of Sciences of the United States of America, 99*, 8448–8453.

Bishop, S. J., Cohen, J. D., Fossella, J., Casey, B. J., & Farah, M. J. (2006). COMT genotype influences prefrontal response to emotional distraction. *Cognitive, Affective and Behavioral Neuroscience*, *6*, 62–70.

Blair, R. J. (2001). Neurocognitive models of aggression, the antisocial personality disorders, and psychopathy. *Journal of Neurology, Neurosurgery and Psychiatry, 71*, 727–731.

Blair, R. J. (2004). The roles of orbital frontal cortex in the modulation of antisocial behavior. *Brain and Cognition*, *55*, 198–208.

Blair, R. J. (2005). Applying a cognitive neuroscience perspective to the disorder of psychopathy. *Development and Psychopathology*, *17*, 865–891.

Blair, R. J., & Cipolotti, L. (2000). Impaired social response reversal. A case of 'cquired sociopathy'. *Brain*, *123*(6), 1122–1141.

Blasi, G., Goldberg, T. E., Weickert, T., Das, S., Kohn, P., Zoltick, B., *et al.* (2006). Brain regions underlying response inhibition and interference monitoring and suppression. *The European Journal of Neuroscience*, *23*, 1658–1664.

Book, A. S., Starzyk, K. B., & Quinsey, V. L. (2001). The relationship between testosterone and aggression: a meta-analysis. *Aggressive and Violent Behavior*, *6*, 579–599.

Bouchard Jr., T. J., Lykken, D. T., Mcgue, M., Segal, N. L., & Tellegen, A. (1990). Sources of human psychological differences: the Minnesota Study of Twins Reared Apart. *Science*, *250*, 223–228.

Brown, G. L., & Linnoila, M. I. (1990). CSF serotonin metabolite (5-HIAA) studies in depression, impulsivity, and violence. *Journal of Clinical Psychiatry*, *51*(Suppl), 31–41; discussion 42–43.

Brown, S. M., Peet, E., Manuck, S. B., Williamson, D. E., Dahl, R. E., Ferrell, R. E., *et al.* (2005). A regulatory variant of the human tryptophan hydroxylase-2 gene biases amygdala reactivity. *Molecular Psychiatry*, *10*, 884–888, 805.

Brunner, H. G., Nelen, M., Breakefield, X. O., Ropers, H. H., & van Oost, B. A. (1993). Abnormal behavior associated with a point mutation in the structural gene for monoamine oxidase A. *Science*, *262*, 578–580.

Brunner, H. G., Nelen, M. R., van Zandvoort, P., Abeling, N. G., van Gennip, A. H., Wolters, E. C., *et al.* (1993). X-linked borderline mental retardation with prominent behavioral disturbance: phenotype, genetic localization, and evidence for disturbed monoamine metabolism. *American Journal of Human Genetics*, *52*, 1032–1039.

Buckholtz, J. W., Callicott, J. H., Kolachana, B., Hariri, A. R., Goldberg, T. E., Genderson, M., *et al.* (2008). Genetic variation in MAOA modulates ventromedial prefrontal circuitry mediating individual differences in human personality. *Molecular Psychiatry*, *13*, 313–324.

Buckholtz, J. W., & Meyer-Lindenberg, A. (2008). MAOA and the neurogenetic architecture of human aggression. *Trends Neurosci*, *31*(3), 120–129.

Buckholtz, J. W., Meyer-Lindenberg, A., Honea, R. A., Straub, R. E., Pezawas, L., Egan, M. F., *et al.* (2007). Allelic variation in RGS4 impacts functional and structural connectivity in the human brain. *Journal of Neuroscience*, *27*, 1584–1593.

Bueller, J. A., Aftab, M., Sen, S., Gomez-Hassan, D., Burmeister, M., & Zubieta, J. K. (2006). BDNF Val66Metallele is associated with reduced hippocampal volume in healthy subjects. *Biological Psychiatry*, *59*, 812–815.

Bufkin, J. L., & Luttrell, V. R. (2005). Neuroimaging studies of aggressive and violent behavior: current findings and implications for criminology and criminal justice. *Trauma, Violence and Abuse*, *6*, 176–191.

Butter, C. M., & Snyder, D. R. (1972). Alterations in aversive and aggressive behaviors following orbital frontal lesions in rhesus monkeys. *Acta Neurobiologiae Experimentalis (Wars)*, *32*, 525–565.

Callicott, J. H., Straub, R. E., Pezawas, L., Egan, M. F., Mattay, V. S., Hariri, A. R., *et al.* (2005). Variation in DISC1 affects hippocampal structure and function and increases risk for schizophrenia. *Proceedings of the National Academy of Sciences of the United States of America*, *102*, 8627–8632.

Canli, T., Congdon, E., Gutknecht, L., Constable, R. T., & Lesch, K. P. (2005). Amygdala responsiveness is modulated by tryptophan hydroxylase-2 gene variation. *Journal of Neural Transmission*, *112*, 1479–1485.

Carmichael, S. T., & Price, J. L. (1995). Limbic connections of the orbital and medial prefrontal cortex in macaque monkeys. *The Journal of Comparative Neurology*, *363*, 615–641.

Carmichael, S. T., & Price, J. L. (1996). Connectional networks within the orbital and medial prefrontal cortex of macaque monkeys. *The Journal of Comparative Neurology*, *371*, 179–207.

Cases, O., Seif, I., Grimsby, J., Gaspar, P., Chen, K., Pournin, S., *et al.* (1995). Aggressive behavior and altered amounts of brain serotonin and norepinephrine in mice lacking MAOA. *Science*, *268*, 1763–1766.

Cases, O., Vitalis, T., Seif, I., de Maeyer, E., Sotelo, C., & Gaspar, P. (1996). Lack of barrels in the somatosensory cortex of monoamine oxidase A-deficient mice: role of a serotonin excess during the critical period. *Neuron*, *16*, 297–307.

Caspi, A., McClay, J., Moffitt, T. E., Mill, J., Martin, J., Craig, I. W., *et al.* (2002). Role of genotype in the cycle of violence in maltreated children. *Science*, *297*, 851–854.

Cavada, C., Company, T., Tejedor, J., Cruz-Rizzolo, R. J., & Reinoso-Suarez, F. (2000). The anatomical connections of the macaque monkey orbitofrontal cortex. *A review. Cerebral Cortex*, *10*, 220–242.

Chakravorty, S. G., & Halbreich, U. (1997). The influence of estrogen on monoamine oxidase activity. *Psychopharmacology Bulletin*, *33*, 229–233.

Chen, K., Cases, O., Rebrin, I., Wu, W., Gallaher, T. K., Seif, I., *et al.* (2007). Forebrain-specific expression of monoamine oxidase A reduces neurotransmitter levels, restores the brain structure, and rescues aggressive behavior in monoamine oxidase A-deficient mice. *The Journal of Biological Chemistry*, *282*, 115–123.

Clark, L., & Manes, F. (2004). Social and emotional decision-making following frontal lobe injury. *Neurocase*, *10*, 398–403.

Cleckley, H. (1988). The psychopath in history. In *The Mask of Sanity*, 5 edn. C.V. Mosby Co.

Cloninger, C. R. (1987). A systematic method for clinical description and classification of personality variants. *A proposal. Archives of General Psychiatry*, *44*, 573–588.

Cloninger, C. R., Svrakic, D. M., & Przybeck, T. R. (1993). A psychobiological model of temperament and character. *Archives of General Psychiatry*, *50*, 975–990.

Coccaro, E. F. (1989). Central serotonin and impulsive aggression. *British Journal of Psychiatry* (Suppl), 52–62.

Coccaro, E. F., Kavoussi, R. J., Cooper, T. B., & Hauger, R. L. (1997). Central serotonin activity and aggression: inverse relationship with prolactin response to d-fenfluramine, but not CSF 5-HIAA concentration, in human subjects. *American Journal of Psychiatry*, *154*, 1430–1435.

Coccaro, E. F., McCloskey, M. S., Fitzgerald, D. A., & Phan, K. L. (2007). Amygdala and orbitofrontal reactivity to social threat in individuals with impulsive aggression. *Biological Psychiatry*, *62*(2), 168–178.

Coccaro, E. F., Siever, L. J., Klar, H. M., Maurer, G., Cochrane, K., Cooper, T. B., *et al.* (1989). Serotonergic studies in patients with affective and personality disorders. *Correlates with suicidal and impulsive aggressive behavior. Archives of General Psychiatry*, *46*, 587–599.

Coccaro, E. F., Silverman, J. M., Klar, H. M., Horvath, T. B., & Siever, L. J. (1994). Familial correlates of reduced central serotonergic system function in patients with personality disorders. *Archives of General Psychiatry*, *51*, 318–324.

Contini, V., Marques, F. Z., Garcia, C. E., Hutz, M. H., & Bau, C. H. (2006). MAOA-uVNTR polymorphism in a Brazilian sample: further support for the association with impulsive behaviors and alcohol dependence. *American Journal of Medical Genetics: Part B, Neuropsychiatric Genetics*, *141*, 305–308.

Costa, P. T., & McCrae, R. R. (1992). *Professional Manual: Revised NEO Personality Inventory (NEO-PI-R) and NEO Five-Factor Inventory (NEO-FFI).* Odessa, FL: Psychological Assessment Resources.

Crick, N. R., & Dodge, K. A. (1996). Social information-processing mechanisms in reactive and proactive aggression. *Child Development, 67,* 993–1002.

Daderman, A. M., & Lidberg, L. (2002). Relapse in violent crime in relation to cerebrospinal fluid monoamine metabolites (5-HIAA, HVA and HMPG) in male forensic psychiatric patients convicted of murder: a 16-year follow-up. *Acta Psychiatrica Scandinavica* (Suppl), 71–74.

Davidson, R. J. (2002). Anxiety and affective style: role of prefrontal cortex and amygdala. *Biological Psychiatry, 51,* 68–80.

Davis, M., & Whalen, P. J. (2001). The amygdala: vigilance and emotion. *Molecular Psychiatry, 6,* 13–34.

Deckert, J., Catalano, M., Syagailo, Y. V., Bosi, M., Okladnova, O., di Bella, D., *et al.* (1999). Excess of high activity monoamine oxidase A gene promoter alleles in female patients with panic disorder. *Human Molecular Genetics, 8,* 621–624.

Delongis, A., & Holtzman, S. (2005). Coping in context: the role of stress, social support, and personality in coping. *Journal of Personality, 73,* 1633–1656.

Drabant, E. M., Hariri, A. R., Meyer-Lindenberg, A., Munoz, K. E., Mattay, V. S., Kolachana, B. S., *et al.* (2006). Catechol O-methyltransferase val158met genotype and neural mechanisms related to affective arousal and regulation. *Archives of General Psychiatry, 63,* 1396–1406.

Ducci, F., Enoch, M. A., Hodgkinson, C., Xu, K., Catena, M., Robin, R. W., *et al.* (2008). Interaction between a functional MAOA locus and childhood sexual abuse predicts alcoholism and antisocial personality disorder in adult women. *Molecular Psychiatry, 13,* 334–347.

Ducci, F., Newman, T. K., Funt, S., Brown, G. L., Virkkunen, M., & Goldman, D. (2006). A functional polymorphism in the MAOA gene promoter (MAOA-LPR) predicts central dopamine function and body mass index. *Molecular Psychiatry, 11,* 858–866.

Egan, M. F., Goldberg, T. E., Kolachana, B. S., Callicott, J. H., Mazzanti, C. M., Straub, R. E., *et al.* (2001). Effect of COMT Val108/158 Met genotype on frontal lobe function and risk for schizophrenia. *Proceedings of the National Academy of Sciences of the United States of America, 98,* 6917–6922.

Egan, M. F., Kojima, M., Callicott, J. H., Goldberg, T. E., Kolachana, B. S., Bertolino, A., *et al.* (2003). The BDNF val66met polymorphism affects activity-dependent secretion of BDNF and human memory and hippocampal function. *Cell, 112,* 257–269.

Egan, M. F., Straub, R. E., Goldberg, T. E., Yakub, I., Callicott, J. H., Hariri, A. R., *et al.* (2004). Variation in GRM3 affects cognition, prefrontal glutamate, and risk for schizophrenia. *Proceedings of the National Academy of Sciences of the United States of America, 101,* 12604–12609.

Eisenberger, N. I., Way, B. M., Taylor, S. E., Welch, W. T., & Lieberman, M. D. (2007). Understanding genetic risk for aggression: clues from the brain's response to social exclusion. *Biological Psychiatry, 61,* 1100–1108.

Fan, J., Fossella, J., Sommer, T., Wu, Y., & Posner, M. I. (2003). Mapping the genetic variation of executive attention onto brain activity. *Proceedings of the National Academy of Sciences of the United States of America, 100,* 7406–7411.

Fishbein, D. H., Lozovsky, D., & Jaffe, J. H. (1989). Impulsivity, aggression, and neuroendocrine responses to serotonergic stimulation in substance abusers. *Biological Psychiatry, 25,* 1049–1066.

Foley, D. L., Eaves, L. J., Wormley, B., Silberg, J. L., Maes, H. H., Kuhn, J., *et al.* (2004). Childhood adversity, monoamine oxidase a genotype, and risk for conduct disorder. *Archives of General Psychiatry, 61,* 738–744.

Fowler, J. S., Alia-Klein, N., Kriplani, A., Logan, J., Williams, B., Zhu, W., *et al.* (2006). Evidence that brain MAO A activity does not correspond to MAO A genotype in healthy male subjects. *Biological Psychiatry, 62*(4), 355–358.

Fowler, J. S., MacGregor, R. R., Wolf, A. P., Arnett, C. D., Dewey, S. L., Schlyer, D., *et al.* (1987). Mapping human brain monoamine oxidase A and B with 11C-labeled suicide inactivators and PET. *Science, 235,* 481–485.

Frankle, W. G., Lombardo, I., New, A. S., Goodman, M., Talbot, P. S., Huang, Y., *et al.* (2005). Brain serotonin transporter distribution in subjects with impulsive aggressivity: a positron emission study with [11C]McN 5652. *American Journal of Psychiatry, 162,* 915–923.

Frazzetto, G., di Lorenzo, G., Carola, V., Proietti, L., Sokolowska, E., Siracusano, A., *et al.* (2007). Early trauma and increased risk for physical aggression during adulthood: the moderating role of MAOA genotype. *PLoS ONE, 2*, e486.

Garpenstrand, H., Norton, N., Damberg, M., Rylander, G., Forslund, K., Mattila-Evenden, M., *et al.* (2002). A regulatory monoamine oxidase a promoter polymorphism and personality traits. *Neuropsychobiology, 46*, 190–193.

Ghashghaei, H. T., & Barbas, H. (2002). Pathways for emotion: interactions of prefrontal and anterior temporal pathways in the amygdala of the rhesus monkey. *Neuroscience, 115*, 1261–1279.

Ghashghaei, H. T., Hilgetag, C. C., & Barbas, H. (2007). Sequence of information processing for emotions based on the anatomic dialogue between prefrontal cortex and amygdala. *Neuroimage, 34*, 905–923.

Gingrich, J. A., Ansorge, M. S., Merker, R., Weisstaub, N., & Zhou, M. (2003). New lessons from knockout mice: the role of serotonin during development and its possible contribution to the origins of neuropsychiatric disorders. *CNS Spectrum, 8*, 572–577.

Good, C. D., Lawrence, K., Thomas, N.S., Price, C.J., Ashburner, J., Friston, K. J., *et al.* (2003). Dosage-sensitive X-linked locus influences the development of amygdala and orbitofrontal cortex, and fear recognition in humans. *Brain, 126*(Pt 11), 2431–2446.

Gothelf, D., Eliez, S., Thompson, T., Hinard, C., Penniman, L., Feinstein, C., *et al.* (2005). COMT genotype predicts longitudinal cognitive decline and psychosis in 22q11.2 deletion syndrome. *Nature Neuroscience, 8*, 1500–1502.

Gottesman, I., & Gould, T. D. (2003). The endophenotype concept in psychiatry: etymology and strategic intentions. *American Journal of Psychiatry, 160*, 636–645.

Goursaud, A. P., & Bachevalier, J. (2007). Social attachment in juvenile monkeys with neonatal lesion of the hippocampus, amygdala and orbital frontal cortex. *Behavioural Brain Research, 176*, 75–93.

Grimsby, J., Chen, K., Wang, L. J., Lan, N. C., & Shih, J. C. (1991). Human monoamine oxidase A and B genes exhibit identical exon-intron organization. *Proceedings of the National Academy of Sciences of the United States of America, 88*, 3637–3641.

Grimsby, J., Toth, M., Chen, K., Kumazawa, T., Klaidman, L., Adams, J. D., *et al.* (1997). Increased stress response and beta-phenylethylamine in MAOB-deficient mice. *Nature Genetics, 17*, 206–210.

Gross, C., & Hen, R. (2004). The developmental origins of anxiety. *Nature Reviews. Neuroscience, 5*, 545–552.

Grove, W. M., Eckert, E. D., Heston, L., Bouchard Jr., T. J., Segal, N., & Lykken, D. T. (1990). Heritability of substance abuse and antisocial behavior: a study of monozygotic twins reared apart. *Biological Psychiatry, 27*, 1293–1304.

Gullone, E., & Moore, S. (2000). Adolescent risk-taking and the five-factor model of personality. *Journal of Adolescence, 23*, 393–407.

Gundlah, C., Lu, N. Z., & Bethea, C. L. (2002). Ovarian steroid regulation of monoamine oxidase-A and -B mRNAs in the macaque dorsal raphe and hypothalamic nuclei. *Psychopharmacology (Berl), 160*, 271–282.

Guo, G., Ou, X. M., Roettger, M., & Shih, J. C. (2008). The VNTR 2 repeat in MAOA and delinquent behavior in adolescence and young adulthood: associations and MAOA promoter activity. *European Journal of Human Genetics, 16*, 626–634.

Haberstick, B. C., Lessem, J. M., Hopfer, C. J., Smolen, A., Ehringer, M. A., Timberlake, D., *et al.* (2005). Monoamine oxidase A (MAOA) and antisocial behaviors in the presence of childhood and adolescent maltreatment. *American Journal of Medical Genetics: Part B, Neuropsychiatric Genetics, 135*, 59–64.

Hariri, A. R., Drabant, E. M., Munoz, K. E., Kolachana, B. S., Mattay, V. S., Egan, M. F. , *et al.* (2005). A susceptibility gene for affective disorders and the response of the human amygdala. *Archives of General Psychiatry, 62*, 146–152.

Hariri, A. R., Goldberg, T. E., Mattay, V. S., Kolachana, B. S., Callicott, J. H., Egan, M. F., *et al.* (2003). Brain-derived neurotrophic factor val66met polymorphism affects human memory-related hippocampal activity and predicts memory performance. *Journal of Neuroscience, 23*, 6690–6694.

Hariri, A. R., Mattay, V. S., Tessitore, A., Kolachana, B., Fera, F., Goldman, D., *et al.* (2002). Serotonin transporter genetic variation and the response of the human amygdala. *Science, 297*, 400–403.

Hashimoto, R., Numakawa, T., Ohnishi, T., Kumamaru, E., Yagasaki, Y., Ishimoto, T., *et al.* (2006). Impact of the DISC1 Ser704Cys polymorphism on risk for major depression, brain morphology and ERK signaling. *Human Molecular Genetics*, *15*, 3024–3033.

Heinz, A., Braus, D. F., Smolka, M. N., Wrase, J., Puls, I., Hermann, D., *et al.* (2005). Amygdala-prefrontal coupling depends on a genetic variation of the serotonin transporter. *Nature Neuroscience*, *8*, 20–21.

Higley, J. D., & Linnoila, M. (1997). Low central nervous system serotonergic activity is trait-like and correlates with impulsive behavior. *A nonhuman primate model investigating genetic and environmental influences on neurotransmission. Annals of the New York Academy of Sciences*, *836*, 39–56.

Higley, J. D., Mehlman, P. T., Poland, R. E., Taub, D. M., Vickers, J., Suomi, S. J., *et al.* (1996). CSF testosterone and 5-HIAA correlate with different types of aggressive behaviors. *Biological Psychiatry*, *40*, 1067–1082.

Ho, B. C., Milev, P., O'Leary, D. S., Librant, A., Andreasen, N. C., & Wassink, T. H. (2006). Cognitive and magnetic resonance imaging brain morphometric correlates of brain-derived neurotrophic factor Val66Met gene polymorphism in patients with schizophrenia and healthy volunteers. *Archives of General Psychiatry*, *63*, 731–740.

Ho, B. C., Wassink, T. H., O'Leary, D. S., Sheffield, V. C., & Andreasen, N. C. (2005). Catechol-O-methyl transferase Val158Met gene polymorphism in schizophrenia: working memory, frontal lobe MRI morphology and frontal cerebral blood flow. *Molecular Psychiatry*, *10*, 287–298.

Holschneider, D. P., Kumazawa, T., Chen, K., & Shih, J. C. (1998). Tissue-specific effects of estrogen on monoamine oxidase A and B in the rat. *Life Sciences*, *63*, 155–160.

Huang, Y. Y., Cate, S. P., Battistuzzi, C., Oquendo, M. A., Brent, D., & Mann, J. J. (2004). An association between a functional polymorphism in the monoamine oxidase a gene promoter, impulsive traits and early abuse experiences. *Neuropsychopharmacology*, *29*, 1498–1505.

Hubbard, J. A., Dodge, K. A., Cillessen, A. H., Coie, J. D., & Schwartz, D. (2001). The dyadic nature of social information processing in boys' reactive and proactive aggression. *Journal of Personality and Social Psychology*, *80*, 268–280.

Hudley, C., & Friday, J. (1996). Attributional bias and reactive aggression. *American Journal of Preventive Medicine*, *12*, 75–81.

Huizinga, D., Haberstick, B. C., Smolen, A., Menard, S., Young, S. E., Corley, R. P., *et al.* (2006). Childhood maltreatment, subsequent antisocial behavior, and the role of monoamine oxidase A genotype. *Biological Psychiatry*, *60*, 677–683.

Jacob, C. P., Muller, J., Schmidt, M., Hohenberger, K., Gutknecht, L., Reif, A., *et al.* (2005). Cluster B personality disorders are associated with allelic variation of monoamine oxidase A activity. *Neuropsychopharmacology*, *30*, 1711–1718.

Jahng, J. W., Houpt, T. A., Wessel, T. C., Chen, K., Shih, J. C., & Joh, T. H. (1997). Localization of monoamine oxidase A and B mRNA in the rat brain by in situ hybridization. *Synapse*, *25*, 30–36.

Jonsson, E. G., Norton, N., Gustavsson, J. P., Oreland, L., Owen, M. J., & Sedvall, G. C. (2000). A promoter polymorphism in the monoamine oxidase A gene and its relationships to monoamine metabolite concentrations in CSF of healthy volunteers. *Journal of Psychiatric Research*, *34*, 239–244.

Keightley, M. L., Seminowicz, D. A., Bagby, R. M., Costa, P. T., Fossati, P., & Mayberg, H. S. (2003). Personality influences limbic-cortical interactions during sad mood induction. *Neuroimage*, *20*, 2031–2039.

Kim, J. J., Shih, J. C., Chen, K., Chen, L., Bao, S., Maren, S., *et al.* (1997). Selective enhancement of emotional, but not motor, learning in monoamine oxidase A-deficient mice. *Proceedings of the National Academy of Sciences of the United States of America*, *94*, 5929–5933.

Kim, S. J., Kim, Y. S., Kim, S. Y., Lee, H. S., & Kim, C. H. (2006). An association study of catechol-O-methyltransferase and monoamine oxidase A polymorphisms and personality traits in Koreans. *Neuroscience Letters*, *401*, 154–158.

Kim-Cohen, J., Caspi, A., Taylor, A., Williams, B., Newcombe, R., Craig, I. W., *et al.* (2006). MAOA, maltreatment, and gene-environment interaction predicting children's mental health: new evidence and a meta-analysis. *Molecular Psychiatry*, *11*, 903–913.

Koenig, L. B., McGue, M., Krueger, R. F., & Bouchard Jr., T. J. (2007). Religiousness, antisocial behavior, and altruism: genetic and environmental mediation. *Journal of Personality*, *75*, 265–290.

Koller, G., Bondy, B., Preuss, U. W., Bottlender, M., & Soyka, M. (2003). No association between a polymorphism in the promoter region of the MAOA gene with antisocial personality traits in alcoholics. *Alcohol and Alcoholism*, *38*, 31–34.

Krakowski, M. (2003). Violence and serotonin: influence of impulse control, affect regulation, and social functioning. *Journal of Neuropsychiatry and Clinical Neuroscience*, *15*, 294–305.

Krawczyk, D. C. (2002). Contributions of the prefrontal cortex to the neural basis of human decision making. *Neuroscience and Biobehavioral Reviews*, *26*, 631–664.

Lee, B. T., & Ham, B. J. (2008). Monoamine oxidase A-uVNTR genotype affects limbic brain activity in response to affective facial stimuli. *Neuroreport*, *19*, 515–519.

Lee, R., & Coccaro, E. (2001). The neuropsychopharmacology of criminality and aggression. *Canadian Journal of Psychiatry*, *46*, 35–44.

Levitt, P., Pintar, J. E., & Breakefield, X. O. (1982). Immunocytochemical demonstration of monoamine oxidase B in brain astrocytes and serotonergic neurons. *Proceedings of the National Academy of Sciences of the United States of America*, *79*, 6385–6389.

Likhtik, E., Pelletier, J. G., Paz, R., & Pare, D. (2005). Prefrontal control of the amygdala. *Journal of Neuroscience*, *25*, 7429–7437.

Linnoila, M., Virkkunen, M., George, T., Eckardt, M., Higley, J. D., Nielsen, D., *et al.* (1994). Serotonin, violent behavior and alcohol. *Exs*, *71*, 155–163.

Linnoila, M., Virkkunen, M., Scheinin, M., Nuutila, A., Rimon, R., & Goodwin, F. K. (1983). Low cerebrospinal fluid 5-hydroxyindoleacetic acid concentration differentiates impulsive from nonimpulsive violent behavior. *Life Sciences*, *33*, 2609–2614.

Lynam, D. R., & Widiger, T. A. (2001). Using the five-factor model to represent the DSM-IV personality disorders: an expert consensus approach. *Journal of Abnormal Psychology*, *110*, 401–412.

Machado, C. J., & Bachevalier, J. (2006). The impact of selective amygdala, orbital frontal cortex, or hippocampal formation lesions on established social relationships in rhesus monkeys (Macaca mulatta). *Behavioral Neuroscience*, *120*, 761-786.

Maclusky, N. J., Naftolin, F., & Goldman-Rakic, P. S. (1986). Estrogen formation and binding in the cerebral cortex of the developing rhesus monkey. *Proceedings of the National Academy of Sciences of the United States of America*, *83*, 513–516.

Manuck, S. B., Flory, J. D., Ferrell, R. E., Mann, J. J., & Muldoon, M. F. (2000). A regulatory polymorphism of the monoamine oxidase-A gene may be associated with variability in aggression, impulsivity, and central nervous system serotonergic responsivity. *Psychiatry Research*, *95*, 9–23.

Manuck, S. B., Flory, J. D., McCaffery, J. M., Matthews, K. A., Mann, J. J., & Muldoon, M. F. (1998). Aggression, impulsivity, and central nervous system serotonergic responsivity in a nonpatient sample. *Neuropsychopharmacology*, *19*, 287–299.

Maunder, R. G., & Hunter, J. J. (2001). Attachment and psychosomatic medicine: developmental contributions to stress and disease. *Psychosomatic Medicine*, *63*, 556–567.

Mayberg, H. S., Liotti, M., Brannan, S. K., Mcginnis, S., Mahurin, R. K., Jerabek, P. A., *et al.* (1999). Reciprocal limbic-cortical function and negative mood: converging PET findings in depression and normal sadness. *American Journal of Psychiatry*, *156*, 675–682.

McIntosh, A. M., Baig, B. J., Hall, J., Job, D., Whalley, H. C., Lymer, G. K., *et al.* (2006). Relationship of catechol-O-methyltransferase variants to brain structure and function in a population at high risk of psychosis. *Biological Psychiatry*, *61*(10), 1127–1134.

Mehlman, P. T., Higley, J. D., Faucher, I., Lilly, A. A., Taub, D. M., Vickers, J., *et al.* (1994). Low CSF 5-HIAA concentrations and severe aggression and impaired impulse control in nonhuman primates. *American Journal of Psychiatry*, *151*, 1485–1491.

Mesulam, M. M. (1998). From sensation to cognition. *Brain*, *121*(6), 1013–1052.

Meyer-Lindenberg, A., Buckholtz, J. W., Kolachana, B., Pezawas, L., Blasi, G., Wabnitz, A., *et al.* (2006). Neural mechanisms of genetic risk for impulsivity and violence in humans. *Proceedings of the National Academy of Sciences of the United States of America*, *103*, 6269–6274.

Meyer-Lindenberg, A., Hariri, A. R., Munoz, K. E., Mervis, C. B., Mattay, V. S., Morris, C. A., *et al.* (2005). Neural correlates of genetically abnormal social cognition in Williams syndrome. *Nature Neuroscience*, *8*, 991–993.

Meyer-Lindenberg, A., Kohn, P. D., Kolachana, B., Kippenhan, S., Mcinerney-Leo, A., Nussbaum, R., *et al.* (2005). Midbrain dopamine and prefrontal function in humans: interaction and modulation by COMT genotype. *Nature Neuroscience, 8*, 594–596.

Meyer-Lindenberg, A., Straub, R. E., Lipska, B. K., Verchinski, B. A., Goldberg, T., Callicott, J., *et al.* (2007). Genetic evidence implicating DARPP-32 in human frontostriatal structure, function, and cognition. *The Journal of Clinical Investigation, 117*, 672–682.

Meyer-Lindenberg, A., & Weinberger, D. R. (2006). Intermediate phenotypes and genetic mechanisms of psychiatric disorders. *Nature Reviews. Neuroscience, 7*, 818–827.

Miller, J. D., Lynam, D. R., Widiger, T. A., & Leukefeld, C. (2001). Personality disorders as extreme variants of common personality dimensions: can the Five-Factor Model adequately represent psychopathy? *Journal of Personality, 69*, 253–276.

Moffitt, T. E. (2006). Life-course-persistent versus adolescent-limited antisocial behavior. In D. Cicchetti, & D. Cohen (eds), *Developmental Psychopathology*. New York: John Wiley & Sons, Inc.

Moffitt, T. E., Caspi, A., Rutter, M., & Silva, P. (2001). *Sex Differences in Antisocial Behavior: Conduct Disorder, Delinquency and Violence in the Dunedin Longitudinal Study*. New York: Cambridge University Press.

Most, S. B., Chun, M. M., Johnson, M. R., & Kiehl, K. A. (2006). Attentional modulation of the amygdala varies with personality. *NeuroImage, 31*(2), 934–944.

Neumann, S. A., Brown, S. M., Ferrell, R. E., Flory, J. D., Manuck, S. B., & Hariri, A. R. (2006). Human choline transporter gene variation is associated with corticolimbic reactivity and autonomic-cholinergic function. *Biological Psychiatry, 60*, 1155–1162.

Newman, T. K., Syagailo, Y. V., Barr, C. S., Wendland, J. R., Champoux, M., Graessle, M., *et al.* (2005). Monoamine oxidase A gene promoter variation and rearing experience influences aggressive behavior in rhesus monkeys. *Biological Psychiatry, 57*, 167–172.

Nicotra, A., Pierucci, F., Parvez, H., & Senatori, O. (2004). Monoamine oxidase expression during development and aging. *Neurotoxicology, 25*, 155–165.

Nilsson, K. W., Sjoberg, R. L., Damberg, M., Leppert, J., Ohrvik, J., Alm, P. O., *et al.* (2006). Role of monoamine oxidase a genotype and psychosocial factors in male adolescent criminal activity. *Biological Psychiatry, 59*, 121–127.

Ochsner, K. N., Bunge, S. A., Gross, J. J., & Gabrieli, J. D. (2002). Rethinking feelings: an fMRI study of the cognitive regulation of emotion. *Journal of Cognitive Neuroscience, 14*, 1215–1229.

Ochsner, K. N., Ray, R. D., Cooper, J. C., Robertson, E. R., Chopra, S., Gabrieli, J. D., *et al.* (2004). For better or for worse: neural systems supporting the cognitive down- and up-regulation of negative emotion. *NeuroImage, 23*, 483–499.

Ohnishi, T., Hashimoto, R., Mori, T., Nemoto, K., Moriguchi, Y., Iida, H., *et al.* (2006). The association between the Val158Met polymorphism of the catechol-O-methyl transferase gene and morphological abnormalities of the brain in chronic schizophrenia. *Brain, 129*, 399–410.

Ongur, D., & Price, J. L. (2000). The organization of networks within the orbital and medial prefrontal cortex of rats, monkeys and humans. *Cerebral Cortex, 10*, 206–219.

Ou, X. M., Chen, K., & Shih, J. C. (2006). Glucocorticoid and androgen activation of monoamine oxidase A is regulated differently by R1 and Sp1. *The Journal of Biological Chemistry, 281*, 21512–21525.

Passamonti, L., Fera, F., Magariello, A., Cerasa, A., Gioia, M. C., Muglia, M., et al. (2006). Monoamine oxidase-A genetic variations influence brain activity associated with inhibitory control: new insight into the neural correlates of impulsivity. *Biological Psychiatry, 59(4)*, 334–340

Pezawas, L., Meyer-Lindenberg, A., Drabant, E. M., Verchinski, B. A., Munoz, K. E., Kolachana, B. S., *et al.* (2005). 5-HTTLPR polymorphism impacts human cingulate-amygdala interactions: a genetic susceptibility mechanism for depression. *Nature Neuroscience, 8*, 828–834.

Pezawas, L., Verchinski, B. A., Mattay, V. S., Callicott, J. H., Kolachana, B. S., Straub, R. E., *et al.* (2004). The brain-derived neurotrophic factor val66met polymorphism and variation in human cortical morphology. *Journal of Neuroscience, 24*, 10099–10102.

Phelps, E. A. (2006). Emotion and cognition: insights from studies of the human amygdala. *Annual Review of Psychology, 57*, 27–53.

Phelps, E. A., Delgado, M. R., Nearing, K. I., & Ledoux, J. E. (2004). Extinction learning in humans: role of the amygdala and vmPFC. *Neuron, 43*, 897–905.

Pinsonneault, J. K., Papp, A. C., & Sadee, W. (2006). Allelic mRNA expression of X-linked monoamine oxidase a (MAOA) in human brain: dissection of epigenetic and genetic factors. *Human Molecular Genetics, 15*, 2636–2649.

Price, J. L. (2005). Free will versus survival: brain systems that underlie intrinsic constraints on behavior. *The Journal of Comparative Neurology, 493*, 132–139.

Prichard, Z., Mackinnon, A., Jorm, A. F., & Easteal, S. (2008). No evidence for interaction between MAOA and childhood adversity for antisocial behavior. *American Journal of Medical Genetics: Part B, Neuropsychiatric Genetics, 147*, 228–232.

Quirk, G. J., & Beer, J. S. (2006). Prefrontal involvement in the regulation of emotion: convergence of rat and human studies. *Current Opinion in Neurobiology, 16*, 723–727.

Quirk, G. J., Likhtik, E., Pelletier, J. G., & Pare, D. (2003). Stimulation of medial prefrontal cortex decreases the responsiveness of central amygdala output neurons. *Journal of Neuroscience, 23*, 8800–8807.

Raine, A., Buchsbaum, M., & Lacasse, L. (1997). Brain abnormalities in murderers indicated by positron emission tomography. *Biological Psychiatry, 42*, 495–508.

Raine, A., Buchsbaum, M. S., Stanley, J., Lottenberg, S., Abel, L., & Stoddard, J. (1994). Selective reductions in prefrontal glucose metabolism in murderers. *Biological Psychiatry, 36*, 365–373.

Raine, A., Meloy, J. R., Bihrle, S., Stoddard, J., Lacasse, L., & Buchsbaum, M. S. (1998). Reduced prefrontal and increased subcortical brain functioning assessed using positron emission tomography in predatory and affective murderers. *Behavioral Sciences and the Law, 16*, 319–332.

Ramirez, J. M., & Andreu, J. M. (2006). Aggression, and some related psychological constructs (anger, hostility, and impulsivity); some comments from a research project. *Neuroscience and Biobehavioral Review, 30*, 276–291.

Rosenberg, S., Templeton, A. R., Feigin, P. D., Lancet, D., Beckmann, J. S., Selig, S., etal (2006). The association of DNA sequence variation at the MAOA genetic locus with quantitative behavioural traits in normal males. Human Genetics, 120, 447–459,

Rosenkranz, J. A., & Grace, A. A. (2001). Dopamine attenuates prefrontal cortical suppression of sensory inputs to the basolateral amygdala of rats. *Journal of Neuroscience, 21*, 4090–4103.

Rosenkranz, J. A., Moore, H., & Grace, A. A. (2003). The prefrontal cortex regulates lateral amygdala neuronal plasticity and responses to previously conditioned stimuli. *Journal of Neuroscience, 23*, 11054–11064.

Sabol, S. Z., Hu, S., & Hamer, D. (1998). A functional polymorphism in the monoamine oxidase A gene promoter. *Human Genetics, 103*, 273–279.

Samochowiec, J., Lesch, K. P., Rottmann, M., Smolka, M., Syagailo, Y. V., Okladnova, O., *et al.* (1999). Association of a regulatory polymorphism in the promoter region of the monoamine oxidase A gene with antisocial alcoholism. *Psychiatry Research, 86*, 67–72.

Samochowiec, J., Syrek, S., Michal, P., Ryzewska-Wodecka, A., Samochowiec, A., Horodnicki, J., *et al.* (2004). Polymorphisms in the serotonin transporter and monoamine oxidase A genes and their relationship to personality traits measured by the Temperament and Character Inventory and NEO Five-Factor Inventory in healthy volunteers. *Neuropsychobiology, 50*, 174–181.

Samuels, J., Bienvenu, O. J., Cullen, B., Costa Jr., P. T., Eaton, W. W., & Nestadt, G. (2004). Personality dimensions and criminal arrest. *Comprehensive Psychiatry, 45*, 275–280.

Saura, J., Bleuel, Z., Ulrich, J., Mendelowitsch, A., Chen, K., Shih, J. C., *et al.* (1996). Molecular neuroanatomy of human monoamine oxidases A and B revealed by quantitative enzyme radioautography and in situ hybridization histochemistry. *Neuroscience, 70*, 755–774.

Saura, J., Nadal, E., van den Berg, B., Vila, M., Bombi, J. A., & Mahy, N. (1996). Localization of monoamine oxidases in human peripheral tissues. *Life Sciences, 59*, 1341–1349.

Schoenbaum, G., Setlow, B., & Ramus, S. J. (2003). A systems approach to orbitofrontal cortex function: recordings in rat orbitofrontal cortex reveal interactions with different learning systems. *Behavioural Brain Research, 146*, 19–29.

Schwartz, D., Dodge, K. A., Coie, J. D., Hubbard, J. A., Cillessen, A. H., Lemerise, E. A., *et al.* (1998). Social-cognitive and behavioral correlates of aggression and victimization in boys' play groups. *Journal of Abnormal Child Psychology, 26*, 431–440.

Shih, J. C. (2004). Cloning, after cloning, knock-out mice, and physiological functions of MAO A and B. *Neurotoxicology, 25*, 21–30.

Shih, J. C., Chen, K., & Ridd, M. J. (1999). Monoamine oxidase: from genes to behavior. *Annual Review of Neuroscience*, *22*, 197–217.

Shih, J. C., Ridd, M. J., Chen, K., Meehan, W. P., Kung, M. P., Seif, I., *et al.* (1999). Ketanserin and tetrabenazine abolish aggression in mice lacking monoamine oxidase A. *Brain Research*, *835*, 104–112.

Sjoberg, R. L., Ducci, F., Barr, C. S., Newman, T. K., Dell'osso, L., Virkkunen, M., *et al.* (2007). A non-additive interaction of a functional MAO-A VNTR and testosterone predicts antisocial behavior. *Neuropsychopharmacology*, *33*, 425–430.

Smith, T. W., Glazer, K., Ruiz, J. M., & Gallo, L. C. (2004). Hostility, anger, aggressiveness, and coronary heart disease: an interpersonal perspective on personality, emotion, and health. *Journal of Personality*, *72*, 1217–1270.

Smolka, M. N., Buhler, M., Schumann, G., Klein, S., Hu, X. Z., Moayer, M., *et al.* (2007). Gene-gene effects on central processing of aversive stimuli. *Molecular Psychiatry*, *12*, 307–317.

Smolka, M. N., Schumann, G., Wrase, J., Grusser, S. M., Flor, H., Mann, K., *et al.* (2005). Catechol-O-methyltransferase val158met genotype affects processing of emotional stimuli in the amygdala and prefrontal cortex. *Journal of Neuroscience*, *25*, 836–842.

Soderstrom, H., Blennow, K., Manhem, A., & Forsman, A. (2001). CSF studies in violent offenders. *I. 5-HIAA as a negative and HVA as a positive predictor of psychopathy. Journal of Neural Transmission*, *108*, 869–878.

Sotres-Bayon, F., Bush, D. E., & Ledoux, J. E. (2004). Emotional perseveration: an update on prefrontal-amygdala interactions in fear extinction. *Learn and Memory*, *11*, 525–535.

Sotres-Bayon, F., Cain, C. K., & Ledoux, J. E. (2006). Brain mechanisms of fear extinction: historical perspectives on the contribution of prefrontal cortex. *Biological Psychiatry*, *60*(4), 329–336.

Stadler, C., Sterzer, P., Schmeck, K., Krebs, A., Kleinschmidt, A., & Poustka, F. (2007). Reduced anterior cingulate activation in aggressive children and adolescents during affective stimulation: association with temperament traits. *Journal of Psychiatric Research*, *41*, 410–417.

Stanley, B., Molcho, A., Stanley, M., Winchel, R., Gameroff, M. J., Parsons, B., *et al.* (2000). Association of aggressive behavior with altered serotonergic function in patients who are not suicidal. *American Journal of Psychiatry*, *157*, 609–614.

Stefanacci, L., & Amaral, D. G. (2002). Some observations on cortical inputs to the macaque monkey amygdala: an anterograde tracing study. *The Journal of Comparative Neurology*, *451*, 301–323.

Sterzer, P., Stadler, C., Krebs, A., Kleinschmidt, A., & Poustka, F. (2005). Abnormal neural responses to emotional visual stimuli in adolescents with conduct disorder. *Biological Psychiatry*, *57*, 7–15.

Strolin Benedetti, M., Dostert, P., & Tipton, K. F. (1992). Developmental aspects of the monoamine-degrading enzyme monoamine oxidase. *Developmental Pharmacology and Therapeutics*, *18*, 191–200.

Szeszko, P. R., Lipsky, R., Mentschel, C., Robinson, D., Gunduz-Bruce, H., Sevy, S., *et al.* (2005). Brain-derived neurotrophic factor val66met polymorphism and volume of the hippocampal formation. *Molecular Psychiatry*, *10*, 631–636.

Tochigi, M., Otowa, T., Hibino, H., Kato, C., Otani, T., Umekage, T., *et al.* (2006). Combined analysis of association between personality traits and three functional polymorphisms in the tyrosine hydroxylase, monoamine oxidase A, and catechol-O-methyltransferase genes. *Neuroscience Research*, *54*, 180–185.

Tsang, D., Ho, K. P., & Wen, H. L. (1986). Ontogenesis of multiple forms of monoamine oxidase in rat brain regions and liver. *Developmental Neuroscience*, *8*, 243–250.

Varnas, K., Halldin, C., & Hall, H. (2004). Autoradiographic distribution of serotonin transporters and receptor subtypes in human brain. *Human Brain Mapping*, *22*, 246–260.

Viding, E., Blair, R. J., Moffitt, T. E., & Plomin, R. (2005). Evidence for substantial genetic risk for psychopathy in 7-year-olds. *Journal of Child Psychology and Psychiatry*, *46*, 592–597.

Viding, E., Frick, P. J., & Plomin, R. (2007). Aetiology of the relationship between callous-unemotional traits and conduct problems in childhood. *British Journal of Psychiatry*, *190*, s33–s38.

Virkkunen, M., Goldman, D., Nielsen, D. A., & Linnoila, M. (1995). Low brain serotonin turnover rate (low CSF 5-HIAA) and impulsive violence. *J Psychiatry and Neuroscience*, *20*, 271–275.

Virkkunen, M., & Linnoila, M. (1990). Serotonin in early onset, male alcoholics with violent behaviour. *Annals of Medicine*, *22*, 327–331.

Virkkunen, M., & Linnoila, M. (1993). Brain serotonin, type II alcoholism and impulsive violence. *Journal of Studies on Alcohol Supplement*, *11*, 163–169.

Volz, K. G., Schubotz, R. I., & von Cramon, D. Y. (2006). Decision-making and the frontal lobes. *Current Opinion in Neurology*, *19*, 401–406.

Weaver, I. C., Cervoni, N., Champagne, F. A., D'alessio, A. C., Sharma, S., Seckl, J. R., *et al.* (2004). Epigenetic programming by maternal behavior. *Nature Neuroscience*, *7*, 847–854.

Wendland, J. R., Hampe, M., Newman, T. K., Syagailo, Y., Meyer, J., Schempp, W., *et al.* (2006). Structural variation of the monoamine oxidase A gene promoter repeat polymorphism in nonhuman primates. *Genes, Brain and Behavior*, *5*, 40–45.

Wendland, J. R., Lesch, K. P., Newman, T. K., Timme, A., Gachot-Neveu, H., Thierry, B., *et al.* (2006). Differential functional variability of serotonin transporter and monoamine oxidase A genes in macaque species displaying contrasting levels of aggression-related behavior. *Behavior Genetics*, *36*, 163–172.

Westlund, K. N., Denney, R. M., Kochersperger, L. M., Rose, R. M., & Abell, C. W. (1985). Distinct monoamine oxidase A and B populations in primate brain. *Science*, *230*, 181–183.

Westlund, K. N., Denney, R. M., Rose, R. M., & Abell, C. W. (1988). Localization of distinct monoamine oxidase A and monoamine oxidase B cell populations in human brainstem. *Neuroscience*, *25*, 439–456.

Westlund, K. N., Krakower, T. J., Kwan, S. W., & Abell, C. W. (1993). Intracellular distribution of monoamine oxidase A in selected regions of rat and monkey brain and spinal cord. *Brain Research*, *612*, 221–230.

Whalen, P. J., Shin, L. M., McInerney, S. C., Fischer, H., Wright, C. I., & Rauch, S. L. (2001). A functional MRI study of human amygdala responses to facial expressions of fear versus anger. *Emotion*, *1*, 70–83.

Widiger, T. A., & Lynam, D. R. (1998). Psychopathy as a variant of common personality traits: implications for diagnosis, etiology and pathology. In T. Millon (ed), *Psychopathy: Antisocial, Criminal and Violent Behavior*. New York: Guilford.

Widom, C. S., & Brzustowicz, L. M. (2006). MAOA and the 'cycle of violence': childhood abuse and neglect, MAOA genotype, and risk for violent and antisocial behavior. *Biological Psychiatry, 60*, 684–689,

Williams, R. B., Marchuk, D. A., Gadde, K. M., Barefoot, J. C., Grichnik, K., Helms, M. J., *et al.* (2003). Serotonin-related gene polymorphisms and central nervous system serotonin function. *Neuropsychopharmacology*, *28*, 533–541.

Willoughby, J., Glover, V., & Sandler, M. (1988). Histochemical localisation of monoamine oxidase A and B in rat brain. *Journal of Neural Transmission*, *74*, 29–42.

Zald, D. H. (2003). The human amygdala and the emotional evaluation of sensory stimuli. *Brain Research Reviews*, *41*, 88–123.

Zald, D. H., Mattson, D. L., & Pardo, J. V. (2002). Brain activity in ventromedial prefrontal cortex correlates with individual differences in negative affect. *Proceedings of the National Academy of Sciences of the United States of America*, *99*, 2450–2454.

Zalsman, G., Huang, Y. Y., Harkavy-Friedman, J. M., Oquendo, M. A., Ellis, S. P., & Mann, J. J. (2005). Relationship of MAO-A promoter (u-VNTR) and COMT (V158M) gene polymorphisms to CSF monoamine metabolites levels in a psychiatric sample of caucasians: A preliminary report. *American Journal of Medical Genetics: Part B, Neuropsychiatric Genetics*, *132*, 100–103.

Zubieta, J. K., Heitzeg, M. M., Smith, Y. R., Bueller, J. A., Xu, K., Xu, Y., *et al.* (2003). COMT val158met genotype affects mu-opioid neurotransmitter responses to a pain stressor. *Science*, *299*, 1240–1243.

15

Reducing personal violence: Risk factors and effective interventions

James McGuire

Objectives

The principal objectives of this chapter are to survey research on the outcomes of interventions designed to reduce personal violence, and to summarize what has emerged from that work with a view to identifying the most effective approaches to the problem that have been discovered to date. The emphasis will be primarily on aggression and violent behaviour among adolescents and adults, and although work with younger children will also be discussed, it is not the central focus of the chapter.

To facilitate the principal task, a series of initial, but subsidary objectives will be addressed: first, to consider some issues that arise in defining violence, in order to obtain a clearer appraisal of the subject under discussion; second, to survey the nature of personal violence as a social and public health problem; and third, to discuss some difficulties that arise when conducting research in this area, as a partial explanation of why there is not as yet a consolidated body of knowledge concerning it. This will focus particularly on the problem of evaluating interventions. It will be followed by an overview of the principal factors that have emerged as contributing to personal violence. A final objective, addressed later in the chapter, is to forward an integrative perspective on the factors that influence the occurrence of violence acts, in a probabilistic causal model.

There is a useful distinction that is often made in studying interventions designed to reduce recurrent problem behaviours such as criminal conduct in general or violent offending in particular. This is a classification forwarded by Guerra *et al.* (1994) between *primary*, *secondary*, and *tertiary* prevention of antisocial activity in adolescence.

The first of these refers to general population or community-level initiatives designed to alleviate or eradicate a social problem. In criminology this may consist of situational prevention: for example, 'target hardening', increased security, improvements in street lighting or other environmental modifications, installation of closed-circuit television, neighbourhood watch, or other efforts to make crimes less likely to occur. Alternatively, it may consist of investment in additional resources: for example, improved family welfare, education, or other social provision that will lower the socio-economic deprivation associated with some types of crime (Farrington & Coid, 2003).

The second denotes any type of intervention that 'targets individuals who show preclinical manifestations of some type of problem, whether it be physical, psychological, or social' (Fields & McNamara, 2003; p. 66). This entails work with designated 'at-risk' groups, such as children truanting from school, or involved in bullying or other aggression that is not strictly classed as illegal (because of the perpetrator's age or other characteristics; Goldstein, 2002).

The third level, tertiary prevention, describes work undertaken with adjudicated offenders, those already convicted by the courts (usually more than once), and intended to reduce their subsequent rates of criminal recidivism (Gendreau & Andrews, 1990). Although some reference will be made to the first two of these classifications in what follows, the primary focus of this chapter is on interventions in the criminal justice system, in youth justice, probation, prison, and related agencies.

The nature of violence

Violence is not a unitary phenomenon: it takes many different forms. It is important to identify its principal manifestations and if possible to distinguish various types within them.

Definitional problems

The central focus of this chapter is upon what is generally termed *personal violence*, committed by one individual against another, in a context in which such actions are specifically proscribed by societal norms and usually codified in formal law. Under the legal framework of England and Wales, for example, numerous statutes, perhaps most notably the Offences Against the Person Act (1861) define the nature of actions that are considered to constitute different forms of violent crime (e.g., assault occasioning actual bodily harm, grievous bodily harm, malicious wounding, threats to kill). Although this might appear straightforward, the task of describing and classifying violent behaviour in legal terms is a complex and challenging one (Carter & Harrison, 1991). English law discerns numerous other discrete types of violence: for example, harassment, racially or religiously aggravated assault, public disorder, sexual assault, infanticide, homicide, and complicity in another's suicide (Cook *et al.*, 2006). The associated complexities notwithstanding, one way to define violence is to do so in terms of what is described as such in the criminal law. Much research in social science adopts that approach.

Definitions of violence have been described as varying along six dimensions (Jackson *et al.*, 2004): (1) the level of action of the behaviour (individual, interpersonal, collective), (2) the nature and degree of force, (3) the outcome including extent of injury, (4) the type of injury (e.g., physical harm, emotional degradation, interpersonal dominance), (5) the nature and significance of the target(s), and (6) whether or not the actions were intentional. Given the multiple possibilities so generated, there is as yet no agreed benchmark regarding how violence should be conceptualized.

Thus, violent offences can be defined restrictively in terms of physical harm, possibly (as done in the Denver Youth Survey) subdividing them to denote 'those acts in which someone was hurt or injured, but perhaps only in a minor way. Thus, hitting, getting into fights, and so on are included. Serious violent offences, however, include only acts that resulted in serious injury (requiring medical treatment: cut, bleeding, unconscious, etc.) or in which a weapon was used' (Thornberry *et al.*, 1995; p. 224). In the field of developmental psychopathology by contrast, violence is generally conceptualized more broadly, to encompass acts committed by children below the age of criminal responsibility and to study continuities in behavioural patterns across successive maturational periods. For example, in forwarding a model of the development of antisocial behaviour and conduct problems, Dodge and Pettit (2003) defined the target variables as including 'recurrent problem behaviours that lead to injury to others or arrest' (2002; p. 350), so referring not only to violent crimes in the sense delineated in the preceding, but also '... verbal assault, vandalism, delinquency, destruction of another's social standing (as in relational aggression), and physical abuse of one's offspring' (2003; p. 350) These actions have interpersonal targets and are distinguished from self-destructive behaviours such as substance abuse, suicide, and internalizing problems. Given the observed continuities in these behaviours across developmental stages, in the present chapter, this broader definition will be employed, to include research on interventions designed to reduce any repeated manifestations of interpersonally harmful behaviour.

Spatial and temporal variations

Personal violence as defined in criminal law typically constitutes a smaller fraction of all crimes than offences against property (such as theft, burglary, or criminal damage). For example, in England and Wales in 2006–07 it formed 22% of recorded crime (Home Office, 2007). Although officially recorded violent crime doubled between 1998–99 and 2006–07, there is evidence that the underlying rate of total and of violent crime has been generally declining. Since 1995, incidents of wounding have fallen by 37%, of assaults with minor injury by 58%, and assaults resulting in no injury by 36%. Nevertheless, according to British Crime Survey estimates, there were still nearly 2.5 million incidents of violence against adults in 2006–07 (Jansson *et al.*, 2007).

The amounts and levels of seriousness of personal violence show considerable international variations (Bureau of Justice Statistics, 2003). Table 15.1 shows selected extracts from data collected by the United Nations Office on Drugs and Crime (2008), showing recorded rates of intentional homicide, serious assault, and rape in 15 UN member countries for the year 2002 (the latest year for which comparative figures are available). Those listed are designed to illustrate the sizeable disparities in officially recorded rates. Victim surveys where available tend to show lower rates of reporting for violent than for other types of crimes (van Kesteren *et al.*, 2000; del Frate 2003; Naudé *et al.*, 2006). For some types of crime, notably domestic sexual violence towards women or children (Grubin, 1998; Hadi, 2000), discrepancies between officially recorded rates and likely 'real' underlying rates may be particularly large.

Table 15.1 International variations in selected crimes of personal violence (police statistics, year 2002, rates per 100 000 population).

Intentional homicide	Major assault	Rape
South Africa: 47.53	South Africa: 587.32	South Africa: 115.61
El Salvador: 31.54	Argentina: 343.39	Canada: 77.64
Mexico: 13.04	United States: 310.14	United States: 32.99
Belarus: 9.96	Mexico: 186.68	United Kingdom[a]: 22.62
Argentina: 9.47	Tunisia: 152.22	Mexico: 14.26
Lithuania: 8.45	Uruguay: 137.28	El Salvador: 13.12
Uruguay: 6.46	El Salvador: 70.78	Denmark: 9.30
Albania: 5.68	United Kingdom[a]: 43.70	Uruguay: 9.02
United States: 5.62	Poland: 39.03	Belarus: 8.59
United Kingdom[a]: 2.03	Denmark: 25.38	Argentina: 8.32
Poland: 1.87	Morocco: 23.33	Poland: 6.13
Canada: 1.67	Albania: 13.97	Lithuania: 5.42
Tunisia: 1.22	Lithuania: 13.14	Morocco: 3.42
Denmark: 1.04	Canada: 8.56	Tunisia: 3.13
Morocco: 0.48	Belarus: 3.71	Albania: 1.43

[a]Per-capita values for England and Wales were considered a proxy for the entire United Kingdom.
Source: United Nations Office on Drugs and Crime (2008).

A separate series of surveys is reported by the World Health Organisation (WHO; Krug *et al.*, 2002). Focusing on deaths caused by violence, as a broad initial categorization, this first of all distinguishes deaths due to suicide, military conflicts, and homicide, respectively. Surveying data on a global scale, Krug *et al.* estimated that in the year 2000, there were approximately 1.66 million deaths due to violence. Of this total, just under half (815 000) consisted of suicides, roughly one-fifth (310 000) were war-related, and one-third (510 000) were homicides. The last figure corresponds to one approximately every 60 seconds.

As Table 15.1 shows, however, the homicide rate is only the 'tip of the iceberg' as far as crimes of violence are concerned. Non-fatal assaults are far more numerous (those shown are only the most serious). The WHO report (Krug *et al.*, 2002) also cites figures on domestic violence, and on fighting in schools. For partner assault, rates ranged from 10% in Paraguay and the Philippines to 22.1% in the United States and 34.4% in Egypt. For fighting among adolescent males, self-reported rates varied from 22% in Sweden to 44% in the United States and 76% in Israel.

There are also marked temporal variations in the occurrence of violent deaths. For example, during the 40 months between March 2003 and July 2006, there were an estimated 654 965 additional deaths (above the expected natural rate) in Iraq (Burnham *et al.*, 2006). Between 1998 and 2004, an estimated 3.9 million people died due to military conflict in the Congo (Coughlan *et al.*, 2006). Apart from war, episodes of genocide have produced very large numbers of fatalities at recurrent intervals over much of the last 100 years: such as the Turkish genocide in Armenia (1915), enforced starvation in Russia (1930–34), the Nazi holocaust (1941–45), the Khmer Rouge regime in Cambodia (1975–78), more recent brutalities in the Balkans (1991–95), Rwanda (1994), and the still unfolding events in Darfur (Power, 2003; Totten & Parsons, 2008). Cumulatively, these and similar events are estimated to have led to over 100 million deaths. Staub (1989) developed a framework for understanding the factors that combine to create the conditions for genocide, basing this on an historical and socio-psychological analysis of four of the most extensively documented occurrences in the twentieth century. More recently Waller (2007) has forwarded a more elaborate framework based on evidence concerning a range of genocidal events, synthesizing historical, political, psychological, and other types of evidence and theory in an integrative casual account.

Historical data thus suggest that there are some circumstances, such as intergroup conflict, in which many people resort to collective violence. Hence, childhood externalizing behaviours or later criminality that are the focus of most research represent only a small proportion of the phenomena of human violence considered in broader terms. Although all human activity can be understood as at some level being a function of neurobiological processes, models that are derived from studies of brain function are likely to be somewhat limited in their explanatory scope and power. To develop a comprehensive explanatory model of violence will require integration of evidence from a wide array of fields, including anthropology, neurobiology, psychology, sociology, politics, and history.

Individual continuity

With reference to the more regularly occurring types of aggression and violence as conventionally defined, many studies indicate (as is found with most other types of offence) that a relatively small proportion of the population is responsible for a comparatively large proportion of recorded violent crimes (Surgeon General, 2001). For example, in the Rochester Youth Development Study, it was found that 15% of the sample accounted for 75% of the violent offences (Thornberry *et al.*, 2003). According to Tremblay (2003), the proportion of children identified in longitudinal studies as exhibiting *chronic physical aggression* is approximately 5%. According to Blair *et al.* (2005), the proportion of adults repeatedly engaging in violence as a function of psychopathy is also approximately 5%.

Thus, there are measurable individual differences in *aggressiveness*, which has been conceptualized as '... a relatively persistent readiness to become aggressive in a variety of different situations' (Berkowitz, 1993; p. 21).Concerning individuals likely to act frequently or repeatedly in this way, there is evidence of relative stability in patterns of aggressiveness between infancy, middle childhood, adolescence, and adulthood, comparable to that shown for general intellectual functioning. For example, the presence of aggressive classroom behaviour in the early school years has been shown to be a good predictor of delinquency in adolescence (Spivack & Cianci, 1987). Across a more limited timescale of five or six years, studies have shown that aggressive behaviour in middle childhood is strongly predictive of conduct problems during the teenage years (Loeber & Stouthamer-Loeber, 1987; Farrington & West, 1993). A recent study has shown moderate stability in assessments of psychopathy across an 11-year period, between ages 13 and 24 (Lynam *et al.*, 2007).

Data of these kinds have been consolidated in two independent analyses of correlations over time. Olweus (1979, 1988) reported a review of 16 longitudinal studies examining levels of consistency in aggressive behaviour over periods ranging from one to 21 years. The dependent variables in the studies were nominations or ratings of aggressiveness provided by peers, teachers, or other observers. From these findings, Olweus extracted a total of 24 correlation coefficients and plotted their interrelationships on a regression line. Although unsurprisingly the correlations decreased with increasing time intervals, there was nevertheless a striking degree of consistency. For example, mean correlations across 12 and 24 months were 0.76 and 0.69, respectively, but fell to 0.36 in one 21 year follow up. In a subsequent review, Zumkley (1994) analysed an additional 10 studies, confirming the pattern found by Olweus. The levels of continuity discovered in these studies may be a function of the subgroup of those engaging in antisocial behaviour who can be depicted as manifesting *life-course-persistent* delinquent conduct, as hypothesized by Moffitt (1993, 2003).

Expressive and instrumental aggression

Attempts to identify subtypes of aggression are particularly important with reference to the small proportion of individuals likely to manifest persistently high levels of it over a prolonged segment of the life course (Hodgins, 2007). Researchers and clinicians have found it useful to make a distinction between two types of aggression: *expressive* and *instrumental*. In the former, also variously called reactive, angry, emotional, hostile, or impulsive aggression, harm to a victim decreases an unpleasant internal feeling state in the aggressor, possibly through the reduction of physiological arousal or tension (Berkowitz, 1993; Blackburn, 1993). In the latter, threats or injury facilitate achievement of non-injurious goals, as for example in robbery; violence works proactively as a means to an end rather than an end in itself. Although some researchers have expressed reservations over the rigour with which this distinction can be maintained, given that many aggressive acts have mixed motives (Bushman & Anderson, 2001; Anderson & Bushman, 2002), there is both psychometric and neuropsychological evidence that supports its meaningfulness (Blair *et al.*, 2005). In addition, the distinction appears vital when allocating individuals to intervention programmes, given the importance of linking interventions to a functional understanding of violence motivation.

Challenges of violence intervention research

There are several major obstacles to pursuing a systematic scientific study of violent behaviour, and additional difficulties arise in research designed to evaluate the impact of tertiary interventions. First, as already described, defining violence is a precarious and unsatisfactory process. There is consequently a fundamental and recurrent problem of recording and measurement in this field. When studying aggression or other behaviour labelled as 'antisocial' in children, it is recognized that many acts though superficially similar are functionally very dissimilar (Tremblay, 2000). The experience of an interpersonal event such as an assault and how it is described, respectively, by protagonists and observers is a product of both individual, subjective perceptions, and of wider, socially constructed interpretative frameworks. This brings to mind the distinction outlined by Searle (1995) between 'brute' and 'institutional' facts, the former independent of human institutions or mentality, the latter a function of human interaction and communication.

Second, notwithstanding the data presented in the preceding section on the numbers of violent crimes, relative to other human activities violence is a comparatively rare event. Even the most frequently aggressive individual is unlikely to act violently in every encounter. That serious and violent offending manifests an 'episodic or intermittent nature ... has important implications for research' (Huizinga et al., 2003; p. 55). The low base rate of assault can make it very difficult to isolate a group of individuals who can be reliably identified as violence-prone: most individuals who commit such offences are criminally 'versatile'. When evaluating the impact of interventions, the low frequency of violent reoffences may result in studies being statistically underpowered.

Third, most assaults are a product of an intricate sequence of events and processes of separate but interconnected types (neurobiological, hormonal, cognitive, attitudinal, experiential, interactional). Hostile exchanges resulting in violence are influenced by the interplay of dispositional and situational factors. These in turn are a function of participants' temperaments, developmental histories, socialization experiences, interpersonal skills, attitudes, and self-concepts (Toch, 1969; Tremblay, 2000). Identifying causal pathways and developing integrative explanatory models pose major challenges.

Fourth, commensurate with the level of complexity of violence causation, when individuals who are frequently aggressive are assessed by criminal justice or other practitioners, they are usually found to have multiple criminogenic needs. Interventions devised to address several problems in combination have been termed *multimodal* (Lipsey, 1995). However, their implementation leaves a significant residual problem of disentangling the most likely 'active ingredients' and of developing appropriate methods for maximizing treatment impact. Research projects in which such components are dismantled and evaluated separately remain relatively exceptional, leaving many issues concerning effectiveness unresolved.

Fifth, in outcome research, there are often competing demands between practical need and service delivery on the one hand and rigorous evaluation for the purposes of hypothesis testing on the other. Allocation to different levels or types of services in social welfare and criminal justice is customarily in the hands of decision makers (sentencers, case managers) whose priorities are in the realms of public protection or of meeting client needs. Typically, evaluation projects are unlikely to attain the standards of good experimental designs, most importantly in ensuring the equivalence of experimental and control samples with respect to key variables that may be conflated with measured outcomes. An additional difficulty arises from the recurrently high levels of attrition found among offender samples. These factors often reduce the methodological quality of evaluations with important consequences for hypothesis testing regarding treatment effects.

Factors influencing personal violence

As previously indicated, the occurrence of violent acts is typically a function of several factors interacting in complex multilayered patterns, and although many of the associated factors have been identified, the manner in which they interact is so far only poorly understood. Indeed it is possible that such interactions can themselves take several forms, suggesting that a general model of violence causation may remain hard to articulate, requiring researchers to develop a set of interconnected models applicable to different categories of aggression or violence. The following provides a general outline of the types of factors that have been shown to contribute to the occurrence of violent acts and to the establishment of a pattern of repeated violent conduct.

Temperament

It is in this area that neurobiological findings are potentially of prime importance. In behavioural terms, inherited factors are manifested in the form of a set of dispositions that are collectively called *temperament*. This term refers to '... substantially heritable and relatively persistent individual differences in global aspects of socio-emotional responding that emerge early in childhood and constitute the foundation for many personality traits later in life' (Lahey & Waldman, 2003; p. 80). Measurable variables include general activity level, attentiveness, adaptiveness to new situations, quality and intensity of mood expression, relative proneness to distress, and distractibility (Chess & Thomas, 1990; Rothbart *et al.*, 1994).

Individual differences in these variables appear very soon after birth and before any significant learning experiences. There is evidence that they are maintained into the first few months and perhaps first few years of life. As with other factors studied longitudinally, however, the differentiation of dimensions becomes less clear and their predictive validity weaker over lengthier timescales. Thus, regarding the long term consistency of those variables identified in neonates, even using a relatively broad 'easy-difficult' continuum, findings have been less reliable (Chess & Thomas, 1990).

Nevertheless, some longitudinal studies have uncovered noteworthy consistencies in temperament variables over extended periods. For example, Caspi *et al.* (1995) compared observations of children when aged 3 with independent descriptions of them at age 15, and their descriptions of themselves at age 18. Three-year-olds described as undercontrolled, and who manifested irritability and impulsiveness (as rated by observers), were more likely to be described as having *externalizing* problems when aged 15. This pattern held for both girls and boys. When aged 18, they were more likely than others to describe themselves as reckless, careless, and rebellious, and more prepared to cause discomfort or harm to others.

Lahey and Waldman (2003) propose that there are three dimensions of temperament most relevant to the development of conduct problems: negative emotionality, daring, and prosociality; and adduce evidence in support of them as fundamental factors in the emergence of persistent antisocial behaviour. Such stability as has been discovered is almost certainly a function of genotype-environmental interactions, and a *transactional* model such as that proposed by Dodge and Pettit (2003; p. 357), incorporating the possibility that 'certain predispositions elicit particular reactions' from others, appears the best account of the data currently available.

Socialization: family processes

A considerable volume of research links observed patterns of continuity in aggressiveness to socialization experiences within families (Rutter *et al.*, 1998). The predominant factors at work in this context, and which contribute to the development of longer-term aggressive-ness and the risk of violence, are found in child rearing, parenting, and other social learning processes (Farrington, 1995; Snyder *et al.*, 2003). In general terms, the larger the number of these factors that are present in adverse form earlier in life, the greater the likelihood that a young person will later become involved in offending.

Problems of this kind are more likely to accumulate in unfavourable circumstances entail-ing social deprivation, low incomes, and poor housing, which place families under signifi-cant stress. This is likely to affect the enduring mood and demeanour of parents or other caregivers, their interactions with each other, and the manner in which they respond to chil-dren. Some studies have illuminated the intermediate links in a chain of processes through which economic hardship may be associated with problem behaviour and in due course adjudicated delinquency.

Dodge *et al.* (1994) studied a set of 585 children over a four-year period between the ages of 4 and 7. Information was also obtained from their parents concerning economic circum-stances, socialization practices, and other conditions in the family home, and from teachers and classmates concerning the children's behaviour in school. The latter was described mainly in terms of the presence or absence of externalizing problems, which included the extent to which a child was involved in fighting, or threatening other people. The best pre-diction of the level of a child's externalizing or aggressive problems came not from direct socio-economic indicators, but from a set of pathways involving intermediate events: pat-terns of interaction within the family. They included harshness of discipline, exposure to violence, maternal support, maternal warmth, maternal endorsement of aggressive values, having only transient contacts with people outside the family, and level of cognitive stimula-tion. Thus, the association between family hardship and the child's behaviour could be best understood through a model that included a set of interactional processes inside the family as mediating variables.

Parental conflict, poor or inconsistent supervision, and physical or emotional neglect are associated in general terms with later overall risks for delinquency. With reference more specifically to aggression, there is evidence that within intact families, some parents provide little reinforcement of children's prosocial behaviours, while giving direct reinforcement of coercive behaviours. This has been shown in numerous studies carried out over a 40-year period in the Oregon Social Learning Center. This research has demonstrated, for example, how parental reactions that reduce the likelihood of an aversive behaviour (such as aggres-sion) in the short term can serve to increase its likelihood in the long term. Thus, children can progressively learn that their own belligerent behaviour 'works', either in securing atten-tion of parents or in terminating unwanted intrusions by them (Snyder *et al.*, 2003).

According to the social learning approach (Bandura, 2001), a large portion of the vari-ance in behaviour is a function of situational factors. Hence, much aggression is accounted for by time-specific determinants: '... what appears to be trait-like may in fact be situational, relationship-specific, and 'functional'' (Snyder *et al.*, 2003; p. 30). Furthermore '... social contingencies and experiences that foster antisocial behaviour often simultaneously mitigate the acquisition of capacities to self-regulate emotions, deploy attention, problem solve, engage in autonomous rule following, and relate effectively to others. Antisocial and skilled behaviours are 'opposite sides of the same coin'' (Snyder *et al.*, 2003; p. 31).

Social learning also occurs as a function of wider communal influences such as exposure to media violence, which has effects independent of initial interest in or proneness towards externalizing aggression. Huesmann *et al.* (2003) examined the strength of this influence with the effects of predispositions taken into account. They reinterviewed a group of

557 participants in a television-viewing study originally begun in 1977. At that stage, members of their sample were in the age ranges 6–7 and 8–9; at the time of follow-up, they were young adults with mean ages of 21 and 23, respectively. Data were collected on background characteristics, educational level, evidence of aggressiveness as children, perceived realism of violence in TV programmes, and extent of identification with characters seen in programmes containing violence. Results suggest strongly that television is an agent of socialization for developing children that may influence their likelihood of being violent as adults. 'For both male and female participants, more childhood exposure to TV violence, greater childhood identification with same-sex aggressive TV characters, and a stronger childhood belief that violent shows tell about life "just like it is" predicted more adult aggression regardless of how aggressive participants were as children' (Huesmann *et al.*, 2003; p. 216).

Cognition and information processing

Other research findings draw attention to the importance of *social information processing* in contributing to the likelihood of aggression. According to this proposal, the meanings individuals attribute to events are prime determinants of their subsequent behavioural responses. The emergence or maintenance of aggressive behaviour depends on cognitive appraisal and other internal mediating processes (Dodge, 2003).

In an information-processing model, reactions to an external event are analysed in terms of a sequence of cognitive events, comprising six stages: encoding, representation, goal clarification, response construction, response decision, and enactment. Several researchers (Akhtar & Bradley, 1991; Crick & Dodge, 1994; Dodge, 2003) have reviewed studies comparing frequently aggressive children with non aggressive control groups, and have developed models integrating these findings with other types of variables (Dodge & Pettit, 2003; Dodge & Schwartz, 1997). General trends found are such that, compared to their less aggressive peers, frequently aggressive children encode a narrower range of environmental cues or sources of information; they selectively attend to aggressive cues; are more likely to attribute hostile intent to others, especially in ambiguous situations; more readily label internal states of arousal as anger; generate fewer potential alternative solutions to problems; select action-oriented rather than reflective solutions; possess a more limited range of interactive skills; and manifest an 'egocentric' perspective in social problem solving.

Cognitive processing may influence the tendency to use aggression at both conscious and non-conscious levels. In terms of conscious events, which individuals can easily access, there is evidence that the process of *neutralization* (use of self-statements that permit or justify behaviour otherwise considered objectionable) is important in facilitating engagement in violent behaviour or in enabling individuals to excuse it afterwards. Agnew (1994) analysed data concerning this from the US National Youth Survey, conducted in annual waves in the late 1970s with a large representative sample (>1600) of young people in the age range 11-17. Agnew found first that the overwhelming majority (93%) of respondents stated that it is wrong to hit people; only 0.5% took the view that it is not wrong at all. Even those who admitted to having acted violently in the previous year expressed disapproval of hitting. However, more than half (54%) of the sample accepted one or more of a series of statements justifying the use of violence. Endorsement of these statements was a significant predictor of involvement in violence cross-sectionally (at a specific moment in time) and also longitudinally (one year following). Neutralizations were equivalent in their effects to the influence of delinquent peers, and considerably more so than attitudes generally approving of violence.

There are several channels through which an individual's non-conscious information processing might be 'primed' with constructs associated with aggression. Todorov and Bargh (2000) have reviewed evidence pertaining to this. For example, if individuals are subliminally exposed to aggressive words, they subsequently describe another person as more aggressive than individuals similarly exposed to neutral words. In other studies, priming was shown to automatically predispose individuals to express more hostility when interacting with others, even where there was no immediate situational source of tension. With repeated use, aggression-related constructs may become 'chronically accessible', intermittently disposing individuals to pre-emptive aggression in the absence of any provocative event.

Situational and contextual influences

The research findings discussed so far demonstrate the existence of some kinds of continuity in socialization, which is linked to the appearance of aggression and violence in young people. To obtain a fuller understanding of this behaviour, we have to supplement this background with information on the immediate precursors of aggression. This has come from laboratory and field research in social psychology (Berkowitz, 1993). That work shows that there is an enormous range of situational influences on aggression. They include basic stimulus conditions such as levels of heat and noise, a wide array of personal frustrations and stresses, as well as critical events such as provocations or threats.

Other factors superimposed on these include audience or self-image enhancement effects, and local group norms concerning aggression. Certain categories of events are potential precursors of aggressive acts. They may be subtle non-verbal exchanges, momentary eye contact or glances, facial expressions, gestures or bodily movements that convey hostility, or are simply interpreted as hostile by perceivers. Aggressive signals usually instil fear and escape reactions in observers. In a study by Ellsworth *et al.* (1972), researchers waited by traffic lights, either sitting on a scooter or standing on the street corner. When motorists or pedestrians stopped at red signals, the experimenters either stared straight at them or looked at them but without staring. They then measured the time taken to cross the intersection when the lights changed to green. Those who were stared at sped off significantly faster. Results supported the hypothesis that the stare constituted a 'stimulus to flight'. Clinical assessment of individuals who have committed homicides or serious assaults often yield scenarios in which violence was triggered by apparently ephemeral exchanges the impact of which was grossly magnified in the circumstances.

Cultural influences

Culture is extremely difficult to define in a way that will allow the testing of hypotheses concerning its associations with behaviour at the individual level. Nevertheless, some researchers have accomplished this, through the device of comparing different states or regions of the United States.

Nisbett and Cohen (1996) focused on rates of violent crimes, including homicide. Their starting point was the finding that, excluding the largest urban areas, cities of comparable sizes in different parts of the United States have markedly different murder rates. The highest rates are in the states of the South and South-West, the lowest in the New England and Mid-Atlantic regions. In the South and South-West, their research discovered that homicides were more likely to result from arguments than to be committed in the course of other crimes such as robberies. In surveys of social attitudes, there was greater endorsement of a 'shoot to kill' policy in law enforcement, for the exercise of violence in the defence of a man's reputation, a greater tendency to ruminate over personal insults, more support for physical discipline of children, and significant increases in cortisol and testosterone levels following an experimentally contrived insult, than was the case for citizens from other parts of the United States. The researchers forwarded the view that these differences are a function of an historical attachment to values that flow from a 'herding' culture, in which the economy of a community is dependent on the rearing and control of animals, and the need to be perceived as tough and willing to resort to violence for the protection of property and of self-image.

Using a similar comparative method, Baron *et al.* (1988) investigated the relationship between society-wide attitudes concerning sexual aggression and the rates of serious sexual crimes. To do this, they developed a composite measure entitled the Legitimate Violence Index. This combined various indicators of the extent to which it could be inferred that there was social approval of violence in a community. The variables measured within it included (a) the level of violent content in television programmes, (b) rates of readership of magazines with a high violence content, (c) existence of laws permitting corporal punishment in schools, (d) the numbers of hunting licenses issued, (e) levels of National Guard enrolment, and (f) the numbers of lynchings per million population in the period 1882–1927. Combining these data, the level of support for violence was assessed in all 50 US states. Several types of demographic information (level of urbanization, degree of income inequality, age distribution, and numbers of single and divorced males in the population) were also collected and entered into a path analysis.

Scores on the Index were then compared with recorded rates of rape in each state, which differed by a ratio of 8:1. Broadly speaking, mountain and central states (e.g., Wyoming, Montana, Mississippi, Utah, and Idaho) had high scores on the Index. Eastern and northeastern states (e.g., Rhode Island, Massachusetts, New Jersey, Maryland, and New York) came at the bottom of the scale.

A parallel analysis was conducted using separate attitudinal measure, the Violence Approval Index, based on a survey in which citizens' views were sought regarding the use of violence in certain situations: for example, whether they thought it permissible to punch an adult male stranger under certain circumstances (e.g., someone who is drunk and bumps into you in the street).

In both analyses, demographic variables including the level of urbanization and percentage of divorced males in the population were strong predictors of the rate of rape. But, so also were the Legitimate Violence Index and the Violence Approval Index; the former highly significant, the second significant but less markedly. This provided support for the authors' conclusion that '… the social approval of nonsexual and noncriminal violence has a significant relationship to rape, independently of those effects contributed by the control variables' (Baron *et al.*, 1988; p. 95). Such findings are convergent with those of Sanday (2003). Although rape occurs in almost all societies, there are reported exceptions. Sanday (2003) has described its almost complete absence among the Minangkabau people of Western Sumatra, which she ascribes to the pattern in that society of symmetrical male-female status and relationships.

Summary

In seeking to comprehend violent offending, it is essential to construct a model that has a wide range of components. There are evolutionary predispositions to aggression in some interpersonal circumstances, for which everyone carries the potential. There are also individual differences in temperament at birth, which have a moderate degree of heritability.

Socialization influences, notably parenting skills and styles, interact with these tendencies to shape the course of development in the early years. The level of economic stress and adversity to which parents or other caregivers are subjected will significantly influence the environment they create for their children. Basic learning processes are overlaid with the transmission of attitudes and expectations that growing children absorb, and which in turn shape their own perceptions of their surroundings and their styles and habits when interpreting the actions of others. All these factors will influence the way someone deals with interpersonal conflict. Within each category of events, it is possible to identify specific patterns that are associated with tendencies to respond with aggression, and ultimately physical violence, in conflict situations. Anderson and Bushman (2002) have forwarded an integrative General Aggression Model of how the foregoing sets of variables may interact. Importantly, for the purposes of intervention research, their model and others include some variables that are (at least in principle) susceptible to change, and this provides the basis for what has been called the 'risk factors' approach.

Reducing criminal recidivism

The feasibility of implementing effective tertiary prevention in criminal justice has been the subject of sometimes fierce debate for several decades. The associated controversies have been summarized elsewhere (e.g., Gaes, 1998; McGuire, 2004; Andrews & Bonta, 2006). Whereas until approximately the late 1990s there was a widely held assumption that persistent offending behaviour was not susceptible to change, the growing volume of positive research findings eventually achieved a sufficient critical mass to engender the pursuit of a variety of evidence-based practice in criminal justice services (Raynor, 2004). The background evidence relevant to this will first be briefly summarized before turning attention to the findings more closely related to aggression and violence.

General findings

The usage of meta-analysis has had a considerable impact in criminology with particular reference to offender treatment (Wilson, 2001), and between 1985 and mid 2007, 70 meta-analyses were published or presented in this and adjacent fields. These reviews are listed in Table 15.2, which shows authors and dates of publication, the number of effect-size tests (k) conducted within each meta-analysis, and the mean effect size obtained either across all studies reviewed or from specified subsets within them. The table includes basic information from meta-analytic reviews of interventions with adjudicated offenders or in some instances pre-delinquents (e.g., those exhibiting antisocial behaviour in school or home settings). Reviews are tabulated chronologically by year of publication and in alphabetic order of first-named authors within each year.

   This list excludes reviews of (a) evaluations of changes in penal policy or practice such as the introduction of curfews, drug courts, or new sentencing guidelines; (b) studies of psychological therapy conducted exclusively with children outside the age range of criminal responsibility; and (c) reviews of anger management and allied interventions to be discussed separately later.

   The number of tests as listed in column 3 may not correspond to the number of studies that were subsumed in a review. Rather, it is the number of effect sizes used to compute a mean effect relevant to the primary focus of the review. Where more than one effect size is given in column 4, this corresponds to major categories reported in a review. Not all reviews

Table 15. 2 Summary information from 70 meta-analyses of offender treatment-outcome studies, 1985–2007.

Review	Focus	Number of effect-size tests (k)	Mean effect size(s) reported
Garrett (1985)	Young offenders in residential placements	121	+0.18
Gensheimer et al. (1986)	Diversion schemes for young offenders	31	+0.26
Mayer et al. (1986)	Social learning-based interventions with youth	17	+0.33
Gottschalk et al. (1987a)	Community-based interventions with youth	61	+0.22
Gottschalk et al. (1987b)	Behavioural interventions with youth	14	+0.25
Lösel and Koferl 1989	Socio-therapeutic prison regimes in Germany	16	+0.12
Whitehead and Lab (1989)	Young offenders: general	50	+0.13
Andrews et al. (1990)	Testing model of 'human service principles'	Types of service: 'Appropriate' 54 'Unspecified' 32 'Inappropriate' 38 Deterrence 30	+0.30 +0.13 –0.06 –0.07
Izzo and Ross (1990)	Cognitive versus non-cognitive interventions	46	Ratio of mean effect sizes = 2.5:1
Roberts and Camasso (1991)	Young offenders: general	46	na
Lipsey (1992)	Offenders aged 12–21	397	+0.10
Hall (1995)	Sexual offending	12	+0.12
Wells-Parker et al. (1995)	Drink–driving offences	215	8–9% reduction
Gendreau and Goggin (1996)	Deterrence and intermediate punishment	138	0.00
Cleland et al. (1997)	Impact of age as moderator variable	659	na
Pearson et al. (1997)	CDATE Project: comprehensive review	846	na
Redondo et al. (1997)	European structured programmes	57	+0.12
Lipsey and Wilson (1998)	Serious violent and sexual offending by youth	Institutional 83; Community 117	+0.10; +0.14
Marsch (1998)	Methadone maintenance for opiate dependence	24	$r = +0.23$; $d = +0.54$
Alexander (1999)	Sexual offending	79	+0.10
Dowden and Andrews (1999a)	Programmes for women offenders	24	na
Dowden and Andrews (1999b)	Young offenders: general	229	+0.09
Gallagher et al. (1999)	Sexual offending	25	$d = +0.43$
Pearson and Lipton (1999)	Substance abuse treatment and offending	30	na
Polizzi et al. (1999)	Sexual offending	13	na
Redondo et al. (1999)	European structured programmes	32	+0.12
Dowden and Andrews (2000)	Interventions for violent offenders	52	+0.07

continued

Table 15. 2 (Continued) Summary information from 70 meta-analyses of offender treatment-outcome studies, 1985–2007.

Review	Focus	Number of effect-size tests (k)	Mean effect size(s) reported
Egg *et al.* (2000)	Treatment programmes in Germany	25	$r = +0.12$; OR = 1.9
Petrosino *et al.* (2000)	Scared straight programmes	9	−0.01
Prendergast *et al.* (2000)	Treatment of drug dependence (treatment-comparison studies only)	28; 17	Drug use +0.29; crime +0.17
Wilson *et al.* (2000)	Educational and vocational programmes, adults	53	OR = 1.52
Wilson and Lipsey (2000)	Wilderness challenge programmes	22	+0.18
Gendreau *et al.* (2001)	Intermediate punishment	140	0.00
Latimer (2001)	Family treatment	50	+0.15
Lipsey *et al.* (2001)	Cognitive-behavioural interventions	14	OR = 0.66
MacKenzie *et al.* (2001)	Correctional boot camps	44	OR = 1.02
Wilson *et al.* (2001)	School-based interventions	40	$d = +0.04$
Hanson *et al.* (2002)	Sexual offending	43	OR = 0.81
Lipton *et al.* (2002a)	Therapeutic communities	35	+0.14
Lipton *et al.* (2002b)	Cognitive-behavioural interventions	68	+0.12
Prendergast *et al.* (2002)	Programme factors in treating drug dependence	78; 25	Drug use g +0.33; crime g +0.13
Redondo *et al.* (2002)	European structured programmes	23	+0.21
Salekin (2002)	Treatment of personality disorders	42	na
Woolfenden *et al.* (2002)	Family-based interventions	5	OR = 0.66
Andrews and Bonta (2006)	Restorative justice	67	+0.07
Dowden and Andrews (2003)	Family-based interventions	53	+0.21
Dowden *et al.* (2003)	Effectiveness of relapse prevention	40	+0.15
Farrington and Welsh (2003)	Family-based interventions	40	+0.32
Lösel and Beelman (2003)	Child skills training	135	Post-test d +0.38; follow-up d +0.28
Wilson, Lipsey, Derzon (2003)	School-based intervention programmes	522	+0.25
Wilson, Lipsey, Soydan (2003)	Impact of ethnicity as moderator variable	305	na
Babcock *et al.* (2004)	Domestic violence/programmes for abusers	36	na
Dowden and Andrews (2004)	Influence of staff practice and related variables	273	na
Nugent *et al.* (2004)	Victim-offender mediation (young offenders)	15	OR = 0.70
Andrews and Dowden (2005)	Programme and treatment integrity as moderator	273	na
Landenberger and Lipsey (2005)	Treatment factors, cognitive-behavioural programmes	58	OR = 1.53
Latimer *et al.* (2005)	Restorative justice	32	+0.07
Lösel and Schmucker (2005)	Sexual offending	80	+0.29

continued

Table 15. 2 (Continued) Summary information from 70 meta-analyses of offender treatment-outcome studies, 1985–2007.

Review	Focus	Number of effect-size tests (k)	Mean effect size(s) reported
Visher et al. (2005)	Employment programmes (community)	10	+0.03
Wilson, Bouffard, MacKenzie (2005)	Cognitive-behavioural group programmes	74	Range: +0.16 to +0.49
Wilson, MacKenzie, Mitchell (2005)	Correctional boot camps	43	OR = 1.02
Andrews and Dowden (2006)	'Risk–Needs' principles of case classification	374	Significant support
Bradshaw et al. (2006)	Victim offender mediation (juveniles)	15	+0.34
French and Gendreau (2006)	Reducing prison misconducts	104	+0.14
Holloway et al. (2006)	Impact of drug treatment on criminal recidivism	28	OR 1.41–1.56
McCart et al. (2006)	Relative effects of behavioural parent training (BPT) and cognitive-behavioural therapy (CBT)	BPT 32; CBT 45	+0.47; +0.35
Mitchell et al. (2006)	Incarceration-based drug treatment	66	OR = 1.37
Tong and Farrington (2006)	Reasoning and rehabilitation programme	25	OR = 1.16
Garrido and Morales (2007)	Institutionally-based interventions, violent youth	Recidivism 30; serious offence 15	OR = 1.13; OR = 1.35
Tanasichuk and Wormith (2007)	Comparison between treated and untreated psychopaths	3	Criminality −0.10; violence +0.03

were designed to test hypotheses about whether treatment 'worked'; several are focused on the importance of moderator variables (age, gender, ethnicity, treatment integrity), some are evaluations of interventions for specific types of offence (violent, sexual, drink-driving, substance abuse), and others of the impact of interventions conducted in different settings (prison, community, school, family).

Most effect sizes reported are standardized mean difference (d or g) or correlation coefficients (r or phi). In these cases, a '+' sign indicates that the outcome favoured the experimental sample (i.e., its level of recidivism was lower than that of controls). However, where odds ratios (OR) are reported, the direction varies according to the method of analysis used in the denoted review. Where column 4 reads *na* (not available or not applicable) this is where, for varying reasons, no average effect size was computed, or alternatively, the overall result is not a comparison between treated and untreated groups but a mean correlation between either an independent or moderator variable and recidivism outcomes.

As can be seen from the table, almost all effect sizes are positive, and although some are close to zero, the majority are in the small or moderate range, following the conventions proposed by Cohen (1992). The only negative mean effect sizes reported to date are those obtained from criminal sanctions or deterrence, or treatment of offenders classified as psychopaths. One outcome of the generally encouraging pattern regarding psychosocial intervention has been the development and dissemination of structured programmes (Andrews, 2001; McGuire, 2001): pre-planned and reproducible sequences of focused activities, typically delivered in group formats, and supported by a manual and other accompanying materials.

Limitations of studies and reviews

A degree of caution is warranted when scrutinizing the output from a large array of meta-analytic reviews such as that shown in Table 15.2. Some researchers have been sceptical about the use of meta-analysis on a variety of grounds. First, if the quality of the original research is poor, regrettably a not infrequent occurrence, it will be neither feasible nor permissible to draw any firm conclusions even from the most carefully conducted review of it. Second and as noted above, given the circumstances in which most research of this kind takes place, the design of some evaluation studies is very weak. It can be difficult to use random allocation to experimental and comparison samples, and the members of these groups are often not well matched, as researchers may have no control over who is placed under what conditions. As this activity often takes place in the daily routines of the criminal justice system, neatly designed experimental trials are difficult to carry out, and most evaluations are of a less robust nature (Lipsey, 1999). Third, follow-up periods have often been very short: six to nine months is not uncommon. However, there are also studies with 12- and 24-month follow-up, and a proportion where data have been collected for five years or more (e.g., a mean of 46 months in the review by Hanson *et al.*, 2002). Fourth, sample sizes in some studies are small and if there is a further loss due to attrition, or attempts are made to subdivide samples for particular analyses, it may be difficult to draw clear conclusions. Fifth, despite there being hundreds of primary studies in this field, when examined more closely, the number in any given category can be disappointingly small (Lösel, 2001). Thus, when attempting to review studies, it can be difficult to draw anything other than the most 'broad brush' conclusions (Lipsey, 1995). Sixth, it has been claimed that positive outcomes are merely a product of self-selection effects: if offenders participating in treatment are observed to change, it is primarily because they were motivated to do so, and would do well anyway (Simon, 1998; but see Hollin, 2006). Finally, an awkward interpretative problem arises due to publication bias. If research studies with non-significant findings are less likely to be submitted and/or published, those that are publicly available may be unrepresentative of the research actually done. Drawing conclusions from published work alone may give a distorted picture.

Many of these factors can be corrected or taken into account in properly conducted meta-analysis. Studies with larger samples can be given more weight, and well-designed and poorly-designed experiments can be evaluated separately to check whether they demonstrate broadly similar effects. Although publication bias cannot be eradicated, it can be minimized by making every possible effort to locate unpublished studies, or by computing the *fail-safe* or *file-drawer n*, the number of unpublished studies with zero or negative effect sizes that would be needed to discount or overturn an observed positive effect.

Violence meta-analyses

Of particular interest for present purposes are those reviews that have focused specifically on interventions designed to reduce aggression and violence. With reference to young offenders, this area has been subject to narrative review (Fields & McNamara, 2003) and findings of several meta-analyses concerning the impact of residential treatment on young offenders' general delinquency have also been collated (Grietens & Hellinckx, 2004). To the present author's knowledge, however, no previous review has synthesized findings across available meta-analyses focused on outcomes of interventions designed to reduce aggression and violence among both adolescents and adults.

Most intervention studies, and consequently many meta-analyses, describe work with samples of offenders with varied criminal histories, a proportion of whom are likely to have committed assaults, robberies, or other violent crimes in the midst of a pattern of 'generalist' offending. Most individuals with multiple convictions for violent offending have committed other types of offence in addition (Surgeon General, 2001). Unfortunately, many studies give insufficient details of the criminal backgrounds of treatment participants, and the number reporting the differential impact of interventions on violent as opposed to other types of reconviction is not large. Where such data have been assembled, meta-analysis has revealed a trend towards larger effect sizes for personal (violent and sexual) offences than for property (theft, burglary, criminal damage) or drug-related offences (Redondo et al., 2002). Fortunately, several meta-analytic reviews among the tabulated list are of particular note with reference to obtaining a fuller picture of the impact of interventions in reducing violent recidivism.

Dowden and Andrews (2000) integrated a series of 34 evaluations of interventions to reduce violence, yielding 52 effect-size tests. The target offence behaviours included general violence, sexual, and domestic assaults. Most (70%) of the studies included in this review focused primarily on work with adults. The overall mean effect size (r) was relatively low at +0.07, although there was enormous heterogeneity in the findings: effect sizes ranged from a low of −0.22 to a high of +0.63. The effect size for 'human service interventions', based on combining the principles defined by Gendreau and Andrews (1990) and now reconfigured as the Risk-Needs-Responsivity model (Andrews et al., 2006) was +0.12. Using the binomial effect size display devised by Rosenthal and Rubin (1982), this corresponds to recidivism rates of 44% for experimental and 56% for control groups. Another important finding to emerge from this review was evidence of a close correspondence between the number of criminogenic needs targeted in interventions and the associated effect size: a correlation coefficient of +0.69 (p <0.001).

More specific results have emerged from review of outcome studies with younger offenders, including those who have committed serious violent or sexual offences, as discovered in a more detailed meta-analysis by Lipsey and Wilson (1998). These authors integrated findings from a total of 200 studies, 83 of the interventions delivered in residential settings and 117 delivered in the community. Lipsey and Wilson grouped types of interventions in broad categories defined by a combination of mean effect size (ES) and the consistency with which it was obtained. Intervention programmes in the most consistently effective category were found to have an average impact in reducing recidivism by 40% in community settings and 30% in custodial settings (Lipsey & Wilson, 1998).

For community-based interventions, Lipsey and Wilson (1998) found the largest mean effect sizes (d) were for structured individual counselling (+0.46), interpersonal skills training (+0.44), and behavioural programmes (+0.42). For institutionally based methods, the largest mean effect sizes were for interpersonal skills training (+0.39) and teaching family homes (+0.34). Positive effects were obtained, but with less consistency, for the provision of 'multiple services' (sometimes called 'service brokerage', d = +0.29) in the community, and for behavioural programmes (+0.33), community residential facilities (+0.28), and multiple services (+0.20) in institutional settings. Other types of intervention were either weaker or less consistent in their effects, or both. For a few interventions, notably deterrence-based initiatives, both this and the preceding review found effect sizes close to zero or negative.

There are three other meta-analyses of interventions to reduce aggressive or violent behaviour among youth. Wilson, Lipsey, and Derzon (2003) reviewed findings from 221 studies of interventions designed to reduce aggression in schools. The selected studies were carried out with participant samples ranging from preschool to 13th grade (age 17–18 years), resulting in an aggregate sample of almost 56 000. Of the 522 comparisons possible between experimental and control groups, 34% were derived from randomized designs. The methods employed included competence training, with and without cognitive-behavioural components, classroom management techniques, counselling, separate streaming within schools, peer mediation, academic interventions, and varied combinations of the foregoing. Among randomized designs, there was an overall ES difference between experimental and control samples of 0.31 in favour of the former; the corresponding figure for non-randomized designs was 0.16. There were larger mean effect sizes for groups at opposite ends of the age distribution (≤5 and ≥14 years) than for those in the middle age ranges. Social competence training (with or without cognitive-behavioural components) and counselling both yielded positive effect sizes in the 0.24–0.36 range.

McCart et al. (2006) compared the relative effectiveness of behavioural parent training (BPT) and cognitive-behavioural therapies (CBT) in reducing aggression and other antisocial behaviour among young people under the age of 18. They found 41 studies of the former and 30 of the latter. The dependent variables were physical or verbal aggression, or delinquency. There was a mean effect size across all studies of +0.40 at post-test and +0.22 at follow-up (although the latter was based on only 17 studies). A direct comparison between the two approaches proved difficult as the mean age of those provided BPT was much lower than that of those provided CBT (5.44 years versus 11.28 years). The comparison was thus restricted to seven studies using the former and 21 using the latter that focused on the 6–12 year age group: corresponding mean effect sizes were +0.45 and +0.23. Across the full sets of studies, the weighted post-treatment means were +0.47 and +0.35 for BPT and CBT, respectively, and in the 13 CBT studies for which follow-up data could be analysed, there was a mean effect size of +0.31.

Garrido and Morales (2007) updated aspects of the Lipsey and Wilson (1998) review, although with a narrower focus on interventions provided in secure institutions only and confining the analysis to studies of groups defined as violent and chronic delinquents. Outcome measures included both general ($k = 30$) and serious ($k = 15$) recidivism, the later defined as comprising offences that led to re-incarceration. There was a cumulative sample size of 6658 and a median follow-up period of 18 months. The odds ratios for general and serious recidivism were 1.235 and 1.354, respectively, in favour of experimental and treatment groups. The latter effect size showed a surprising homogeneity. The authors sought to take account of sample attrition by conducting an intent-to-treat analysis, yielding an odds ratio of 1.307. All effect sizes are statistically significant.

For domestic violence, primarily consisting of assaults by males on female partners (designated *intimate partner violence*; Polaschek, 2006), a meta-analysis has been reported by Babcock et al. (2004). These authors examined findings from 22 studies yielding (after elimination of outliers) 36 effect size tests; 17 of the studies were quasi-experiments and the remaining 5 'true' experimental designs. For the Duluth model, using police reports as the outcome variable, the mean effect size (*d*) was +0.32 for quasi-experimental and +0.12 for experimental designs. For cognitive-behavioural methods, the mean effect size was +0.12 for quasi-experiments (no effect size could be computed for experimental designs). For partner reports, Duluth interventions had a mean effect size of +0.35 and CBT of +0.29. Nevertheless, Babcock et al. (2004; p. 1044) concluded that '… there is great room for improvement in our batterers' treatment interventions'. It should be borne in mind that this is a singularly sensitive area in which to provide interventions, and high attrition rates are common.

There have been six meta-analyses conducted to date of the effectiveness of interventions to reduce sexual recidivism (all listed in Table 15.2). The most recent and comprehensive review (Lösel & Schmucker, 2005) synthesized findings from 69 studies, covering a cumulative sample of 22 181 participants, and including both medical and psychosocial treatments. From these findings Lösel & Schmucker were able to compute a total of 80 effect size tests. A majority (60%) of the studies consisted of non-equivalent group designs, for a further 19 equivalence was assumed, seven used statistical controls, and six involved random allocation. Mean effect sizes across interventions, expressed as odds ratios (OR), were +1.70 for reductions in sexual recidivism, equivalent to a 37% reduction relative to comparison samples; +1.90 for violent recidivism (44% reduction); and +1.67 for general recidivism (31% reduction). The largest effects were for physical treatments (surgical castration, eight studies, OR = 15.34; hormonal medication, six studies, OR = 3.08). Some psychosocial interventions achieved significant effects (behavioural, seven studies, OR = 2.19; cognitive-behavioural, 35 studies, OR = 1.45), whereas others (insight-oriented and therapeutic community approaches) had odds ratios not significantly different from 1. The mean effect size for cognitive-behavioural methods is lower than the OR of 1.67 found in another review of sex offender treatment that focused solely on psychologically based interventions (Hanson *et al.*, 2002).

Given the close association between violence and traits of callousness, low empathy, impulsivity, and irresponsibility, a further set of meta-analytic reviews pertains to the effects of interventions with individuals classified as psychopathic. Unfortunately, the findings of the two available reviews in this area have not resolved the long-debated issue of treatability with this population. Salekin (2002) reviewed a series of 42 outcome studies; however, only eight involved group comparison designs, and many others were single case reports. So, although the latter may be clinically instructive, any firmer conclusions must remain tentative at present. Of those studies that could be regarded as more robust, there were five of CBT incorporating a cumulative sample of 246 individuals. There were high effect sizes on intermediate outcome variables for several therapeutic approaches, including CBT, personal construct therapy, and other approaches which '… addressed patients' thoughts about themselves, others and society. Thus, they tended to directly treat some psychopathic traits' (Salekin, 2002; p. 93). Salekin also observed that there was a strong association between effect size and duration and intensity of treatment: interventions lasting less than 6 months were less likely to produce benefits than longer ones: where attendance was maintained for more than a year, or delivered at a rate of more than four sessions per week, a considerably higher fraction of the samples benefited. Working with civil psychiatric patients, Skeem *et al.* (2002) reported that those assessed as either psychopathic or 'potentially psychopathic' who received higher dosages of treatment (attended seven or more sessions) were approximately three times less likely to be involved in subsequent violence than those who receive little or no treatment. This difference remained after controlling both for a number of background and clinical variables, and for treatment assignment.

The studies reviewed by Salekin (2002) predominantly reported increased levels of engagement in treatment, rather than treatment outcomes. More recently, Tanasichuk and Wormith (2007) have reported a meta-analysis of outcome trials in this area. They located an initial total of 21 studies yielding 50 effect-size estimates (cumulative sample $n = 5550$). In comparisons between those designated as psychopaths and samples of non-psychopaths, the former consistently showed higher general, violent, and sexual recidivism, more antisocial behaviour, higher levels of substance abuse, and spent significantly less time in treatment.

In three studies where comparisons were possible between treated and untreated psychopaths, there were no significant differences in general or violent recidivism; other types of comparisons were not feasible given the available data. However, contrary to the findings of some earlier researchers (Rice *et al.*, 1992), there was no evidence that treatment made psychopaths worse, and a study by Wong *et al.* (2006) found that psychopaths completing Aggressive Behavioural Control, a violence risk reduction programme at the Saskatoon Regional Psychiatric Centre, subsequently committed less serious offences than matched controls. Although there was no significant difference in total reconvictions, 'the mean length of the sum of the aggregate sentences was halved & the longest aggregated sentence was more than halved' (Wong *et al.*, 2006; p. 3).

Outcome studies in this area are relatively few in number and suffer from poor designs, leading Tanasichuk and Wormith (2007) to recommend that more matched control group studies should be conducted. Other authors researching this area have remained unconvinced that evidence concerning therapeutic change among diagnosed psychopaths is likely to be forthcoming (Harris & Rice, 2006). Against such 'therapeutic nihilism', as it has been called, it is equally plausible that appropriate interventions adopting 'best practice' formulae have not yet been devised for working with this group. Long-term monitoring of the diagnostic status of those classified as suffering from personality disorders, including psychopathy, indicates that reductions in symptom severity occur. Serin (1995) noted longitudinal evidence concerning decreasing portions of study samples retaining diagnostic features. This is amplified by Sanislow and McGlashan (1998) who reviewed 44 studies of the 'natural course' of personality disorders including ASPD. Rather than finding a fixed, immutable pattern as was previously expected, this review showed a pattern of changeability over time.

If individuals are assessed as having more extreme scores on measures of various criminogenic risk factors, it is not surprising to find that more complex, intensive, multimodal methods are required to engender attitudinal or behavioural change. Furthermore, two studies have shown that it is possible to improve the ability of children and adolescents with callous-unemotional traits (considered a precursor component of the emergence of psychopathy) to recognize facial expressions of fear, by redirecting their attention to other people's eyes (Richell *et al.*, 2003; Dadds *et al.*, 2006). If this is feasible for children thought to be at long-term risk of developing psychopathy, it suggests that the variables associated with aggression can be ameliorated. It also indicates a possible method of doing so that could be modified and incorporated in multimodal treatments.

Finally, Leitner *et al.* (2006) reported a systematic review of risk assessment and violence prevention in the field of forensic mental health. Of 228 182 citations initially retrieved, 299 evaluations that employed some form of between-groups statistical analyses were retained after screening. Among these studies, 54.5% were of pharmacological agents, 29.8% of psychosocial interventions, 6.7% some combination of the former two, and 9% were classed as 'other interventions' (e.g., organizational changes in ward management procedures). Within these general categories, the proportions of studies with unequivocally positive outcomes were 80.4%, 79.8%, 85% and 66.7%, respectively. Hence, in general, there were fairly high success rates of interventions of a variety of types for reducing violence in this client group.

Currently, Whittington *et al.* (in preparation) are undertaking meta-analysis of the best controlled trials in this data set, to be reported in a future paper. Of 112 studies of psychosocial interventions that were located, only 28 employed randomized designs. This differs somewhat from the results of a scoping survey (Cure *et al.*, 2005), which suggested that over

700 interventions to reduce aggression have been tested in 300 controlled trials, including 328 'named talking therapies'. The target populations in the studies are very varied, and include diagnoses of schizophrenia, attention deficit hyperactivity disorder (ADHD), individuals who have committed domestic violence or child abuse, prisoners, and social care residents or offenders with learning disabilities. Similarly, there is a wide variety of intervention methods, including socialization games, social skills training, relaxation training, anger management, behaviour modification, CBT, motivational interviewing, parental skills training, family therapy, group psychotherapy, and psychodynamic therapy. Unfortunately, most methods are represented by a single study only, and studies also employ a miscellany of outcome measures, including self-report and psychometric scales, observational measures, and official data sources such as criminal reconvictions. Initial effect-size analyses (using Cohen's d) show variations from +0.01 to +1.40.

Overall, on the basis of the series of 11 meta-analyses just discussed, addressing violent behaviour in general or specific forms of it, there are numerous positive outcomes. These permit reasonable confidence in the broad conclusion that it is possible to reduce violent recidivism by systematic and carefully designed intervention. As with offender treatment considered more broadly, and apart from the findings obtained for physical treatment of sexual offending, the most consistent outcome effects are for a collection of methods derived from the cognitive social learning model (behavioural, cognitive, interpersonal, and problem-solving training methods). However, a considerable need remains for further, better controlled outcome studies to test more refined hypotheses concerning the relationships between intervention methods, offence typologies, participant characteristics, delivery settings, and other variables, and to address the enduring problem of transfer of findings to routine practice in criminal justice or mental health services.

Illustrative applications and outcomes

Meta-analyses of treatment studies are, of course, to some extent abstractions; subsuming information from various sources, they are removed from the direct clinical work or service delivery that is being evaluated in each of the studies. In order to portray more accurately the nature of interventions tested in these reviews, this section provides some illustrative outlines of specific programmes and methods and in some cases corresponding results.

Reactive (emotional) aggression: anger management

Numerous behavioural and cognitive methods have been applied to angry aggression, perhaps most notably the model of anger reactions and their management developed by Novaco (1975, 1997, 2007), which has had a seminal effect in many clinical locations, including work with offenders. The model describes the interdependence of cognitive appraisal, emotional arousal, and angry response in a manner that enables individuals both to understand their experiences of anger, and acquire a framework and techniques for regaining control where they may have lost it.

There are several meta-analytic reviews of anger management or anger control, covering work with a wide range of populations. In an early review, Edmondson and Conger (1996) carried out a synthesis of 18 studies. Most had small samples and the total contact time (session length multiplied by number of sessions) was fairly limited, usually amounting to only 6–8 hours. The effect sizes were remarkably high, although they varied according to the outcome target. The authors suggested that the choice of anger treatment should depend on the specific types of anger problems experienced by participants.

More recently, DiGuiseppe and Tafrate (2003) reported a meta-analysis of 50 studies (with a total sample of 1841 adult participants and 81 effect size tests). Many different types of therapy were evaluated in the studies reviewed: including self-instructional training, cognitive restructuring, problem solving, relaxation training, systematic desensitization, exposure therapy, behavioural self-management, anxiety management training, and various combinations of the foregoing. Their review found positive effects of interventions on both expression of anger and on aggressive behaviour, and the maintenance of gains over time. The mean effect size for anger control was +0.71 and for aggression-related outcomes +1.16, a large effect.

A separate review has also been reported, focusing on anger-based interventions for children and adolescents ranging in age from 6 to 18 years (Sukhodolsky *et al.*, 2004). There were 40 studies included, 80% of which involved random assignment, generating 173 outcome tests and a cumulative sample of 1953. The mean effect size (*d*) for anger experience was +0.47 and for physical aggression +0.63.

Additional reviews have followed. Gansle (2005) synthesized findings from 20 studies conducted in schools: 75% used random assignment. The mean effect size across studies for externalizing anger problems was +0.54 at post-test and +0.53 at follow-up. Another review was restricted to randomized trials only (del Vecchio & O'Leary, 2004). There were 23 studies with a total sample of 1730 participants. Mean effect sizes for four categories of intervention represented were: for relaxation training alone, +0.90; for cognitive therapy alone, +0.82; for CBT, +0.68; and for a mixed group of other treatments, +0.61. The effect sizes were such that '… as per this analysis, hundreds of additional studies averaging negligible results would be needed to reduce these findings to negligible levels, alleviating the effect of the file drawer problem' (del Vecchio & O'Leary, 2004; pp. 25–26).

Overall, the results for interventions designed to reduce anger or to render it more manageable, and decrease resultant aggression, appear impressive. Effect sizes are in the moderate-to-large range and there is a healthy representation of well-controlled trials. However, with some notable exceptions, the majority of the participants in the studies reviewed are general population samples reporting anger as a problem and seeking help to manage it. In work with violent offenders, although there have been some valuable outcomes, overall results are less consistent. It should be emphasized that although some violent offences may be directly caused by loss of control over anger, it is difficult to ascertain how much this contributes to violent behaviour in general (Polaschek & Reynolds, 2004). It appears essential to assess a pattern of offending (using functional analysis, case formulation) prior to allocating individuals to programmes. Polaschek (2006) has noted the inappropriateness of anger management alone for individuals exhibiting either overcontrolled or instrumental aggression, although it could constitute an element in a multimodal programme focused on such problems.

In penal settings, one of the most extensive applications of anger control programmes was carried out in Canadian prisons. The programme consisted of 25 two-hour sessions, offered between two and five times per week, for groups varying between 4 and 10 prisoners. Dowden *et al.* (1999) reported a three-year follow-up of 110 programme participants and matched controls. For lower-risk cases, there was no impact on levels of reoffending. For high-risk cases, however, there was a 69% reduction in general recidivism and an 86% reduction in violent reoffending, one of the largest effects reported in the literature. Dowden and Serin (2001) reported a more searching analysis of the follow-up data taking account of performance measures (indicators of extent of participation in the programme). There was a correlation of +0.32 between these measures and recidivism outcomes, making them the strongest predictor of recidivism. At the follow-up point, there were significant differences (p , 0.001) between treatment completers, untreated comparisons, and programme dropouts, with respective rates of general recidivism being 10%, 30%, and 52%, and of violent recidivism 5%, 17%, and 40%. These findings suggest there may be an underlying treatment effect, but this cannot be ascertained with confidence given the higher rate of recidivism among the dropouts than among the controls.

Implementation of anger management training in penal settings has not proved to be uniformly successful. In some instances, treatment gains have been marginal. Howells *et al.* (2002) carried out a large-scale evaluation of anger management programmes in several prisons in Australia. On the basis of their study, the authors made a number of observations: while arguing that anger management interventions should be continued, they recommended moving away from 'blanket delivery' of programmes. The same authors have also drawn attention to the importance of readiness for change in assigning prisoners to anger control sessions (Howells & Day, 2003).

Interventions with young offenders

In the extensive meta-analytic review reported by Lipsey and Wilson (1998) described earlier, several intervention methods emerged as most consistently yielding positive outcomes with regard to reduced rates of violent and sexual recidivism among young offenders.

Interpersonal skills training
This comprises a series of exercises designed to improve participants' skills in interacting with others. Working in a small group, individuals identify situations in which they are uncertain how to act or which they sometimes mishandle. Suitable ways of behaving in the situation are discussed, practised using role-play, and shaped via behavioural rehearsal and feedback. An example of this is a study by Chandler (1973) on training in 'perspective taking' skills.

Structured individual counselling
The most widely used format of counselling as a relatively unstructured, person-centred, non-directive activity has not emerged as an effective means of reducing offender recidivism. However, more structured approaches, based for example on reality therapy, problem-solving, or multimodal frameworks, have yielded positive effects, especially in community settings. For example, a very large effect size was reported for Multi-Systemic Therapy (MST; Borduin *et al.*, 1995) in a four-year follow-up of serious young offenders, including significant reductions in violence. Although effects have been smaller in subsequent studies, this intervention has generally demonstrated positive outcomes with very challenging young people.

Behavioural interventions
In work with offenders, this has included contingency contracts in which individual offenders and their supervisors compose a list of problem behaviours and a system of rewards for progress towards modifying them, in conjunction with behavioural training procedures such as modelling and graduated practice, and cognitive and problem-solving skills training. For example, using behavioural methods in work with families, large reductions in

juvenile offending were obtained over follow-ups of 2.5–3.5 years (Klein *et al.*, 1977; and see Gordon, 2002).

Teaching family homes

These are residential units or group homes in which specially trained adults work in pairs as 'teaching parents'. Their role is to develop positive working alliances with residents, impart a range of interpersonal and self-management skills, and provide counselling and advocacy services. Young people can continue to attend school and return to their homes of origin at weekends (see Kirigin *et al.*, 1982).

'Decompression' with difficult-to-manage youth

Several more recent studies have reported on the effect of an institutional regime that is designed to put into reverse the downward spiral in which young people who have shown repeated violence are subject to maximal control but respond with increased defiance, and may remain resistant to intervention efforts for lengthy periods. Caldwell and Van Rybroek (2005) have described the application and the effects of a 'decompression' regime, designed to counter this pattern, which incorporates additional training programmes (notably Aggression Replacement Training) in a 'clinical-correctional hybrid' (2005, p. 625) at the Mendota Juvenile Treatment Center, Wisconsin. This group of young people, who had committed their first offences at an average age of nine years, had been considered unmanageable in other institutional settings. A sample of 101 programme participants was followed up after discharge for an average of 4.5 years alongside a matched untreated comparison group of 147. As random allocation was difficult to implement with this population, propensity scores were used to take account of possible selection effects. Members of the treatment group were six times less likely than controls to be re-convicted of a violent offence. Economic analysis of the intervention showed a cost-benefit ratio of 1:7 for the Center (Caldwell, Vitacco & Van Rybroek 2006). Of note, a sizeable proportion of these young people met criteria for classification as having 'psychopathic' personalities, assessed using the Psychopathy Check List: Youth Version (PCL:YV). Nevertheless, this group too showed a response to treatment, with significant changes in behaviour ratings between commencement and completion of the programme. The latter scores proved more accurate predictors of future success or failure than scores on the PCL:YV (Caldwell, McCormick, Unstead & Van Rybroek 2007).

Cognitive skills programmes for adults

Cognitive skills programmes are so called because their objectives and the methods they employ are directed towards helping participants to acquire new capacities for thinking about and solving their problems, particularly in the interpersonal domain. They draw on earlier work such as that of Chandler (1973) or Platt *et al.* (1980) (for background, see McGuire, 2005).

Programmes of this type are derived from the *cognitive model of offender rehabilitation* proposed by Ross and Fabiano (1985), a variant of the social learning theory placing a particular accent on cognitive skills. These denote the capacity when faced with a personal difficulty to engage in a sequence of activities including problem identification, generating alternative solutions, means-end thinking, anticipating consequences of actions, and perspective taking. Ordinarily, such skill acquisition occurs naturally during development, but that process is a function of appropriate learning opportunities. Conversely, the absence of such skills is held to constitute a risk factor for antisocial behaviour including resorting to aggression.

The most widely disseminated programme derived from the model, entitled Reasoning and Rehabilitation (R&R) consists of a series of 38 two-hour sessions delivered on a group basis and led by special trained tutors (Antonowicz, 2005). Its constituent materials are organized into a sequence of interlinked modules focusing on problem solving, social interaction, impulse control and self-management, negotiation and conflict resolution, and critical thinking.

In a large-scale evaluation for Correctional Services Canada, with a sizeable sample of federally sentenced prisoners (n = 1444), there was a reduction in recidivism of 36.4% among those completing the programme compared with controls (Robinson, 1995; Robinson & Porporino, 2001). Of specific relevance here, these effects were moderated by offence type: prisoners with records of violent, sexual, and substance-related offending were less likely to be reconvicted than those with histories of property crimes. Both R&R and other cognitive skills programmes have emerged as beneficial from focused meta-analytic reviews (Wilson et al., 2005; Tong & Farrington, 2006). However, system-wide implementation of R&R along side an associated programme, Enhanced Thinking Skills in prisons in England and Wales yielded mixed and predominantly non-significant results (Friendship et al., 2002; Cann et al., 2003; Falshaw et al., 2003).

Outcomes for probation-based versions of cognitive skills interventions have been generally more positive. There are significant reductions in actual two-year recidivism rates below expected rates across most types of programme (Hollis, 2007). Where it has been possible to enter prior levels of risk of reconviction among programme participants, non-completers, and comparison samples, as variables in logistic regression analyses, offenders completing programmes have been found to have significantly lower rates of subsequent recidivism (Palmer et al., 2007; Hollin et al., 2008). In order to take account of between-group differences in the likelihood of programme non-completion, such data can also be analysed using propensity scores, separating variables likely to influence completion from the potential impact of programmes on recidivism as the dependent variable. Where this has been done, again there is evidence of a link between programme completion and a significant reduction in criminal recidivism (McGuire et al., 2008). Within this, reductions are observed in rates of violence alongside other types of offending, although the relationship between this and programme completion has not been analysed separately.

Cognitive self-change
Cognitive skills programmes are designed to impart to their participants a series of cognitive, interpersonal, and self-management skills, limitations or deficits in which are thought to have contributed to the occurrence of acts of crime. An alternative approach is to consider such acts as arising from cognitive distortions held by the offender; beliefs or assumptions that are directly conducive to antisocial acts.

A programme of this type was developed within an adult prison establishment in the Vermont Department of Corrections, United States. Bush (1995) has described the rationale for the programme and its mode of delivery. Sessions were run within a separate unit inside the prison; groups of between 5 and 10 prisoners with histories of violent offending met three to five times per week. In each session, one prisoner was asked to describe an incident in which he had been involved, and to furnish a *thinking report*. This is a detailed record of thoughts and feelings before, during, and after a violent act, in which participants seek to obtain a fuller understanding of the factors that have influenced them. Groups collaborated in identifying criminogenic thought patterns, then generated new thoughts or practised skills that would make violent behaviour less likely, a procedure entitled *self-risk management*.

Henning and Frueh (1996) reported a two-year follow-up of 55 prisoners who attended this programme for an average of 9.8 months, compared with an appropriately matched sample of 141 non-attenders. There was a significant difference in the respective recidivism rates of the two groups (50% versus 71%). The follow-up analysis also showed that members of the experimental group survived significantly longer in the community before committing new offences.

Other multimodal interventions for violence

A more elaborate, multimodal programme to address violent offending is described by Cortoni *et al.* (2006). The Violence Prevention Program (VPP) consists of many different elements and is based on a model that incorporated motivational enhancement, behavioural change methods, a focus on aggressive beliefs, cognitive distortions, arousal management, impulsivity, conflict resolution, problem solving, empathy enhancement, and relapse prevention (Serin & Preston, 2001).

The evaluation study consisted of two samples: 500 VPP participants and 466 prisoners in a matched comparison group. Members of both groups were in custody during the period 1999–2004; 66.6% of the former group completed the programme. The comparison sample was matched to the experimental group using propensity scores defined with reference to the probability of receiving treatment. Evaluation data included numbers of institutional incidents (disciplinary infractions) as a proximate outcome, with general and violent recidivism as follow-up outcomes after discharge into the community, taking account of time at risk. Those who completed the programme had a uniformly lower failure rate (on all measures) than the comparison sample, notably a violent recidivism rate of 8.5% compared with that for the non-completers of 24.5% and for the comparison group of 21.8%. Expressed as risk ratios using Cox regression, the comparison group had a 1.36 times greater risk of any failure and a 2.10 times higher rate of violent recidivism, than completers. For non-completers, the rate of violent recidivism was 4.25 times that of completers. Similar findings were obtained for Aboriginal offenders when data for that group were analysed separately.

Possible confounding variables included a difference between the groups in terms of motivation for intervention, which was higher among the experimental than the comparison sample, and the fact that a slightly higher proportion of treatment-group members had completed other violence-related programmes prior to embarking on the VPP.

Other multimodal cognitive skills group programmes that have demonstrated success in reducing violence include the Montgomery House Violence Prevention Project and the Violence Prevention Unit (VPU) in New Zealand (Polaschek & Reynolds, 2004; Polaschek *et al.*, 2005; Polascheck, 2006). Although the study of the former was statistically underpowered, there was a large observed reduction in violent reoffending for treated offenders and minimal change in a matched untreated control group. In a five-year follow-up evaluation, of 64 men in the treated group, 33 committed new offences; of the same number in the control group, 51 committed new offences. When the outcomes were adjusted for the rate of pre-programme violence, the recidivism rates were 25% and 42% for the experimental and control samples, respectively (Montgomery House, 2007). For the prison-based VPU, the first 22 completers were compared with a matched untreated sample drawn from a national database. At a minimal two-year follow-up, 32% of the completers had a violent reconviction alongside 63% for the comparison group; survival analysis found an effect-size difference between the two groups of +0.41 in 'days to failure'.

Finally, Aggression Replacement Training (ART) is a multimodal programme designed for individuals who have committed violent offences that employs methods of social skills, anger management, and moral reasoning training in an integrated, 30-session format (Goldstein & Glick, 2001). Evaluations of its use with young offenders, although based on small samples and in non-equivalent designs, have found positive effects, but are reported in terms of general re-arrest rates rather than violent recidivism. Aos *et al.* (2001) summarized four studies with adjusted effect sizes ranging from 0.07 to 0.26. On the basis of unpublished Home Office data concerning the use of ART with adults on probation, McGuire and Clark (2004) reported that programme completers (n = 113) had a significantly lower rate of recidivism at a 12-month follow-up than matched comparison samples allocated to other types of probation supervision. Whereas the predicted and actual reconviction rates for the comparison sample were 37.9% and 34.5% respectively, the corresponding figures for the ART participants were 34.6% and 20.4%. Predicted and actual rates of those allocated to the programme or to other probation interventions, whose probation orders were revoked, were uniformly higher. Thus, the ART completer group was the only one to show a significant reduction in reconviction below predicted levels. Again however, the use of a quasi-experimental design leaves the results open to more than one interpretation.

Using an intent-to-treat analysis, with a comparison sample formed on the basis of one-to-one matching, Hatcher *et al.* (in press) found a reduction of 13.3% in reconviction among those allocated to ART relative to controls. Compared with their matched counterparts, programme completers had a reconviction rate 15.1% lower, and completion of the programme was associated with a 78% improvement in survival times. This was, however, a fairly short follow-up (10 months) and the completion rate for the programme during the study period was rather low; these are nevertheless reasonably promising results.

Conceptualizing violent behaviour

Given the multiplicity of factors shown to influence violent conduct and the variety of interventions with some supportive evidence of effectiveness, the construction of a viable model of causation and intervention remains an elusive goal. Arguably, a great deal is known about separate risk factors and permutations of them that are associated with delinquency and crime in general (Farrington, 2007) or with a repetitive pattern of violence in particular (e.g., Herrenkohl *et al.*, 2000; Surgeon General, 2001; Farrington, 2003). Not unreasonably, some authors (Rutter, 2003; Moffit & Caspi, 2006) have expressed dissatisfaction with the risk factors approach and the absence of coherent accounts of causal pathways confirmed by empirical findings. However, models of functional relationships between factors operating at different levels (biological, psychological, social) and different developmental stages (infancy, middle childhood, adolescence) have been proposed (e.g., Dodge & Pettit, 2003; LeBlanc, 2006) and are capable of accounting at least in general terms for a sizeable proportion of the data currently available.

There is a consensus that violence is only likely to be comprehensible within probabilistic rather than deterministic causal models, an assumption pivotal to the risk factors approach. But the extent to which this can be developed into a formal theory remains questionable. An ineluctable problem arising in all research in this field is that most discrete risk factors or other variables account for only a small proportion of the measured variance in violent behaviours, underlining the necessity of a multifactorial model. What should be the nature of such a model?

Tackling the task of theory construction, some formerly intractable problems are addressed and some fundamental principles are enunciated by Dodge and Pettit (2003). One is that of *equifinality*, whereby '... the same antisocial outcome can accrue from disparate sources' (p. 354). Another is that of *multifinality*, whereby '... specific risk factors can be associated with a variety of outcomes' (p. 354). This is to some extent reminiscent of the problem known in the philosophy of science as 'underdetermination of theory', wherein the available data are potentially compatible with more than one of the theoretical formulations on offer (Klee, 1997).

But it may be that, given the nature of the problem, data that would allow a critical choice between theories, or even allow differential apportioning of causal weight to diverse classes of variable, will not be obtainable. Any theoretical model that is designed to account for the available data at anything other than a macroscopic level may be unlikely to succeed. A possible route out of this dilemma is offered in the philosophical work of Mackie (1980) concerning causality. In addition to the familiar Humean categories of necessary and sufficient causes of events, Mackie specifies a third category of factors entitled *inus* conditions. This acronym refers to an insufficient, non-redundant part of an unnecessary but sufficient condition. The possible meaning of this is represented diagrammatically in Fig. 15.1.

Thus, there are different sets of factors (denoted A, ... D, ... in Fig. 15.1) that influence the likelihood of a violent act (or pattern of perpetrating such acts; denoted P). They are customarily grouped under familiar headings (e.g., neurobiological, cognitive, social) and within each there is a potentially extensive list of defined independent variables (e.g., *MAOA* polymorphism, suppressed amygdala activity, dysexecutive syndrome, callousness, impulsivity, attributions of hostility, coercive family process, peer pressure, social inequality, media images, provocations, intoxication). Given any instance or sample of instances of persistent aggressiveness, there could be different patterns of influence at work yielding the same outcome, operating along multiple pathways (Dahlberg & Potter, 2001). Each of the aforementioned factors alone (or any of numerous others) may be an *insufficient* cause of aggression by itself; but it cannot be dispensed with (it is *non-redundant*) as part of a larger set of causes, each of which is *unnecessary* to the observed outcome (i.e., it could occur in their absence) but may nevertheless collectively be *sufficient* to cause it in some cases. Where the independent variables in a research study account for only a small proportion of the variance in the dependent variable (the standard scenario), or where the findings of different studies contradict each other, it may be that this is due to each of them having measured some *inus* conditions and not others.

Returning to the evidence reviewed in this chapter concerning effective interventions, a core question that remains is how those changes that engender reductions in aggression and

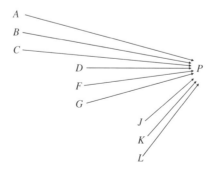

Fig. 15.1 *Inus* conditions and probabilistic models of violence causation

violence occur ('treatment theory'; Polaschek, 2006). Although numerous variables operate during such a process, arguably what they share in common is an increase in the individual's capacity for, and motivation to engage in, *self-regulation* of cognitive and emotional processes and of the interaction between them. Longitudinal research by Bandura and his colleagues (2001, 2003; Caprara *et al.*, 2002) using structural equation models have revealed significant linkages between low perceived self-regulatory efficacy and patterns of violent conduct in young people followed up between the ages of 11 and 19. Working with a different age group in very different circumstances (recidivist offenders who had already served several prison sentences and were re-incarcerated again following a new offence), Zamble and Quinsey (1997) found that poor self-regulation, misdirected attempts at problem solving, and failure to manage negative emotions were connected with the occurrence of reoffences.

There are invaluable integrative frameworks within which these observations might be subsumed in striving towards a properly articulated theory. They include the bio-psychosocial model proposed by Dodge and Pettit (2003), deploying concepts of non-linear, transactional relationships between key variables. Another example is the work of LeBlanc (2006) who draws extensively on control theory in criminology in constructing a developmental model of interactions between personal and social controls in the genesis of deviant behaviour. A still broader conceptual framework (applicable to clinical problems beyond that of violence) is the 'hot/cool system' analysis of Metcalfe and Mischel (1999).

Arguably, within each of these perspectives, however, ultimate behavioural outcomes must be mediated by psychological variables (Kinderman, 2005). Whatever the distal factors may be that lead through multiple developmental pathways to aggressive propensity, in the overwhelming majority of cases these interact with current circumstances and are expressed through experiential (including cognitive and emotional) processes and events. Kinderman (2005) has forwarded a general conceptual scheme depicting these relationships, shown in a modified form in Fig. 15.2.

According to Dodge and Pettit (2003), 'life experiences with parents, peers and social institutions mediate, at least partially, the effects of biological predispositions and sociocultural contexts' (2003; p. 357) in ways that lead to disordered conduct. They also assign a core role to 'agentic emotional and cognitive processes' which are 'posited as the crucial factors that mediate the relation between risk factors and conduct problems' (2003, p. 361). Kinderman (2005) argues that by ascribing equivalent status to biological, psychological, and social factors in causation, the bio-psychosocial model pays insufficient attention to the

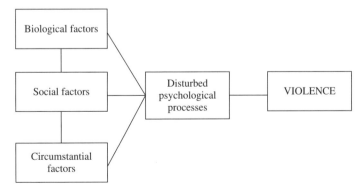

Fig. 15.2 Mediating psychological variables as a 'final common pathway' (Adapted from Kinderman, 2005)

role of psychological processes as a 'final common pathway' in mental disorder. Such a view is equally applicable to understanding violent behaviour, in that regardless of the distal origins of contributory factors, to result in overt actions they must be expressed through psychological processes. Similarly, the basis of effective violence reduction should be grounded in addressing aspects of those processes in intervention efforts.

Conclusions

On the basis of the present review, the following conclusions are offered regarding the prospects of being able to reduce established patterns of aggression and personal violence. First, there are large amounts of evidence showing that it is possible to reduce the rate of occurrence of these problems among individuals who have been identified as manifesting them. There are methodological weaknesses within segments of that evidence, and inconsistencies among reported outcomes, but there are sufficient indications to detect several encouraging trends. Emotional self-management, interpersonal skills, social problem solving, and allied training approaches show mainly positive effects with a reasonably high degree of reliability. Findings are weaker with respect to domestic violence, and less consistent with reference to prison-based programmes. Given our present state of knowledge, findings to date of treatment non-responsiveness among some groups are arguably best interpreted as 'absence of evidence rather than evidence of absence'.

Second, therefore, with regard to almost all issues, there is a need for more and better quality research if this is not to remain an 'underdeveloped corner of offender rehabilitation' (Polaschek, 2006; p. 145). It is important to maintain pluralism of research designs to test both internal and external validity. That is, there need to be more randomized experiments to test specific hypotheses. But it is important not to abandon practical trials that will attest to the usefulness of methods in routine service delivery: quasi-experimental studies can yield valuable information that may be more easily transferred to practical settings, provided researchers adhere to the TREND guidelines (des Jarlais *et al.*, 2004; and see Hollin, 2008). Given the complexity of the problem, it appears advisable to research multimodal interventions only, but the contribution of separate components could be evaluated in dismantling designs.

Third, in relation to practice, for most programmatic interventions in extant use, it is almost certainly necessary to increase the duration and intensity of treatment ('dosage') above presently inadequate levels if intended effects are to be obtained. In criminal justice services, there is a need to improve targeting, preferably applying the Risk-Needs-Responsivity framework (Andrews *et al.*, 2006) as currently the best-validated model. In implementing this at an individual case management level, it is imperative to employ functional analysis or case formulation for treatment allocation decisions.

References

Agnew, R. (1994). The techniques of neutralization and violence. *Criminology, 34*, 555–580.
Akhtar, N., & Bradley, E. J. (1991). Social information processing deficits of aggressive children: present findings and implications for social skills training. *Clinical Psychology Review, 11*, 621–644.
Alexander, M. A. (1999). Sexual offender treatment efficacy revisited. *Sexual Abuse: Journal of Research and Treatment, 11*, 101–116.

Anderson, C. A., & Bushman, B. J. (2002). Human aggression. *Annual Review of Psychology*, *53*, 27–51.

Andrews, D. A. (2001). Principles of effective correctional programs. In L. L. Motiuk, & R. C. Serin (eds), *Compendium 2000 on Effective Correctional Programming* (pp. 9–17). Ottawa: Correctional Service Canada.

Andrews, D. A., & Bonta, J. (2006). *The Psychology of Criminal Conduct*, 4th edn. Cincinnati, OH: LexisNexis/Anderson Publishing Co.

Andrews, D. A., Bonta, J., & Wormith, J. S. (2006). The recent past and near future of risk and/or need assessment. *Crime and Delinquency*, *52*, 7–27.

Andrews, D. A., & Dowden, C. (2005). Managing correctional treatment for reduced recidivism: a meta-analytic review of programme integrity. *Legal and Criminological Psychology*, *10*, 173–187.

Andrews, D. A., & Dowden, C. (2006). Risk principle of case classification in correctional treatment: a meta-analytic investigation. *International Journal of Offender Therapy and Comparative Criminology*, *50*, 88–100.

Andrews, D. A., Zinger, I., Hoge, R. D., Bonta, J., Gendreau, P., & Cullen, F. T. (1990). Does correctional treatment work? A clinically relevant and psychologically informed meta-analysis. *Criminology*, *28*, 369–404.

Antonowicz, D. H. (2005). The Reasoning and Rehabilitation programme: outcome evaluations with offenders. In M. McMurran, & J. McGuire (eds), *Social Problem Solving and Offending: Evidence, Evaluation and Evolution* (pp. 163–181). Chichester, UK: John Wiley & Sons.

Aos, S., Phipps, P., Barnoski, R., & Lieb, R. (2001). *The Comparative Costs and Benefits of Programs to Reduce Crime*. [Online], Olympia, WA: Washington State Institute for Public Policy. Available at: http://www.wsipp.wa.gov/rptfiles/costbenefit.pdf

Babcock, J. C., Green, C. E., & Robie, C. (2004). Does batterers' treatment work? A meta-analytic review of domestic violence treatment. *Clinical Psychology Review*, *23*, 1023–1053.

Bandura, A. (2001). Social learning theory: an agentic perspective. *Annual Review of Psychology*, *52*, 1–26.

Bandura, A., Caprara, G. V., Barbaranelli, C., Gerbino, M., & Pastorelli, C. (2003). Role of affective self-regulatory efficacy in diverse spheres of psychosocial functioning. *Child Development*, *74*, 769–782.

Bandura, A., Caprara, G. V., Barbaranelli, C., Pastorelli, C., & Regalia, C. (2001). Sociocognitive self-regulatory mechanisms governing transgressive behaviour. *Journal of Personality and Social Psychology*, *80*, 125–135.

Baron, L., Straus, M. A., & Jaffee, D. (1988). Legitimate violence, violent attitudes, and rape: a test of the Cultural Spillover Theory. In R. A. Prentky, & V. L. Quinsey (eds), *Human Sexual Aggression: Current Perspectives. Annals of the New York Academy of Sciences*, *528*, 79–110.

Berkowitz, L. (1993). *Aggression: Its Causes, Consequences, and Control*. New York: McGraw-Hill.

Blackburn, R. (1993). *The Psychology of Criminal Conduct*. Chichester, UK: John Wiley & Sons.

Blair, J., Mitchell, D., & Blair, K. (2005). *The Psychopath: Emotion and the Brain*. Oxford: Blackwell Publishing.

Borduin, C. M., Mann, B. J., Cone, L. T., Henggeler, S. W., Fucci, B. R., Blaske, D. M., *et al.* (1995). Multisystemic treatment of juvenile offenders: long-term prevention of criminality and violence. *Journal of Consulting and Clinical Psychology*, *63*, 569–578.

Bradshaw, W., Roseborough, D., & Umbreit, M. (2006). The effect of victim offender mediation on juvenile offender recidivism: a meta-analysis. *Conflict Resolution Quarterly*, *24*, 87–98.

Bureau of Justice Statistics (2003). *World Factbook of Criminal Justice Systems*. [Online], Washington, DC: Office of Justice Programs, US Department of Justice. Available at: http://www.ojp.usdoj.gov/bjs/abstract/wfcj.htm

Burnham, G., Lafta, R., Doocy, S., & Roberts, L. (2006). Mortality after the 2003 invasion of Iraq: a cross-sectional cluster sample survey. *Lancet*, *368*, 1421–1428.

Bush, J. (1995). Teaching self-risk management to violent offenders. In J. McGuire (ed), *What Works: Reducing Re-offending: Guidelines from Research and Practice* (pp. 139–154). Chichester, UK: John Wiley & Sons.

Bushman, B. J., & Anderson, C. A. (2001). Is it time to pull the plug on the hostile versus instrumental aggression dichotomy? *Psychological Review*, *108*, 273–279.

Caldwell, M. F., McCormick, D. J., Umstead, D., & Van Rybroek, G. J. (2007). Evidence of treatment progress and therapeutic outcomes among adolescents with psychopathic features. *Criminal Justice and Behavior*, *34*, 573–587.

Caldwell, M. F., & Van Rybroek, G. J. (2005). Reducing violence in serious juvenile offenders using intensive treatment. *International Journal of Law and Psychiatry*, *28*, 622–636.

Caldwell, M. F., Vitacco, M., & Van Rybroek, G. J. (2006). Are violent delinquents worth treating? a cost-benefit analysis. *Journal of Research in Crime and Delinquency*, *43*, 148–168.

Cann, J., Falshaw, L., Nugent, F., & Friendship, C. (2003). Understanding What Works: Accredited Cognitive Skills Programmes for Adult Men and Young Offenders. Research Findings No. 226. London: Home Office Research, Development and Statistics Directorate.

Caprara, G. V., Regalia, C., & Bandura, A. (2002). Longitudinal impact of perceived self-regulatory efficacy on violent conduct. *European Psychologist*, *7*, 63–69.

Carter, P., & Harrison, R. (1991). *Carter and Harrison on Offences of Violence*. London: Waterlow Publishers.

Caspi, A., Henry, B., McGee, R. O., Moffitt, T. E., & Silva, P. A. (1995). Temperamental origins of child and adolescent behavior problems: from age three to age fifteen. *Child Development*, *66*, 55–68.

Chandler, M. J. (1973). Egocentrism and anti-social behavior: the assessment and training of social perspective-taking skills. *Developmental Psychology*, *9*, 326–332.

Chess, S., & Thomas, A. (1990). Continuities and discontinuities in temperament. In L. Robins, & M. Rutter (eds), *Straight and Devious Pathways from Childhood to Adulthood* (pp. 205–220). Cambridge: Cambridge University Press.

Cleland, C. M., Pearson, F. S., Lipton, D. S., & Yee, D. (1997). Does age make a difference? A meta-analytic approach to reductions in criminal offending for juveniles and adults. Paper presented at the Annual Meeting of the American Society of Criminology, San Diego, California, November.

Cohen, J. (1992). A power primer. *Psychological Bulletin*, *112*, 155–159.

Cook, K., James, M., & Lee, R. (2006). *Core Statutes on Criminal Law*. Exeter, UK: Law Matters Publishing.

Cortoni, F., Nunes, K., & Latendresse, M. (2006). *An Examination of the Effectiveness of the Violence Prevention Program*. Research Report R-178. Ottawa: Correctional Service Canada.

Coughlan, B., Brennan, R. J., Ngoy, P., Dofara, D., Otto, B., Clements, M., *et al.* (2006). Mortality in the Democratic Republic of Congo: a nationwide survey. *Lancet*, *367*, 44–51.

Crick, N. R., & Dodge, K. A. (1994). A review and reformulation of social information-processing mechanisms in children's social adjustment. *Psychological Bulletin*, *115*, 74–101.

Cure, S., Chua, W. L., Duggan, L., & Adams, C. (2005). Randomised controlled trials relevant to aggressive and violent people, 1955-2000: a survey. *British Journal of Psychiatry*, *186*, 185–189.

Dadds, M. R., Perry, Y., Hawes, D. J., Merz, S., Riddell, A. C., Haines, D. J., *et al.* (2006). Attention to the eyes and fear-recognition deficits in child psychopathy. *British Journal of Psychiatry*, *189*, 280–281.

Dahlberg, L. L., & Potter, L. B. (2001). Youth violence: developmental pathways and prevention challenges. *American Journal of Preventive Medicine*, *20*, 3–14.

Del Frate, A. A. (2003). The voice of victims of crime: estimating the true level of conventional crime. *Forum on Crime and Society*, *3*, 127–140.

Del Vecchio, T., & O'Leary, K. D. (2004). Effectiveness of anger treatments for specific anger problems: a meta-analytic review. *Clinical Psychology Review*, *24*, 15–34.

Des Jarlais, D. C., Lyles, C., Crepaz, N., & the TREND Group. (2004). Improving the reporting quality of nonrandomized evaluations of behavioural and public health interventions: The TREND statement. *American Journal of Public Health*, *94*, 361–366.

DiGiuseppe, R., & Tafrate, R. C. (2003). Anger treatment for adults: a meta-analytic review. *Clinical Psychology: Science and Practice*, *10*, 70–84.

Dodge, K. A. (2003). Do social information-processing patterns mediate aggressive behavior? In B. B. Lahey, T. E. Moffitt, & A. Caspi (eds), *Causes of Conduct Disorder and Juvenile Delinquency* (pp. 254–274). New York & London: Guilford Press.

Dodge, K. A., & Pettit, G. S. (2003). A biopsychosocial model of the development of chronic conduct problems in adolescence. *Developmental Psychology*, *39*, 349–371.

Dodge, K. A., & Schwartz, D. (1997). Social information processing mechanisms in aggressive behavior. In D. M. Stoff, J. Breiling, & J. D. Maser (eds), *Handbook of Antisocial Behavior* (pp. 171–180). New York: John Wiley & Sons.

Dowden, C., & Andrews, D. A. (1999a). What works for female offenders: a meta-analytic review. *Crime and Delinquency*, *45*, 438–452.

Dowden, C., & Andrews, D. A. (1999b). What works in young offender treatment: a meta-analysis. *Forum on Corrections Research*, *11*, 21–24.

Dowden, C., & Andrews, D. A. (2000). Effective correctional treatment and violent reoffending: a meta-analysis. *Canadian Journal of Criminology and Criminal Justice*, *42*, 449–467.

Dowden, C., & Andrews, D. A. (2003). Does family intervention work for delinquents? Results of a meta-analysis. *Canadian Journal of Criminology and Criminal Justice*, *45*, 327–342.

Dowden, C., & Andrews, D. A. (2004). The importance of staff practice in delivering effective correctional treatment: a meta-analytic review of core correctional practice. *International Journal of Offender Therapy and Comparative Criminology*, *48*, 203–214.

Dowden, C., Antonowicz, D., & Andrews, D. A. (2003). The effectiveness of relapse prevention with offenders: a meta-analysis. *International Journal of Offender Therapy and Comparative Criminology*, *47*, 516–528.

Dowden, C., Blanchette, K., & Serin, R. C. (1999). *Anger Management Programming for Federal Male Inmates: An Effective Intervention*. Research Report R-82. Ottawa: Correctional Service Canada.

Dowden, C., & Serin R. C. (2001). *Anger Management Programming for Offenders: The Impact of Program Performance Measures*. Research Report R-106. Ottawa: Correctional Service Canada.

Edmondson, C. B., & Conger, J. C. (1996). A review of treatment efficacy for individuals with anger problems: conceptual, assessment, and methodological issues. *Clinical Psychology Review*, *16*, 251–275.

Egg, R., Pearson, F. S., Cleland, C. M., & Lipton, D. S. (2000). Evaluations of correctional treatment programs in Germany: a review and meta-analysis. *Substance Use and Misuse*, *35*, 1967–2009.

Ellsworth, P. C., Carlsmith, J. M., & Henson, A. (1972). The stare as a stimulus to flight in human subjects: a series of field experiments. *Journal of Personality and Social Psychology*, *21*, 302–311.

Falshaw, L., Friendship, C., Travers, R., & Nugent, F. (2003). *Searching for 'What Works': An Evaluation of Cognitive Skills Programmes*. Research Findings No. 206. London: Home Office Research, Development and Statistics Directorate.

Farrington, D. P. (1995). The development of offending and antisocial behaviour from childhood: key findings from the Cambridge Study in Delinquent Development. *Journal of Child Psychology and Psychiatry*, *36*, 929–964.

Farrington, D. P. (2003). Key results from the first forty years of the Cambridge Study in Delinquent development. In T. P. Thornberry, & M. D. Krohn (eds), *Taking Stock of Delinquency: An Overview of Findings from Contemporary Longitudinal Studies* (pp. 137–183). New York: Kluwer Academic/ Plenum Publishers.

Farrington, D. P. (2007). Childhood risk factors and risk-focused prevention. In M. Maguire, R. Morgan, & R. Reiner (eds), *The Oxford Handbook of Criminology*, 4th edn (pp. 602–640). Oxford: Oxford University Press.

Farrington, D. P., & Coid, J. W. (eds) (2003). *Early Prevention of Adult Antisocial Behaviour*. Cambridge: Cambridge University Press.

Farrington, D. P., & Welsh, B. C. (2003). Family-based prevention of offending: a meta-analysis. *The Australian and New Zealand Journal of Criminology*, *36*, 127–151.

Farrington, D. P., & West, D. (1993). Criminal, penal and life histories of chronic offenders: risk and protective factors and early identification. *Criminal Behaviour and Mental Health*, *3*, 492–523.

Fields, S. A., & McNamara, J. R. (2003). The prevention of child and adolescent violence: a review. *Aggression and Violent Behavior*, *8*, 61–91.

French, S. A., & Gendreau, P. (2006). Reducing prison misconducts: What Works! *Criminal Justice and Behavior*, *33*, 185–218.

Friendship, C., Blud, L. Erikson, M., & Travers, R. (2002). *An Evaluation of Cognitive Behavioural Treatment for Prisoners*. Research Findings No. 161. London: Home Office Research, Development and Statistics Directorate.

Gaes, G. G. (1998). Correctional treatment. In M. Tonry (ed), *The Handbook of Crime and Punishment* (pp. 712–738). Oxford: Oxford University Press.

Gallagher, C. A., Wilson, D. B., Hirschfield, P., Coggeshall, M. B., & MacKenzie, D. L. (1999). A quantitative review of the effects of sexual offender treatment on sexual reoffending. *Corrections Management Quarterly*, *3*, 19–29.

Gansle, K. A. (2005). The effectiveness of school-based anger interventions and programs: a meta-analysis. *Journal of School Psychology*, *43*, 321–341.

Garrett, C. G. (1985). Effects of residential treatment on adjudicated delinquents: a meta-analysis. *Journal of Research in Crime and Delinquency*, *22*, 287–308.

Garrido, V., & Morales, L.A. (2007). Serious (violent and chronic) juvenile offenders: a systematic review of treatment effectiveness in secure corrections. Philadelphia, PA: Campbell Collaboration Reviews of Intervention and Policy Evaluations (C2-RIPE). [Online], Available at: http://www.campbellcollaboration.org/doc-pdf/Garrido_seriousjuv_review.pdf

Gendreau, P., & Andrews, D. A. (1990). Tertiary prevention: what the meta-analyses of the offender treatment literature tell us about 'what works'. *Canadian Journal of Criminology*, *32*, 173–184.

Gendreau, P., & Goggin, C. (1996). Principles of effective correctional programming. *Forum on Corrections Research*, *8*, 38–41.

Gendreau, P., Goggin, C., Cullen, F. T., & Paparozzi, M. (2001). The effects of community sanctions and incarceration on recidivism. In L. L. Motiuk, & R. C. Serin (eds), *Compendium 2000 on Effective Correctional Programming* (pp. 18–21). Ottawa: Correctional Services Canada.

Gensheimer, L. K., Mayer, J. P., Gottschalk, R., & Davidson, W. S. (1986). Diverting youth from the juvenile justice system: a meta-analysis of intervention efficacy. In S. A. Apter, & A. P. Goldstein (eds), *Youth Violence: Program and Prospects* (pp. 39–57). Elmsford, NJ: Pergamon Press.

Goldstein, A. P. (2002). Low-level aggression: definition, escalation, intervention. In J. McGuire (ed), *Offender Rehabilitation and Treatment: Effective Programmes and Policies to Reduce Re-offending* (pp. 169–192). Chichester, UK: John Wiley & Sons.

Goldstein, A. P., & Glick, B. (2001). Aggression Replacement Training: application and evaluation management. In G. A. Bernfeld, D. P. Farrington, & A. W. Leschied (eds), *Offender Rehabilitation in Practice: Implementing and Evaluating Effective Programs* (pp. 121–148). Chichester, UK: John Wiley & Sons.

Gottschalk, R., Davidson, W. S., Gensheimer, L. K., & Mayer, J. P. (1987a). Community-based interventions. In H. C. Quay (ed), *Handbook of Juvenile Delinquency* (pp. 266–289). New York: John Wiley & Sons.

Gottschalk, R., Davidson, W. S., Mayer, J., & Gensheimer, L. K. (1987b). Behavioral approaches with juvenile offenders: a meta-analysis of long-term treatment efficacy. In E. K. Morris, & C. J. Braukmann (eds), *Behavioral Approaches to Crime and Delinquency* (pp. 399–422). New York: Plenum Press.

Grietens, H., & Hellinckx, W. (2004). Evaluating effects of residential treatment for juvenile offenders by statistical metaanalysis: a review. *Aggression and Violent Behavior*, *9*, 401–415.

Grubin, D. (1998) *Sex Offending Against Children: Understanding the Risk*. Police Research Series Paper 99. London: Home Office Policing and Reducing Crime Unit.

Guerra, N. G., Tolan, P. H., & Hammond, W. R. (1994). Prevention and treatment of adolescent violence. In L. D. Eron, J. H. Gentry, & P. Schlegel (eds), *Reason to Hope: A Psychosocial Perspective on Violence and Youth* (pp. 383–403). Washington, DC: American Psychological Association.

Hadi, A. (2000). Prevalence and correlates of the risk of marital sexual violence in Bangladesh. *Journal of Interpersonal Violence*, *15*, 787–805.

Hall, G. C. N. (1995). Sexual offender recidivism revisited: a meta-analysis of recent treatment studies. *Journal of Consulting and Clinical Psychology*, *63*, 802–809.

Hanson, R. K., Gordon, A., Harris, A. J. R., Marques, J. K., Murphy, W., Quinsey, V. L., *et al.* (2002). First report of the Collaborative Outcome Data Project on the effectiveness of psychological treatment for sex offenders. *Sexual Abuse: A Journal of Research and Treatment*, *14*, 169–194.

Harris, G. T., & Rice, M. E. (2006). Treatment of psychopathy: a review of empirical findings. In C. J. Patrick (ed), *Handbook of Psychopathy* (pp. 555–572). New York & London: Guilford Press.

Hatcher, R. M., Palmer, E. J., McGuire, J., Hounsome, J. C., Bilby, C. A. L., & Hollin, C. R. (2008). Aggression Replacement Training with adult male offenders within community settings: a reconviction analysis. *Journal of Forensic Psychiatry and Psychology*, in press.

Henning, K. R., & Frueh, B. C. (1996). Cognitive-behavioral treatment of incarcerated offenders: an evaluation of the Vermont Department of Corrections' Cognitive Self-Change Program. *Criminal Justice and Behavior, 23,* 523–542.

Herrenkohl, T. I., Maguin, E., Hill, K. G., Hawkins, J. D., Abbott, R. D., & Catalano, R. F. (2000). Developmental risk factors for youth violence. *Journal of Adolescent Health, 26,* 176–186.

Hodgins, S. (2007). Persistent violent offending: What do we know? *British Journal of Psychiatry, 190,* s12–s14.

Hollin, C. R. (2006). Offending behaviour programmes and contention: evidence-based practice, manuals, and programme evaluation. In C. R. Hollin, & E. J. Palmer (eds), *Offending Behaviour Programmes: Development, Application, and Controversies* (pp. 33–67). Chichester, UK: John Wiley & Sons.

Hollin, C. R. (2008). Evaluating offender programmes: does only randomization glister? *Criminology and Criminal Justice, 8,* 89–106.

Hollin, C. R., McGuire, J., Hatcher, R. M., Bilby, C. A. L., Hounsome, J., & Palmer, E. J. (2008) Cognitive skills offending behavior programs in the community: a reconviction analysis. *Criminal Justice and Behavior, 34,* 269–283.

Hollis, V. (2007). *Reconviction Analysis of Interim Accredited Programmes Software (IAPS) Data.* London: Research Development Statistics, National Offender Management Service.

Holloway, K. R., Bennett, T. H., & Farrington, D. P. (2006). The effectiveness of drug treatment programmes in reducing criminal behaviour: a meta-analysis. *Psichothema, 18,* 620–629.

Home Office (2007). *Crime in England and Wales 2006/2007: A Summary of the Main Figures.* London: Home Office Research, development and Statistics. [Online], Available at: http://www.homeoffice.gov.uk/rds/pdfs07/crime0607summ.pdf

Howells, K., & Day, A. (2003). Readiness for anger management. *Clinical Psychology Review, 23,* 319–337.

Howells, K., Day, A., Bubner, S., Jauncey, S., Parker, A., Williamson, P., *et al.* (2002). *Anger Management and Violence Prevention: Improving Effectiveness.* Trends and Issues in Crime and Criminal Justice, No. 227. Canberra: Australian Institute of Criminology. [Online], Available at: http://www.aic.gov.au/publications/tandi/tandi227.html

Huesmann, R. L., Moise-Titus, J., Podolski, C. L., & Eron, L. P. (2003). Longitudinal relations between children's exposure to TV violence and their aggressiveness and violent behaviour in young adulthood: 1977-1992. *Developmental Psychology, 39,* 201–221.

Huizinga, D., Weiher, A. W., Espitiru, R., & Esbensen, F. (2003). Delinquency and crime: some highlights from the Denver Youth Study. In T. P. Thornberry, & M. D. Krohn (eds), *Taking Stock of Delinquency: An Overview of Findings from Contemporary Longitudinal Studies* (pp. 47–91). New York: Kluwer Academic/Plenum Publishers.

Izzo, R. L., & Ross, R. R. (1990). Meta-analysis of rehabilitation programmes for juvenile delinquents. *Criminal Justice and Behavior, 17,* 134–142.

Jackson, S. L., Brownstein, H. H., & Zahn, M. A. (2004). The need for a theory of violence. In M. A. Zahn, H. H. Brownstein, & S. L. Jackson (eds), *Violence: From Theory to Research* (pp. 251–261). Cincinnati, OH: LexisNexis/Anderson Publishing Co.

Jansson, K., Povey, D., & Kaiza, P. (2007). Violent and sexual crime. In S. Nicholas, C. Kershaw, & A. Walker (eds), *Crime in England and Wales 2006/07* (pp. 49–72). London: Home Office Research, Development and Statistics Directorate. [Online], Available at: http://www.homeoffice.gov.uk/rds/pdfs07/hosb1107.pdf.

Kinderman, P. (2005). A psychological model of mental disorder. *Harvard Review of Psychiatry, 13,* 206–217.

Kirigin, K. A., Braukmann, C. J., Atwater, J. D., & Wolf, M. M. (1982). An evaluation of teaching-family (achievement place) group homes for juvenile offenders. *Journal of Applied Behavior Analysis, 15,* 1–16.

Klee, R. (1997). *Introduction to the Philosophy of Science: Cutting Nature at its Seams.* New York: Oxford University Press.

Klein, N. C., Alexander, J. F., & Parsons, B. V. (1977). Impact of family systems intervention on recidivism and sibling delinquency: a model of primary prevention and program evaluation. *Journal of Consulting and Clinical Psychology, 45,* 469–474.

Krug, E. G., Dahlberg, L. L., Mercy, J. A., Zwi, A. B., & Lozano, R. (eds) (2002). *World Report on Violence and Health*. Geneva: World Health Organization.

Lahey, B. B., & Waldman, I. D. (2003). A developmental propensity model of the origins of conduct problems during childhood and adolescence. In B. B. Lahey, T. E. Moffitt, & A. Caspi (eds), *Causes of Conduct Disorder and Juvenile Delinquency* (pp. 76–117). New York & London: Guilford Press.

Landenberger, N. A., & Lipsey, M. W. (2005). The positive effects of cognitive-behavioral programs for offenders: a meta-analysis of factors associated with effective treatment. *Journal of Experimental Criminology*, *1*, 451–476.

Latimer, J. (2001). A meta-analytic examination of youth delinquency, family treatment, and recidivism. *Canadian Journal of Criminology*, *43*, 237–253.

Latimer, J., Dowden, C., & Muise, D. (2005). The effectiveness of restorative justice practices: a meta-analysis. *The Prison Journal*, *85*, 127–144.

LeBlanc, M. (2006). Self-control and social control of deviant behaviour in context: development and interactions along the life course. In P-O. H. Wikström, & R. J. Sampson (eds), *The Explanation of Crime: Context, Mechanisms and Development* (pp. 195–242). Cambridge: Cambridge University Press.

Leitner M., Jones, S., Barr, W., Whittington, R., & McGuire, J. (2006). Systematic review of prevention and intervention strategies for populations at high risk of engaging in violent behaviour. Final project report to the NHS National Forensic Mental Health R&D Programme.

Lipsey, M. W. (1992). Juvenile delinquency treatment: a meta-analytic inquiry into the variability of effects. In T. Cook, D. Cooper, H. Corday, H. Hartman, L. Hedges, R. Light, *et al.* (eds), *Meta-analysis for Explanation: A Casebook* (pp. 83–127). New York: Russell Sage Foundation.

Lipsey, M. W. (1995). What do we learn from 400 studies on the effectiveness of treatment with juvenile delinquents? In J. McGuire (ed), *What Works: Reducing Re-offending: Guidelines from Research and Practice* (pp. 63–78). Chichester, UK: John Wiley & Sons.

Lipsey, M. W. (1999). Can rehabilitative programs reduce the recidivism of juvenile offenders? An inquiry into the effectiveness of practical programs. *Virginia Journal of Social Policy and the Law*, *6*, 611–641.

Lipsey, M. W., Chapman, G. L., & Landenberger, N. A. (2001). Cognitive-behavioral programs for offenders. *Annals of the American Academy of Political and Social Science*, *578*, 144–157.

Lipsey, M. W., & Wilson, D. B. (1998). Effective intervention for serious juvenile offenders: a synthesis of research. In R. Loeber, & D. P. Farrington (eds), *Serious and Violent Juvenile Offenders: Risk Factors and Successful Interventions* (pp. 313–345). Thousand Oaks, CA: Sage Publications.

Lipton, D. S., Pearson, F. S., Cleland, C. M., & Yee, D. (2002a). The effects of therapeutic communities and milieu therapy on recidivism: meta-analytic findings from the Correctional Drug Abuse Treatment Effectiveness (CDATE) study. In J. McGuire (ed), *Offender Rehabilitation and Treatment: Effective Programmes and Policies to Reduce Re-Offending* (pp. 39–77). Chichester, UK: John Wiley & Sons.

Lipton, D. S., Pearson, F. S., Cleland, C. M., & Yee, D. (2002b). The effectiveness of cognitive-behavioural treatment methods on offender recidivism: meta-analytic outcomes from the CDATE project. In J. McGuire (ed), *Offender Rehabilitation and Treatment: Effective Programmes and Policies to Reduce Re-Offending* (pp. 79–112). Chichester, UK: John Wiley & Sons.

Loeber, R., & Stouthamer-Loeber, M. (1987). Prediction. In H. C. Quay (ed), *Handbook of Juvenile Delinquency* (pp. 325–328). New York: John Wiley & Sons.

Lösel, F. (2001). Evaluating the effectiveness of correctional programs: bridging the gap between research and practice. In G. A. Bernfeld, D. P. Farrington, & A. W. Leschied (eds), *Offender Rehabilitation in Practice: Implementing and Evaluating Effective Programs* (pp. 67–92). Chichester, UK: John Wiley & Sons.

Lösel, F., & Beelman, A. (2003). Effects of child skills training in preventing antisocial behaviour: a systematic review of randomized evaluations. *Annals of the American Academy of Political and Social Science*, *587*, 84–109.

Lösel, F., & Koferl, P. (1989). Evaluation research on correctional treatment in West Germany: a meta-analysis. In H. Wegener, F. Lösel, & J. Haisch (eds), *Criminal Behavior and the Justice System: Psychological Perspectives* (pp. 334–355). New York: Springer-Verlag.

Lösel, F., & Schmucker, M. (2005). The effectiveness of treatment for sexual offenders: a comprehensive meta-analysis. *Journal of Experimental Criminology*, *1*, 117–146.

Lynam, D., Caspi, A., Moffitt, T. E., Loeber R., & Stouthamer-Loeber, M. (2007). Longitudinal evidence that psychopathy scores in early adolescence predict adult psychopathology. *Journal of Abnormal Psychology*, *116*, 155–165.

MacKenzie, D. L., Wilson, D. B., & Kider, S. B. (2001). Effects of correctional boot camps on offending. *Annals of the American Academy of Political and Social Science*, *578*, 126–143.

Mackie, J. L. (1980). *The Cement of the Universe*. Oxford: Clarendon Press.

Marsch, L. A. (1998). The efficacy of methadone maintenance interventions in reducing illicit opiate use, HIV risk behaviour and criminality: a meta-analysis. *Addiction*, *93*, 515–532.

Mayer, J. P., Gensheimer, L. K., Davidson, W. S., & Gottschalk, R. (1986). Social learning treatment within juvenile justice: a meta-analysis of impact in the natural environment. In S. A. Apter, & A. P. Goldstein (eds), *Youth Violence: Programs and Prospects* (pp. 24–38). Elmsford, NJ: Pergamon Press.

McCart, M. R., Priester, P. E., Davies, W. H., & Azen, R. (2006). Differential effectiveness of behavioural parent-training and cognitive-behavioral therapy for antisocial youth: a meta-analysis. *Journal of Abnormal Child Psychology*, *34*, 527–543.

McGuire, J. (2001). Defining correctional programs. In L. L. Motiuk, & R. C. Serin (eds), *Compendium 2000 on Effective Correctional Programming* (pp. 1–8). Ottawa: Correctional Service Canada.

McGuire, J. (2004). *Understanding Psychology and Crime: Perspectives on Theory and Action*. Maidenhead, UK: Open University Press/McGraw-Hill Education.

McGuire, J. (2005). Social problem solving: basic concepts, research and applications. In M. McMurran, & J. McGuire (eds), *Social Problem-solving and Offending: Evidence, evaluation and evolution* (pp. 3–29). Chichester, UK: John Wiley & Sons.

McGuire, J., Bilby, C. A. L., Hatcher, R. M., Hollin, C. R. Hounsome, J., & Palmer, E. J. (2008). Evaluation of structured cognitive-behavioural treatment programmes in reducing criminal recidivism. *Journal of Experimental Criminology*, *5*, 21–40.

McGuire, J., & Clark, D. (2004). A national dissemination program. In A. P. Goldstein, R. Nensén, B. Daleflod, & M. Kalt (eds), *New Perspectives on Aggression Replacement Training* (pp. 139–150). Chichester, UK: John Wiley & Sons.

Metcalfe, J., & Mischel, W. (1999). A hot/cool-system analysis of delay of gratification: dynamics of willpower. *Psychological Review*, *106*, 3–19.

Mitchell, O., Wilson, D. B., & MacKenzie, D. L. (2006). *The Effectiveness of Incarceration-based Drug Treatment on Criminal Behaviour*. Philadelphia, PA: Campbell Collaboration systematic review. [Online], Available at: http://www.campbellcollaboration.org/doc-pdf/Incarceration-Based Drug TxSept06final.pdf

Moffitt, T. E. (1993). Adolescence-limited and life-course-persistent antisocial behavior: a developmental taxonomy. *Psychological Review*, *100*, 674–701.

Moffitt, T. E. (2003). Life-course-persistent and adolescence-limited antisocial behaviour: a 10-year research review and a research agenda. In B. B. Lahey, T. E. Moffitt, & A. Caspi (eds), *Causes of Conduct Disorder and Juvenile Delinquency* (pp. 49–75). New York & London: Guilford Press.

Moffitt, T. E., & Caspi, A. (2006). Evidence from behavioural genetics for environmental contributions to antisocial conduct. In P-O. H. Wikström, & R. J. Sampson (eds), *The Explanation of Crime: Context, Mechanisms and Development* (pp. 108–152). Cambridge: Cambridge University Press.

Montgomery House (2007). Violence Prevention Programme. [Online], Available at: http://corrections. govt.nz/public/research/effectiveness-treatment/montgomery-house.html#

Naudé, C. M. B., Prinsloo, J. H., & Ladikos, A. (2006). *Experiences of Crime in Thirteen African Countries: Results from the International Crime Victim Survey*. Turin, Italy: United Nations Office on Drugs and Crime. [Online], Available at: www.unicri.it/wwd/analysis/icvs/pdf_files/ICVS%20 13%20African%20countries.pdf

Nisbett, R. E., & Cohen, D. (1996). *Culture of Honor: The Psychology of Violence in the South*. Oxford: Westview Press.

Novaco, R. W. (1975). *Anger Control: Development and Evaluation of an Experimental Treatment*. Lexington, KT: D. C. Heath.

Novaco, R. W. (1997). Remediating anger and aggression with violent offenders. *Legal and Criminological Psychology*, *2*, 77–88.

Novaco, R. W. (2007). Anger dysregulation. In T. A. Cavell, & K. T. Malcolm (eds), *Anger, Aggression and Interventions for Interpersonal Violence* (pp. 3–54). Mahwah, NJ: Lawrence Erlbaum Associates.

Nugent, W. R., Williams, M., & Umbreit, M. S. (2004). Participation in victim-offender mediation and the prevalence of subsequent delinquent behaviour: a meta-analysis. *Research on Social Work Practice*, *14*, 408–416.

Olweus, D. (1979). Stability of aggressive reaction patterns in males: a review. *Psychological Bulletin*, *86*, 852–875.

Olweus, D. (1988). Environmental and biological factors in the development of aggressive behaviour. In W. Buikhuisen, & S. A. Mednick (eds), *Explaining Criminal Behaviour* (pp. 90–120). Leiden, the Netherlands: E. J. Brill.

Palmer, E. J., McGuire, J., Hounsome, J., Hatcher, R. M., Bilby, C. A. L., & Hollin, C. R. (2007). Offending behaviour programmes in the community: the effects on reconviction of three programmes with adult male offenders. *Legal and Criminological Psychology*, *12*, 251–264.

Pearson, F., S. & Lipton, D. S. (1999). A meta-analytic review of the effectiveness of corrections-based treatments for drug abuse. *The Prison Journal*, *79*, 384–410.

Pearson, F. S., Lipton, D. S., & Cleland, C. M. (1997). Rehabilitative programs in adult corrections: CDATE meta-analyses. Paper presented at the Annual Meeting of the American Society of Criminology, San Diego, California, November.

Petrosino, A., J., Turpin-Petrosino, C., & Finckenauer, J. O. (2000). Well-meaning programs can have harmful effects! Lessons from experiments of programs such as Scared Straight. *Crime and Delinquency*, *46*, 354–379.

Platt, J. J., Perry, G., & Metzger, D. (1980). The evaluation of a heroin addiction treatment program within a correctional environment. In R. R. Ross, & P. Gendreau (eds), *Effective Correctional Treatment* (pp. 419–437). Toronto, Canada: Butterworths.

Polaschek, D. (2006). Programmes for violent offenders. In C. R. Hollin, & E. J. Palmer (eds), *Offending Behaviour Programmes: Development, Application, and Controversies* (pp. 131–147). Chichester, UK: John Wiley & Sons.

Polaschek, D., & Reynolds, N. (2004). Assessment and treatment: violent offenders. In C. R. Hollin (ed), *The Essential Handbook of Offender Assessment and Treatment* (pp. 201–218). Chichester, UK: John Wiley & Sons.

Polaschek, D. L. L., Wilson, N. J., Townsend, M. R., & Daly, L. R. (2005). Cognitive-behavioural rehabilitation for violent offenders: an outcome evaluation of the Violence Prevention Unit. *Journal of Interpersonal Violence*, *20*, 1611–1627.

Polizzi, D. M., MacKenzie, D. L., & Hickman, L. J. (1999). What works in adult sex offender treatment? A review of prison- and non-prison-based treatment programs. *International Journal of Offender Therapy and Comparative Criminology*, *43*, 357–374.

Power, S. (2003). *'A Problem from Hell': America and the Age of Genocide*. London: Flamingo/HarperCollins.

Prendergast, M. L., Podus, D., & Chang, E. (2000). Program factors and treatment outcomes in drug dependence treatment: an examination using meta-analysis. *Substance Use and Misuse*, *35*, 1931–1965.

Prendergast, M. L., Podus, D., Chang, E., & Urada, D. (2002). The effectiveness of drug abuse treatment: a meta-analysis of comparison group studies. *Drug and Alcohol Dependence*, *67*, 53–72.

Raynor, P. (2004). Seven ways to misunderstand evidence-based probation. In D. Smith (ed), *Social Work and Evidence-Based Practice* (pp. 161–178). London & Philadelphia: Jessica Kingsley Publishers.

Redondo, S., Garrido, V., & Sánchez-Meca, J. (1997). What works in correctional rehabilitation in Europe: a meta-analytical review. In S. Redondo, V. Garrido, J. Pérez, & R. Barberet (eds), *Advances in Psychology and Law: International Contributions* (pp. 499–523). Berlin: Walter de Gruyter.

Redondo, S., Sánchez-Meca, J., & Garrido, V. (1999). The influence of treatment programmes on the recidivism of juvenile and adult offenders: an European meta-analytic review. *Psychology, Crime and Law*, *5*, 251–278.

Redondo, S., Sánchez-Meca, J., & Garrido, V. (2002). Crime treatment in Europe: a review of outcome studies. In J. McGuire (ed), *Offender Rehabilitation and Treatment: Effective Programmes and Policies to Reduce Re-Offending* (pp. 113–141). Chichester, UK: John Wiley & Sons.

Rice, M. E., Harris, G. T., & Cormier, C. A. (1992). An evaluation of a maximum security therapeutic community for psychopaths and other mentally disordered offenders. *Law and Human Behaviour*, *16*, 399–412.

Richell, R. A., Mitchell, D. G. V., & Newman, C. (2003). Theory of mind and psychopathy: Can psychopathic individuals read the 'language of the eyes'? *Neuropsychologia*, *41*, 523–526.

Roberts, A. R., & Camasso, M. J. (1991). The effect of juvenile offender treatment programs on recidivism: a meta-analysis of 46 studies. *Notre Dame Journal of Law, Ethics and Public Policy*, *5*, 421–441.

Robinson, D. (1995). *The Impact of Cognitive Skills Training on Post-release Recidivism Among Canadian Federal Offenders*. Research Report R-41. Ottawa: Correctional Service Canada.

Robinson, D., & Porporino, F. J. (2001). Programming in cognitive skills: the reasoning and rehabilitation programme. In C. R. Hollin (ed), *Handbook of Offender Assessment and Treatment* (pp. 179–193). Chichester, UK: John Wiley & Sons.

Rosenthal, R., & Rubin, D. B. (1982). A simple, general purpose display of magnitude of experimental effect. *Journal of Educational Psychology*, *74*, 166–169.

Ross, R. R., & Fabiano, E. A. (1985). *Time to Think: A Cognitive Model of Delinquency Treatment and Offender Rehabilitation*. Ottawa: Institute of Social Sciences and Arts

Rothbart, M. K., Derryberry, D., & Posner, M. I. (1994). A psychobiological approach to the development of temperament. In J. E. Bates, & T. D. Wachs (eds), *Temperament: Individual Differences at the Interface of Biology and Behavior* (pp. 83–116). Washington, DC: American Psychological Association.

Rutter, M. (2003). Crucial paths from risk indicator to causal mechanism. In B. B. Lahey, T. E. Moffitt, & A. Caspi (eds), *Causes of Conduct Disorder and Juvenile Delinquency* (pp. 3–24). New York & London: Guilford Press.

Rutter, M., Giller, H., & Hagell, A. (1998). *Antisocial Behavior by Young People*. Cambridge: Cambridge University Press.

Salekin, R. T. (2002). Psychopathy and therapeutic pessimism: Clinical lore or clinical reality? *Clinical Psychology Review*, *22*, 79–112.

Sanday, P. R. (2003). Rape-free versus rape-prone: how culture makes a difference. In C. B. Travis (ed), *Evolution, Gender, and Rape* (pp. 337–362). Cambridge, MA: MIT Press.

Sanislow, C. A., & McGlashan, T. H. (1998). Treatment outcomes of personality disorders. *Canadian Journal of Psychiatry*, *43*, 237–250.

Searle, J. R. (1995). *The Construction of Social Reality*. London: Penguin Books.

Serin, R. C. (1995). Treatment responsivity in criminal psychopaths. *Forum on Corrections Research*, *7*, 23–26.

Serin, R. C., & Preston, D. L. (2001). Violent offender programming. In L. L. Motiuk, & R. C. Serin (eds), *Compendium 2000 on Effective Correctional Programming* (pp. 146–157). Ottawa: Correctional Service Canada.

Simon, L. M. J. (1998). Does criminal offender treatment work? *Applied and Preventive Psychology*, *7*, 137–159.

Skeem, J. L., Monahan, J., & Mulvey, E. P. (2002). Psychopathy, treatment involvement, and subsequent violence among civil psychiatric patients. *Law and Human Behavior*, *26*, 577–603.

Snyder, J., Reid, J., & Patterson, G. (2003). A social learning model of child and adolescent antisocial behaviour. In B. B. Lahey, T. E. Moffitt, & A. Caspi (eds), *Causes of Conduct Disorder and Juvenile Delinquency* (pp. 27–48). New York & London: Guilford Press.

Spivack, G., & Cianci, N. (1987). High risk early behavior pattern and later delinquency. In J. D. Burchard, & S. N. Burchard (eds), *Prevention of Delinquent Behavior* (pp. 44–74). Newbury Park, CA: Sage Publications.

Staub, E. (1989). *The Roots of Evil: The Origins of Genocide and Other Group Violence*. New York: Plenum Press.

Sukhodolsky, D. G., Kassinove, H., & Gorman, B. S. (2004). Cognitive-behavioral therapy for anger in children and adolescents: a meta-analysis. *Aggression and Violent Behavior*, *9*, 247–269.

Surgeon General (2001). *Youth Violence: A Report of the Surgeon General*. Washington, DC: US Department of Health and Human Services. [Online], Available at: www.surgeongeneral.gov/library/youthviolence/youvioreport.htm.

Tanasichuk, C. L., & Wormith, J. S. (2007). Does treatment makes psychopaths worse? A meta-analytic review. Paper delivered at the North American Criminal Justice and Correctional Psychology Conference, The Westin, Ottawa, Canada.

Thornberry, T. P., Huizinga, D., & Loeber, R. (1995). The prevention of serious delinquency and violence: implications from the Program of Research on the Causes and Correlates of Delinquency. In J. C. Howell, B. Krisberg, J. D. Hawkins, & J. J. Wilson (eds), *Sourcebook on Serious, Violent and Chronic Juvenile Offenders* (pp. 213–237). Thousand Oaks, CA: Sage Publications.

Thornberry, T. P., Lizotte, A. J., Krohn, M. D., Smith, C. A., & Porter, P. K. (2003). Causes and consequences of delinquency: findings from the Rochester Youth Development Study. In T. P. Thornberry, & M. D. Krohn (eds), *Taking Stock of Delinquency: An Overview of Findings from Contemporary Longitudinal Studies* (pp. 11–46). New York: Kluwer Academic/Plenum Publishers.

Toch, H. (1969). *Violent Men: An Inquiry into the Psychology of Violence*. Harmondsworth, UK: Penguin Books.

Todorov, A. & Bargh, J. A. (2002). Automatic sources of aggression. *Aggression and Violent Behavior*, 7, 53–68.

Tong, L. S. J., & Farrington, D. P. (2006). How effective is the 'Reasoning and Rehabilitation' programme in reducing re-offending? A meta-analysis of evaluations in three countries. *Psychology, Crime and Law*, 12, 3–24.

Totten, S., & Parsons, W. (eds) (2008). *A Century of Genocide: Critical Essays and Eyewitness Accounts*, 2nd edn. London: Routledge.

Tremblay, R. E. (2000). The development of aggressive behaviour during childhood: What have we learned in the past century? *International Journal of Behavioral Development*, 24, 129–141.

Tremblay, R. E. (2003). Why socialisation fails: the case of chronic physical aggression. In B. B. Lahey, T. E. Moffitt, & A. Caspi (eds), *Causes of Conduct Disorder and Juvenile Delinquency* (pp. 182–224). New York & London: Guilford Press.

United Nations Office on Drugs and Crime (2008). *Eighth United Nations Survey of Crime Trends and Operations of Criminal Justice Systems*. Vienna: United Nations Office on Drugs and Crime. [Online], Available at: www.unodc.org/unodc/en/data-and-analysis/Eighth-United-Nations-Survey-on-Crime-Trends-and-the-Operations-of-Criminal-Justice-Systems.html

Van Kesteren, J. N., Mayhew, P., & Nieuwbeerta, P. (2000). *Criminal Victimisation in Seventeen Industrialised Countries: Key Findings from the 2000 International Crime Victims Survey*. The Hague: Ministry of Justice. [Online], Available at: www.unicri.it/wwd/analysis/icvs/pdf_files/key2000i/index.htm

Visher, C. A., Winterfield, L., & Coggeshall, M. B. (2005). Ex-offender employment programs and recidivism: a meta-analysis. *Journal of Experimental Criminology*, 1, 295–315.

Waller, J. (2007). *Becoming Evil: How Ordinary People Commit Genocide and Mass Killing*. 2nd edition. Oxford: Oxford University Press.

Wells-Parker, E., Bangert-Drowns, R., McMillen, R., & Williams, M. (1995). Final results from a meta-analysis of remedial interventions with drink/drive offenders. *Addiction*, 9, 907–926.

Whitehead, J. T., & Lab, S. P. (1989). A meta-analysis of juvenile correctional treatment. *Journal of Research in Crime and Delinquency*, 26, 276–295.

Whittington, R., Leitner, M., Barr, W., Jones, S., & McGuire, J. (in preparation). Psychosocial interventions and the reduction of violent behaviour: a meta-analysis.

Wilson, D. B. (2001). Meta-analytic methods for criminology. *Annals of the American Academy of Political and Social Science*, 578, 71–89.

Wilson, D. B., Bouffard, L. A., & Mackenzie, D. L. (2005). A quantitative review of structured, group-oriented, cognitive-behavioral programs for offenders. *Criminal Justice and Behavior*, 32, 172–204.

Wilson, D. B., Gallagher, C. A., & MacKenzie, D. L. (2000). A meta-analysis of corrections-based education, vocation and work programs for adult offenders. *Journal of Research in Crime and Delinquency*, 37, 568–581.

Wilson, D. B., Gottfredson, D. C., & Najaka, S. S. (2001). School-based prevention of problem behaviors: a meta-analysis. *Journal of Quantitative Criminology*, 17, 247–272.

Wilson, D. B., MacKenzie, D. L., & Mitchell, F. N. (2005). Effects of correctional boot camps on offending. Campbell Collaboration systematic review. Philadelphia, PA. Campbell Collaboration systematic review. [Online], Available at: www.campbellcollaboration.org/doc-pdf/Wilson_boot-camps_rev.pdf

Wilson, S. J., & Lipsey, M. W. (2000). Wilderness challenge programs for delinquent youth: a meta-analysis of outcome evaluations. *Evaluation and Program Planning, 23*, 1–12.

Wilson, S. J., Lipsey, M. W., & Derzon, J. H. (2003). The effects of school-based intervention programs on aggressive behaviour: a meta-analysis. *Journal of Consulting and Clinical Psychology, 71*, 136–149.

Wilson, S. J., Lipsey, M. W., & Soydan, H. (2003). Are mainstream programs for juvenile delinquency less effective with minority youth than majority youth? A meta-analysis of outcomes research. *Research on Social Work Practice, 13*, 3–26.

Wong, S. C. P., Witte, T. D., Gordon, A., Gu, D., & Lewis, K. (2006). Can a treatment program designed primarily for violent risk reduction reduce recidivism in psychopaths? Poster Presentation at the Annual Convention of the Canadian Psychological Association, Calgary, Alberta.

Woolfenden, S. R., Williams, K., & Peat J. K. (2002). Family and parenting interventions for conduct disorder and delinquency: a meta-analysis of randomised controlled trials. *Archives of Disease in Childhood, 86*, 251–256.

Zamble, E., & Quinsey, V. L. (1997). *The Criminal Recidivism Process.* Cambridge: Cambridge University Press.

Zumkley, H. (1994). The stability of aggressive behavior: a meta-analysis. *German Journal of Psychology, 18*, 273–281.

16

Effective psychological interventions for child conduct problems: Current evidence and new directions

Eamon McCrory and Elly Farmer

Introduction

Conduct Disorder (CD) is a diagnostic category defined by a persistent pattern of antiso-cial and aggressive externalizing behaviours, including fighting, lying, stealing, cruelty, and a variety of violations of other people's rights. Often, the disorder is preceded by the Oppositional Defiant Disorder (ODD). This chapter uses the term conduct problems to span the array of child behaviour problems that might be regarded as 'undercontrolled' (Achenbach, 1985). The societal impact of CD is enormous. Children presenting with CD are often impaired across multiple domains, showing poor social skills, educational underachievement, and psychopathology (Frick, 1998). These personal costs occur along-side the significant economic costs to society in relation to residential care, policing, pros-ecution, and poor social, educational, and health outcomes (Scott *et al.*, 2001). These factors do not take into account either lost productivity nor the emotional and psychologi-cal impact of antisocial behaviour on victims.

In this chapter, we review evidence-based psychological interventions for conduct prob-lems and then consider several ways in which such interventions may be developed. In the first section, we present the evidence in relation to parent management training (PMT), systemic interventions, and cognitive-behavioural therapy (CBT). The review is necessarily selective, focusing on those treatments that have received adequate research evaluation. Other forms of evidence, such as that from non-randomized trials and cohort studies, are discussed when more reliable sources are unavailable. Preventative interventions are beyond this chapter's remit (see Tremblay, Chapter 18), although a firm distinction between preven-tion and treatment is at times difficult to draw, given that all interventions are aimed at the prevention of future, often more serious, conduct problems. In the second section, we con-sider three key areas that are likely to significantly inform and advance approaches to psy-chological intervention. Firstly, we briefly review the evidence for the mechanisms of treatment; this incorporates a consideration of those factors believed to mediate treatment effectiveness as well as potential moderating factors that can augment or attenuate out-comes. Secondly, we present the case for future psychological intervention approaches to explicitly consider outcome data in relation to subgroups of children with CD. Developmental theories have distinguished between early and late onset types, and a subgroup of children with callous-unemotional (CU) traits, each of whom may show differential treatment responses to traditional intervention approaches. Finally, we touch on the potential contri-bution of neuroscience and genetics to inform and improve intervention for conduct prob-lems. We propose that multilevel perspectives provide the potential for an integrated and developmentally informed understanding that is of increasing relevance to clinical practice.

Review of psychological interventions

Parent management training

Overview
Historically, parent management training (PMT) began as an approach founded on behavioural theory. The key tenet of the theory posits that antisocial behaviour is initiated and maintained by contingencies in the child's social environment. Since the 1960's, the work of Patterson and colleagues at the Oregon Social Learning Centre has played a central role in establishing the principles of PMT. It was observed that parents of conduct-disordered children often unwittingly reinforced child aversive behaviour, firstly by giving in to child protest—the 'reinforcement trap' (Patterson, 1982)—and secondly by being inconsistent and unresponsive to both positive and negative behaviours (Patterson, 1976). PMT aims to teach parenting styles that shift social contingencies so that only children's prosocial behaviours are positively reinforced; later stages of PMT may also involve negative reinforcement for aversive behaviours.

Typically, treatment involves direct weekly work with parents for anything between 6 and 25 weeks. Programmes also vary along a number of other dimensions, such as their method of teaching (e.g., video instruction, discussion, role-play, guided interactions); their inclusion of other treatment objectives (e.g., modifying parental attributions of their child's behaviour); the age range for the identified child (although usually between 2 and 12 years); and their format (group, individual, or self-directed). Central to all PMT approaches, however, is the principle that a systematic shift is required in how parents respond to positive and aversive behaviours in their child. In this way, they contrast with parenting programmes that have a more generic focus on promoting positive relationship factors (such as problem solving and empathy) without specific attention being directed to environmental contingencies. These treatments are promising, but their effectiveness has not yet been adequately explored (Lundahl *et al.*, 2006) and so they are not considered here.

PMT effectiveness
Three main meta-analytic studies have evaluated the overall effectiveness of PMT. Serketich and Dumas (1996) meta-analysed the results from 26 controlled studies examining child behavioural outcomes for PMT provided to parents of preschool and elementary school-aged children. They found post-treatment effect sizes (ES)[1] of 0.86 in relation to overall child outcome, with comparable figures for parent report and observer ratings. They also found a more modest ES of 0.44 for the impact of these programmes on parental adjustment (in relation, for example, to marital satisfaction, depression, stress, etc.) These results suggest that PMT has a large impact on children's conduct problems. McCart *et al.* (2006) addressed a number of methodological limitations in this study and benefited from the inclusion of more recent studies in their comparative meta-analysis of controlled evaluations of PMT and cognitive-behavioural therapy (CBT) for children up to the age of 18 years. They reported a PMT post-treatment weighted ES of 0.47 overall, again with similar estimates according to parent report (0.38), observer rating (0.45), and teacher report (0.38). Their reported ES of 0.33 for parental adjustment is, however, comparable.

---

[1] The most common effect size used to estimate treatment outcome is Cohen's d. Effect sizes close to 0.2 indicate a small effect, those close to 0.5 a medium effect, and those close to 0.8 a large effect (Cohen, 1992).

McCart and colleagues (2006) adopted two inclusion criteria (use of a no-treatment/placebo control condition and the inclusion of studies with only significant findings) not used in another recent meta-analysis by Lundahl *et al.* (2006). Nevertheless, the latter study reported similar effect sizes; collapsing across forms of measurement, they reported a post-treatment ES of 0.42 for child behaviour and 0.45 for parental behaviour. These two most recent meta-analyses converge to suggest that PMT has a medium post-treatment effect, with limited evidence of maintenance of gains at one-year follow-up (Lundahl *et al.*, 2006). There are a range of established PMT programmes, which vary significantly in their content and evidence-base; we consider three main approaches here in more detail.

The incredible years programme

The Incredible Years Programme (IYP; Webster-Stratton & Reid, 2003) is a parent training programme based on video-based instruction, modelling, and group discussion, which primarily aims to reduce conduct problems and enhance social competence in young children typically aged between 2 and 7 years. The programme is planned around two-hour weekly sessions held with the parents, with structured homework between sessions. The 'BASIC' programme lasts for 12–14 weeks and has three phases: an initial stage facilitating positive parent-child relationships through child-directed play, praise, and incentive programmes; a second stage focusing on non-violent discipline strategies, such as the consistent use of monitoring, ignoring, and commanding; and a final phase in which the parent is taught how to teach their child problem-solving skills. An additional 'ADVANCE' programme focuses on adult relationships and problem-solving skills.

A large number of well-controlled randomized controlled trials (RCTs) have demonstrated the effectiveness of the IYP in reducing conduct problems (e.g., Webster-Stratton & Hammond, 1997; see Webster-Stratton *et al.*, 2004 for a review). These studies have largely found effect sizes in the medium range. Although follow-up studies have shown some lasting improvements (up to 3 years post-treatment), as yet there have been no control group follow-up comparisons. Recent research has demonstrated positive effects with socially disadvantaged families, in community settings, and in several countries. For example, a recent RCT of a community-based IYP in the United Kingdom (Gardner *et al.*, 2006) with low-income families reported post-treatment ESs of 0.48 for parent-reported behaviour and 0.78 for observed behaviour, alongside increases in positive parenting and parental self-efficacy. Gains were still evident at 18-month follow-up. Similarly, moderate to large ESs were reported at one-year follow-up in a UK-based RCT of IYP conducted with a large community sample (Scott *et al.*, 2001).

Triple P: the positive parenting programme

Triple P is a multitiered intervention designed in Australia by Sanders and colleagues (Sanders, 1999) that aims to increase parenting skills and knowledge, and promote positive family relationships as well as child competencies. Levels of intervention range from a media-based, population-focused campaign (Level One) to an intensive, individually tailored programme for families where both the child and parents present with difficulties (Level Five). Level Four, which has received the most research evaluation, is typically for children showing severe behaviour problems. Treatment in the form of didactic teaching, discussion, and homework practice is provided over 10 weekly sessions in the form of individual, group, or self-directed therapy. Differential reinforcement, communication skills, and consistent non-violent discipline strategies are emphasized with a key goal being to promote self-efficacy.

In a meta-analysis of eight controlled trials of Triple P, Thomas and Zimmer-Gembeck (2007) found generally medium parent-report ESs for the individual and group forms on child behaviour, and medium to large parent-report ESs for the self-directed and enhanced versions. However, on observational measures only the enhanced form yielded a medium ES. The impact of Triple P has been supported by more recent studies (Markie-Dadds & Sanders, 2006), and has been shown to extend to Australian indigenous communities with high rates of unemployment and low education (Turner *et al.*, 2007). However, independent RCTs to assess the applicability of Triple P cross-culturally remain outstanding.

Parent-child interaction therapy

Although Parent-Child Interaction Therapy (PCIT; Eyberg *et al.*, 1995) shares its broad theoretical basis with other programmes, it has a unique approach in that the majority of sessions consist of direct interactive guidance: parents play with their children while taking advice from a therapist sitting behind a one-way mirror with a 'bug-in-the-ear' device. As well as the 12-session standard programme, abbreviated and enhanced versions have been developed with the latter incorporating an additional motivational module. A meta-analysis of 11 PCIT outcome studies has found medium to large parent-report ESs for child behaviour compared with waiting list, non-clinical, or matched control groups (Thomas & Zimmer-Gembeck, 2007). Effects based on observational measures were large in studies using non-clinical controls, but negligible in those making waiting list comparisons. Both the abbreviated and enhanced forms appear to be effective (e.g., Nixon *et al.*, 2004), although positive results have not yet been obtained in controlled comparisons using appropriately large samples. Nevertheless, the robust quality of the PCIT outcome studies means that we can be relatively confident that the reported effects are reliable estimates of change.

Other approaches

A number of other well-developed PMT approaches exist. These include those of Kazdin (2003), McMahon and Forehand (2003), Patterson (1976), and Forgatch (1994). They have some unique features: for example, those of Kazdin and Patterson include the individualized implementation of a token reward programme. Although some RCTs have provided initial positive support for these approaches, larger studies with additional follow-up measures are required.

Summary

A substantial body of research now provides compelling evidence that PMT, in a variety of forms, is an effective approach in reducing conduct problems in preschool and elementary-aged children. Techniques and protocols vary across programmes although all share a common focus on modifying patterns of child-parent interactions by enhancing parents' responsiveness and skills with the aim of increasing positive and reducing negative child behaviours. PMT has shown to be successful, at least in the short term, in clinical and non-clinical settings with families from a variety of backgrounds, and is particularly cost-effective (Edwards *et al.*, 2007).

Systemic Interventions

Overview

Several treatment programmes have been developed that focus on modifying the interconnected family, peer, school, and community systems thought to play a role in influencing
adolescent conduct problems. These interventions assume that such behaviours serve a function within these proximal and distal systems. Acknowledging that each young person's
behaviour might be shaped by unique factors, these programmes take an individualized
approach informed by an assessment of putative systemic influences. As a result, the precise
content of treatment is less easy to quantify than with other approaches—rather than specifying the components of the intervention, the adherence to key principles is at the heart of
maintaining treatment integrity. The three programmes reviewed here have received substantial research attention; their main differences lie in their emphasis on different systems
and the age range they target.

Multi-systemic therapy

Multi-Systemic Therapy (MST; Henggeler *et al.*, 1998) is an intensive intervention involving
approximately 60 hours of therapeutic support spread across 3–5 months. A trained therapist works closely with the family, initially building up a systemic formulation, which then
forms the basis for collaborative decisions to be made with the adolescent and their family
regarding priorities for change. Cognitive-behavioural, behavioural, and strategic and structural family therapy techniques are used flexibly accommodating the family's needs and
include an 'on call' facility. MST is rarely prescriptive in its interventions; rather therapists
attempt to adhere to nine principles including keeping a positive focus, increasing responsibility, clearly defining the problem and solutions within a developmentally appropriate
framework, and continuous evaluation. Improving communication and collaborative work
with the young person's school are also central elements.

Nine RCTs and one quasi-experimental trial for serious juvenile offenders have explored
the impact of MST, often using individual therapy matched for hours as a comparison.
These report medium to large ESs for the three efficacy trials, small to medium ESs for the
three effectiveness trials, and on average, small ESs for transportability trials. As well as
reductions in recidivism (which range from 25% to 70%), behaviour problems and self-
reported criminal offending, MST has been shown to decrease out-of-home placement days,
relationship problems, and school non-attendance. Schaeffer and Borduin (2005) provide
evidence for long-term effectiveness into adulthood in terms of reduced recidivism and days
incarcerated. An additional strength of MST is its low dropout rate (Henggeler *et al.*,
1996).

A more equivocal picture of MST is presented by a recent independent systematic review
(Littell *et al.*, 2005), which evaluated eight of the RCT studies. The authors note that, of
these, seven failed to provide outcome data for an intent-to-treat analysis with necessary
follow-up data. In addition, psychosocial outcome measures were typically obtained by self-
report or from staff not blind to group assignment. They report that the largest study conducted to date, which also meets intention-to-treat criteria (Leschied & Cunningham, 2002),
found no significant benefit of MST relative to usual juvenile services. The remaining studies
were viewed as being of various methodological quality. Littell and colleagues (2005) therefore concluded that the evidence for MST effectiveness remains inconclusive. Findings from
government-funded studies currently underway in the United Kingdom and elsewhere will
provide a broader evidence base to inform future evaluation.

Multidimensional treatment foster care

Multidimensional Treatment Foster Care (MTFC) stems from the behavioural and social learning principles established at the Oregon Social Learning Centre and aims to reduce problem behaviour and promote prosocial behaviours (Chamberlain, 1998). Children and young people are placed for between six and nine months in the care of trained foster carers who apply behavioural management techniques (such as close monitoring, setting boundaries, providing predictable consequences, and supportive mentoring) in the context of an individualized programme that is responsive to the young person's changing needs. Simultaneously, therapists work with the young person in individual weekly therapy sessions and provide family therapy to the natural family, addressing potential barriers to reintegration and teaching structured parenting skills. A case manager acts as coordinator and 'on-call' consultant.

In an initial RCT, Chamberlain and Moore (1998) supported and extended the promising findings of earlier MTFC outcome studies. They found that in a sample of 79 adolescents, those receiving MTFC, compared to those receiving residential care, were more likely to have completed the programme, run away less often, and spent less time in prison (53 versus 129 days) at one-year follow-up. At two-year follow-up, only 5% of the MTFC group had received a criminal referral for a violent offence, compared to 24% of the control group (Eddy et al., 2004). More recent studies report positive results of MTFC in female populations (Chamberlain et al., 2007) and high levels of social acceptability (Westermark et al., 2007).

Functional family therapy

Functional Family Therapy (FFT; Alexander & Parsons, 1973) derives from family systems theory wherein the young person's conduct problems are understood as performing a function in the family (such as obtaining support or increasing interpersonal contact). It aims to increase the level of supportive interactions, promote monitoring and effective discipline, and reduce maladaptive communication patterns. FFT comprises three phases of intervention: the first stage focuses on modifying the understanding of the problem (using positive reframing), the second concentrates on effecting behavioural change, and the third on generalizing these strategies to other settings (Sexton & Alexander, 1999). As with MTFC and MST, FFT focuses on working with families in the community rather than the clinic.

In one RCT, court-referred adolescents were assigned to FFT, no treatment, individual psychotherapy, or client-centred family therapy (Alexander & Parsons, 1973). Recidivism in the FFT group at 6–18-month follow-up was 26% compared with 47–73% in the other groups. This trial also found positive effects of FFT on sibling conduct problems. More recent investigations of matched but not randomly assigned comparison groups have provided further support for the efficacy of the approach (Barton et al., 1985; Gordon et al., 1988). The evidence base suggests that FFT is an effective intervention although a number of limitations (typically small sample sizes, non-randomized comparisons, and a focus on recidivism as the outcome measure) mean that further methodologically robust investigations are warranted.

Summary

Systemic interventions as a whole have an impressive body of evidence supporting their effectiveness. They have relatively low dropout rates (possibly linked to their non-stigmatizing framework), demonstrated cost-effectiveness, and applicability to a wide variety of children and families. These interventions are typically packaged as distinct 'approaches', which can often belie their similarities and common principles, most notably their individualized and collaborative approach in tackling individual, family, and environmental factors linked to the presenting conduct problems. Future independently conducted intervention trials with more methodologically robust protocols and longer-term follow-up periods are required.

Cognitive-behavioural therapy

Overview

Cognitive-behavioural therapy (CBT) is founded on the central tenet that thoughts, beliefs, and established cognitive strategies alongside environmental contingencies shape how we behave. Dodge and colleagues (1990) have cogently argued that cognitive maladaptations in four stages of social information processing (SIP) play a key role in initiating and maintaining children's aggressive behaviour: encoding (selective attention to and recall of hostile cues), interpretation (an increased attribution of hostile intent), response search (limited generation of solutions to social problems), and response decision (positively biased valuation of aggression outcomes). Aggressive problems have been shown to be correlated (and to a degree causally related) to these maladaptations (Dodge *et al.*, 1990; see Dodge, 2003 for a review). CBT for child conduct problems typically aims to address these social cognitive deficits in an attempt to reduce antisocial behaviour. More broadly, CBT has included techniques to improve emotional and behavioural regulation. Treatments include social skills training, enhancing problem-solving abilities, anger management strategies, and cognitive restructuring. They tend to use a group format and an active therapist to build skills through psychoeducation, role-playing, group discussion, reinforcement of appropriate skills, and modelling.

CBT effectiveness

Four recent meta-analyses have addressed the effectiveness of CBT for reducing conduct problems in young people (Bennett & Gibbons, 2000; Sukhodolsky *et al.*, 2004; McCart *et al.*, 2006; Armelius & Andreassen, 2007). Bennett and Gibbons (2000) identified 30 controlled CBT outcome studies that targeted antisocial behaviour in school-aged children and adolescents. They reported a small to moderate post-treatment ES of 0.23, and a larger follow-up ES of 0.51. Arguably, these significant but modest effects may partly reflect the rather conservative criteria adopted by the authors when computing the overall ES. McCart and colleagues (2006) found broadly consistent findings in their meta-analysis of the results of 41 studies of CBT despite using somewhat different methods and inclusion criteria. CBT was defined as any treatment containing cognitive restructuring, social skills training, conflict resolution, or anger management. They reported a weighted post-treatment ES of 0.35 for CBT. Although the ESs were broadly similar across forms of measurement, it is perhaps pertinent to note that the observational post-treatment ES of 0.51 was larger than those computed from reported measures. Adolescents appeared to respond better than pre-adolescents. However, McCart and colleagues (2006) note that these adolescents likely represent a heterogeneous group comprising childhood- and adolescent-onset types. It is suggested that these groups may be responding differentially to CBT such that combining them potentially waters down the aggregated results.

In their meta-analytic review, Sukhodolsky and colleagues (2004) specifically considered CBT interventions for anger-related problems in young people. They categorized treatments as one of four types and reported a wide range of ESs for physical aggression post-treatment: skills training (ES: 0.67), problem solving (ES: 0.57), affective education (ES: 0.36), and multimodal approaches (ES: 0.75). Armelius and Andreassen (2007) also conducted a focused meta-analysis in relation to CBT for adolescents placed in secure or non-secure residential settings. For these young people, family and systemic approaches are often simply not an option. The authors reported that CBT was significantly better than control conditions at 12-month follow-up (odds ratio = 0.69) and recidivism was reduced by about 10% on average.

As a general principle, multimodal interventions appear to be more beneficial. One RCT has reported that systematically addressing each of the four stages of Dodge's SIP model is more effective than social skills training alone (van Manen *et al.*, 2004). This finding is consistent with previous studies demonstrating the impact of CBT at each cognitive stage (e.g., Lochman, 1992); by contrast, CBT programmes that address a more limited range of skills often do not appear to significantly reduce conduct problems (e.g., Lipman *et al.*, 2006). It might be argued, however, that even multimodal CBT programmes have a limited efficacy if concurrent changes are not made to the child's social and environmental context and if the latent internalized meanings the child holds about the world are not addressed. We now examine in turn the significance of these two factors for treatment.

Combined treatments

Guerra *et al.* (2005) state that: 'Ecologies must change *in tandem with individual skills* to support the emergence and crystallization of new cognitions' (p. 283, italics in original). Indeed a number of contextual factors, such as peer rejection, coercive parenting, and maltreatment, appear to have a direct influence independent of cognitive factors (Dodge, 2003). With this in mind, a number of interventions have combined CBT with parent training interventions to good effect. In an initial study, Kazdin and colleagues (1992) compared the effects of PMT, problem-solving skills training, and a combination of the two on levels of antisocial behaviour. On parental rating measures, 64% of those who received the combined treatments moved into the normal range of functioning, compared with approximately a third of those in either of the other two groups. Other CBT programmes have also been shown in controlled studies to benefit from the addition of PMT (Webster-Stratton & Hammond, 1997), and the two combined appear to have a powerful impact on later delinquency when offered before adolescence (Vitaro *et al.*, 2001). Evidence is also emerging for the added value of other systemic interventions, such as teacher training programmes (Webster-Stratton *et al.*, 2004).

Scripts, schemas, internal working models

In a revision to the original SIP theory, Crick and Dodge (1994) outlined the role of latent mental structures, containing meanings about the self and others, which organize and guide SIP via feedback loops at each stage of processing. These are similar in concept to the schemas, core beliefs, internal working models, and scripts described in other models of psychopathology. In essence, therefore, cognitive theory identifies the reciprocal interaction between maladaptive cognitive processes and maladaptive cognitive meanings. Children with aggressive behaviour appear to hold more negative and aggressive understandings of themselves and others. Although challenging core beliefs and cognitive restructuring are routine CBT approaches for other psychological difficulties, they have not played a prominent role in the treatment of CD. At the very least, the two appear to converge at the interpretation stage of the SIP model, such that methods that address a child's hostile attributional bias may result in shifts in his or her core beliefs regarding the self and their relation to the world. However, CBT strategies that target latent meaning structures, such as continuum work, Socratic questioning, and narrative techniques are rarely used explicitly. We currently know little regarding the potential for meaning-focused CBT techniques to reduce conduct problems (e.g., by modifying maladaptive core beliefs or by constructing a more adaptive self-narrative) nor how they might be adapted to work with young people with CD.

Summary

CBT approaches to child conduct problems are empirically supported and theoretically motivated. Group or individual CBT draws on a wide variety of techniques typically focused on modifying cognitive biases, developing problem-solving skills, and cultivating new cognitive-behavioural strategies. Relatively little explicit emphasis has been placed to date on cognitive restructuring in relation to the assumptions and core beliefs that may characterize a child's internal working model. An emphasis on developing a positive self-schema may represent a powerful complement to current CBT approaches. ESs have been variable, although the potential of combining CBT with PMT is particularly promising.

Advancing clinical practice

Mechanisms of intervention

The extant evidence base in relation to the efficacy of interventions for conduct problems in children is impressive. However, relatively little attention has been paid to the specific therapeutic factors that drive change and to the mechanisms through which change actually occurs. Nock (2003) has argued convincingly that an increased understanding of how and for whom treatments work will allow researchers, clinicians, and services to adapt interventions to best therapeutic effect. The identification of 'active ingredients' of given interventions is an important endeavour if we are to understand which components contribute to therapeutic change. Here, we focus on the evidence pointing to possible mediators of change (factors that are changed by the treatment that cause change in conduct problems) as well as moderators of change (characteristics of the child and their system that influence the success of therapy).

Mediators

Although PMT has been shown to reduce negative and increase positive parenting behaviours (Dishion *et al.*, 1992; Thomas & Zimmer-Gembeck, 2007), the question arises whether these changes actually mediate change in conduct problem behaviour. Two recent studies have addressed this question. Beauchaine *et al.* (2005) used latent growth-curve analysis to examine mediators and moderators of treatments for conduct problems. After controlling for baseline levels, a reduction in negative parenting (critical, harsh, and/or ineffective parenting) but not an increase in positive parenting mediated the effect of treatment on conduct problems. However, Gardner *et al.* (2006) reported that observed positive parenting in the IYP statistically mediated treatment effects.

Similarly, a small number of studies have identified likely mediators of change in relation to systemic intervention. In a study of MST, Huey *et al.* (2000) reported convincing evidence to support the core therapeutic assumption that improvement in family functioning contributes to reductions in problem behaviour. The authors also report that reduced deviant peer association and therapist adherence to MST were important mediators of change. Similar findings have been reported in relation to MTFC (Eddy & Chamberlain, 2000). These two studies taken together suggest that reduced deviant peer affiliation and enhanced parent-child interaction are key factors in the change process.

CBT theory posits that it is primarily changes in cognitive processing patterns (e.g., in hostile attributions or problem-solving ability) that account for observed reductions in problematic behaviour. Although evidence now exists demonstrating that CBT leads to changes in such patterns (e.g., Guerra & Slaby, 1990), we do not yet know whether such changes *precede* reductions in antisocial behaviour, or account for the impact of the intervention on this behaviour. It is necessary to demonstrate such contingencies if the role of cognitive mechanisms is to be supported. It is perfectly plausible, for example, that CBT reduces antisocial behaviours by facilitating the child's experience of new social contingencies.

Moderators

Client, family, and environmental moderators of treatment efficacy have been studied as well as moderators that pertain to therapist characteristics and how the intervention is delivered. Low socio-economic status has been reported to be associated with poorer PMT outcome, as has family dysfunction and complexity, as measured by factors such as single-parent structure, low social support, substance misuse, and marital discord (e.g., Lundahl *et al.*, 2006). However, a large prospective study examining the impact of complexity failed to find an effect of socio-economic disadvantage on treatment responsiveness (Kazdin & Whitley, 2006) and other contradictory findings have been reported (e.g., Beauchaine *et al.*, 2005). Similarly, no consistent finding has emerged regarding whether a child's age impacts on treatment outcome (Dishion & Patterson, 1992; Beauchaine *et al.*, 2005; Lundahl *et al.*, 2006). A similar pattern emerges in relation to systemic interventions: no effect of family and child complexity or co-morbidity has been found on mediating variables or outcomes for MTFC (Smith, 2004) and studies of MST (e.g., Schaeffer & Borduin, 2005) have not found socio-economic status, ethnicity, age, or the severity or violence of the offending to be significant moderators. Some studies of PMT suggest that aspects of the child's personality may influence treatment response (e.g., Hawes & Dadds, 2005); this is discussed in more detail in the next section.

Because CBT employs techniques that tend to be verbal, abstract, and at times complex, investigators have considered whether such an approach would be as effective with younger or intellectually impaired children. A number of studies have now shown that older and more cognitively able children tend to benefit more from CBT (Kazdin & Crowley, 1997; McCart *et al.*, 2006). In addition, the severity of the child's behavioural problem and level of contextual risk (e.g., poor parenting) have been associated with poorer CBT outcomes (Kazdin & Crowley, 1997). Arguably, children with more severe and persistent problems would require both an enhanced package of individual therapy (increased number of sessions, follow-up sessions, etc.) alongside systemic interventions that aim to promote a shared understanding of the problem, motivation to change, and a reduction in environmental contingencies maintaining the problem behaviours.

Mixed findings have been reported regarding whether group or individual therapy is more effective for both PMT (Cunningham *et al.*, 1995; Lundahl *et al.*, 2006) and CBT. For the latter, a concern has been raised about the possibility of 'peer deviancy training' whereby interventions that group antisocial adolescent peers have an iatrogenic effect (Poulin *et al.*, 2001).

However, this may only occur in CBT groups where individuals with and without conduct problems are combined (Mager *et al.*, 2005); indeed, CBT groups solely containing adolescents with conduct problems may have a positive rather than iatrogenic influence (e.g., van Manen *et al.*, 2004).

Heterogeneity in CD: the case for distinct trajectories

Patterns of serious or violent offending behaviour in adolescents and adults are generally preceded by histories of earlier conduct problems in childhood (Marshall & Cooke, 1999; Vermeiren, 2003). However, in those children with early conduct problems, we know that only a minority, typically about one third, manifest a persistent pattern of antisocial behaviour later in life (Robins, 1978, Robbins *et al.*, 1991). Theoretical models of CD have made significant strides in postulating distinct causal pathways to characterize those children at the most risk (Moffit, 1993; Frick & Ellis, 1999). Such advances are an attempt to move beyond simply identifying general risk factors associated with CD (of which there are a prolific number; see Bassarath, 2001 for a review) and instead delineate specific pathways and subtypes of children among those who at a surface behavioural level may have similar presentations at a given point in time. The argument that a more heterogeneous understanding of CD is required to inform models of clinical formulation and treatment is made here in relation to two postulated groups who are at risk for serious and persistent offending.

Early onset CD

An influential contribution to the conceptualization of CD has been the distinction between those children who present with conduct problems prior to or during adolescence (Patterson, 1986; Moffitt, 1993). Moffitt's developmental taxonomy of antisocial behaviour has endeavoured to describe these distinct pathways theoretically and empirically. According to this model, it is hypothesized that children showing an early onset of problem behaviours are more likely to show persistent antisocial behaviour later in life. In line with their hypothesis, Moffitt and colleagues (2002) report that of 45 men from a birth cohort of 539 males who displayed significant conduct problems in pre-adolescence, 38% were subsequently convicted in adulthood for violent offences compared with 14% in the adolescent-onset group and 5% in the control group of individuals with no history of conduct problems. It is postulated that this differential outcome derives from the presence of a set of early internal (relating to neuropsychological vulnerabilities and temperament) and external (relating to family dysfunction) risk factors in the early onset group. This contrasts with adolescent-onset risk factors, which relate to a time-limited drive to gain maturity and adult status through delinquent rather than prosocial strategies, learned via deviant peer affiliation. Clinically, this taxonomy has reinforced the need for early targeted intervention; it has been suggested that for a minority of children aggressive tendencies may crystallize by the time they reach their eighth birthday (Webster-Stratton & Taylor, 2001). In addition, it highlights the important role a child's developmental history should play in informing clinical formulation and treatment as comparable patterns of adolescent conduct problems may in fact conceal distinct sets of aetiological risk and maintaining factors.

What is manifestly missing from the intervention studies reported here is a consideration of the potential differential outcome in adolescence for those children on early onset and adolescent-onset trajectories. For younger children, there is a need to develop criteria to identify those at the most risk, such that relatively transient and normative externalizing aggressive behaviours can be distinguished from more serious patterns. In this regard,

Campbell (1990) has proposed a number of criteria: namely, the presence of a constellation of problems impacting different levels of functioning (e.g., social and cognitive), different situations (e.g., home and school), and manifest with different people such that they can be described as frequent and severe. A context of family dysfunction or stress may represent an additional key criterion (Patterson *et al.*, 1989; Campbell *et al.*, 2000).

CU traits

A second approach to conceptualize and differentiate distinct trajectories in CD has been a focus on empathic functioning. It has been proposed that children with high levels of 'callous-unemotional' or CU traits, referring to limited empathy, guilt, and emotional expression, can be distinguished from other children of a similar age with comparable problem behaviours. It is argued that these children are characterized by a particular set of features that have a strong genetic basis (Viding *et al.*, 2005), are primarily neurobiological in origin (Blair *et al.*, 2006; Viding *et al.*, 2007), and are associated with lower levels of fearfulness and anxiety (see Frick and Petitclerc, Chapter 4, this volume). From the perspective of identifying early features of children at the most risk, the presence of conduct problems and high-CU traits are associated with a more severe, aggressive, and persistent pattern of antisocial behaviour (Oxford *et al.*, 2003). At the present time, longitudinal evidence is sparse; however, preliminary findings suggest that features of CU traits are not immutable, and are amenable to intervention (Frick, Kimonis *et al.*, 2003; Hawes & Dadds, 2007).

Conceptually, children with conduct problems and high-CU traits would be hypothesized to respond differentially to current treatment approaches given, for example, their known punishment insensitivity and tendency to instrumental aggression. Few treatment studies have been conducted to address this question. In a more general context, it has been shown that children with a relatively fearless temperament may respond preferentially to a more reward-focused parenting style (Kochanska & Murray, 2000). Preliminary studies have examined the efficacy of parent training in children specifically in relation to their levels of CU traits and point to an attenuated treatment response for these children, particularly in relation to punishment-related components such as time-out (Hawes & Dadds, 2007). These findings can be considered alongside more generic studies that suggest that co-morbid Attention Deficit/Hyperactivity Disorder (ADHD), anxiety, and depression are associated with improved treatment outcomes (Beauchaine *et al.*, 2006; Kazdin & Whitley, 2006). Children with low levels of CU traits have a more impulsive and emotionally laden style of aggression (Frick, Cornell *et al.*, 2003). This is thought to be linked to deficits in emotional and behavioural regulation that are aggravated by environmental adversity (Oxford *et al.*, 2003). As such, children with high and low levels of CU traits may respond differentially to different forms of intervention; this requires systematic investigation.

The contribution of neuroscience and a multilevel perspective to clinical intervention

Can genetics and neuroscience help advance effective clinical practice for CD? We suggest that a multiple-levels approach is likely to provide a significant contribution to this endeavour in at least four ways. In essence, such an approach provides the framework and the tools to advance our understanding of the putative developmental trajectories to CD and a basis to identify mechanisms by which intervention can lead to more adaptive functioning.

Firstly, a consideration of the genetic, neural, and cognitive underpinnings of a developmental disorder is necessary to provide the framework for a truly integrated and causal theory (Morton & Frith, 1995). As we have just seen, it is very plausible that there are distinct subgroups of children with CD who are likely to be characterized by specific sets of neurocognitive, genetic, and environmental features that generate different developmental patterns of risk. This possibility is presented schematically in Fig. 16.1, which illustrates how two trajectories, A and B, may present with similar behavioural characteristics but have only partly shared risk factors. For example, Pathway A is potentiated by a greater number of specific environmental risk factors, whereas for Pathway B, increased risk emerges from the interaction between greater genetic vulnerability and a more limited exposure to environmental risk. Different factors (illustrated by the shaded circles) are likely to play different roles for each trajectory. Underlying differences for each trajectory may have implications for intervention as different genetic, neurocognitive, and environmental factors are likely to interact with therapeutic mechanisms that drive change. Currently, we know little about what such interactions might look like. By understanding the make-up of distinct trajectories, we will be in a position to begin to differentiate those treatments effective for one trajectory but which are of limited effectiveness (or even iatrogenic) for another. From the perspective of formulation, the clinician will be well placed to consider how two identical behavioural presentations may in fact be underpinned by different patterns of neurocognitive, genetic, and environmental vulnerabilities. In essence, a delineated multilevel framework for CD will provide a theoretical rationale to empirically explore specific ways in which treatment outcomes differ for delineated groups of children (e.g., those with and without CU traits).

A second contribution of a multiple-levels approach will be to identify clusters of genetic vulnerabilities that may make some children more susceptible to poor outcomes as a function of their exposure to adverse environmental experiences. We know already that allelic variation in the gene that regulates monoamine oxidase A (MAOA) activity influences the

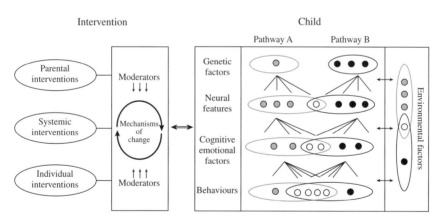

Fig. 16.1 This schematic shows two hypothetical pathways (Pathway A: grey ellipses; Pathway B: black ellipses) that illustrate how different subgroups of children with conduct problems may present with different risk factors at different levels of explanation. Thus, although the example pathways shown may have a high level of similarity in terms of shared features at the behavioural level, this in fact conceals underlying differences at the genetic, neurocognitive, and environmental levels (Coloured circles: pathway-specific risk factors; open circles: shared risk factors).

likelihood of conduct problems later in life, an effect that relates only to those individuals who have experienced childhood maltreatment (Capsi *et al.*, 2002). In other words, it is the *interaction* between genes and environment that is crucial, not the effect of either in isolation. This highlights the fact that a genetic (or indeed any other) account is not primary—the role of genes is not a reductionistic one, rather forms part of a complex interacting system. Genes predispose to certain neural features that endow resilience and vulnerability to different kinds of environmental experience, from early parenting, to diet, and even therapeutic intervention, as well as predisposing the child to behave in ways that will evoke patterns of responses in their caregivers. Understanding how children with particular clusters of genetic markers may benefit from one kind of treatment compared to another or may be more susceptible to one form of early adversity can help progress clinical formulation and the development of interventions that suit the child (and the system) they treat.

The third contribution of a multiple-levels approach will be to make links between genes on the one hand and behaviour on the other. The crucial intervening levels relate to neural and cognitive function. The same allelic variation for MAOA is also known to be associated with differences in the structure and functionality of the amygdala and the prefrontal and cingulate cortices in normal individuals (Meyer-Lindenberg *et al.*, 2006; Buckholtz *et al.*, 2007). Male carriers of the low-expressing genetic variant have been reported to show atypical amygdala activation and increased functional coupling with the ventromedial prefrontal cortex (vmPFC). These neural markers have been associated with differences at the cognitive level in terms of increased harm avoidance and decreased reward dependence scores. These findings suggest that a genotype codes for a particular neural circuitry that is associated with biases in information processing. What will be informative to the clinician is a better understanding of the direct links between these features (potentially characterized as endophenotypes) and environmental experiences such as poor parenting and maltreatment in the trajectory to antisocial behaviour.

Finally, a multiple-levels approach may, in the longer term, provide a framework to better understand the processes of behavioural and emotional dysregulation that are at the heart of conduct problems, and allow the investigation of how interventions serve to alter the functionality of regulatory systems. Poor self-regulation is a well-established risk factor associated with CD (Riggs *et al.*, 2006), although there is still little agreement as to how self-regulation should be measured and conceptualized. Neuroscientific studies have begun a systematic investigation of appraisal, planning, response selection, inhibition, and monitoring as putative components of behavioural and emotional regulatory systems. These have been variously associated with dorsal and ventral regions of the anterior cingulate cortex, dorsolateral prefrontal cortex, and medial and orbital frontal cortices in the frontal lobes (see Ochsner & Gross, 2005 for a review). There have been attempts to both localize sets of processes in specific regions as well as to understand how these regions interact with each other and with subcortical limbic structures.

To date, few developmental studies have been conducted. Sterzer and colleagues, however, have investigated brain structure and function in adolescents with CD (Sterzer *et al.*, 2005; Stadler *et al.*, 2007; Sterzer *et al.*, 2007; see Sterzer & Stadler, Chapter 9, this volume) and have reported that compared with their peers, these young people show atypical amygdala activation and anterior cingulate cortex activation when viewing negatively valenced pictures (of animals and humans) compared to neutral pictures, and reduced grey matter volume in the bilateral anterior insular cortex. These neural differences are linked to temperamental differences as well as to empathic functioning. These findings are preliminary clues in the construction of an integrated model of atypical processing in the regulatory system associated with CD. Cognitive-behavioural interventions that aim to promote a child's ability to reflect, plan, and inhibit their behaviour may be seen as a 'top-down' intervention designed to increase the capacity of a behaviour and emotion regulatory system subserved by the prefrontal and anterior cingulate cortices. Interventions external to the child that improve the quality, warmth, and predictability of the environment (e.g., parenting responses) and reduce negative influences (e.g., deviant peer affiliation) may also help to improve social and emotional competence by facilitating development of this regulatory system. On the other hand, tackling maladaptive core beliefs, increasing self-esteem, and processing prior trauma—in other words, addressing meaning and appraisal rather than functional capacity—might represent a 'bottom-up' process whereby reactivity to emotional stimuli is modified (potentially implicating subcortical structures and the insula). Understanding the components and interaction of such a regulatory system at the neural level will provide tools to explore the mechanism of change during treatment and may pinpoint previously overlooked areas of vulnerability and targets for intervention.

Conclusions

We have reviewed those core clinical interventions shown to be effective in addressing conduct problems across childhood and adolescence; these clinical approaches intervene variously at the child, parent, and system levels. Although there is now good evidence that these approaches have a modest efficacy, we suggest that much still needs to be done to advance their effectiveness. Firstly, more methodologically robust evaluations are required in order to develop the quality of the current evidence base. Secondly, an increased focus on the active ingredients of each intervention alongside the investigation of mediating and moderating factors is essential if we are to understand the mechanisms of change and drive clinical progress. Thirdly, intervention studies need to take account of the possible underlying subgroups within CD, as these may (or may not) show differential responses to current interventions; we have highlighted in particular children with an early onset of conduct problems and those with high levels of CU traits. Finally, clinical interventions will increasingly require a multilevel framework in order to make use of the tools necessary to advance clinical intervention. Such a framework will help us differentiate and characterize distinct developmental trajectories with their associated genetic, neurocognitive, and environmental features. This in turn will provide a developmentally informed basis to understand how and through what mechanisms factors at each level interact to influence responsiveness to treatment.

References

Achenbach, T. M. (1985). *Assessment and Taxonomy of Child and Adolescent Psychopathology.* Thousand Oaks, CA: Sage.

Alexander, J. F., & Parsons, B. V. (1973). Short-term behavioural intervention with delinquent families: impact on family process and recidivism. *Journal of Abnormal Psychology, 81*(3), 219–225.

Armelius, B. A., & Andreassen, T. H. (2007). Cognitive-behavioral treatment for antisocial behavior in youth in residential treatment. [Online], *Cochrane Database of Systematic Reviews, 17*(4).

Barton, C., Alexander, J. F., Waldron, H., & Turner, C. W. (1985). Generalizing treatment effects of functional family therapy: three replications. *American Journal of Family Therapy, 13*(3), 16–26.

Bassarath, L. (2001). Conduct Disorder: a biopsychosocial review. *Canadian Journal of Psychiatry*, *46*(7), 609–616.

Beauchaine, T. P., Webster-Stratton, C., & Reid, M. J. (2005). Mediators, moderators and predictors of 1-year outcomes among children treated for early-onset conduct problems: a latent growth curve analysis. *Journal of Consulting and Clinical Psychology*, *73*(3), 371–388.

Bennett, D. S., & Gibbons, T. A. (2000). Efficacy of child cognitive-behavioral interventions for anti-social behavior: a meta-analysis. *Child and Family Behavior Therapy*, *22*(1), 1–15.

Blair, J. R., Peschardt, K. S., Budhani, S., Mitchell, D. G. V., & Pine, D. S. (2006). The development of psychopathy. *Journal of Child Psychology and Psychiatry*, *47*(3/4), 262–275.

Buckholtz, J. W., Callicott, J. H., Kolachana, B., Hariri, A. R., Goldberg, T. E., Genderson, M., *et al.* (2007). Genetic variation in MAOA modulates ventromedial prefrontal circuitry mediating individual differences in human personality. *Molecular Psychiatry*, *33*, 313–324.

Campbell, S. B. (1990). *Behaviour Problems in Preschool Children: Clinical and Developmental Issues.* New York: Guilford Press.

Campbell, S. B., Shaw, D. S., & Gilliom, M. (2000). Early externalizing behavior problems: toddlers and preschoolers at risk for later maladjustment. *Developmental Psychopathology*, *12*(3), 467–488.

Caspi, A., McClay, J., Moffitt, T. E., Mill, J., Martin, J., Craig, I. W., *et al.* (2002). Role of genotype in the cycle of violence in maltreated children. *Science*, *297*(5582), 851–854.

Chamberlain, P. (1998). *Blueprints for Violence Prevention: Multidimensional Treatment Foster Care.* Colorado: Institute of Behavioral Science.

Chamberlain, P., Leve, L. D., & DeGarmo, D. S. (2007). Multidimensional treatment foster care for girls in the juvenile justice system: two year follow-up of a randomized clinical trial. *Journal of Consulting and Clinical Psychology*, *75*(1), 187–193.

Chamberlain, P., & Moore, K. (1998). A clinical model for parenting juvenile offenders: a comparison of group care versus family care. *Clinical Child Psychology and Psychiatry*, *3*(3), 375–386.

Crick, N. R., & Dodge, K. A. (1994). A review and reformulation of social information-processing mechanisms in children's social adjustment. *Psychological Bulletin*, *115*(1), 74–101.

Cunningham, C. E., Bremner, R., & Boyle, M. (1995). Large group community-based parenting programs for families of preschoolers at risk for disruptive behaviour disorders: utilization, cost effectiveness, and outcome. *Journal of Child Psychology and Psychiatry*, *36*(7), 1141–1159.

Dishion, T. J., Patterson, G. R., & Kavanagh, K.A. (1992). An experimental test of the coercion model: Linking theory, measurement, and intervention. In R. E. Tremblay, & J. McCord (eds), *Preventing Antisocial Behavior: Interventions from Birth through Adolescence* (pp. 253–282). New York: Guilford Press.

Dishion, T. J., & Patterson, G. R. (1992). Age effects in parent training outcome. *Behavior Therapy*, *23*(4), 719–729.

Dodge, K. A. (2003). Do social information processing patterns mediate aggressive behavior? In B. B. Lahey, T. E. Moffitt, & A. Caspi (eds), *Causes of Conduct Disorder and Juvenile Delinquency* (pp. 254–274). New York: Guilford Press.

Dodge, K. A., Bates, J. E., & Pettit, G. S. (1990). Mechanisms in the cycle of violence. *Science*, *250*(4988), 1678–1683.

Eddy, J. M., & Chamberlain, P. (2000). Family management and deviant peer association as mediators of the impact of treatment condition on youth antisocial behavior. *Journal of Consulting and Clinical Psychology*, *68*(5), 857–863.

Eddy, J. M., Whaley, R. B., & Chamberlain, P. (2004). The prevention of violent behavior by chronic and serious male juvenile offenders: a two year follow up of a randomized clinical trial. *Journal of Emotional and Behavioral Disorders*, *12*(1), 2–8.

Edwards, R. T., Céilleachair, A., Bywater, T., Hughes, D. A., & Hutchings, J. (2007). Parenting programme for parents of children at risk of developing conduct disorder: cost effectiveness analysis. *British Medical Journal*, *334*(7595), 682.

Eyberg, S. M., Boggs, S. R., & Algina, J. (1995). Parent-child interaction therapy: a psychosocial model for the treatment of young children with conduct problem behavior and their families. *Psychopharmacology Bulletin*, *31*(1), 83–91.

Forgatch, M. S. (1994). *Parenting through Change: A Training Manual.* Eugene, OR: Oregon Social Learning Center.

Frick, P. J. (1998). Conduct disorders. In M. Hersen, & T. H. Ollendick, (eds), *Handbook of Child Psychopathology*, 3rd edn (pp. 213–237). New York: Plenum Press.

Frick, P. J., Cornell, A. H., Bodin, S. D., Dane, H., Barry, C. T., & Loney, B. R., (2003). Callous-unemotional traits and developmental pathways to severe conduct problems. *Developmental Psychology, 39*(2), 246–260.

Frick, P. J., & Ellis, M. L. (1999). Callous-unemotional traits and subtypes of conduct disorder. *Clinical Child and Family Psychology Review, 2*(3), 149–168.

Frick, P. J., Kimonis, E. R., Dandreaux, D. M., & Farell, J. M. (2003). The four-year stability of psychopathic traits in non-referred youth. *Behavioral Sciences and the Law, 21*(6), 713–736.

Frick, P. J., & Marsee, M. A. (2006). Psychopathy and developmental pathways to antisocial behavior in youth. In C. J. Patrick (ed), *Handbook of Psychopathy* (pp. 355–374). New York: Guilford Press.

Gardner, F., Burton, J., & Klimes, I. (2006). Randomised controlled trial of a parenting intervention in the voluntary sector for reducing child conduct problems: outcomes and mechanisms of change. *Journal of Child Psychology and Psychiatry, 47*(11), 1123–1132.

Gordon, D. A., Arbuthnot, J., Gustafson, K. E., & McGreen, P. (1988). Home-based behavioral-systems family therapy with disadvantaged juvenile delinquents. *American Journal of Family Therapy, 16*(3), 243–255.

Guerra, N. G., Boxer, P., & Kim, T. E. (2005). A cognitive-ecological approach to serving students with emotional and behavioral disorders: application to aggressive behavior. *Behavioral Disorders, 30*(3), 277–288.

Guerra, N. G., & Slaby, R. G. (1990). Cognitive mediators of aggression in adolescent offenders: II. *Intervention. Developmental Psychology, 26*(2), 269–277.

Hawes, D. J., & Dadds, M. R. (2005). The treatment of conduct problems in children with callous-unemotional traits. *Journal of Consulting and Clinical Psychology, 73*(4), 737–741.

Hawes, D. J., & Dadds, M. R. (2007). Stability and malleability of callous-unemotional traits during treatment for childhood conduct problems. *Journal of Clinical Child and Adolescent Psychology, 36*(3), 347–255.

Henggeler, S. W., Pickrel, S. G., Brondino, M. J., & Crouch, J. L. (1996). Eliminating (almost) treatment dropout of substance abusing or dependent delinquents through home-based multisystemic therapy. *American Journal of Psychiatry, 153*(3), 427–428.

Henggeler, S. W., Schoenwald, S. K., Borduin, C. M., Rowland, M. D., & Cunningham, P. B. (1998). *Multisystemic Treatment of Antisocial Behavior in Children and Adolescents*. New York: Guilford Press.

Huey, S. J., Henggeler, S. W., Brondino, M. J., & Pickrel, S. G. (2000). Mechanisms of change in multisystemic therapy: reducing delinquent behavior through therapist adherence and improved family and peer functioning. *Journal of Consulting and Clinical Psychology, 68*(3), 451–467.

Kazdin, A. E. (2003). Problem-solving skills training and parent management training for conduct disorder. In A. E. Kazdin, & J. R. Weisz (eds), *Evidence-Based Psychotherapies for Children and Adolescents* (pp. 241–262). New York: Guilford Press.

Kazdin, A. E., & Crowley, M. (1997). Moderators of treatment outcome in cognitively based treatment of antisocial behavior. *Cognitive Therapy and Research, 21*(2), 185–207.

Kazdin, A. E., Siegal, T. C., & Bass, D. (1992). Cognitive problem-solving skills training and parent management training in the treatment of antisocial behavior in children. *Journal of Consulting and Clinical Psychology, 60*(5), 733–747.

Kazdin, A. E., & Whitley, M. K. (2006). Comorbidity, case complexity, and effects of evidence-based treatment for children referred for disruptive behavior. *Journal of Consulting and Clinical Psychology, 74*(3), 455–467.

Kochanska, G., & Murray, K. T. (2000). Mother-child mutually responsive orientation and conscience development: from toddler to early school age. *Child Development, 71*(2), 417–431.

Leschied, A. W., & Cunningham, A. (2002). *Seeking Effective Interventions for Young Offenders: Interim Results of a Four-Year Randomized Study of Multi-Systemic Therapy in Ontario, Canada*. London, ON: Centre for Children and Families in the Justice System.

Lipman, E. L., Boyle, M. H., Cunningham, C., Kenny, M., Sniderman, C., Duku, E., *et al.* (2006). Testing effectiveness of a community based aggression management program for children 7 to 11 years old and their families. *Journal of the American Academy of Child and Adolescent Psychiatry, 45*(9), 1085–1093.

Littell, J. H., Popa, M., & Forsythe, B. (2005). Multisystemic therapy for social, emotional and behavioral problems in youth aged 10-17. [Online], *The Cochrane Database of Systematic Reviews, 4.*

Lochman, J. E. (1992). Cognitive behavioral intervention with aggressive boys: three year follow-up and preventive effects. *Journal of Consulting and Clinical Psychology, 60*(3), 426–432.

Lundahl, B., Risser, H. J., Lovejoy, & M. C. (2006). A meta-analysis of parent training: moderators and follow-up effects. *Clinical Psychology Review, 26*(1), 86–104.

Mager, W., Milich, R., Harris, M. J., & Howard, A. (2005). Intervention groups for adolescents with conduct problems: is aggregation harmful or helpful? *Journal of Abnormal Child Psychology, 33*(3), 349–362.

Markie-Dadds, C., & Sanders, M. R. (2006). A controlled evaluation of an enhanced self-directed behavioural family intervention for parents of children with conduct problems in rural and remote areas. *Behaviour Change, 23*(1), 55–72.

Marshall, L., & Cooke, D. J. (1999). The childhood experiences of psychopaths: a retrospective study of familial and societal factors. *Journal of Personality Disorders, 13*(33), 211–225.

McCart, M. R., Priester, P. E., Davies, W. H., & Azen, R. (2006). Differential effectiveness of behavioral parent training and cognitive behavioral therapy for antisocial youth: a meta-analysis. *Journal of Abnormal Child Psychology, 34*(4), 527–543.

McMahon, R. J., & Forehand, R. L. (2003). *Helping the Noncompliant Child: Family-Based Treatment for Oppositional Behavior*, 2nd edn. New York: Guilford Press.

Meyer-Lindenberg, A., Buckholtz, J. W., Kolachana, B. R., Hariri, A., Pezawas, L., Blasi, G., *et al.* (2006). Neural mechanisms of genetic risk for impulsivity and violence in humans. *Proceedings of the National Academy of Sciences of the United States of America, 103*(16), 6269–6274.

Moffitt, T. E. (1993). 'Life-course-persistent' and 'adolescence-limited' antisocial behavior: a developmental taxonomy. *Psychological Review, 100*(4), 674–701.

Moffitt, T. E., Caspi, A., Harrington, H., & Milne, B. J. (2002). Males on the life-course persistent and adolescence-limited pathways: follow-up at age 26 years. *Developmental Psychopathology, 14*(1), 179–207.

Morton, J., & Frith, U. (1995). Causal modelling: a structural approach to developmental psychology. In D. Cicchetti, & D. J. Cohen (eds), *Manual of Developmental Psychopathology* (pp. 357–390). New York: Wiley & Sons.

Nixon, R. D. V., Sweeney, L., Erickson, D. B., & Touyz, S. W. (2004). Parent-child interaction therapy: one- and two-year follow-up of standard and abbreviated treatments for oppositional preschoolers. *Journal of Abnormal Child Psychology, 32*(3), 263–271.

Nock, M. K. (2003). Progress review of the psychosocial treatment of child conduct problems. *Clinical Psychology: Science and Practice, 10*(1), 1–28.

Ochsner, K. N., & Gross, J. J. (2005). The cognitive control of emotion. *Trends in Cognitive Science, 9*(5), 242–249.

Oxford, M., Cavell, T. A., & Hughes, J. N. (2003). Callous-unemotional traits moderate the relation between ineffective parenting and child externalizing problems: a partial replication and extension. *Journal of Clinical Child and Adolescent Psychology, 32*(4), 577–585

Patterson, G. R. (1976). *Living with Children: New Methods for Parents and Teachers*, 2nd edn. Champaign, IL: Research Press.

Patterson, G. R. (1982). *Coercive Family Processes*. Eugene, OR: Castalia.

Patterson, G. R. (1986). Performance models for antisocial boys. *American Psychologist, 41*(4), 432–444.

Patterson, G. R., de Baryshe, B. D., & Ramsey, E. (1989). A developmental perspective on antisocial behaviour. *American Psychologist, 44*(2), 329–335.

Poulin, F., Dishion, T. J., & Burraston, B. (2001). Three-year iatrogenic effects associated with aggregating high-risk adolescents in cognitive-behavioral preventive interventions. *Applied Developmental Science, 5*(4), 214–224.

Riggs, N. R., Greenberg, M. T., Kusché, C. A., & Pentz, M. A. (2006). The mediational role of neurocognition in the behavioral outcomes of a social-emotional prevention program in elementary school students: effects of the PATHS Curriculum. *Prevention Science, 7*(1), 91–102.

Robins, L. N. (1978). Sturdy childhood predictors of adult antisocial behaviour: replications from longitudinal studies. *Psychological Medicine, 8*(4), 611–622.

Robins, L. N., Tipp, J., & Przybeck, T. R. (1991). Antisocial personality. In L. N. Robins, & D. A. Regier (eds), *Psychiatric Disorders in America* (pp. 258–290). New York: Free Press.

Sanders, M. R. (1999). Triple P positive parenting program: towards an empirically validated multi-level parenting and family support strategy for the prevention of behaviour and emotional problems in children. *Clinical Child and Family Psychology Review, 2*(2), 71–90.

Schaeffer, C. M., & Borduin, C. M. (2005). Long-term follow-up to a randomized clinical trial of multisystemic therapy with serious and violent juvenile offenders. *Journal of Consulting and Clinical Psychology, 73*(3), 445–453

Scott, S., Spender, Q., Doolan, M., Jacobs, B., & Aspland, H. C. (2001). Multicentre controlled trial of parenting groups for childhood antisocial behavior in clinical practice. *British Medical Journal, 323*(7306), 194.

Serketich, W. J., & Dumas, J. E. (1996). The effectiveness of behavioral parent training to modify antisocial behavior in children: a meta-analysis. *Behavior Therapy, 27*(2), 171–186.

Sexton, T. L., & Alexander, J. F. (1999). *Functional Family Therapy: Principles of Clinical Assessment and Implementation.* Henderson, NV: RCH Enterprises.

Smith, D. K. (2004). Risk, reinforcement, retention in treatment and reoffending for boys and girls in multidimensional treatment foster care. *Journal of Emotional and Behavioral Disorders, 12*(1), 38–48.

Stadler, C., Sterzer, P., Schmeck, K., Krebs, A., Kleinschmidt, A., & Poustk, F. (2007). Reduced anterior cingulate activation in aggressive children and adolescents during affective stimulation: association with temperament traits. *Journal of Psychiatry Research, 41*(5), 410–417.

Sterzer, P., Stadler, C., Krebs, A., Kleinschmidt, A., & Poustka, F. (2005). Abnormal neural responses to emotional visual stimuli in adolescents with conduct disorder. *Biological Psychiatry, 57*(1), 7–15.

Sterzer, P., Stadler, C., Poustka, F., & Kleinschmidt, A. (2007). A structural neural deficit in adolescents with conduct disorder and its association with lack of empathy. *Neuroimage, 37*(1), 335–342.

Sukhodolsky, D. G., Kassinove, H., & Gorman, B. S. (2004). Cognitive-behavioral therapy for anger in children and adolescents: a meta-analysis. *Aggression and Violent Behavior, 9*(3), 247–269.

Thomas, R., & Zimmer-Gembeck, M. J. (2007). Behavioral outcomes of parent-child interaction therapy and Triple P-positive parenting program: a review and meta-analysis. *Journal of Abnormal Child Psychology, 35*(3), 475–495.

Turner, K. M. T., Richards, M., & Sanders, M. R. (2007). Randomised clinical trial of a group parent education programme for Australian indigenous families. *Journal of Paediatrics and Child Health, 43*(6), 429–437.

Van Manen, T. G., Prins, P. J. M., & Emmelkamp, P. M. G. (2004). Reducing aggressive behavior in boys with a social cognitive group treatment: results of a randomized controlled trial. *Journal of the American Academy of Child and Adolescent Psychiatry, 43*(12), 1478–1487.

Vermeiren, R. (2003). Psychopathology and delinquency in adolescents: a descriptive and developmental perspective. *Clinical Psychology Review, 23*(2), 277–318.

Viding, E., Blair, J. R., Moffitt, T. E., & Plomin, R. (2005). Evidence for substantial genetic risk for psychopathy in seven year olds. *Journal of Child Psychology and Psychiatry, 46*(6), 592–597.

Viding, E., Frick, P. J., & Plomin, R. (2007). Aetiology of the relationship between callous-unemotional traits and conduct problems in childhood. *British Journal of Psychiatry, 190*(49), s33–s38.

Vitaro, F., Brendgen, M., & Tremblay, R. E. (2001). Preventative intervention: assessing its effects on its trajectories of delinquency and testing for mediational processes. *Applied Developmental Science, 5*(4), 201–213.

Webster-Stratton, C., & Hammond, M. (1997). Treating children with early-onset conduct problems: a comparison of child and parent training interventions. *Journal of Consulting and Clinical Psychology, 65*(1), 93–109.

Webster-Stratton, C., & Reid, M. J. (2003). The incredible years parents, teachers and children training series: a multifaceted treatment approach for young children with conduct problems. In A. E. Kazdin, & J. R. Weisz (eds), *Evidence-Based Psychotherapies for Children and Adolescents* (pp. 224–240). New York: Guilford Press.

Webster-Stratton, C., Reid, M. J., & Hammond, M. (2004). Treating children with early onset conduct problems: intervention outcomes for parent, child and teacher training. *Journal of Clinical Child and Adolescent Psychology*, *33*(1), 105–124.

Webster-Stratton, C., & Taylor, T. (2001). Nipping early risk factors in the bud: Preventing substance abuse, delinquency, and violence in adolescence through interventions targeted at young children (0 to 8 Years). *Prevention Science*, *2*(3), 165–192.

Westermark, P. K., Hanssson, K., & Vinnerljung, B. (2007). Foster parents in multidimensional treatment foster care: How do they deal with implementing standardized treatment components? *Children and Youth Services Review*, *29*(4), 442–459.

17

Why are programmes for offenders with personality disorder not informed by the relevant scientific findings?

Conor Duggan

'It is a characteristic of the design of scientific research that exquisite attention is devoted to methodological problems that can be solved, while the pretense is made that the ones that cannot be solved are really nothing to worry about.' (Lewontin, 1995)

Introduction

One of my most striking memories from this meeting was the discontinuity between the sophistication of many of the scientific papers-especially those from a developmental perspective-and the failure to translate these findings into clinical practice. This was best illustrated by one of the speakers when, after a very erudite exposition on the developmental origins of psychopathy, seemed at a loss to explain how his findings might inform the management of a difficult, out of control, teenager when questioned by a clinician.

The rhetorical nature of my title underscores this dissonance between the research evidence and clinical practice. Clearly, as the excerpt demonstrates, there is a significant gap between what is known and what we need to know if we are to conduct clinical practice based on scientific evidence in this area. Despite this gap, clinicians will still have to deliver a service even though this will always be playing 'catch-up' with the scientific evidence. This chapter has two purposes: (i) to answer the question posed in the title and (ii) to come up with some practical recommendations to fill the 'gap' between the scientific evidence and clinical practice.

Returning to my title, even if the proposition implied is true, it poses a question that can be answered at a number of levels. In this chapter, I will consider each of the following in turn:

(a) What is the nature of the scientific evidence for effective interventions in offenders with personality disorder?
(b) If such evidence exists, under which conditions can mental health professionals ignore such evidence?
(c) Even when such evidence exists and is accepted by the professionals, can it still be ignored by policymakers and politicians?

In order to focus this endeavour, I will consider these questions in relation to Antisocial Personality Disorder (ASPD)-specifically, as it is defined in the *Diagnostic and Statistical Manual of Mental Disorders* (DSM). Apart from the self-evident relationship between ASPD and violent offending, there may be surprise that I have chosen to concentrate on ASPD, rather than psychopathy. After all, psychopathy has been the focus of many of the presentations at this meeting. It is also much more sharply defined than ASPD and has been studied at much greater depth with much neuropsychological evidence identifying one or more of mechanisms that might explain it. ASPD, in contrast, is a much less credible diagnostic construct as it is poorly researched and has little theoretical underpinning (see, Hare *et al.*, 1991; Ogloff, 2006 for a review of the overlap between these constructs). Nonetheless, I believe that this focus on ASPD, rather than that psychopathy, is justified for the following reasons.

Reasons for taking ASPD seriously

Epidemiology

Estimates of the lifetime prevalence of ASPD in the general population vary with rates in North America of 4.5% in men and 0.8% in women (Robins *et al.*, 1991), 6.8% among men and 0.8% in women (Swanson *et al.*,1994) being significantly higher than in Europe having corresponding figures of 1.3% in men and 0% in women (Torgensen *et al.*, 2001) and 1% in men and 0.2 % in women (Coid *et al.*, 2006). Whether these differences are real differences in rates or are a consequence of different methodologies is unclear; nonetheless, we can draw two conclusions. First, despite these relative differences, the rates of ASPD reported suggest that it is a prevalent personality disorder whereas psychopathy (as defined by the *Psychopathy Checklist-Revised* [PCL-R]) is a much less prevalent. For instance, although 50% of those in prison will meet criteria for ASPD, the prevalence of psychopathy among UK prisoners is only 4.5% using a PCL-R score of more than 30 and 13% using a score of greater than 25 (Hare *et al.*, 2000). Hence, the greater prevalence of ASPD indicates that it is much more important than psychopathy, from a public health perspective.

Second, even with the most conservative estimates, ASPD in men has the same prevalence as major mental illnesses such as schizophrenia and bipolar disorder. However, these conditions receive the greatest attention and resources from mental health professionals whereas those with ASPD receive very little. I make this point not in anyway to downplay the often-times devastating consequences of these disorders; rather, it is to highlight that the high prevalence of ASPD suggests that it deserves our attention especially if it is associated with some impairment for the individual. Moreover, even for those with schizophrenia, it is often their co-morbid ASPD that makes them difficult to manage, particularly as regards their violent behaviour (Bloom *et al.*, 2000).

Evidence of an associated biological disadvantage for those with ASPD

Identifying a disorder as being prevalent is not sufficient to justify the allocation of scarce human resources unless it is also associated with obvious disadvantages. The respiratory physician John Scadding (1967), for instance, defined a disease in biomedical terms as a condition that would place the individual at a biological disadvantage compared to other members of the species. The two obvious criteria by which this could be judged are either an increase in mortality or an increase in morbidity in the individual being so affected. Regarding the former, Martin *et al.*'s (1985) follow-up of 500 psychiatric outpatients with a range of psychiatric conditions in St Louis found that those with ASPD had the second highest standardized mortality rate (SMR = 8.57, $p = 0.01$), exceeded only by drug addiction. This increased mortality was not only due to an increased rate of suicide but was also a consequence of reckless behaviour such as drug misuse and aggression. An even more striking finding was provided by Black *et al.* (1996) in their follow-up of men with ASPD: they found that young men with ASPD in particular had a high rate of premature death with those under the age of 40 having an SMR of 33 and the risk diminishing with increasing age.

As regards an increase in morbidity, ASPD is often co-morbid with several other Axis 1 disorders, with the Swanson *et al.* (1994) community study showing that those with ASPD had an increased prevalence of '... nearly every other psychiatric disorder with 90.4% having at least one other psychiatric disorder'. Co-morbidity with substance misuse is especially common. For instance, in the Epidemiological Catchment Area study, when men with and without ASPD were compared, those with ASPD were 3 and 5 times more likely to abuse alcohol and illicit drugs (Robins *et al.*, 1991). It is also important to note that, although women have a significantly lower prevalence of ASPD than men, those women with ASPD have an even higher prevalence of substance misuse compared with the men (Robins *et al.*, 1991; Compton *et al.*, 2005). In addition, ASPD has been found to co-occur with anxiety disorders in 54% (Goodwin & Hamilton, 2003) and 47.5% (Lenzenweger *et al.*, 2007). The latter also found that 28% of those with ASPD also suffered from any mood disorder. One point that I will return to later is that the presence of ASPD is often a negative moderator when these co-morbid conditions are treated with conventional approaches. As ASPD has also been shown to frequently co-occur with other Axis 11 conditions (Moran, 1999), it is reasonable to conclude that ASPD is a condition with high morbidity.

ASPD is associated with increased costs, not only to the individual but also to society more generally

ASPD is associated with fractured families, low educational attainment, a poor occupational history, and a significant association with criminality. Hence, one of the important reasons for intervening in those with ASPD is that it has not only a high cost to the individual but also a high cost to society. This arises both as a direct cost on public services and the indirect cost of lost economic productivity. An example of the former is provided by Scott *et al.*'s (2001) comparison of the lifetime public costs of three groups of 27-year-olds (those who were normal in childhood, those with some Conduct Disorder (CD) traits, and those with CD in childhood). They found a tenfold difference in the costs between those adults with and without CD in childhood. This will be important when I shall argue later that these high costs provide a justification for using expensive interventions in this group.

Early prevention

ASPD is unique in that it is the only personality disorder (at least within the DSM) that requires an antecedent criterion from childhood (i.e., CD) in order to make a diagnosis. The criticism of this requirement has been made sharply by Millon *et al.* (1998; p. 8) in an often cited quotation that 'the DSM-111 Task Force voted to base its diagnostic guidelines on this single, albeit well-designed, follow-up study of delinquent cases referred to one child guidance clinic in a large mid-western city'. In addition, it has been difficult to distinguish those with adult criteria for ASPD only (so-called 'late bloomers') from those with CD and adult criteria when they are compared across a range of characteristics independent of the diagnosis (Black & Braun, 1998; Perdiouri *et al.*, 2007).

Despite these criticisms, Robins' earlier finding has now been replicated by several prospective longitudinal follow-up studies identifying a substantial number of children where their CD with aggressive behaviour persists into adulthood (Robins, *et al.*, 1991; Moffit *et al.*, 2001; Loeber *et al.*, 2002; Simonoff *et al.*, 2004; De Brito and Hodgins, in press). Moreover, males with CD go on to commit more violent crimes in adultdhood (Loeber *et al.*, 2002). The important implication of the presence of this childhood criterion in the diagnosis of adult ASPD is that prevention at an early stage may be possible. Indeed, I take this to be the leitmotiv of this meeting with several of the presentations (i.e., by Hodgins and Loeber & Pardini) emphasizing (and providing evidence) that early identification and intervention is both possible and desirable.

ASPD and criminality are not the same (or are they?)

One of the major criticisms of ASPD is its apparent emphasis on criminal behaviour in its definition. This has led to the belief that ASPD and its variants may be overdiagnosed in certain settings, such as prison, and underdiagnosed in the community (Lilienfeld, 1998; Ogloff, 2006). However, if ASPD was synonymous with criminal behaviour and vice versa, this would imply that all of those in custodial settings would meet criteria for ASPD and that ASPD would be rare in those without a criminal history. However, this is not the case. For instance, the prevalence of ASPD among prisoners is slightly less than 50% (Hart & Hare, 1989; Singleton *et al.*, 1998; Fazel & Danesh, 2002). Even Robins, who has empha-sized aberrant behaviour as key to the diagnosis of ASPD, pointed out that only 47% of those who met the DSM-111 APD in the Epidemiological Catchment Area study (i.e., in the community) had significant arrest records with aggression, job problems, and promiscuity being more common than serious crimes (Robins, 1987; Robins *et al.*, 1991). Thus, although there is an important relationship between ASPD and criminal behaviour, this relationship is not straightforward, with half of those convicted not meeting the criteria for ASPD and half of those in the community with ASPD never having had a conviction.

Moreover, the majority of the mental health practitioners do not regard the criminal focus for ASPD as defined by DSM-IV or one of the other diagnostic systems as being especially helpful in their clinical practice. Rather, they focus on unstable interpersonal rela-tionships, disregard for the consequences of one's behaviour, a failure to learn from experi-ence, egocentricity, and a disregard for the feelings of others (Livesley *et al.*, 1987, Tennant *et al.*, 1990). Clearly, therefore, there is more to ASPD than criminal behaviour, as to what is the underlying personality construct I will discuss later.

What is the nature of the scientific evidence for effective interventions among offenders with ASPD?

There is now general agreement that there is a hierarchy of evidence that one can call upon in deciding which intervention to use in a clinical case. This hierarchy places meta-analyses that summarize the results of relevant randomized controlled trials (RCTs) at the peak, followed by the results of well-conducted individual RCTs, in turn followed by other forms of evidence (e.g., controlled studies, cohort studies, case series, etc.) Although these weaker forms of design are regarded as less persuasive, their contribution ought not to be dismissed out of hand as RCTs do not arise *de novo*. In addition, it has been argued that, as interven-tions in this group are what have been termed as 'complex interventions', different criteria apply (Anon, 2000).

This has been ably reviewed for offender programmes by Hollin (2006) who points out that, as many of the interventions for offenders (and for those with ASPD) are complex interventions, it would be foolhardy to rely on any one methodology to provide the necessary evidence in this field. Hollin concludes with a quotation from Slade and Priebe (2001) that provides an argument for a diverse set of methodologies given the heterogeneity in the area:

'Mental health research needs to span both the natural and social sciences. Evidence based on RCTs has an important place, but to adopt concepts from only one body of knowledge is to neglect the contribution that other, well-established methodologies can make ... RCTs can give better evidence about some contentious research questions, but it is an illusion that the development of increasingly rigorous and sophisticated RCTs will ultimately provide a complete evidence base.' (Slade & Priebe, 2001; p. 287)

Although one might accept the trust of Slade and Priebe's argument, this carries a danger. If, for instance, one assumes that interventions in mental health are somehow different and more complex than other health areas so that alternative criteria in assessing their efficacy apply, this could easily result in they being treated differently (i.e., more disadvantageously) than other areas of health care where its arguments may be seen as a form of 'special pleading'. In the next section, therefore I shall concentrate exclusively in describing those RCTs that met the Cochrane criteria for those with ASPD.

Systematic reviews of treatments for ASPD

Similar scientific imperatives apply in conducting a systematic review as designing a RCT (i.e., to avoid bias and to have a methodology that can be replicated). This is achieved by specifying the following in advance of reviewing any of the literature: the criteria by which trials are to be included/excluded on the basis of the **P**opulations studied, the **I**nterventions offered, the **C**ontrol population against which the intervention is compared, and finally, the **O**utcomes that are relevant. It needs to be understood that making decisions on each of the components of the acronym PICO are based on common sense assumptions and not on the science itself. Of especial relevance to this discussion is whether or not to include the offending literature in evaluating the effectiveness of interventions for those with ASPD?

There is an argument both for and against considering this literature. The argument in favour is that, unless there is a specific process that might exclude them, it is likely that half of the inmates involved in correctional programmes will meet criteria for ASPD (i.e., it is unlikely that they would be specifically excluded as an ASPD diagnosis is not an inclusion/exclusion criterion in such programmes.) Hence, there is an argument for including the results from this offending literature. The argument against is that as a diagnosis of ASPD has not been made, it is impossible to know who is being treated in these trials and so it would be foolhardy to draw any inferences as to their relevance for ASPD.

In the systematic reviews to be described, we took a conservative position and restricted the review to studies in which an explicit diagnosis of ASPD had been made, a decision that effectively excluded the criminological literature. We leave it to others as to whether or not this was the correct decision, but the point to note here is that this could not be regarded as a decision based on scientific evidence alone; rather, it depended on value judgements and common sense. The reasons which guided our reviews are discussed at length in two companion papers (Duggan *et al.*, 2007, 2008).

Findings from our review

Although this review largely supported the findings from the two earlier reviews by Dolan and Coid (1993) and Warren *et al.* (2003) in that there was very little evidence for intervening in ASPD in particular, our review extended the previous searches to 31st December 2006. In this review, we were able to include only five trials on ASPD that meet the Cochrane criteria (see Table 17.1). Although overall, there were as many trials for personality disorder of any kind between our previous review up to 2002 (Duggan *et al.*, 2006) as between 2002 and 2006, it is noteworthy that there had been no new trials for ASPD between 2002 and 2006.

The second significant finding was that all five trials (three of which involved a psychological and two a drug intervention) used, as their outcome measure, a reduction in substance misuse. Granted that substance misuse is a serious problem in those with ASPD, yet none of these trials addressed the core psychological problem in those with ASPD. However, as I have previously mentioned that this core disturbance is difficult to describe, perhaps this is not too surprising.

Table 17.1a ASPD: psychological interventions.

Type of analysis	Study	Comparison	Outcome measure	Results	Favours
Individual study	Brooner *et al.* (1998)	CMI versus standard methadone substitution	**Transferred to routine care after 3 months**	**0.50 (0.26,0.97) (RR)**	**CMI**
Individual study	Brooner *et al.* (1998)	CMI versus standard methadone substitution	Treatment dropout	1.38 (0.50,3.84) (RR)	n/s
Individual study	Messina *et al.* (2003)	CM+MM versus CBT+CM+MM	Cocaine free urine sample; during treatment (16 weeks)	1.70 (−9.72,13.12) (WMD)	n/s
Skewed data	Messina *et al.* (2003)	CBT+MM versus CM+MM	**Substance use: cocaine-free urine sample, post treatment (16 weeks)**	*p*<0.05	**CM+MM**
Skewed data	Messina *et al.* (2003)	CBT+MM versus CBT+CM+MM	Substance use: cocaine-free urine sample, post treatment (16 weeks)	n/s	n/s
Skewed data	Messina *et al.* (2003)	CBT+MM versus MM	**Substance use: cocaine-free urine sample, post treatment (16 weeks)**	*p*<0.05	**CBT+MM**
Skewed data	Messina *et al.* (2003)	CM+MM versus MM	**Substance use: cocaine-free urine sample, post treatment (16 weeks)**	*p*<0.05	**CM+MM**
Skewed data	Messina *et al.* (2003)	CBT+CM+MM versus MM	**Substance use: cocaine-free urine sample, post treatment (16 weeks)**	*p*<0.05	**CBT+CM**

CMI, contingency management intervention; MM, methadone maintenance; CBT, cognitive behavioural therapy; WMD,; RR, relative risk; n/s, not significant.

Table 17.1b   ASPD: pharmacological interventions

Type of analysis	Study	Comparison	Outcome measure	Results	Favours
Meta-analysis	Leal *et al.* (1994)Powell *et al.*(1995)	Dopaminergic (amantadine) versus placebo	Leaving study early	1.18 (0.72,1.94) (RR)	n/s
Meta-analysis	Leal *et al.* (1994)Powell *et al* (1995)	Tricyclic (desipramine) versus dopaminergic (amantadine)	Leaving study early	0.74 (0.45,1.23) (RR)	n/s
Meta-analysis	Leal *et al.* (1994)Powell *et al.*(1995)	Tricyclic (desipramine) versus placebo	Leaving study early	0.90 (0.52,1.55) (RR)	n/s
Individual study	Arndt *et al.* (1992, 1994)	Desipramine + standard methadone treatment versus placebo + standard methadone treatment	Days with medical problems in past 30 days; ASI: at 12 weeks	0.67 (0.21,2.13) (RR)	n/s
Individual study	Arndt *et al.* (1992, 1994)	Desipramine + standard methadone treatment versus placebo + standard methadone treatment	Days worked in past 30 days; ASI: at 12 weeks	0.90 (0.43,1.90) (RR)	n/s
Individual study	Arndt *et al.* (1992, 1994)	Desipramine + standard methadone treatment versus placebo + standard methadone treatment	Days of opiate use in past 30 days; ASI: at 12 weeks	1.00 (0.15,6.64) (RR)	n/s
Individual study	Arndt *et al.* (1992, 1994)	Desipramine + standard methadone treatment versus placebo + standard methadone treatment	Days of cocaine use in past 30 days; ASI: at 12 weeks	1.13 (0.50,2.52) (RR)	n/s
Individual study	Arndt *et al.* (1992, 1994)	Desipramine + standard methadone treatment versus placebo + standard methadone treatment	Days of illegal activity in past 30 days; ASI: at 12 weeks	2.00 (0.40,10.11) (RR)	n/s
Individual study	Arndt *et al.* (1992, 1994)	Desipramine + standard methadone treatment versus placebo + standard methadone treatment	Days with family or social problems in past 30 days; ASI: at 12 weeks	1.00 (0.54,1.86) (RR)	n/s
Individual study	Arndt *et al.* (1992, 1994)	Desipramine + standard methadone treatment versus placebo + standard methadone treatment	Days with psychological problems in past 30 days; ASI: at 12 weeks	1.25 (0.37,4.21) (RR)	n/s
Individual study	Leal *et al.* (1994)	Desipramine versus placebo	Leaving the study early	1.14 (0.15,8.99) (RR)	n/s
Individual study	Leal *et al.* (1994)	Amantadine versus placebo	Leaving the study early	2.50 (0.42,14.83) (RR)	n/s
Individual study	Leal *et al.* (1994)	Desipramine versus amantadine	Leaving the study early	0.46 (0.13,1.66) (RR)	n/s
Individual study	Powell *et al.* (1995)	Nortriptyline versus bromocriptine	Leaving the study early	0.85 (0.49,1.46) (RR)	n/s

continued

Table 17.1b (Continued) ASPD: pharmacological interventions

Type of analysis	Study	Comparison	Outcome measure	Results	Favours
Individual study	Powell *et al.* (1995)	Nortriptyline versus bromocriptine	Substance use: not abstinent from alcohol, by 6 months	0.79 (0.57,1.10) (RR)	n/s
Individual study	Powell *et al.* (1995)	Nortriptyline versus placebo	Leaving the study early	0.88 (0.50,1.53) (RR)	n/s
Individual study	Powell *et al.* (1995)	Nortriptyline versus placebo	**Substance use: not abstinent from alcohol, by 6 months**	**0.72 (0.53,0.97) (RR)**	**Nortriptyline**
Individual study	Powell *et al.* (1995)	Bromocriptine versus placebo	Leaving the study early	1.03 (0.62,1.72) (RR)	n/s
Individual study	Powell *et al* (1995)	Bromocriptine versus placebo	Substance use: not abstinent from alcohol, by 6 months	0.91 (0.75,1.10) (RR)	n/s
Skewed data	Coccaro & Kavoussi (1997)	Fluoxetine versus placebo	**Mental state: anxiety score; HARS-14, by 12 weeks**	**$F = 5.5$ (ANCOVA) $P = 0.03$**	**Fluoxetine**
Skewed data	Coccaro & Kavoussi (1997)	Fluoxetine versus placebo	Behaviour: depression; HDRS-21, by 12 weeks	n/s	n/s
Skewed data	Coccaro & Kavoussi (1997)	Fluoxetine versus placebo	Quality of life: HASSLES score, by 12 weeks	n/s	n/s
Skewed data	Coccaro & Kavoussi (1997)	Fluoxetine versus placebo	Quality of life: uplift scores; HUS, by 12 weeks	n/s	n/s
Skewed data	Leal *et al.* (1994)	Desipramine versus placebo	Drug use: $ spent per week on cocaine, by 12 weeks	n/s	n/s
Skewed data	Leal *et al.* (1994)	Amantadine versus placebo	Drug use: $ spent per week on cocaine, by 12 weeks	n/s	n/s
Skewed data	Leal *et al.* (1994)	Amantadine versus desipramine	Drug use: $ spent per week on cocaine, by 12 weeks	n/s	n/s

Given the persistent problems in trying to produce the relevant evidence and our failure to do so, this begs the question as to why this is so. The reasons are not difficult to determine. Returning to the PICO acronym, one can see difficulties in each of these areas that are relevant to ASPD. For the population (**P**) component, there is no unanimity of approach with many questioning the whole construct of ASPD, in particular seeing it in the DSM as being too wedded to criminality (Widiger & Corbitt, 1993). Similarly, there are problems for the selection of the intervention (**I**) as, in the absence of a good theory of personality disorder (Epstein, 1987), there is no clear steer as to which of a wide range of interventions might be used.

As a consequence, it is difficult to make comparisons across studies as few use the same intervention. For the comparator (**C**), those trials that we reviewed were frequently underpowered. For instance, the mean number of participants in the pharmacological trials was 22, which is far too low a number to have any confidence in the findings. An additional caveat is the choice of the comparator, as in many trials this choice was likely to favour the experimental treatment. This has been a problem in other areas of mental health where attempts at replicating earlier trials with a large effect size in the experimental treatment failed when a more effective comparator was used in subsequent trials. For instance, when assertive outreach services were first compared against conventional services for those with serious and enduring mental illness in the United States, a large effect size was found in favour of the assertive outreach service (Stein & Test, 1998). However, when an attempt was made to replicate this in the United Kingdom, it failed (Burns *et al.*, 1999). One of the reasons to explain this discrepancy is that routine services in the United Kingdom (i.e. the comparator) are already reasonably effective; so, the magnitude of the benefit of an enhanced (and more expensive) service is unlikely to match the earlier US results where conventional services were poorly resourced and organized (Tyrer, 2000).

Finally, to consider outcomes (**O**). A major criticism of existing trials of personality disorder in general is that there are far too many outcome measures used, a feature that makes cross-study comparison difficult, if not impossible. However, the criticism goes deeper than this technical consideration in systematic reviews as a recent review of outcomes in psychiatric practice condemned the many and varied outcome measures used as being useful neither to clinical practitioners nor to patients (Gilbody *et al.*, 2003). Here, the excessive number of outcomes in mental health contrasted unfavourably with the minimalist approach of rheumatology and oncology. Although mental health can legitimately claim to have conditions that are more complex in their outcome than, say, oncology, there is nonetheless a sense that mental health trialists are self-indulgent in measuring too many outcomes, and that exercising greater restraint would serve themselves (and those who attempt to interpret their data) well.

In summary, I believe that any fair reading of the current literature on the efficacy of intervening in those with ASPD from a mental health perspective is that we have very little evidence to justify any intervention. However, there is evidence (described in the following) from the criminological literature that may justify intervening provided that the outcome is a reduction in reoffending.

Currently, therefore, we find ourselves in a curious predicament: namely, when ASPD is diagnosed in a mental health context, there is little evidence to justify intervening from the mental health literature. Conversely, when ASPD is not diagnosed, there may be some justification in providing interventions from the criminological or correctional literature. I will return to identifying the conditions required to 'square this circle' towards the end of this chapter, but I first make a brief digression to examine scientific evidence more generally from a philosophical or, perhaps, more appropriately a historiographic perspective.

If such evidence exists, under which conditions can mental health professionals ignore it?

To answer this question requires us to examine the nature of scientific inquiry itself. In the early to mid part of the last century, the nature of scientific inquiry was dominated by the Viennese Logical Positivist inductivist tradition suggesting that science advanced through an accumulation of valid facts (e.g., Carnap, 1962). This view of scientific advance was subsequently challenged by a number of philosophers including Hanson (1958) and Polanyi (1958) who saw this view as being too simplistic as these scientific 'facts' were always viewed through a prism of an assumptive world that directed their inquiry.

For brevity, and to summarize this debate, I shall focus on the work of Thomas Kuhn who wrote an influential work entitled *The Structure of Scientific Revolutions* (Kuhn, 1970). Kuhn was a student of theoretical physics who, during his late graduate career, shifted to the history, sociology, and philosophy of science. In his work, Kuhn also challenged the accepted notion that advancement in science was a result of an incremental process of accumulating more and more valid 'facts'-the so-called 'scientific development as a process of accretion' (p. 3).

In his exploration of scientific discovery, Kuhn observed that the kind of disagreements on fundamentals that appeared to pervade the social and psychological sciences (and I suspect that of mental health also) were not evident in such sciences as astronomy, physics, or biology. To explain this difference in approach, Kuhn introduced the notion of the 'paradigm' in scientific research. This, a now much overused term in general discourse, he defined as '… universally recognized scientific achievements that for a time provide model problems and solutions to a community of practitioners' (Kuhn; viii). As a paradigm implicitly defined the legitimate problems and methods of a research field for a succeeding generations of practitioners, 'normal science' was understood as scientists working on puzzles generated by the paradigm, without having to consider fundamentals. Thus, for Kuhn, (normal) science is '… like an accepted judicial decision in the common law, it is an object for further articulation and specification under new or more stringent conditions.' (Kuhn, p. 23)

Kuhn lays great stress-surprisingly for many scientists-that science is not a process of discovery; rather, it is a process to confirm through 'puzzle solving' that which might already be anticipated. Because the questions that might be answered are already predefined by the paradigm, they need to be '… firmly embedded in the educational initiation that prepares and licenses the student for professional practice. Because that education is both rigorous and rigid, these answers come to exert a deep hold on the scientific mind'. (p. 5)

This 'deep hold on the scientific mind' plays a crucial role in determining the kinds of questions asked, the methods used to answer them, the answers that might be deemed acceptable, and so on, but the crucial aspect is that practitioners buy into these assumptions in their training and by doing so no longer have to concern themselves with fundamentals in the field (that are now taken as 'given'). Hence, the scientist can focus on precise work that ultimately may generate anomalies. This ability to disregard 'fundamental questions' has an enormous advantage for the practitioner as it provides a consensual view of the world so that his or her function as a scientist is to confirm this through a series of more and precise measurements and technical accomplishments.

Training and membership to the scientific community is crucial to the functioning of paradigms. Kuhn writes, for instance, that 'The study of paradigms … is what mainly prepares the student for membership in a particular scientific community with which he will later practice. Because he there joins men who learnt the bases of their field from the same concrete models, his subsequent practice will seldom evoke overt disagreement. Men whose research is based on shared paradigms are committed to the same rules and standards for scientific practice.' (Kuhn, p. 11) Moreover, it is exclusive, as professional researchers no longer write for the public. 'Instead, they (i.e., his research articles) will appear as brief articles addressed only to professional colleagues, the men whose knowledge of a shared paradigm can be assumed and who prove to be the only ones able to read the papers addressed to them.' (Kuhn, p. 20)

This commitment to greater precision demanded in the practice of 'normal science' is critical in explaining how science advances, for this focused activity inevitably leads to 'anomalies' that stretch the paradigm and eventually leads to its replacement (i.e., a scientific revolution). Hence, Kuhn challenged the progress of science as an incremental process of gathering valid facts, observing that science advanced through a series of paradigmatic shifts (or revolutions) in which old phenomena (or 'facts') were viewed in new ways. Hence, 'progress' in science is best portrayed by a discontinuous process in which 'normal' scientific endeavours are punctuated by extraordinary change (i.e., revolutions). Examples are the Copernican Revolution, the overthrow of the Phlogiston Theory, and so on. However, according to Kuhn, these revolutions depended on scientists accepting the necessity of a shared paradigm in the first place.

Although Kuhn's views have been criticized (e.g., Lakatos & Musgrave, 1970), they do provide us with a possible answer as to why it is difficult to develop a science in the area of mental health in general and in forensic mental health in particular. Clearly, this latter task is difficult as it would require bringing together a broad range of disciplines-mental health, law, criminology, sociology, and so on-all of which have a legitimate interest in the area but which also are likely to have different priorities and ways of working. Indeed, as Kuhn himself acknowledges, 'history suggests that the road to a firm research consensus is extraordinarily arduous' (Kuhn, 1970; p. 15), and '... it remains an open question what parts of social science have yet acquired such paradigms at all.' Unfortunately, without an agreement on fundamentals, it is easy for practitioners to choose whichever 'facts' support their position and disregard those that contradict it. This, I believe, is one of the reasons why forensic mental health practice is slow to advance: that is, those who work within it are not working from a common paradigm.

I am arguing, therefore, that the challenge facing mental health practitioners if they wish their area to become a science (à la Kuhn) is to achieve a consensus on fundamentals so that 'normal science' can develop and prosper. And, there is some evidence that this is beginning to occur. Consider, for instance, how mental health professionals altered their view on whether mental disorder was (or was not) associated with violent offending. In the 1970s, the prevailing view was that mental disorder was not associated with violent offending; yet, within a decade, this view was reversed and replaced by its opposite (i.e., the mental disorder was related to violent offending; Beck & Wechel, 1998). This change of view was motivated by evidence that found increased rates of offending in those with mental disorder compared with that in the general population in several large cohorts (e.g., Hodgins *et al*, 1996) so that this evidence could not easily be discounted.

Once this association was accepted (I suggest that this represented a paradigmatic shift because of the fundamental nature of the assumptions), it legitimized a large endeavour to develop more and more precise measurements of this association. Hence, over the past two decades, there has been a concentration on the development of new risk measures to detect the relationship between the mental disorder and an offending history. For instance, this has seen the development of HCR-20, VRS, and so on, this technological development being exactly the kind of activity that might be predicted by Kuhn's theory. Those who developed these instruments were no longer concerned as to whether or not mental disorder was associated with offending. For them, the answer was clear and positive; so their role was to articulate this with greater and greater precision by developing the appropriate technology to measure this association.

Hence, there is evidence–supported by much of the developmental and experimental neuropsychological presentation at this meeting–that 'science' is beginning to develop in this area. Notwithstanding these developments, as the first paragraph makes clear, there is a considerable gap between what the science is able to tell us and what we need to know to respond to clinical demands. As this response cannot wait until all the 'science' is in, do we have anything sensible to recommend to those who are required to intervene in those with ASPD in their current day-to-day practice?

A possible way forward in the treatment of those with ASPD

Although I have pointed out that there are very few RCT data to justify intervening in those with ASPD, this condition has two advantages over other types of personality disorder to legitimize intervening in this group. First, there is a very large correctional literature that may have some relevance to those with ASPD, given that 50% of those in correctional settings meet the criteria for ASPD. Second, ASPD is associated not merely with personal costs (although that is indeed the case) but oftentimes has additional societal costs. These added costs need to be taken into account in any determination of the costs and benefits in intervening in this group.

Returning to the first point, I accept that the inclusion of the correctional literature reverses our earlier decision to exclude this in our systematic review; but I see this as being justified for the purposes of this chapter. The correctional literature with interventions to reduce reoffending is considerable, and although it parallels that in the mental health, there is little overlap between them. This correctional or 'what works' literature has already been discussed at length elsewhere (Blackburn, 2004; McGuire, 2004; Andrews & Bonta, 2006), so I will merely refer to McGuire's (2004) summary table in Fig. 17.1. The figure shows effect sizes for selected types of interventions from meta-analytic reviews, to illustrate the range of findings obtained. In the graph, the vertical line represents zero change (no difference between experimental and control samples), bars extending to the right represent *increases* in recidivism among experimental samples relative to controls, and bars to the left represent *reductions* in recidivism.

This table allows us to draw two important conclusions. Criminogenic programmes (on the right) that have a punitive intent either have no effect or increase the likelihood of subsequent reoffending; conversely, criminogenic programmes (on the left) with a therapeutic ethos have a positive effect in reducing future reoffending. Many of these positive programmes are based on cognitive behavioural principles and on the **R**isk-**N**eed-**R**esponsivity (RNR) principle (Andrews & Bonta, 2006): the principles of this programme are to match the programme with the offender's risk to reoffend (the **R** component), to assess criminogenic needs and target these with treatment (the **N** component), and finally, to tailor the intervention to the capacity of the offender to benefit from them (the **R** component). It is interesting to note in passing that in their more recent work, Bonta and Andrews (2007) distinguish between a general and a specific responsivity. They describe the latter as a 'fine tuning' of the cognitive behavioural therapy (CBT) approach so that it takes into account the personality characteristics of the individual-a point that we will return to in the following. Although criminogenic programmes have been criticized by mental health professionals as sometimes being too formulaic, this is often a result of inadequate resources rather then anything inherently in the programme as the 'responsivity' element makes clear.

The importance of estimating the costs and benefits of treatments for those with ASPD

Although some of these correctional programmes are effective, compared to the (usually) no treatment control, the decision to invest in them also needs to consider the costs of implementing the programme versus the money saved as a consequence. Although cost-effectiveness in

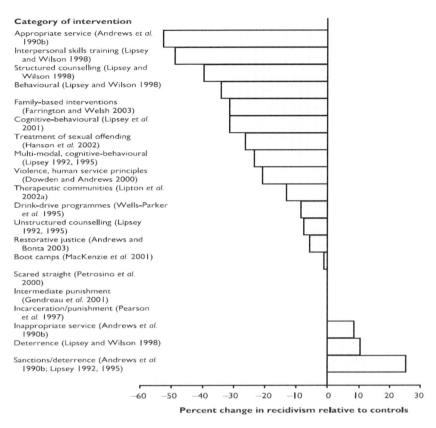

Fig. 17.1 Variations in effect sizes (*From* McGuire, 2004)

studies is only now becoming commonplace in the evaluation of mental health interventions (for instance, only four of the 27 trials [15%] reported a cost-effectiveness component in our systematic review described earlier), these are more commonplace in a correctional setting, but are again not without their critics (Welsh & Farrington, 2000; McDougall *et al.*, 2003). Nonetheless, I believe that correctional programmes lead the way in that they have a simple dichotomous outcome measure (reoffended or not?) and hence can provide data on costs that can usefully be interrogated.

As an example, I will briefly describe a study by Aos *et al.* (2001) who provided a report on the cost-effectiveness of different programmes to reduce reoffending in Washington State. They systematically analysed different programmes to determine whether their benefits (as measured by the value to the taxpayer, and to the victim as a result of subsequent crime reduction) were likely to outweigh their costs. The purpose of this exercise was clear: '… to help decision makers in directing scarce public resources *toward* economically successful programs and *away from* unsuccessful programs …' (my italics). Thus, the imperative to policymakers and those who controlled the public purse was clear: invest in those programmes that show a positive cost benefit and disinvest in programmes with a negative cost benefit.

The findings of Aos *et al.* are reported in Fig. 17.2 and Table 17.2. In the figure, the vertical line of no effect separates programmes that have a net cost benefit (on the right) with those with a negative benefit on the left. The programme evaluations are sequenced by age with the earliest interventions in childhood at the top proceeding to interventions for juveniles and finally for those for adults. A summary of the conclusions from the table is as

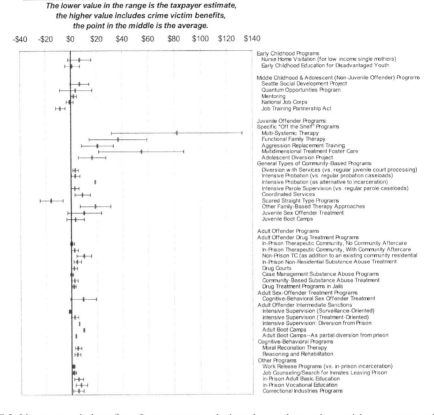

Fig. 17.2 Net economic benefits of programmes designed to reduce crime, with monetary values in 2000 dollars (*From* Aos *et al.*, 2001).

follows: (a) the greatest cost-benefit advantage is intervening in juveniles, (b) the greatest cost benefit is to the victim (not surprisingly) rather than society at large, (c) and programmes of the same effect size (e.g., Quantum Opportunities Programme and Multi-Systemic Therapy, both of which had an effect size of –0.31) may have very different benefits when their costs are taken into account.

No doubt, there is much with Aos *et al.*'s analysis that is deficient and will be contested. The reason, however, for reporting it here is to illustrate that this is a level that mental health

Table 17.2

Type of programme	Effect size	Cost of programme/head $	Net benefit for taxpayer $	Net benefit for taxpayer and victim $
Quantum opportunities programme	−0.31	18.964	−8 855	16 428
Multi-Systemic therapy	−0.31	4 743	31 681	131 918
In-prison therapeutic community	−0.05	2 804	−899	5 230
CBT sex offender treatment	−0.11	6 246	−778	19 534
Intensive supervision	−0.03	3 296	−2 250	−384
Reasoning and rehabilitation	−0.07	308	2 202	7 104

CBT, cognitive behavioural therapy.*Source*: From Aos *et al.*, 2001.

programmes need to attain if they are to remain competitive in attracting funding from the public purse to support their services.

In summary, I believe that one can draw the following conclusions from the McGuire and Aos *et al.* data: (a) interventions that are therapeutic, rather than punitive, are more likely to be beneficial in reducing reoffending; (b) the magnitude of this effect is age-dependent (i.e., the greatest impact is on juvenile offenders with a reduced effect on young children or adults); and (c) for some crimes (especially those involving violence), the cost benefits in favour of the intervention are often considerable as the costs of these types of crimes are often very high.

Although, overall, the effect of these criminogenic programmes in reducing reoffending is positive, their overall effect size is not massive. Losel (1998), for instance, has calculated that their mean effect size as 0.10–0.12 (i.e., a 10–12% reduction of the active intervention over the control). Further, despite the theoretical power of the RNR model, it is not without its critics, who argue for its reconstruction (Ward *et al.*, 2007). If we assume, and I accept it is an unproven but I believe nonetheless reasonable assumption, that

(a) Fifty per cent of those in prisons have ASPD;
(b) Those with ASPD are as likely as not to be treated in correctional programmes (as there is no explicit attempt to exclude them because the presence or absence of ASPD is not an entry criterion to treatment); and
(c) The presence of ASPD itself but moreover its co-occurrence with many other Axis 1 and Axis 11 conditions is likely to have a detrimental effect on the effectiveness of correctional programmes (Newton-Howes *et al.*, 2006)

Then, these assumptions have a number of therapeutic implications.

One could argue, for instance, that this modest effect of current correctional programmes might be enhanced if the specific psychological vulnerabilities of the subset of ASPD offenders were addressed during programme development (as suggested by Bonta & Andrews, 2007). This might include a need to address a high level of impulsivity, treating co-occurring Axis 1 disorders, substance misuse, non-compliance with treatment, and so on, many of which feature in those with ASPD. For instance, Tyrer *et al.* (2003) subdivided those with personality disorder into treatment seekers and treatment rejecters, with those with ASPD having several features suggesting that they would reject treatment (e.g., hostility, poor education, etc.). Consequently, there is much that mental health services can to contribute to already existing programmes for offenders.

For this to be a meaningful, however, we need a mechanism that links convincingly the features of ASPD to their poor response to interventions; for this we need a theory of personality disorder. Unfortunately, we currently lack such a theory for personality in general and for ASPD in particular. This echoes Epstein's (1987) observation made 30 years ago on the absence of a good theory for personality disorder: 'The joker in the deck is how to get a good theory.' Clearly, the essence of a scientific enterprise is a continuous interaction between observation and conceptualization, or expressed otherwise, between empiricism and theory construction.

Although much of Epstein's plea still remains the case, I believe that we are now in possession of a sufficient number of 'empirical' facts to begin developing such a theory. For instance, this conference, and others like it, has identified a prototypic ASPD individual as someone with development trajectory who, as a result of innate temperamental difficulties interacting with a harsh and inconsistent parenting style, results in a '… child [who] never acquires the social skills and regulatory mechanisms necessary to navigate the world of adolescence. The child consistently fails to attend to relevant social cues, readily makes hostile attributions about peers and adults, accesses aggressive responses in social situations, and either impulsively performs these responses, without thinking about their consequences or evaluates their likely outcomes as acceptable and selects them.' (Dodge, 2000)

The clinician dealing with those with ASPD will recognize many of these features (i.e., the lack of social skills, the paranoid thinking that leads to hostile attributions, aggression in social situations and impulsivity without thought as to the consequences, etc.) The problem with this description is that it merely a collection of undesirable traits. What is required therefore is a unifying theory that brings these disparate elements together to produce a personality construct.

What, then, are the core psychological characteristics of those with ASPD that could aid theory development? I believe that these are best captured by Benjamin (1993) in the following quotation:

'There is a pattern of inappropriate and unmodulated desire *to control others*, implemented in a *detached manner*. There is a strong need to be independent, to resist being controlled by others, who are usually held in contempt. There is a willingness to use untamed aggression to back up the need for control or independence. The ASP[D] usually presents in a friendly, sociable manner, but that friendliness is always accompanied by a baseline position of detachment. He or she doesn't care what happens to self or others.' (p. 198; my italics)

My interpretation of Benjamin's quotation is as follows. First, the core personality characteristics of ASPD are described as both (a) a need to be in control and (b) also to be detached. (This resonates with the 'callous-unemotional behaviour' ascribed to the psychopath.) Second, there are secondary consequences of these primary characteristics of (a) using 'untamed aggression' to maintain control and (b) a carelessness (or thoughtlessness) about what happens to self or others, thereby leading to risky behaviour. Thus, although the surface phenomena of violent and irresponsible behaviour may be the most visible aspects of ASPD, Benjamin draws to our attention that this behaviour is a consequence of a deeper psychological need to be in control while remaining detached. This need to be in control explains why those with ASPD are largely 'treatment resisting' so that they are (a) difficult to engage in treatment and (b) difficult to maintain in treatment once engaged. Correctional programmes for those with ASPD need to be informed by this thinking and enhanced accordingly if their current level of effectiveness is to be improved.

Is the problem that the evidence exists but is ignored by policymakers and politicians?

In light of the foregoing, it is difficult to argue that policymakers and politicians ignore evidence offered to them as it is clear that there is little evidence to start with. Muir-Gray (2001) indeed makes the point that politicians are often blamed unfairly for ignoring scientific evidence when, in fact, the real issue is that this evidence does not exist. He provides an example where the Government made a decision to reject mass screening for carcinoma of the prostrate on the evidence from two high-quality meta-analyses. The implication is clear: there is an imperative for scientists and clinicians to provide decision makers with the appropriate evidence to allow the latter to arrive at the best decision.

Muir-Gray goes on to distinguish between 'decision making' and 'decision taking'. The former involves (and indeed ought to involve) contributions from scientists and clinicians so that those who ultimately have to make decisions on behalf of the public are properly informed. However, when these decisions are finally 'taken', additional considerations that go beyond the 'evidence' professionals seek and ought to make a contribution, as such 'values' and 'resources' have also to be considered by those who have charge of the public purse. As the trust of this contribution is that we have failed at the 'decision-making' phase (i.e., in not being able to provide evidence for the reasons given in the preceding), we can hardly blame politicians and policymakers in not 'taking' the correct decision when they have to do so.

Conclusion

To answer the question in the title, my response is the following:

(a) We have very limited scientific evidence for effective interventions in offenders with ASPD from the mental health field. However, the evidence from correctional pro-grammes does exist and it is likely that these interventions are being offered to those with ASPD-both in custodial settings and in the community by probation services. The effectiveness of these interventions is likely to be enhanced if the core psychological characteristics of those with ASPD are taken into account.
(b) The failure to develop a consensus on some crucial aspects of ASPD and its interven-tions has severely hampered the field and limited its progress. This failure to agree on fundamentals is partly a result of the several different disciplines in this field, but this absence of consensus inhibits its 'scientific' development and needs to be overcome if it is to produce high-quality scientific evidence.
(c) In the light of (a) and (b), we are in a weak position to influence the political process in the allocation of funds; so, unless and until these areas are addressed, interventions for those with ASPD are likely to continue to remain in scientific limbo.

Acknowledgements

I wish to acknowledge the contributions of my fellow reviewers Nick Huband, Nadja Smailagic, Mike Ferriter, and Clive Adams for their assistance in the preparation of the systematic reviews and a special thanks to Nick Huband for his help in chasing up innumerable references.

References

Anon (2000). *A Framework for Development and Evaluation of RCTs for Complex Interventions to Improve Health*. London: Medical Research Council.

Andrews, D. A., & Bonta, J. (2006). *The Psychology of Criminal Conduct*, 4th edn. Newark, NJ: LexisNexis.

Aos, S., Phipps, P., Barnoski, R., & Leib, R. (2001). *The Comparative Costs and Benefits of Programs to Reduce Crime*. [Online], Olympia, WA: Washington State Institute for Public Policy. Available at: http://www.wa.gov/wsipp

Arndt, I. O., Dorozynski, L., McLellan, A. T., Woody, G. E., & O'Brien, C. P. (1992). Controlled study of desipramine treatment of cocaine dependence in methadone treated patients. *Archives of General Psychiatry, 49*, 888–893.

Arndt, I. O., McClellan, A. T., Dorozynsky, L., Woody, G. E., & O'Brien, C. P. (1994). Desipramine treatment for cocaine dependence: role of antisocial personality disorder. *Journal of Nervous and Mental Disease, 182*(3), 151–156.

Beck, J., & Wechel, H. (1998). Violent crime and Axis 1 psychopathology. In A. E. Skodol (ed), *Psychopathology and Violent Crime* (pp. 1–13). Washington, DC: American Psychiatric Association.

Benjamin, L. S. (1993). *Interpersonal Diagnosis and the Treatment of Personality Disorders*. New York: Guilford Press.

Black, D. W., Baumgard, C. H., Bell, S. E., & Kao, C. (1996). Death rates in 71 men with antisocial personality disorder. *Psychomatics, 37*, 131–136.

Black, D. W., & Braun, D. (1998). A comparison of those with and without childhood conduct disorder. *Annals of Clinical Psychiatry, 10*, 53–57.

Blackburn, R. (2004). 'What works' with mentally disordered offenders. *Psychology*, Crime and Law, 10, 297–308.

Bloom, J. D., Meuser, K. T., & Müller-Isberner, R. (2000). Treatment implications of the antecedents of criminality and violence in schizophrenia and major affective disorders. In S. Hodgins (ed), *Violence among the Mentally Ill* (pp. 145–165). Dordrecht, the Netherlands: Kluwer Academic.

Brooner, R. K., Kidorf, M., King, V. L., & Stoller, K. (1998). Preliminary evidence of good treatment response in antisocial drug abusers. *Drug and Alcohol Dependence, 49*(3), 249–260.

Burns, T., Creed, F., Fahy, T., Thompson, S., Tyrer, P., & White, I. for the UK 700 Group. (1999). Intensive versus standard case management for severe psychotic illness: a randomised trial. *Lancet, 353*(9171), 2185–2189.

Carnap, R. (1962). *Logical Foundations of Probability*, 2nd edn. Chicago, IL: University of Chicago Press.

Coccaro, E. F., & Kavoussi, R. J. (1997). Fluoxetine and impulsive aggressive behaviour in personality-disordered subjects. *Archives of General Psychiatry, 54*, 1081–1088.

Coid, J., Yang, M., Tyrer, P., Roberts, A., & Ullrich, S. (2006). Prevalence and correlates of personality disorder in Great Britain. *British Journal of Psychiatry, 188*, 423–431.

Compton, W. M., Conway, K. P., Stinson, F. S., Colliver, J. D., & Grant B. F. (2005). Prevalence, correlates and comorbidity of DSM-1V antisocial personality syndromes and alcohol and specific drug use disorders in the United States: results from the National Epidemiological Survey on Alcohol and Related Conditions. *Journal of Clinical Psychiatry, 66*, 677–685.

De Brito, S., & Hodgins, S. (in press). Antisocial personality disorder. In M. McMurran, & R. Howard (eds), *Personality, Personality Disorders, and Risk of Violence*. Chichester, UK: Wiley.

Dodge, K. A. (2000). Conduct disorder. In A. Sameroff, M. Lewis, & S. M. Miller (eds), *Handbook of Developmental Psychopathology* (pp. 447–463). New York: Guilford.

Dolan, B., & Coid, J. (1993). *Psychopathic Personality and Antisocial Personality Disorders: Treatment and Research Issues*. London: Gaskell.

Duggan, C., Adams, C., McCarthy, L., Fenton, M., Lee, T., Binks, C., *et al.* (2006). A systematic review of the effectiveness of pharmacological and psychological treatments for those with personality disorder. National Forensic Mental Health Research and Development Programme [Online], Available at: http://www.nfmhp.org.uk/MRD%2012%2033%20%final%20%Report.pdf

Duggan, C., Huband, N., Smailagic, N., Ferriter, N, & Adams, C. (2007). The use of psychological treatments for people with personality disorder: a systematic review of randomized controlled trials. *Personality and Mental Health, 1*, 95–125.

Duggan, C., Huband, N., Smailagic, N., Ferriter, N., & Adams, C. (under review). The use of pharmacological treatments for people with personality disorder: a systematic review of randomized controlled trials. *Personality and Mental Health* (due 2008).

Epstein, S. (1987). The relative value of theoretical and empirical approaches for establishing a psychological diagnostic system. *Journal of Personality Disorders, 1*, 100–109.

Fazel, S., & Danesh, J. (2002). Serious mental disorder in 23,000 prisoners: a systematic review of 62 surveys. *Lancet, 359*, 545–550.

Gilbody, S., House, A., & Sheldon, T.A. (2003). *Outcome Measurement in Psychiatry: A Critical Review of Outcome Measurement in Psychiatric Research and Practice*. York, UK: The University of York Centre for Reviews and Dissemination.

Goodwin, R. D., & Hamilton, S. P. (2003). Lifetime comorbidity of antisocial personality disorder and anxiety disorders among adults in the community. *Psychiatry Research, 117*, 159–166.

Hanson, N. R. (1958). *Patterns of Discovery*. Cambridge: Cambridge University Press.

Hare, R. D., Clark, D., Grann, M., & Thornton, D. (2000). Psychopathy and the predictive validity of the PCL-R: an international perspective. *Behavioral Sciences and the Law, 18*, 623–645.

Hare, R. D., Hart, S. D., & Harper, T. J. (1991). Psychopathy and the DSM-IV criteria for antisocial personality disorder. *Journal of Abnormal Psychology, 100*, 391–398.

Hart, S. D., & Hare, R. D. (1989). Discriminant validity of the Psychopathy Checklist in a forensic psychiatric population. *Psychological Assessment: A Journal of Consulting and Clinical Psychology, 1*, 211–218.

Hodgins, S., Mednick, S., Brennan, A., Schulsinger, F., & Engberg, M. (1996). Mental disorder and crime: evidence from a Danish birth cohort. *Archives of General Psychiatry, 53*, 489–496.

Hollin, C. (2006). Offending behaviour programmes and contenuation: evidence-based practice, manuals, and programme evaluation. In C. R. Hollin, & E. J. Palmer (eds), *Offending Behaviour Programme: Development, Application and Controversies*. Chichester, UK: Wiley.

Kuhn, T. S. (1970). *The Structure of Scientific Revolutions*, 2nd edn. Chicago, IL: University of Chicago Press.

Lakatos, I., & Musgrave, A. (eds) (1970). *Criticism and the Growth of Knowledge*. Cambridge: Cambridge University Press.

Leal, J., Ziedonis, D., & Kosten, T. (1994). Antisocial personality disorder as a prognostic factor for pharmacotherapy of cocaine dependence. *Drug and Alcohol Dependence, 35*, 31–35.

Lenzenweger, M. F., Lane, M. C., Loranger, A. W., & Kessler, R. C. (2007). DSM-1V personality disorders in the National Comorbidity Survey replication. *Biological Psychiatry, 62*, 553–564.

Lewontin, R. C. (1995). Sex, lies and social science. *New York Review of Books, 42*, 7.

Lilienfeld, S. O. (1998). Methodological advances and developments in the assessment of psychopathy. *Behaviour Research and Therapy, 36*, 99–125.

Livesley, W. J., Reiffer, L. I., Sheldon, A. E. R., & West, M. (1987). Prototypicality ratings of DSM-III criteria for personality disorders. *Journal of Nervous and Mental Disease, 175*, 395–401.

Loeber, R., Burke, J. D., & Lahey, B. B. (2002). What are the adolescent antecedents to antisocial personality disorder? *Criminal Behaviour and Mental Heath, 12(1)*, 24–36.

Losel, F. (1998). Treatment and management of psychopaths. In D. J. Cooke, A. E. Forth, & R. D. Hale. (eds), *Psychopathy, Theory, Research and Implications for Society* (pp. 303–354). Dordrecht, the Netherlands: Kluwer Academic.

Martin, R. L., Cloninger, R., Guze, S. B., & Clayton, P. J. (1985). Mortality in a follow-up of 500 psychiatric outpatients. *Archives of General Psychiatry, 42*, 47–54; 58–66.

McDougall, C., Cohen, M. A., Swaray, R., & Perry, A. (2003). The costs and benefits of sentencing: a systematic review. *Annals of the American Academy of Political and Social Sciences, 587*, 160–177.

McGuire, J. (2004). *Understanding Psychology and Crime: Perspectives on Theory and Action*. Maidenhead, UK: Open University Press/McGraw Hill Education.

Millon, T., Simonsen, E., & Birket-Smith, M. (1998). Historical conceptions of psychopathy in the United States and Europe. In T. Millon, E. Simonsen, M. Birket-Smith, & R.Davis (eds), *Psychopathy, Antisocial, Criminal and Violent Behaviour* (pp. 3–31). New York: Guilford Press.

Moffit, T. E., Caspi, A., Rutter, M., & Silva, P.A. (2001). *Sex Differences in Antisocial Behaviour: Conduct Disorder, Delinquency, and Violence in the Dunedin Longitudinal Study*. New York: Cambridge University Press.

Moran, P. (1999). *Antisocial Personality Disorder: An Epidemiological Perspective*. London: Gaskell.

Muir-Gray, J. A. (2001). Using systematic reviews for evidence based policy making. In. M. Egger, G. Davey-Smith, & D. Altman (eds), *Systematic Reviews in Health Care* (pp. 410–418). London: BMJ Books.

Newton-Howes, G., Tyrer, P., & Johnston, T. (2006). Personality disorder and the outcome of depression: meta- analysis of published studies. *British Journal of Psychiatry, 188*, 13–20.

Ogloff, J. R. P. (2006). Psychopathy/antisocial personality disorder conundrum. *Australian and New Zealand Journal of Psychiatry, 40*, 519–528.

Perdiouri, M., Rathbone, G., Huband, N., & Duggan C. (2007). A comparison of adults with antisocial personality traits with and without childhood conduct disorder. *Annals of Clinical Psychiatry*, *19*(1), 17–23.

Polanyi, M. (1958). *Personal Knowledge*. Chicago, IL: Chicago University Press.

Robins, L. N. (1987). Epidemiology of antisocial personality. In R. Michels *et al.* (eds), *Psychiatry, Vol 3* (pp. 1–14). Philadelphia, PA: J. B. Lippincott Company.

Robins, L. N., Tipp, J., & Przybeck, T. (1991). Antisocial personality. In L. N. Robins, & D. A. Regier (eds), *Psychiatric Disorders in America* (pp. 258–290). New York: Free Press.

Scadding, J. C. (1967). Diagnosis: the clinician and the computer. *Lancet, ii*, 877–882.

Scott, S., Knapp, M., Henderson, J., & Maughan, B. (2001). Financial cost of social exclusion: follow-up study of antisocial children into adulthood. *British Medical Journal*, *323*, 191–195.

Simonoff, E., Elander, J., Holmshaw, J, Pickles, A., Murray, R., & Rutter, M. (2004). Predictors of antisocial personality disorder. *Continuities from childhood to adult life. British Journal of Psychiatry*, *184*, 118–127.

Singleton, N., Meltzer, H., & Gatward, R. (1998). *Psychiatric Morbidity among Prisoners in England and Wales*. London: Stationary Office.

Slade, M., & Priebe, S. (2001). Are randomised controlled trials the only gold that glitters? *British Journal of Psychiatry*, *179*, 286–287.

Stein, L. I., & Test, M. A. (1980). Alternatives to mental hospital treatment. 1: Conceptual model, treatment programme and clinical evaluation. *Archives of General Psychiatry, 37*, 392–397.

Swanson, M. C., Bland, R. C., & Newman, S. C. (1994). Epidemiology of psychiatric disorders in Edmonton. *Antisocial personality disorders. Acta Psychiatrica Scandinavica, 376*(Supplementum), 63–70.

Tennant, G., Tennant, D., Prins, H., & Bedford, A. (1990). Psychopathic disorder—a useful clinical concept? *Medicine, Science, and Law, 30*, 39–44.

Torgensen, S., Kringlen, E., & Cramer, V. (2001). The prevalence of personality disorders in a community sample. *Archives of General Psychiatry, 58*, 590–596.

Tyrer, P. (2000). Are small case-loads beautiful in severe mental illness? *British Journal of Psychiatry, 177*, 386–287.

Tyrer, P., Mitchard, S., Methuen, C., & Ranger M. (2003). Treatment-rejecting and treatment-seeking personality disorders: type R and type S. *Journal of Personality Disorders, 17*(3), 268–270.

Ward, T., Melser, J., & Yates, P. M. (2007). Reconstructing the Risk-Need-Responsivity model: a theoretical elaboration and evaluation. *Aggression and Violent Behaviour, 12*, 208–228.

Warren, F., McGauley, G., Norton, K., Dolan, B., Preedy-Fayers, K., Pickering, A., *et al.* (2003). *Review of Treatment for Severe Personality Disorder*. Home Office Report 30/03. London: Home Office.

Welsh, B. C., & Farrington, D. P. (2000). Correctional intervention programs and cost-benefit analysis. *Criminal Justice and Behaviour, 27*, 115–133.

Widiger, T. A., & Corbitt, E. M. (1993). Antisocial personality disorder: proposals for DSM-IV. *Journal of Personality Disorders, 7*(1), 63–77.

Widiger, T. A., & Frances, A. J. (1985). Axis 11 personality disorders: diagnostic and treatment issues. *Hospital and Community Psychiatry, 36*, 619–627.

18

Understanding development and prevention of chronic physical aggression: Towards experimental epigenetic studies

Richard E. Tremblay

> '[Both] the lack of regularity in the succession of living beings, [and] the variation in species which produces monsters with reference to the typical being, must come from either the germ or an external cause. The first doctrine was still tenable at a time when we could believe in the pre-existence of germs; but nowadays I admit, with everybody, the doctrine of epigenesis. Every normal egg which gives birth to an abnormal individual is influenced by external agents whatever they are; this is what I call action of the milieu.' (Quatrefages, 1863[1])

Introduction

The preceding citation comes from a heated debate that Quatrefages had with one of his colleagues at the Anthropological Society in Paris after he read a letter he had solicited from Charles Darwin in July 1863. The nature-nurture debate has always been a central issue among naturalists, but it was also central to moral philosophers. The first phrase of Rousseau's masterpiece on children's education is a good example: 'Everything is good as it leaves the hands of the author of things; everything degenerates in the hands of man.' (Rousseau, 1762, 1762/1979) A century later, Charles Darwin took a diametrically opposite view. In his autobiography, he writes: *'I can say in my own favour that I was as a boy humane, but I owed this entirely to the instruction and example of my sisters. I doubt indeed whether humanity is a natural or innate quality.'* (Darwin, 1876/1983; p. 11)

The social learning theorists who dominated research on the development of aggression during the last half of the twentieth century were clearly siding with Rousseau rather than Darwin. The main thrust of their argument was that children learned to aggress from their environment-that is, family, peers, neighbourhoods, and the media (e.g., Bandura, 1973; Reiss & Roth, 1993; Human Capital Initiative Coordinating Committee, 1997; Anderson *et al.*, 2003; NIH, 2004;).

The learning of aggression hypothesis led to the idea that some children learn to aggress early in life whereas others learn later. In its report 'Violence and Health', the World Health Organization concluded: 'The majority of young people who become violent are

---

[1] 'Pour que la succession des êtres ne soit pas régulière, pour que l'espèce varie et produise des êtres qui par rapport au type sont des monstres, il faut que cela provienne ou du germe ou d'une cause extérieure. La première doctrine était encore soutenable à l'époque où l'on pouvait croire à la préexistence des germes; mais de nos jours j'admets, avec tout le monde, la doctrine de l'épigénèse. Tout œuf normal qui donne naissance à un individu anormal est influencé par les agents extérieurs quels qu'ils soient; c'est là ce que j'appelle actions de milieu.'

adolescent-limited offenders who, in fact, show little or no evidence of high levels of aggression or other problem behaviours during their childhood.' (WHO, 2002; p. 31) The citation at the end of that phrase suggests that the WHO experts came to the conclusion that violent behaviour is learned de novo during adolescence based on a 2001 report from the US Surgeon General written by a committee of US experts on the development of aggression (US Surgeon General, 2001).

Determining when violent individuals learn to aggress is critical for finding means of preventing chronic physical aggression (CPA). Before summarizing the state of knowledge on this issue, a definition is needed for the term *prevention*. The traditional classification of disease prevention efforts is useful here (Mrazek & Haggerty, 1994): (a) primary prevention attempts to prevent the onset of the disease, (b) secondary prevention attempts to prevent progression of the disease, and (c) tertiary prevention attempts to prevent the negative consequences of the disease.

The focus of this chapter is primary prevention of CPA, and hence prevention of its onset. Two other terms need to be defined to clear any misunderstanding: *physical aggression* and *chronic*. *Physical aggression* is the use of behaviours, such as the following, in antagonistic interactions with other humans: hitting, slapping, kicking, biting, pushing, grabbing, pulling, shoving, throwing objects, beating, twisting, or choking. *Chronic* physical aggression is defined as use of physical aggressions at a significantly higher rate than ones' birth cohort members over an extended period of time. The time period needs to be defined according to the study objectives.

I stress the importance of definitions because research on aggression has long been handicapped by misunderstandings concerning the behaviour being studied. (Hartup & Dewit, 1974; Tremblay *et al.*, 1991; Tremblay, 2000, 2003). A recent example comes from an exhaustive meta-analysis of prevention experiments. In an article titled 'School-Based Interventions for Aggressive and Disruptive Behaviour', Wilson and Lipsey (2007) compiled results of 249 experimental and quasi-experimental prevention studies in schools (pre-kindergarten to 12th grade) published in English. The authors reported that 'positive overall intervention effects were found on aggressive and disruptive behaviour and other relevant outcomes' and concluded: 'Schools seeking prevention programmes may choose from a range of effective programmes with some confidence that whatever they pick will be effective'. This meta-analysis published in one of the leading prevention journal appears to be extremely good news for the prevention of physical violence among our youth and for society in general. Unfortunately, a footnote in the methodology section tempers our enthusiasm. The authors write: 'Ideally, we would have liked to examine programme effects only on aggressive behaviour. However, almost none of the measures that call themselves aggressive behaviour measures focus solely on physically aggressive interpersonal behaviour. Many include disruptiveness, acting out, and other forms of behaviour problems that are negative, but not necessarily aggressive.' (Wilson & Lipsey, 2007; p. 134)

This article is extremely important because it leads us to the conclusion that after 249 preventive experiments, over more than half a century, we have little evidence of the extent to which we can prevent CPA by interventions with school-age children. In fact, it is unclear what we can prevent when investigators use total scores of deviant behaviours, which have different developmental trajectories and different causal mechanisms. For example, Barker *et al.* (2007) recently showed that physical aggression and theft during adolescence have different developmental trajectories and are inversely correlated to neurocognitive performance.

Do we need to start all over again the last 50 years of research with a slight modification to our evaluation design, that is, ensuring that we do assess CPA after preventive interventions with school-age children?

If CPA onset is during adolescence, as claimed by the US Surgeon General and the WHO, one would expect that the best time to implement preventive interventions would be during the elementary and early secondary school years. This clearly appears to be what prevention researchers have been thinking over the past 50 years if we rely on Wilson and Lipsey's meta-analysis. They reported that 49% of the interventions targeted youth who were older than 10 years of age, 43% targeted children who were between 6 and 10 years of age, whereas only 8% targeted 4-5-year-old children. Interestingly, when a random sample of the Canadian population was asked the best age for preventing physical aggression, the opinion matched almost perfectly what the researchers have been doing over the past half century (Tremblay *et al.*, 2003). However, recent longitudinal studies of physical aggression from infancy to adulthood suggest that we need to revisit the traditional beliefs of the general public and the prevention researchers.

When should we attempt to prevent the onset of chronic physical aggression?

The public's focus on violence during adolescence and its prevention during the school years is easy to understand because physical dangerousness, defined as the potential physical harm to a victim, increases with age in young humans and reaches its peak in late adolescence. The most obvious reason for this increase in dangerousness with age is that physical growth from birth to late adolescence increases height, weight, and the power of muscles needed for physical aggression. With the advent of puberty, and a spectacular increase in testosterone levels, the change of magnitude in muscle power is especially noteworthy for adolescent males. In other words, it is less dangerous for a teacher or a neighbour to gain control of a physically aggressive 6-year-old boy than a 17-year-old adolescent.

Research on antisocial behaviour has also focused on the school years because schools are a convenient place to recruit samples of youth, interview them, and experiment interventions. Furthermore, pre-adolescents and adolescents are more likely to understand written questionnaires than younger children. Thus, most longitudinal studies on the development of behaviour problems over the past half century focused on pre-adolescents and adolescents. Our understanding of the origin and development of physical aggression was further handicapped by 'aggression' studies focusing on disruptive behaviours or antisocial behaviour in general rather than on physical aggression (Tremblay *et al.*, 1991; Tremblay, 2000; Wilson & Lipsey, 2007)

The first long-term prospective annual assessment of children's physical aggression development was published at the end of the 1980s by Cairns and his collaborators (1989). Results were far from confirming that children learn to physically aggress during adolescence. The mean frequency of physical aggressions by boys and girls from poor areas in North Carolina was shown to decrease substantially from 10 to 18 years of age. This was true whether teacher reports or self-reports were used to monitor the development of physical aggression.

The main argument offered to explain the discrepancy between the observed developmental data and the popular developmental theories was that although the mean level of physical aggression decreases with age, there is a group of children who eventually start to physically aggress chronically during adolescence without having used physical aggression during childhood. Although some suggested that this would be a small group of individuals (Loeber & Stouthamer-Loeber, 1998), most reviews of the literature still conclude that physical aggression is learned from one's environment, especially peers and the media, during adolescence (DHHS, 2001; WHO, 2002; Anderson *et al.*, 2003; NIH, 2004; Tremblay, 2006). Declining mean levels of physical aggression from 10 to 18 years of age were not sufficient to convince aggression specialists that physical aggression is not learned during adolescence. Analyses of the variability in developmental trajectories of physical aggression with long-term prospective repeated assessments were needed to challenge the traditional learning hypothesis. The first analysis of physical aggression trajectories from 6 to 15 years of age used a sample of males from low socio-economic areas in a large North-American city (see Fig. 18.1; Nagin & Tremblay, 1999). Results led to three important conclusions: (i) frequency of physical aggressions reported by the teachers peaked at the start of the study when the boys were in kindergarten, (ii) the frequency of physical aggressions reported by the teachers decreased from 6 to 15 years of age for 96% of the boys, and (iii) the boys on the high-frequency physical aggression trajectory (4%) were most likely to report high frequency of physical violence at 17 years of age. Similar results were obtained with other large samples of males in New Zealand and the United States (Broidy *et al.*, 2003).

The results of these developmental trajectory analyses were clearly showing that the postulated 'learning' of physical aggression by males as well as the onset of CPA was either occurring during the kindergarten year or before kindergarten, not during the elementary school years, and certainly not during adolescence.

It became very clear that we needed to describe the development of physical aggression during the preschool years to understand the onset of physical aggression as well as the onset of CPA. However, none of the longitudinal birth cohorts initiated between the 1940s and the 1980s had made repeated assessments of physical aggression during the preschool years. New longitudinal studies of birth cohorts were needed. The results from four of these studies in Canada (Tremblay *et al.*, 1999; Tremblay *et al.*, 2004; Côté *et al.*, 2006; Côté *et al.*, 2007), in the Netherlands (Alink *et al.*, 2006), and in the United States (NICHD & ECCR Network, 2004) led to the same observations (see Fig. 18.2): (i) physical aggression starts

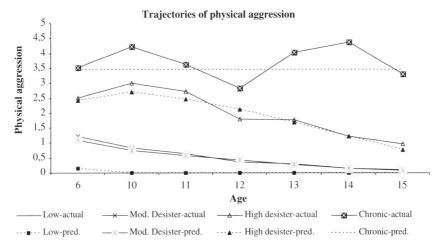

Fig. 18.1 Trajectories of physical aggression between 6 and 15 years of age (N = 1037 males). (*From* Nagin & Tremblay, 1999).

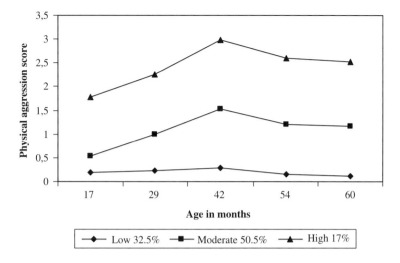

Fig. 18.2 Trajectories of physical aggression between 17 and 60 months (n = 1758 females and males). (*From* Côté *et al.*, 2007)

between the end of the first and second year after birth, (ii) the frequency peaks between the end of the third and fourth year, (iii) females desist earlier than males, and (iv) CPA onsets with onset of physical aggression in infancy. These observations lead to three conclusions that are at odds with the traditional view that humans learn to use physical aggression and that they do so by imitation, especially of the media (Reiss & Roth, 1993; Human Capital Initiative Coordinating Committee, 1997; Anderson *et al.*, 2003): (i) children spontaneously use physical aggression, (ii) rather than learn to physically aggress they learn not to physically aggress, and (iii) children learn not to physically aggress mainly during the preschool years.

These three conclusions have important consequences for the prevention of physical aggression. First, there is probably no good reason to prevent onset of physical aggression if it is a normal behaviour that is eventually replaced by more 'civilized' forms of anger expression, resource acquisition, and assertiveness. Second, efforts to prevent CPA should probably target high-risk individuals before or during the developmental period when they are normally learning alternatives to physical aggression. Third, preventive interventions should target factors that increase the risk of frequent physical aggressions as well as factors that increase the probability of learning alternatives to physical aggressions.

What are the risk factors for chronic physical aggression?

Longitudinal studies tracing the developmental trajectories of physical aggression have also identified risk factors that could be used as targets for preventive interventions. For example, results from the Québec Longitudinal Study of Children (Tremblay *et al.*, 2004) showed that two of the classic family risks, parent separation before birth and low income, predicted high physical aggression during early childhood. Mother characteristics before birth were among the best predictors: frequent antisocial behaviour during adolescence, giving birth before 21 years of age, not having finished high school, and smoking during pregnancy. Smoking apparently affects the development of the foetal brain (Wakschlag *et al.*, 1997; Brennan *et al.*, 1999; Maughan *et al.*, 2004; Button *et al.*, 2007; Jacobsen *et al.*, 2007; Huijbregts *et al.*, 2008). As expected, males were more at risk than females of being on the high physical aggression trajectory, even when the assessment started at 17 months of age. After controlling for prenatal assessments, the fifth month after birth assessments revealed two significant predictors: family dysfunction and coercive-hostile parenting by the mothers. Interestingly, a twin study also showed that at 17 months of age more than half of the variation in frequency of physical aggression was explained by genetic factors (Dionne *et al.*, 2003). One would expect that many of the mother characteristics that were identified as risk factors are mediators of mother's genetic characteristics (Maughan *et al.*, 2004) or interact with the child's genetic characteristics (Kim-Cohen *et al.*, 2006).

In summary, the traditional predictors of adolescent antisocial behaviour are predicting CPA during the preschool years. An important finding for planning the timing of preventive interventions is that all of the risk factors are present during pregnancy or soon after birth. Hence, they could be the target of interventions starting during the prenatal and early post-natal periods.

Have early childhood interventions been shown to prevent chronic physical aggression?

As would be expected from the Wilson and Lipsey (2007) meta-analysis, to our knowledge, no preschool preventive intervention assessed long-term impact on CPA. However, two preventive interventions during the preschool years have shown long-term preventive effects on general antisocial behaviour. The Perry Preschool experiment with 3- and 4-year-olds (Schweinhart *et al.*, 2005) was focused on stimulating cognitive development and showed impressive reduction of adult criminal behaviour among males. A home visitation by nurses from pregnancy to 24 months after birth also reported long-term impact on adolescent delinquency. Investigators randomly allocated a nurse home visitation programme to young underprivileged pregnant women from New York State at high risk of child abuse and neglect. These children were obviously also at high risk of CPA. The long-term follow-up of the children from the intervention group showed that they were less frequently abused and neglected; they were also less likely to exhibit delinquent behaviours during adolescence (Olds *et al.*, 1986; Olds *et al.*, 1998).

Finally, an adoption study is of interest here because it may indicate the maximum effect that can be expected from an early intensive intervention. Van Dussen *et al.* (1983) used Danish records to collect the criminal convictions of adopted females (N = 6374) and males (N = 5649) with reference to the biological and adoptive parents' socio-economic status (SES). Males with high SES biological parents were less likely to have a criminal conviction if they were adopted into a high SES family (9.3%) than if they were adopted into a low SES family (13.8%). Similarly, males with low SES biological parents were less likely to have a criminal record if they were adopted into a high SES family (12.98%) than if they were adopted by a family with the low SES of the biological parents (18.04%). Note that the former (low SES biological-high SES adoptive) are as likely to have a criminal record as the high SES biological-low SES adoptive (12.98% versus 13.8%). The largest difference between groups of males was between the high SES biological-high SES adoptive (9.3%) and the low SES biological-low SES adoptive (18.04%); the latter are close to two times more likely to have a criminal conviction. If we were successful in changing the behaviour of high-risk low

SES parents, it would be surprising that we would achieve better results than placing a high SES biological parent male into a high SES adoptive family.

To find which early preventive interventions will be most cost-effective for preventing CPA, we need to compare interventions with different targets (e.g., parent versus child), different intensities (e.g., pregnancy to 2 years versus pregnancy to 5 years), and different timing (e.g., pregnancy to 2 years versus 3-5 years). Such comparisons are also important for understanding the mechanisms leading to or preventing CPA.

Can early preventive interventions benefit from epigenetic studies?

Children have the physical, cognitive, and emotional means of being physically aggressive towards others by 12 months of age (Tremblay, 2008). As described earlier, most children will 'onset' hitting, biting, or kicking another child or even an adult before their second birthday. However, their environment will play an important role in the developmental trajectories of these new acquired skills. If children are surrounded by adults and children who frequently physically aggress, they will probably learn that physical aggression is a useful strategy in everyday social interactions. On the other hand, if a child lives in an environment that does not tolerate physical aggression, it is likely that the he will acquire the habit of using means other than physical aggression to obtain what he or she wants, or for expressing frustration.

Thus, physical aggression is not a behaviour children learn, such as reading or writing, nor an illness children 'catch', such as poliomyelitis or smallpox. It is rather similar to crying, eating, grasping, throwing, and running, which young humans do when the physiological structure is in place. The young human learns to regulate these 'natural' behaviours with age, experience, and brain maturation. The learning to control process implies regulating your needs to adjust to those of others, and this process is generally labelled 'socialization'.

It is not hard to imagine why the evolutionary process would have given humans a genetic programme coding for all the basic mechanisms in order to react to hunger and to threat. Young children activate their muscles to run, push, kick, grab, hit, throw, and yell with extreme force when hungry, when angry, or when they are strongly attracted by something. However, stating that humans are genetically programmed to physically aggress when needed is different from stating that the frequency of the physical aggressions they use is genetically programmed.

From the available data it seems clear that all 18-month-olds who have developed normally use physical aggression out of fear, anger, disgust, curiosity, and greed. However, not all do so at the same frequency and with the same vigour. To what extent are these individual differences due to the genetic programme they have inherited or to the environment in which they have been growing? The trajectories shown in Fig. 18.2 clearly indicate that these individual differences exist at any given point, starting in early childhood, but the most interesting phenotype is described by the developmental trajectories-that is, intra-individual change over time. Most children learn to reduce the frequency of physical aggression, a behaviour which they apparently did not need to learn. However, relatively stable differences remain among individuals.

To understand how we can prevent the development of CPA trajectories, we need to understand the gene-environment mechanisms that explain the change and stability. They are possibly very similar to the mechanisms explaining the developmental trajectories of growth in height. Genes code for the growth mechanisms, but there are individual differences in this coding, as well as environmental differences (e.g., access to food), which lead to stable individual differences. Thus, the individual differences in the frequency of physical aggression at one point in time, and over time, can be due to a large number of 'causes': for example, due to individual differences in the genetic coding for serotonin (e.g., Pihl & Benkelfat, 2005) or testosterone (e.g., van Goozen, 2005), or language development (e.g., Dionne, 2005) and cognitive development (e.g., Séguin & Zelazo, 2005); or due to environmental differences such as mother's tobacco use during pregnancy (e.g., Wakschlag *et al.*, 2002), birth complications (e.g., Arseneault *et al.*, 2002), parental care (e.g., Raine *et al.*, 1997; Gatti & Tremblay, 2005; Zoccolillo *et al.*, 2005), and peer characteristics. (e.g., Boivin *et al.*, 2005). Thus, individual differences in frequency of physical aggression over time are very likely due to interactions between genetic and environmental mechanisms.

These gene-environment interactions have traditionally been studied from a statistical perspective with two types of samples: (i) twin studies by comparing differences between twins who share the same genes (monozygotes) and those who share only half of their genes (dizygotes; e.g., Dionne *et al.*, 2003), and; (ii) molecular genetic studies comparing differences between individuals who share the same or different polymorphic gene and the same or different environment (e.g., Caspi *et al.*, 2002). However, gene-environment interactions are not simply an abstract mathematical concept. A third approach to understanding such interactions is that of epigenetic studies attempting to understand the physiological mechanisms regulating gene expression. Genetic studies attempt to understand the genome, which is identical in different cell types and throughout life. Epigenetic studies attempt to understand the epigenome, which varies between cell type and during development. Numerous studies, especially cancer research, have shown that developmental, physiological, and environmental signals lead to variation of the epigenome; thus, genetic expression is a dynamic phenomenon dependent on these signals (Szyf, 2003).

Unfortunately, our knowledge of gene-environment mechanisms that could explain and prevent the development of CPA is perilously close to zero. The first reason for this gap in our knowledge is that gene-environment interaction studies are recent. The second reason is that genetically informative longitudinal studies generally do not have repeated assessments of physical aggression from early childhood onwards (Rhee & Waldman, 2002). The third reason is that these studies tend to concentrate on global antisocial behaviour phenotypes, often assessed at one point in time (Eley *et al.*, 1999; Arseneault *et al.*, 2003; Kim-Cohen *et al.*, 2006). Genetic studies have simply followed the main trend, which tends to rely on measurement scales constructed by lumping disruptive behaviour items that are shown to correlate at a given point in time.

Many molecular genetic studies have attempted to identify polymorphisms related to adult male aggressive behaviour in animals and antisocial behaviour in humans (Pihl & Benkelfat, 2005). One of the rare study to address the gene-environment interaction issue with humans (Caspi *et al.*, 2002) observed that males maltreated during their youth were at higher risk of being convicted of a violent crime before 27 years of age if they had the short version of the functional polymorphism in the gene coding for monoamine oxidase A (MAOA) activity. Replications of this study with other samples have found the same type of interaction (MAOA-maltreatment) but with different types of outcome. For example, one replication with adults males found the interaction for a composite measure of antisocial behaviour, and only for white subjects (Widom & Brzustowicz, 2006); another replication found the same type of interaction for Conduct Disorder assessed during adolescence with a sample of male twins (Foley *et al.*, 2004); finally, a third replication with 7-year-old male twins

(Kim-Cohen *et al.*, 2006) found the significant gene-environment interaction for a composite mental health problem scale and Attention Deficit/Hyperactivity Disorder (ADHD), but not for a total antisocial problem scale. Typically, physical aggression was not studied. Thus, we do not know if the MAOA-maltreatment statistical interaction found for physical violence assessed during adulthood is present during early childhood, childhood, or adolescence. We also do not know if it is dependent on racial background and societal factors.

These are important questions to answer for finding effective preventive interventions of CPA for specific groups of individuals. Useful answers should come from research on the mechanisms that underpin the statistical interactions (e.g., Kraemer *et al.*, 2008). MAOA activity is believed to be linked to antisocial behaviour because it plays a key role in regulating behaviour by selectively degrading serotonin, norephinephrine, and dopamine following reuptake from the synaptic cleft. Based on the CPA trajectories presented earlier, one would expect that the interaction between MAOA and maltreatment would have its greatest biopsychosocial impact during early childhood when individuals are learning to regulate their behaviour, especially physical aggression.

Knowledge on the underlying mechanisms should help find the best timing for the preventive interventions. Can interventions soon after maltreatment prevent its long-term negative impact or do we need to prevent early maltreatment? Recent experimental evidence suggests that intensive nurse home visitations after maltreatment has been detected does not have a positive impact (Macmillan *et al.*, 2005), whereas intensive nurse home visitation from pregnancy to age two for mothers at risk of maltreatment has been shown to reduce abuse (Olds *et al.*, 1986). However, as mentioned earlier, the latter study did not assess the children's development of physical aggression. We do not know if the reduction of parental abuse and neglect prevented the development of CPA.

An alternative prevention strategy for males with low MAOA activity born in families at risk of abuse would be to give the child a chemical treatment that would correct or compensate for the low MAOA activity. Admittedly, this is a bold suggestion, but animal studies are pointing in that direction, suggesting that we need to go much beyond the simple demonstration of gene-environment statistical interactions (Weaver *et al.*, 2006).

Recent experimental manipulations of early post-natal maternal behaviour effects on brain functioning are indeed showing that the gene-environment mechanisms involved are likely to be at the level of the epigenome (i.e., environmental programming of the genome). For example, Weaver *et al.* (2004) manipulated post-natal mothering behaviour with rat pups showing that frequency of licking has long-term effects on brain functioning because it regulates the expression of genes influencing the development of the hypothalamic-pituitary-adrenal (HPA) axis. Thus, the environment affects long-established epigenetic programmes in the brain. Szyf *et al.* (2007) conclude that 'since epigenetic programming defines the state of expression of genes, epigenetic differences could have the same consequences as genetic polymorphisms'.

Following this work with rats, we postulated that the adverse early environmental characteristics that predict a CPA trajectory for human males should have an impact on gene expression. We used a sample of males from a low socio-economic background who were found to be on a high physical aggression trajectory between 6 and 12 years of age and compared them with boys from the same background who followed a normal physical aggression trajectory (Broidy *et al.*, 2003). Preliminary analyses indicate that males on the CPA trajectory have substantially more methylated alleles when we look at T cells and more specifically at the interleukin (IL)-1B cytokine. The developmental pattern of these immune system differences will be important to study. Are the differences in gene expression at the origin of the behaviour differences or are they the product of the behaviour differences? Our hypothesis from the rat licking model is that early adverse environments negatively affect gene expression, which in turn disturbs brain development and eventually prevents adequate control over aggressive responses. Experimental work with pregnant monkeys has indeed shown that stress and substance use during pregnancy has a negative impact on the off-spring's cognitive and behavioural development as well as on the immune system (Schneider et al., 2002; Coe & Lubach, 2005; Coe et al., 2007).

Towards experimental epigenetic studies of CPA prevention

Twin studies and molecular genetic studies can address the gene-environment interaction issue. However, they fail to address the causal mechanisms leading to CPA because they are limited to a statistical analysis of correlations. To test causal mechanisms, we need the type of true experiments that are being regularly done with rats and monkeys (Foley et al., 2005; Weaver et al., 2006; Kraemer et al., 2008). Such studies are ethically impossible if the manipulation involves stressing healthy pregnant women; however, attempts to prevent stress in high-risk pregnant women are ethical and necessary if we are to find effective preventive interventions. Thus, experimental preventive interventions can kill two birds with one stone: identify basic mechanisms leading to CPA and identify effective preventive interventions. From both perspectives, they are more likely to rapidly provide useful knowledge than traditional longitudinal studies. Randomized preventive control trials that manipulate mother's behaviour prenatally and post-natally are not new (e.g., Olds et al., 1986); however, they are extremely rare and have failed to monitor effects on the development of gene expression, physiological structures, neurocognitive functioning, and behaviour.

I will end this chapter with two examples of research designs that could relatively rapidly provide experimental evidence of the prenatal and early post-natal environmental impact on CPA through gene expression and brain development.

The first research design involves randomly allocating primiparous pregnant women who smoke to a preventive intervention. There is good evidence from human and animal studies that prenatal exposure to nicotine not only affects birth weight but also brain development and behaviour (Vaglenova et al., 2004; Hsu et al., 2007; Huang et al., 2007). On the other hand, we have good evidence from methylation studies in cancer research that smoking has important epigenetic effects (Feinberg, 2007; Haussmann, 2007). From this evidence, we can hypothesize that smoking during pregnancy has negative epigenetic effects on brain development, which eventually leads to problems with regulation of emotions and learning alternatives to physical aggression. A randomized control trial of smoking cessation during pregnancy could be followed by an assessment of differences between experimental and control group in offspring's gene expression at birth, cognitive development, and regulation of physical aggression, taking into account genetic characteristics such as MAOA activity.

The second research design builds on the first to understand the timing of intervention (environmental) effects. The evidence that enriched post-natal environment can prevent preschool CPA (Côté et al., 2007) and adult criminality (Schweinhart et al., 2005) suggests that the adverse effects of the prenatal environment can be substantially attenuated by a cognitively stimulating environment during the preschool years. Using the first research design, we could randomly allocate half of the control group to an enriched environment such as a high-quality daycare environment. Comparing the differences in gene expression at birth to the differences after the post-natal intervention would reveal to what extent a post-natal intervention can have an impact on gene expression, which eventually accompanies changes in cognitive and behavioural development.

Conclusions

The aim of this chapter was to highlight how developmental psychopathology, developmental epigenetics, and prevention experiments are starting to blend together to explain the developmental causes of chronic violent behaviour and, more importantly, to help prevent the serious physical, mental, and social problems associated with chronic violence.

Traditional research on the development and prevention of antisocial behaviour often referred to physical aggression and violence to justify its importance, but rarely reported results on these specific behaviours. Most of the research concentrated on adult and adolescent general antisocial behaviour while arguing that physical violence is learned during adolescence.

By monitoring the development of physical aggression from infancy onwards, recent longitudinal studies show that human infants spontaneously use physical aggression and that humans learn not to physically aggress rather than learn to aggress. These studies underscore the importance of prenatal and early post-natal development for learning to regulate physical aggression. Meanwhile, epigenetic studies of animal behaviour started to show that the quality of the early environment impacts brain development and behaviour through its impact on gene expression.

Altogether, these studies suggest that preventive interventions for violent behaviour need to start as closely as possible to conception. Unfortunately, to our knowledge, no randomized control trial has yet been implemented to specifically prevent early CPA, and none of the general preventive interventions during early childhood monitored the early development of physical aggression.

In conclusion, randomized preventive control trials during pregnancy and early childhood with a specific focus on epigenetic effects are the research designs most likely to advance our understanding of the bio-psychosocial mechanisms leading to CPA, and the only research design that can lead to the identification of interventions that will effectively prevent the development of CPA and thus prevent the serious physical, mental, and social problems associated with chronic violence.

References

Alink, L. R. A., van Zeijl, J., Stolk, M. N., Juffer, F., Koot, H. M., Bakersman-Kranenburg, M. J., et al. (2006). The early childhood aggression curve: development of physical aggression in 10- to 50-months-old children. *Child Development*, 77, 954–966.

Anderson, C. A., Berkowitz, L., Donnerstein, E., Huesmann, L. R., Johnson, J. D., Linz, D., et al. (2003). The influence of media violence on youth. *Psychological Science in the Public Interest*, 4, 81–110.

Arseneault, L., Moffit, T. E., Caspi, A., Taylor, A., Rijsdijk, F. V., Jaffee, S. R., et al. (2003). Strong genetic effects on cross-situational antisocial behaviour among 5-year-old children according to mothers, teachers, examiner-observers, and twins' self-reports. *Journal of Child Psychology and Psychiatry*, 44, 832–848.

Arseneault, L., Tremblay, R. E., Boulerice, B., & Saucier, J-F. (2002), Obstetrical complications and violent delinquency: testing two developmental pathways. *Child Development, 73*, 496–508.

Bandura, A. (1973). *Aggression: A Social Learning Analysis*. New York: Holt.

Barker, E. D., Séguin, J. R., White, H. R., Bates, M., Lacourse, É., Carbonneau, R., *et al.* (2007). Development trajectories of physical violence and theft: relations to neuro-cognitive performance. *Archives of General Psychiatry*, *64*, 592–599.

Boivin, M., Vitaro, F., & Poulin, F. (2005). Peer relationships and the development of aggressive behaviour in early childhood. In R. E. Tremblay, W. W. Hartup, & J. Archer (eds), *Developmental Origins of Aggression*. New York: Guilford.

Brennan, P. A., Grekin, E. R., & Mednick, S. A. (1999). Maternal smoking and criminal outcomes. *Archives of General Psychiatry*, *56*, 215–219.

Broidy, L. M., Nagin, D. S., Tremblay, R. E., Bates, J. E., Brame, B., Dodge, K., *et al.* (2003). Developmental trajectories of childhood disruptive behaviours and adolescent delinquency: a six-site, cross-national study. *Developmental Psychology*, *39*, 222–245.

Button, T. M. M., Maughan, B., & McGuffin, P. (2007). The relationship of maternal smoking to psychological problems in the offspring. *Early Human Development*, *83*, 727–732.

Cairns, R. B., Cairns, B. D., Neckerman, H. J., Ferguson, L. L., & Gariépy, J. L. (1989). Growth and aggression: 1. Childhood to early adolescence. *Developmental Psychology*, *25*, 320–330.

Caspi, A., McClay, J., Moffitt, T., Mill, J., Martin, J., Craig, I. W., *et al.* (2002). Role of genotype in the cycle of violence in maltreated children. *Science*, *297*, 851–854.

Coe, C. L. & Lubach, G. R. (2005). Prenatal origins of individual variation in behaviour and immunity. *Neuroscience and Biobehavioural Reviews*, *29*, 39–49.

Coe, C. L., Lubach, G. R., & Shirtcliff, E. A. (2007). Maternal stress during pregnancy predisposes for iron deficiency in infant monkeys impacting innate immunity. *Pediatric Research*, *61*, 520–524.

Côté, S., Boivin, M., Nagin, D. S., Japel, C., Xu, Q., Zoccolillo, M. *et al.* (2007). The role of maternal education and non-maternal care services in the prevention of children's physical aggression. *Archives of General Psychiatry*, *64*, 1305–1312.

Côté, S., Vaillancourt, T., Leblanc, J. C., Nagin, D. S., & Tremblay, R. E. (2006). The development of physical aggression from toddlerhood to pre-adolescence: a nation-wide longitudinal study of Canadian children. *Journal of Abnormal Child Psychology*, *34*, 71–85.

Darwin, C. (1876/1983). *Autobiography*. Oxford: Oxford University Press.

DHHS (2001). *Youth Violence: A Report of the Surgeon General*. Washington, DC: US Department of Health and Human Services.

Dionne, G. (2005). Language development and aggressive behaviour. In R. E. Tremblay, W. W. Hartup, & J. Archer (eds), *Developmental Origins of Aggression*. New York: Guilford.

Dionne, G., Tremblay, R. E., Boivin, M., Laplante, D., & Pérusse, D. (2003). Physical aggression and expressive vocabulary in 19 month-old twins. *Developmental Psychology*, *39*, 261–273.

Eley, T. C., Lichenstein, P., & Stevenson, J. (1999). Sex differences in the etiology of aggressive and nonaggressive antisocial behaviour: results from two twin studies. *Child Development*, *70*, 155–168.

Feinberg, A. P. (2007). An epigenetic approach to cancer etiology. *Cancer Journal*, *13*, 70–74.

Foley, A. G., Murphy, K. J., & Regan, C. M. (2005). Complex-environment rearing prevents prenatal hypoxia-induced deficits in hippocampal cellular mechanisms necessary for memory consolidation in the adult Wistar rat. *Journal of Neuroscience Research*, *82*, 245–254.

Foley, D. L., Eaves, L. J., Wormley, B., Silberg, J. L., Maes, H. H., Kuhn, J., *et al.* (2004). Childhood adversity, monoamine oxidase A genotype, and risk for conduct disorder. *Archives of General Psychiatry*, *61*, 738–744.

Gatti, U., & Tremblay, R. E. (2005). Social capital and physical violence. In R. E. Tremblay, W. W. Hartup, & J. Archer (eds), *Developmental Origins of Aggression*. New York: Guilford.

Hartup, W. W., & Dewit, J. (1974). The development of aggression: problems and perspectives. In J. Dewit, & W. W. Hartup (eds), *Determinants and Origins of Aggressive Behavior*. The Hague, Netherlands: Mouton.

Haussmann, H. J. (2007). Smoking and lung cancer: future research directions. *International Journal of Toxicology*, *26*, 353–364.

Hsu, H-S., Chen, T-P., Hung, C-H., Wen, C-K., Lin, R-K., Lee, H-C., *et al.* (2007). Characterization of a multiple epigenetic marker panel for lung cancer detection and risk assessment in plasma. *Cancer Journal*, *110*, 2019–2026.

Huang, Z. G., Griffioen, K. J. S., Wang, X., Dergacheva, O., Kamendi, H., Gorini, C., *et al.* (2007). Nicotinic receptor activation occludes purinergic control of central cardiorespiratory network responses to hypoxia/hypercapnia. *Journal of Neurophysiology*, 98, 2429–2438.

Huijbregts, S. C. J., Séguin, J. R., Zoccolillo, M., Boivin, M., & Tremblay, R. E. (2008). Maternal prenatal smoking, parental antisocial behavior, and early childhood physical aggression. *Development and Psychopathology*, 20(2), 437–453.

Human Capital Initiative Coordinating Committee (1997). Reducing violence: a research agenda. *APS Observer*, special issue.

Jacobsen, L. K., Slotkin, T. A., Mencl, W. E., Frost, S. J., & Pugh, K. R. (2007). Gender-specific effects of prenatal and adolescent exposure to tobacco smoke on auditory and visual attention. *Neuropsychopharmacology*, 32, 2453–2464.

Kim-Cohen, J., Caspi, A., Taylor, A., Williams, B., Newcombe, R., Craig, I. W., *et al.* (2006). MAOA, maltreatment, and gene-environment interaction predicting children's mental health: new evidence and a meta-analysis. *Molecular Psychiatry*, 11, 903–913.

Kraemer, G. W., Moore, C. F., Newman, T. K., Barr, C. S., & Schneider, M. L. (2008). Moderate level fetal alcohol exposure and serotonin transporter gene promoter polymorphism affect neonatal temperament and limbic-hypothalamic-pituitary-adrenal axis regulation in monkeys. *Biological Psychiatry*, 63(3), 317–324.

Loeber, R. & Stouthamer-Loeber, M. (1998). Development of juvenile aggression and violence. Some common misconceptions and controversies. *American Psychologist*, 53, 242–259.

Macmillan, H. L., Thomas, B. H., Jamiesson, E., Walsh, J. C. A., Boyle, M. H., Shannan, H. S., *et al.* (2005). Effectiveness of home visitation by public-health nurses in prevention of the recurrence of child physical abuse and neglect: a randomized controlled trial. *Lancet*, 365, 1786–1793.

Maughan, B., Taylor, A., Caspi, A., & Moffit, T. E. (2004). Prenatal smoking and early childhood conduct problems: testing genetic and environmental explanations of the association. *Archives of General Psychiatry*, 61, 836–843.

Mrazek, P. J., & Haggerty, R. J. (eds) (1994). *Reducing Risks for Mental Disorders: Frontiers for Preventive Intervention Research*. Washington, DC: National Academy Press.

Nagin, D., & Tremblay, R. E. (1999). Trajectories of boys' physical aggression, opposition, and hyperactivity on the path to physically violent and non violent juvenile delinquency. *Child Development*, 70, 1181–1196.

NICHD, & ECCR Network (2004). Trajectories of physical aggression from toddlerhood to middle school. *Monographs of the Society for Research in Child Development*, 278, 69–74.

NIH (2004) Preventing violence and related health-risking social behaviors in adolescents: an NIH State-of-the-Science Conference. National Institutes of Health [Online], Available at: http://consensus.nih.gov/2004/2004YouthViolencePreventionSOS023html.htm.

Olds, D., Henderson, C. R., Chamberlin, R., & Talelbaum, R. (1986). Preventing child abuse and neglect: a randomized trial of nurse home visitation. *Pediatrics*, 78, 65–78.

Olds, D., Henderson, C. R., Cole, R., Eckenrode, J., Kitzman, H., Luckey, D., *et al.* (1998). Long-term effects of nurse home visitation on children's criminal and antisocial behavior: fifteen-year follow-up of a randomized controlled trial. *Journal of the American Medical Association*, 280, 1238–1244.

Pihl, R. O., & Benkelfat, C. (2005). Neuromodulators in the development and expression of inhibition and aggression. In R. E. Tremblay, W. W. Hartup, & J. Archer (eds), *Developmental Origins of Aggression*. New York: Guilford.

Quatrefages, A. (1863). Débats du 16 juillet 1863 de la Société d'Anthropologie de Paris. *Bulletins et mémoires de la Société d'Anthropologie de Paris*.

Raine, A., Brennan, P., & Mednick, S. A. (1997). Interaction between birth complications and early maternal rejection in predisposing individuals to adult violence: specificity to serious, early-onset violence. *American Journal of Psychiatry*, 154, 1265–1271.

Reiss, A. J., & Roth, J. A. (eds) (1993). *Understanding and Preventing Violence*. Washington, DC: National Academy Press.

Rhee, S. H., & Waldman, I. D. (2002). Genetic and environmental influences on antisocial behavior: a meta-analysis of twin and adoption studies. *Psychological Bulletin*, 128, 490–529.

Rousseau, J-J. (1762). *Emile: or, On Education*. Institute for Learning Technologies [Online], Available at: http://www.ilt.columbia.edu/pedagogies/rousseau/em_eng_bk1.html

Rousseau, J-J. (1762/1979). *Emile: or, On Education*. New York: Basic Books.

Schneider, M. L., Mooreb, C. F., Kraemera, G. W., Roberts, A. D., & Dejesuse, O. T. (2002). The impact of prenatal stress, fetal alcohol exposure, or both on development: perspectives from a primate model. *Psychoneuroendocrinology, 27*, 285–298.

Schweinhart, L., Montie, J., Xiang, Z., Barnett, W. S., Belfield, C. R., & Nores, M. (2005). *Lifetime Effects: The High/Scope Perry Preschool Study through Age 40*. Ypsilanti, MI: High/Scope Press.

Séguin, J. R., & Zelazo, P. (2005). Executive function in early physical aggression. In R. E. Tremblay, W. H. Hartup, & J. Archer (eds), *Developmental Origins of Aggression*. New York: Guilford.

Szyf, M. (2003). Targeting DNA methylation in cancer. *Ageing Research Reviews, 2*, 299–328.

Szyf, M., Weaver, I., & Meaney, M. (2007). Maternal care, the epigenome and phenotypic differences in behavior. *Reproductive Toxicology, 24*, 9–19.

Tremblay, R. E. (2000). The development of aggressive behaviour during childhood: What have we learned in the past century? *International Journal of Behavioral development, 24*, 129–141.

Tremblay, R. E. (2003). Why socialization fails? The case of chronic physical aggression. In B. B. Lahey, T. E. Moffitt, & A. Caspi (eds), *Causes of Conduct Disorder and JuvenileDdelinquency*. New York: Guilford Publications.

Tremblay, R. E. (2006). Prevention of youth violence: Why not start at the beginning? *Journal of Abnormal Child Psychology, 34*, 481–487.

Tremblay, R. E. (2008). Anger and Aggression. In M. M. Haith, & J. B. Benson (eds), Encyclopedia of *Infant and Early Childhood Development*, 2nd edn (pp. 62–74). Academic Press.

Tremblay, R. E., Barr, R., & Peters, R. D. V. (2003). Public opinion and violence prevention. Montreal, Canada: CEECD Bulletin.

Tremblay, R. E., Japel, C., Pérusse, D., Mcduff, P., Boivin, M., Zoccolillo, M., *et al.* (1999). The search for the age of 'onset' of physical aggression: Rousseau and Bandura revisited. *Criminal Behavior and Mental Health, 9*, 8–23.

Tremblay, R. E., Loeber, R., Gagnon, C., Charlebois, P., Larivée, S., & Leblanc, M. (1991). Disruptive boys with stable and unstable high fighting behavior patterns during junior elementary school. *Journal of Abnormal Child Psychology, 19*, 285–300.

Tremblay, R. E., Nagin, D. S., Séguin, J. R., Zoccolillo, M., Zelazo, P. D., Boivin, M., *et al.* (2004). Physical aggression during early childhood: trajectories and predictors. *Pediatrics, 114*, e43–e50.

US Surgeon General (2001). *Youth Violence: A Report of the Surgeon General*. Washington, DC: Department of Health and Human Services.

Vaglenova, J., Birru, S., Pandiella, N. M., & Breese, C. R. (2004). An assessment of the long-term developmental and behavioral teratogenicity of prenatal nicotine exposure. *Behavioural Brain Research, 150*, 159–170.

Van Dusen, K. T., Mednick, S. A., & Gabrielli, W. (1983). Social class and crime in an adoption cohort. In K. T. V. Dusen, & S. A. Mednick (eds), *Prospective Studies of Crime*. Boston, MA: Kluwer-Nijhoff.

Van Goozen, S. H. M. (2005). Hormones and the developmental origin of aggression. In R. E. Tremblay, W. W. Hartup, & J. Archer (eds), *Developmental Origins of Aggression*. New York: Guilford Press.

Wakschlag, L., Pickett, K. E., Cook, E., Benowitz, N. L., & Leventhal, B. (2002). Maternal smoking during pregnancy and severe antisocial behavior in offspring: a review. *American Journal of Public Health, 92*, 966–974.

Wakschlag, L. S., Lahey, B. B., Loeber, R., Green, S. M., Gordon, R. A., & Leventhal, B. L. (1997). Maternal smoking during pregnancy and the risk of conduct disorder in boys. *Archives of General Psychiatry, 54*, 670–676.

Weaver, I. C., Cervoni, N., Champagne, F. A., D'Alessio, A. C., Sharma, S., Seckl, J. R., *et al.* (2004). Epigenetic programming by maternal behavior. *Nature Neuroscience, 7*, 847–854.

Weaver, I. C., Meaney, M. J., & Szyf, M. (2006). Maternal care effects on the hippocampal transcriptome and anxiety-mediated behaviours in the offspring that are reversible in adulthood. *Proceedings of the National Academy of Sciences of the United States of America, 103*, 3480–3485.

WHO (2002). *World Report on Violence and Health*. Geneva: World Health Organization.

Widom, C., & Brzustowicz, L. (2006) MAOA and the 'cycle of violence': childhood abuse and neglect, MAOA genotype, and risk for violent and antisocial behavior. *Biological Psychiatry, 60*, 684–689.

Wilson, S. J., & Lipsey, M. W. (2007). School-based interventions for aggressive and disruptive behavior. Update of a meta-analysis. *American Journal of Preventive Medicine, 33*, S130–143.

Zoccolillo, M., Paquette, D., & Tremblay, R. E. (2005). Maternal conduct disorder and the risk for the next generation. In D. Pepler, K. Masden, C. Webster, & K. Levene (eds), *Development and Treatment of Girlhood Aggression*. Mahwah, NJ: Lawrence Erlbaum Associates.

Subject Index

A

active rGE, 257

adolescence-limited involvement, in antisocial behaviour, 24

adolescence-limited pathways, on adverse physical health outcomes, 28

adolescent delinquents and schizophrenia, 45

adoption studies, of antisocial behaviour, 251–253

adrenarche, 205

adrenocorticotropic hormone (ACTH), 207

adult violence, 26

'ADVANCE' programme, 331

aetiological chain, 24

age–aggression curve, 4–5

age–antisocial behaviour curves, 4

age–crime curve, 4, 14

aggression, 1. *see also* neurobiological bases, of aggressive behavior
  expressive, 291
  gender differences, 202–203
  HPA axis system, 207–210
  instrumental, 291
  role of prenatal hormonal exposure, 203
  testosterone and, 202–205

Aggression Replacement Training (ART), 313

Aggression scale of Tellegen, 240

Aggressive Behavioural Control project, of Saskatoon Regional Psychiatric Centre, 306

amygdala
  damages and its impact, 138
  decision making function, 138
  dysfunction and conduct disorder, 102–103, 130–131
  hyperactivity, 138
  and low-expressing genetic variant, 342
  overview, 124–125
  processing of emotional expressions, 125

androgens, in emotional processing, 206–207

anger-driven reactive aggression, 102

anger management, 307–309

anterior cingulate cortex (ACC), 126, 171, 177–178
  lesions, 138–139
  P3 response, 237, 239

antisocial behaviour, 1. *see also* health problems and antisocial behaviour
  in adolescence and adulthood, 201
  animal model studies, 211–213
  causal factors of early onset, 201–202

causal models, 65–66
  correlation with callous and unemotional (CU) affective traits, 255–256
  gender differences in aggressive behavior, 202–203
  and HPA axis system, 207–210
  implications of neuroendocrine findings, 214
  relationships between neuroendocrine variables, 213
  role of adrenal androgens, 205–207
  role of cortisol and psychopathic personality traits, 207–208, 211
  role of prenatal hormone exposure, 203
  and self-reported health problems, 28
  testosterone and aggression, 202–205

Antisocial Personality Disorder (ASPD), 123, 137, 142–143, 168–170, 260
  associated biological disadvantages, 350–351
  Benjamin's quotation of core personality characteristics, 364
  cost and cost analysis, 351
  early prevention, 351–352
  Epidemiological Catchment Area study, 351–352
  epidemiology, 350
  Kuhn's study of paradigms, 358–360
  nature of scientific inquiry, 357–360
  pharmacological interventions, 355–356
  role of politicians and policymakers in research, 364–365
  systematic reviews of treatments for, 353–357
  treatments for, 360–364
  vs criminal behavior, 352

appetitive conditioning, 124

Army Individual Test Battery, 174

Arrogant and Deceitful Interpersonal Style behaviour, 169

attacks, with intent to injure, 1

attention deficit/hyperactivity disorder (ADHD), 9, 162, 179, 307, 340
  link with antisocial behaviour, 30
  patterns of antisocial behaviour associated with, 67

autism, 93

aversive-conditioning paradigm, 124, 144

Axis I disorders, 363

Axis I pathology, 140

B

Baddeley's working memory model, 172

basal glucocorticoid concentrations and aggression, 209–210

Author Index